Advances in Eating Disorders

Advances in Eating Disorders

Editors

Zaida Agüera
Susana Jiménez-Murcia

MDPI • Basel • Beijing • Wuhan • Barcelona • Belgrade • Manchester • Tokyo • Cluj • Tianjin

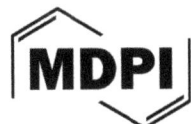

Editors
Zaida Agüera
Instituto de Salud Carlos III Bellvitge
University Hospital-IDIBELL
University of Barcelona
Spain

Susana Jiménez-Murcia
Instituto de Salud Carlos III
Bellvitge University Hospital-IDIBELL
University of Barcelona
Spain

Editorial Office
MDPI
St. Alban-Anlage 66
4052 Basel, Switzerland

This is a reprint of articles from the Special Issue published online in the open access journal *Journal of Clinical Medicine* (ISSN 2077-0383) (available at: https://www.mdpi.com/journal/jcm/special_issues/Eating_Disorders).

For citation purposes, cite each article independently as indicated on the article page online and as indicated below:

LastName, A.A.; LastName, B.B.; LastName, C.C. Article Title. *Journal Name* **Year**, *Volume Number*, Page Range.

ISBN 978-3-0365-0516-9 (Hbk)
ISBN 978-3-0365-0517-6 (PDF)

© 2021 by the authors. Articles in this book are Open Access and distributed under the Creative Commons Attribution (CC BY) license, which allows users to download, copy and build upon published articles, as long as the author and publisher are properly credited, which ensures maximum dissemination and a wider impact of our publications.

The book as a whole is distributed by MDPI under the terms and conditions of the Creative Commons license CC BY-NC-ND.

Contents

About the Editors ix

Zaida Agüera and Susana Jiménez-Murcia
Advances in Eating Disorders
Reprinted from: *J. Clin. Med.* 2020, 9, 4047, doi:10.3390/jcm9124047 1

Mohamed Abdulkadir, Moritz Herle, Bianca L. De Stavola, Christopher Hübel, Diana L. Santos Ferreira, Ruth J. F. Loos, Rachel Bryant-Waugh, Cynthia M. Bulik and Nadia Micali
Polygenic Score for Body Mass Index Is Associated with Disordered Eating in a General Population Cohort
Reprinted from: *J. Clin. Med.* 2020, 9, 1187, doi:10.3390/jcm9041187 7

Howard Steiger and Linda Booij
Eating Disorders, Heredity and Environmental Activation: Getting Epigenetic Concepts into Practice
Reprinted from: *J. Clin. Med.* 2020, 9, 1332, doi:10.3390/jcm9051332 25

Philibert Duriez, Lauralee Robichon, Roland Dardennes, Guillaume Lavoisy, Dominique Grouselle, Jacques Epelbaum, Nicolas Ramoz, Philip Gorwood, Virginie Tolle and Odile Viltart
Unexpected Association of Desacyl-Ghrelin with Physical Activity and Chronic Food Restriction: A Translational Study on Anorexia Nervosa
Reprinted from: *J. Clin. Med.* 2020, 9, 2782, doi:10.3390/jcm9092782 39

Miriam Kemmer, Christoph U. Correll, Tobias Hofmann, Andreas Stengel, Julia Grosser and Verena Haas
Assessment of Physical Activity Patterns in Adolescent Patients with Anorexia Nervosa and Their Effect on Weight Gain
Reprinted from: *J. Clin. Med.* 2020, 9, 727, doi:10.3390/jcm9030727 59

José Ramón Alvero-Cruz, Verónica Parent Mathias and Jerónimo C. García-Romero
Somatotype Components as Useful Predictors of Disordered Eating Attitudes in Young Female Ballet Dance Students
Reprinted from: *J. Clin. Med.* 2020, 9, 2024, doi:10.3390/jcm9072024 75

Kentaro Matsui, Yoko Komada, Katsuji Nishimura, Kenichi Kuriyama and Yuichi Inoue
Prevalence and Associated Factors of Nocturnal Eating Behavior and Sleep-Related Eating Disorder-Like Behavior in Japanese Young Adults: Results of an Internet Survey Using Munich Parasomnia Screening
Reprinted from: *J. Clin. Med.* 2020, 9, 1243, doi:10.3390/jcm9041243 87

Tinne Buelens, Koen Luyckx, Margaux Verschueren, Katrien Schoevaerts, Eva Dierckx, Lies Depestele and Laurence Claes
Temperament and Character Traits of Female Eating Disorder Patients with(out) Non-Suicidal Self-Injury
Reprinted from: *J. Clin. Med.* 2020, 9, 1207, doi:/10.3390/jcm9041207 97

Enrico Collantoni, Christopher R. Madan, Paolo Meneguzzo, Iolanna Chiappini, Elena Tenconi, Renzo Manara and Angela Favaro
Cortical Complexity in Anorexia Nervosa: A Fractal Dimension Analysis
Reprinted from: *J. Clin. Med.* 2020, 9, 833, doi:10.3390/jcm9030833 111

Simon Maier, Kathrin Nickel, Evgeniy Perlov, Alina Kukies, Almut Zeeck,
Ludger Tebartz van Elst, Dominique Endres, Derek Spieler, Lukas Holovics,
Armin Hartmann, Michael Dacko, Thomas Lange and Andreas Joos
Insular Cell Integrity Markers Linked to Weight Concern in Anorexia Nervosa—An MR-Spectroscopy Study
Reprinted from: *J. Clin. Med.* **2020**, *9*, 1292, doi:10.3390/jcm9051292 123

Gloria Villalba Martínez, Azucena Justicia, Purificación Salgado, José María Ginés, Rocío Guardiola, Carlos Cedrón, María Polo, Ignacio Delgado-Martínez, Santiago Medrano, Rosa María Manero, Gerardo Conesa, Gustavo Faus, Antoni Grau, Matilde Elices and Víctor Pérez
A Randomized Trial of Deep Brain Stimulation to the Subcallosal Cingulate and Nucleus Accumbens in Patients with Treatment-Refractory, Chronic, and Severe Anorexia Nervosa: Initial Results at 6 Months of Follow Up
Reprinted from: *J. Clin. Med.* **2020**, *9*, 1946, doi:10.3390/jcm9061946 139

Philibert Duriez, Rami Bou Khalil, Yara Chamoun, Redwan Maatoug, Robertas Strumila, Maude Seneque, Philip Gorwood, Philippe Courtet and Sébastien Guillaume
Brain Stimulation in Eating Disorders: State of the Art and Future Perspectives
Reprinted from: *J. Clin. Med.* **2020**, *9*, 2358, doi:10.3390/jcm9082358 157

Nuria Mallorquí-Bagué, María Lozano-Madrid, Giulia Testa, Cristina Vintró-Alcaraz, Isabel Sánchez, Nadine Riesco, José César Perales, Juan Francisco Navas, Ignacio Martínez-Zalacaín, Alberto Megías, Roser Granero, Misericordia Veciana De Las Heras, Rayane Chami, Susana Jiménez-Murcia, José Antonio Fernández-Formoso, Janet Treasure and Fernando Fernández-Aranda
Clinical and Neurophysiological Correlates of Emotion and Food Craving Regulation in Patients with Anorexia Nervosa
Reprinted from: *J. Clin. Med.* **2020**, *9*, 960, doi:10.3390/jcm9040960 183

María Lozano-Madrid, Danielle Clark Bryan, Roser Granero, Isabel Sánchez,
Nadine Riesco, Núria Mallorquí-Bagué, Susana Jiménez-Murcia, Janet Treasure and
Fernando Fernández-Aranda
Impulsivity, Emotional Dysregulation and Executive Function Deficits Could Be Associated with Alcohol and Drug Abuse in Eating Disorders
Reprinted from: *J. Clin. Med.* **2020**, *9*, 1936, doi:10.3390/jcm9061936 203

Jess Kerr-Gaffney, Luke Mason, Emily Jones, Hannah Hayward, Jumana Ahmad,
Amy Harrison, Eva Loth, Declan Murphy and Kate Tchanturia
Emotion Recognition Abilities in Adults with Anorexia Nervosa are Associated with Autistic Traits
Reprinted from: *J. Clin. Med.* **2020**, *9*, 1057, doi:10.3390/jcm9041057 217

Emma Kinnaird, Yasemin Dandil, Zhuo Li, Katherine Smith, Caroline Pimblett,
Rafiu Agbalaya, Catherine Stewart and Kate Tchanturia
Pragmatic Sensory Screening in Anorexia Nervosa and Associations with Autistic Traits
Reprinted from: *J. Clin. Med.* **2020**, *9*, 1182, doi:10.3390/jcm9041182 233

Julia Philipp, Stefanie Truttmann, Michael Zeiler, Claudia Franta, Tanja Wittek, Gabriele Schöfbeck, Michaela Mitterer, Dunja Mairhofer, Annika Zanko, Hartmut Imgart,
Ellen Auer-Welsbach, Janet Treasure, Gudrun Wagner and Andreas F. K. Karwautz
Reduction of High Expressed Emotion and Treatment Outcomes in Anorexia
Nervosa—Caregivers' and Adolescents' Perspective
Reprinted from: *J. Clin. Med.* **2020**, *9*, 2021, doi:0.3390/jcm9072021 243

Stefanie Truttmann, Julia Philipp, Michael Zeiler, Claudia Franta, Tanja Wittek, Elisabeth Merl, Gabriele Schöfbeck, Doris Koubek, Clarissa Laczkovics, Hartmut Imgart, Annika Zanko, Ellen Auer-Welsbach, Janet Treasure, Andreas F. K. Karwautz and Gudrun Wagner
Long-Term Efficacy of the Workshop Vs. Online SUCCEAT (Supporting Carers of Children and Adolescents with Eating Disorders) Intervention for Parents: A Quasi-Randomised Feasibility Trial
Reprinted from: *J. Clin. Med.* **2020**, *9*, 1912, doi:10.3390/jcm9061912 259

Thorsten Koerner, Verena Haas, Julia Heese, Matislava Karacic, Elmar Ngo, Christoph U. Correll, Ulrich Voderholzer and Ulrich Cuntz
Outcomes of an Accelerated Inpatient Refeeding Protocol in 103 Extremely Underweight Adults with Anorexia Nervosa at a Specialized Clinic in Prien, Germany
Reprinted from: *J. Clin. Med.* **2020**, *9*, 1535, doi:10.3390/jcm9051535 277

Giulia Testa, Isabel Baenas, Cristina Vintró-Alcaraz, Roser Granero, Zaida Agüera, Isabel Sánchez, Nadine Riesco, Susana Jiménez-Murcia and Fernando Fernández-Aranda
Does ADHD Symptomatology Influence Treatment Outcome and Dropout Risk in Eating Disorders? A Longitudinal Study
Reprinted from: *J. Clin. Med.* **2020**, *9*, 2305, doi:10.3390/jcm9072305 291

Bruno Porras-Garcia, Marta Ferrer-Garcia, Eduardo Serrano-Troncoso, Marta Carulla-Roig, Pau Soto-Usera, Helena Miquel-Nabau, Nazilla Shojaeian, Isabel de la Montaña Santos-Carrasco, Bianca Borszewski, Marina Díaz-Marsá, Isabel Sánchez-Díaz, Fernando Fernández-Aranda and José Gutiérrez-Maldonado
Validity of Virtual Reality Body Exposure to Elicit Fear of Gaining Weight, Body Anxiety and Body-Related Attentional Bias in Patients with Anorexia Nervosa
Reprinted from: *J. Clin. Med.* **2020**, *9*, 3210, doi:10.3390/jcm9103210 303

Janet Treasure, Daniel Willmott, Suman Ambwani, Valentina Cardi, Danielle Clark Bryan, Katie Rowlands and Ulrike Schmidt
Cognitive Interpersonal Model for Anorexia Nervosa Revisited: The Perpetuating Factors that Contribute to the Development of the Severe and Enduring Illness
Reprinted from: *J. Clin. Med.* **2020**, *9*, 630, doi:10.3390/jcm9030630 323

About the Editors

Zaida Agüera (Ph.D.), Dr. Zaida Agüera has been a licensed psychologist at the University of Barcelona since 2005. Shortly thereafter, she started conducting research on eating disorders at the department of Psychiatry at the Bellvitge University Hospital-IDIBELL and CIBERobn. She received her Ph.D. from the University of Barcelona in 2014. She is also an Associate Lecturer at the Department of Public health, Mental Health and Perinatal Nursing, at the School of Nursing, University of Barcelona.

Susana Jiménez-Murcia (Ph.D.), Since 2002, Susana Jiménez-Murcia, Specialist in Clinical Psychology, has been the Director of the Pathological Gambling and Behavioral Addictions Unit at the Department of Psychiatry (University Hospital Bellvitge-HUB/IDIBELL), Co-IP of Group CIBERobn (Excellent Spanish Research Network for Obesity and Nutrition), Associate Professor since 2006 (School of Medicine, University of Barcelona). She obtained her Ph.D. in Psychology in 2004, her master's in Clinical Psychology and Behavioral Medicine in 1992 and her BP in 1988 (Clinical Psychology). She has published more than 260 studies in peer review journals with impact factors. She has given more than 100 invited lectures in international/national conferences and more than 800 hours given in different workshops and lectures in officially recognized, by the Psychology and Medical Councils, CBT Institutes, in over 25 competitive research projects achieved in both national and European agencies. She was an invited professor at the Psychiatry and Neurosciences Department, University of North Carolina (UNC, Chapel Hill, USA), in July–August 2005 and at the Douglas Hospital, McGill University (Canada, Montreal), in July–August 2009 and 2015. She received several additional awards on development and innovation (Best European Video Game for Health—2011; Best Spanish Research Ideas—Diario Medico 2011 and 2019).

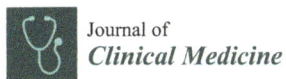 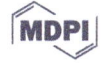

Editorial

Advances in Eating Disorders

Zaida Agüera [1,2,3,*] and Susana Jiménez-Murcia [1,2,4,*]

1. CIBER Fisiopatología Obesidad y Nutrición (CIBERobn), Instituto de Salud Carlos III, 08907 Barcelona, Spain
2. Department of Psychiatry, University Hospital of Bellvitge-IDIBELL, 08907 Barcelona, Spain
3. Department of Public Health, Mental Health and Perinatal Nursing, School of Nursing, University of Barcelona, 08907 Barcelona, Spain
4. Department of Clinical Sciences, School of Medicine and Health Sciences, University of Barcelona, 08907 Barcelona, Spain
* Correspondence: zaguera@bellvitgehospital.cat (Z.A.); sjimenez@bellvitgehospital.cat (S.J.-M.); Tel.: +34-932607227 (Z.A.); +34-932607988 (S.J.-M.)

Received: 8 December 2020; Accepted: 11 December 2020; Published: 15 December 2020

Eating disorders (EDs) are a group of mental disorders characterized by an altered food intake and the presence of inappropriate behaviors for the control of body weight, framed as an excessive concern regarding one's weight and figure. Anorexia nervosa (AN), bulimia nervosa (BN), binge-eating disorder (BED), and other specified feeding or eating disorders (OSFEDs) are the specific EDs defined in the Diagnostic and Statistical Manual of Mental Disorders, 5th Edition (DSM-5) [1]. All EDs lead to physical and psychosocial functioning impairments in the patients which, in turn, may contribute to the persistence of the disease (for example, the effects of starvation on the brain, social isolation or emotional dysregulation, among others) [2]. Furthermore, the severity of EDs has been highlighted by their chronicity [3], medical complications [4], comorbidity [5]), and the high rates of mortality presented by these patients [6].

To address this important health issue, the current Special Issue collected 21 articles examining the most recent and relevant scientific findings regarding advances in ED. The published articles comprised three reviews and 18 research articles focusing on different aspects, such as genetic [7] and epigenetic factors [8], biomarkers [9], comorbidity [10–14], clinical phenotypes [15,16], neurocognition [12,17–21], treatment predictors [22], and treatment models and therapeutic targets [19,23–27]. Altogether, these studies may provide increased knowledge about the pathogenesis, the risk factors, the maintenance factors, and the most appropriate treatments tools for ED. These articles represented contributions from a diverse group of researchers from multiple countries, including France, Austria, Germany, Belgium, Switzerland, Italy, Spain, the United Kingdom, the United States, Canada, and Japan.

Several relevant findings were observed from this collective body of work. Starting with genetics, Abdulkadir et al. [7] found that genetic factors that underlie body mass index (BMI) are associated with disordered eating behaviors and related cognitions, and that this association is also mediated by BMI. These findings suggest that disordered eating and related cognitions should be considered in a broader context that includes anthropometry as well as behavioral and developmental factors. Regarding epigenetic factors, the review carried out by Steiger and Booij [8] highlights that epigenetic processes link malnutrition and life stresses to risk of ED development. Moreover, differences in the direction of methylation effects have been described in recovered and acute patients with AN. Therefore, authors conclude that DNA methylation could serve as a marker of disease staging or therapeutic response.

The identification of biomarkers was also a relevant topic addressed in this issue. Duriez et al. [9], in a translational study, aimed to determine whether some biomarkers, such as acyl-ghrelin (AG) and desacyl-ghrelin (DAG) plasma concentrations, reflect the level of physical activity during food restriction and after renutrition. Authors found that, in experimental models of mice, AG and DAG both increased during food restriction. They also observed that patients with AN showed a rapid decrease of AG and DAG during weight recovery. However, at one-month post-discharge, AG increased, but only DAG plasma concentrations correlated negatively with BMI and positively with physical activity. Overall, the results highlight the potential role of DAG in the recovery process of AN and suggest a potential negative impact of DAG on weight recovery.

Several included studies also focused on identifying clinical phenotypes in ED. For example, Alvero-Cruz et al. [16] aimed to examine whether somatotype components are predictors of disordered eating in female dance students. The risk of presenting disordered eating was higher in the beginner than in the advanced training group. Authors concluded that somatotype components (ectomorphy and mesomorphy) were predictors of disordered eating in the younger dance student group (beginner training). On the other hand, Matsui et al. [15] focused on identifying the factors related to nocturnal eating syndrome (NES) and sleep-related ED in Japanese young adults. Results showed that the prevalence of NES and sleep-related ED was 2% and almost 5%, respectively. The factors associated with both were smoking, sleepwalking, and use of hypnotic medication. In conclusion, NES, but not sleep-related ED, was associated with a delayed sleep-wake rhythm and sleep disturbances. Meanwhile, Kemmer et al. [22] focused on characterizing physical activity patterns and their effect on weight recovery in patients with AN, and concluded that increased light physical activity in AN decreased after inpatient treatment, and was linked to a greater change in the BMI.

As previously noted, comorbidity is one of the factors that is widely related to the severity and prognosis of ED. In this regard, Buelens et al. [10] investigated whether personality may act as a transdiagnostic mechanism underlying both EDs and non-suicidal self-injury (NSSI) behaviors. The findings of this study revealed an alarmingly high prevalence of NSSI in patients with ED. The patients with ED and NSSI lifetime reported low self-directedness and high harm avoidance, and only those who recently engaged in NSSI showed less novelty seeking. Likewise, Lozano-Madrid et al. [12] aimed to examine the clinical features and neuropsychological performance of ED patients with and without substance use disorder (SUD). Authors found that approximately 19% of patients with ED presented SUD symptoms. Patients with ED and comorbid SUD symptoms displayed a specific phenotype characterized by greater impulsive traits, emotional dysregulation, and more impaired executive control. Testa et al. [11] explored whether attention deficit and hyperactivity disorder (ADHD)-related symptoms may influence the treatment outcome in patients with EDs. Authors found poor treatment outcomes in patients with more severe ED symptoms but an indirect effect of ADHD-related symptomatology. In addition, understanding the role that comorbid autistic features play in patients with AN is also interesting. Therefore, Kerr-Gaffney et al. [13] compared the emotion recognition abilities and attention to faces using eye-tracking in patients with AN and healthy control, concluding that difficulties in emotion recognition appear to be associated with high comorbid autistic traits rather than with a phenotypic feature of AN, independent of illness state. In the same vein, Kinnaird et al. [14] explored the use of a brief sensory sensitivity screener in patients with AN, to assess whether self-rated sensory sensitivity is related to autistic traits. The results of this study showed that patients with AN and high autistic traits scored themselves as more sensitive in the areas of smell, vision, texture, and overall total screening scores, compared to those with low autistic traits.

This collection also includes a set of studies that analyze the role of implicit–explicit emotion in patients with ED and their families, supporting the important role of the emotion recognition [13,14], the expressed emotion [27] or the emotion regulation strategies [12,17] in the development and maintenance of these disorders.

The majority of research of this Special Issue focuses on neurosciences and EDs. There are several studies examining and reviewing a variety of relevant topics such as neuropsychology (especially executive functions) [12,17], structural alterations of the brain [18], neurometabolic alterations [20], neuroimaging studies, and the use and efficacy of invasive and non-invasive brain stimulation techniques [19,21]. Specifically, Mallorquí-Bagué et al. [17] used electrophysiological techniques to explore emotion regulation and food craving regulation in patients with AN. The main findings from this study suggest that patients with AN showed reduced P300 amplitudes and exhibited greater food addiction, emotional dysregulation, and greater use of maladaptive techniques (i.e., suppression strategies) to manage negative emotions than healthy controls. Research with neuroimaging techniques to assess morphological complexity of cortical brain structures from Collantoni et al. [18] provided evidence that cortical fractal dimension (FD) may be a feasible and sensitive method to assess the negative effects of severity and duration of malnutrition in patients with AN. In addition, Maier et al. [20] investigated the metabolic signals in the anterior insular cortex by means of magnetic resonance spectroscopy (MRS). Authors analyzed both acute and recovered patients with AN, as well as healthy controls, and found that metabolic alterations in patients with AN (i.e., lower NAA and Glx signals) seem to be state-related symptoms rather than traits. Villaba-Martínez et al. [19] assessed the efficacy and safety of deep brain stimulation (DBS) applied to chronic, severe, and refractory patients with AN. The findings revealed that DBS was effective for some patients with AN and was associated with self-reported improvements in quality of life. However, almost 40% of the patients presented adverse cutaneous complications. In sum, the review from Duriez et al. [21] concluded that there is not sufficient evidence to support the use of brain stimulation in the treatment of EDs, but that further research on this topic is needed.

Lastly, despite having evidence-based treatments for clinical practice that is well recognized by clinical guidelines, these treatments have proven not to be the panacea. Scientific understanding of the treatment of ED has developed significantly in recent years. Some of these advances in the management of ED have included the complementary use of nutritional protocols, new technologies, brain stimulation techniques, and interventions of support for caregivers of adolescents with ED, among others. For example, Koerner at el. [25] describe the effectiveness and safety of a rapid clinical high-caloric refeeding strategy for patients with AN. Regarding the use of new technologies as an adjuvant therapeutic tool, the findings from Porras-García et al. [24] provide evidence about the usefulness of virtual reality-based body exposure to elicit fear of gaining weight and other body-related disturbances in patients with AN. On the other hand, Philipp et al. [27] demonstrated that parental expressed emotion (associated with higher distress and a lack of skills) was reduced after interventions for caregivers (namely the SUCCEAT program), and that this reduction positively influenced patients' outcomes. Likewise, the results from the study of Truttmann et al. [26] provide support for the efficacy of the same interventions for caregivers (i.e., SUCCEAT) reducing parental burden, distress and psychopathology. Last but not least, Treasure et al. [23] reviewed the underpinnings of the Cognitive Interpersonal Model for AN and how this can be targeted to treatment. This model encourages the use of treatments targeting changeable elements, such as: increasing social connection and collaborative recovery, using neuromodulation techniques, and augmenting treatment through digital technology.

The purpose of this Special Issue is to address a wide range of topics and contribute to a greater understanding of advances in ED. We believe that the articles contained in the issue have largely achieved this objective. In addition, we would like to thank the various authors and reviewers for their help in amassing this excellent body of work.

Funding: We thank CERCA Programme/Generalitat de Catalunya for institutional support. This research was supported by Instituto de Salud Carlos III (ISCIII; grant number: PI17/01167), by Ministerio de Economía y Competitividad (grant number: PSI2015-68701-R), by Delegación del Gobierno para el Plan Nacional sobre Drogas (2017I067), by PERIS (Generalitat de Catalunya, SLT006/17/00246), and co-funded by FEDER funds/European Regional Development Fund (ERDF), a way to build Europe. CIBERobn is an initiative of ISCIII.

Conflicts of Interest: The authors declare no conflict of interest.

References

1. American Psychiatric Association. *Diagnostic and Statistical Manual of Mental Disorders*, 5th ed.; American Psychiatric Association: Washington, DC, USA, 2013.
2. Treasure, J.; Claudino, A.M.; Zucker, N. Eating disorders. *Lancet* **2010**, *375*, 583–593. [CrossRef]
3. Broomfield, C.; Stedal, K.; Touyz, S.; Rhodes, P. Labeling and defining severe and enduring anorexia nervosa: A systematic review and critical analysis. *Int. J. Eat. Disord.* **2017**, *50*, 611–623. [CrossRef] [PubMed]

4. Peebles, R.; Sieke, E.H. Medical Complications of Eating Disorders in Youth. *Child Adolesc. Psychiatr. Clin. N. Am.* **2019**, *28*, 593–615. [CrossRef] [PubMed]
5. Keski-Rahkonen, A.; Mustelin, L. Epidemiology of eating disorders in Europe: Prevalence, incidence, comorbidity, course, consequences, and risk factors. *Curr. Opin. Psychiatry* **2016**, *29*, 340–345. [CrossRef] [PubMed]
6. Arcelus, J.; Mitchell, A.J.; Wales, J.; Nielsen, S. Mortality rates in patients with anorexia nervosa and other eating disorders. A meta-analysis of 36 studies. *Arch. Gen. Psychiatry* **2011**, *68*, 724–731. [CrossRef] [PubMed]
7. Abdulkadir, M.; Herle, M.; De Stavola, B.L.; Hübel, C.; Santos Ferreira, D.L.; Loos, R.J.F.; Bryant-Waugh, R.; Bulik, C.M.; Micali, N. Polygenic Score for Body Mass Index Is Associated with Disordered Eating in a General Population Cohort. *J. Clin. Med.* **2020**, *9*, 1187. [CrossRef] [PubMed]
8. Steiger, H.; Booij, L. Eating Disorders, Heredity and Environmental Activation: Getting Epigenetic Concepts into Practice. *J. Clin. Med.* **2020**, *9*, 1332. [CrossRef]
9. Duriez, P.; Robichon, L.; Dardennes, R.; Lavoisy, G.; Grouselle, D.; Epelbaum, J.; Ramoz, N.; Gorwood, P.; Tolle, V.; Viltart, O. Unexpected Association of Desacyl-Ghrelin with Physical Activity and Chronic Food Restriction: A Translational Study on Anorexia Nervosa. *J. Clin. Med.* **2020**, *9*, 2782. [CrossRef]
10. Buelens, T.; Luyckx, K.; Verschueren, M.; Schoevaerts, K.; Dierckx, E.; Depestele, L.; Claes, L. Temperament and Character Traits of Female Eating Disorder Patients with(out) Non-Suicidal Self-Injury. *J. Clin. Med.* **2020**, *9*, 1207. [CrossRef]
11. Testa, G.; Baenas, I.; Vintró-Alcaraz, C.; Granero, R.; Agüera, Z.; Sánchez, I.; Riesco, N.; Jiménez-Murcia, S.; Fernández-Aranda, F. Does ADHD Symptomatology Influence Treatment Outcome and Dropout Risk in Eating Disorders? A longitudinal Study. *J. Clin. Med.* **2020**, *9*, 2305. [CrossRef]
12. Lozano-Madrid, M.; Bryan, D.C.; Sánchez, I.; Riesco, N.; Mallorquí-Bagué, N.; Jiménez-Murcia, S.; Treasure, J.; Fernández-Aranda, F. Impulsivity, Emotional Dysregulation and Executive Function Deficits Could Be Associated with Alcohol and Drug Abuse in Eating Disorders. *J. Clin. Med.* **2020**, *9*, 1936. [CrossRef] [PubMed]
13. Kerr-Gaffney, J.; Mason, L.; Jones, E.; Hayward, H.; Ahmad, J.; Harrison, A.; Loth, E.; Murphy, D.; Tchanturia, K. Emotion Recognition Abilities in Adults with Anorexia Nervosa are Associated with Autistic Traits. *J. Clin. Med.* **2020**, *9*, 1057. [CrossRef] [PubMed]
14. Kinnaird, E.; Dandil, Y.; Li, Z.; Smith, K.; Pimblett, C.; Agbalaya, R.; Stewart, C.; Tchanturia, K. Pragmatic Sensory Screening in Anorexia Nervosa and Associations with Autistic Traits. *J. Clin. Med.* **2020**, *9*, 1182. [CrossRef] [PubMed]
15. Matsui, K.; Komada, Y.; Nishimura, K.; Kuriyama, K.; Inoue, Y. Prevalence and Associated Factors of Nocturnal Eating Behavior and Sleep-Related Eating Disorder-Like Behavior in Japanese Young Adults: Results of an Internet Survey Using Munich Parasomnia Screening. *J. Clin. Med.* **2020**, *9*, 1243. [CrossRef]
16. Alvero-Cruz, J.R.; Parent Mathias, V.; García-Romero, J. Somatotype Components as Useful Predictors of Disordered Eating Attitudes in Young Female Ballet Dance Students. *J. Clin. Med.* **2020**, *9*, 2024. [CrossRef]
17. Mallorquí-Bagué, N.; Lozano-Madrid, M.; Testa, G.; Vintró-Alcaraz, C.; Sánchez, I.; Riesco, N.; César Perales, J.; Francisco Navas, J.; Martínez-Zalacaín, I.; Megías, A.; et al. Clinical and Neurophysiological Correlates of Emotion and Food Craving Regulation in Patients with Anorexia Nervosa. *J. Clin. Med.* **2020**, *9*, 960. [CrossRef]
18. Collantoni, E.; Madan, C.R.; Meneguzzo, P.; Chiappini, I.; Tenconi, E.; Manara, R.; Favaro, A. Cortical Complexity in Anorexia Nervosa: A Fractal Dimension Analysis. *J. Clin. Med.* **2020**, *9*, 833. [CrossRef]
19. Villalba Martínez, G.; Justicia, A.; Salgado, P.; Ginés, J.M.; Guardiola, R.; Cedrón, C.; Polo, M.; Delgado-Martínez, I.; Medrano, S.; Manero, R.M.; et al. A Randomized Trial of Deep Brain Stimulation to the Subcallosal Cingulate and Nucleus Accumbens in Patients with Treatment-Refractory, Chronic, and Severe Anorexia Nervosa: Initial Results at 6 Months of Follow Up. *J. Clin. Med.* **2020**, *9*, 1946. [CrossRef]
20. Maier, S.; Nickel, K.; Perlov, E.; Kukies, A.; Zeeck, A.; Tebartz van Elst, L.; Endres, D.; Spieler, D.; Holovics, L.; Hartmann, A.; et al. Insular Cell Integrity Markers Linked to Weight Concern in Anorexia Nervosa—An MR-Spectroscopy Study. *J. Clin. Med.* **2020**, *9*, 1292. [CrossRef]
21. Duriez, P.; Bou Khalil, R.; Chamoun, Y.; Maatoug, R.; Strumila, R.; Seneque, M.; Gorwood, P.; Courtet, P.; Guillaume, S. Brain Stimulation in Eating Disorders: State of the Art and Future Perspectives. *J. Clin. Med.* **2020**, *9*, 2358. [CrossRef]

22. Kemmer, M.; Correll, C.U.; Hofmann, T.; Stengel, A.; Grosser, J.; Haas, V. Assessment of Physical Activity Patterns in Adolescent Patients with Anorexia Nervosa and Their Effect on Weight Gain. *J. Clin. Med.* **2020**, *9*, 727. [CrossRef] [PubMed]
23. Treasure, J.; Willmott, D.; Ambwani, S.; Cardi, V.; Clark Bryan, D.; Rowlands, K.; Schmidt, U. Cognitive Interpersonal Model for Anorexia Nervosa Revisited: The Perpetuating Factors that Contribute to the Development of the Severe and Enduring Illness. *J. Clin. Med.* **2020**, *9*, 630. [CrossRef]
24. Porras-Garcia, B.; Ferrer-Garcia, M.; Serrano-Troncoso, E.; Carulla-Roig, M.; Soto-Usera, P.; Miquel-Nabau, H.; Shojaeian, N.; de la Montaña Santos-Carrasco, I.; Borszewski, B.; Díaz-Marsá, M.; et al. Validity of Virtual Reality Body Exposure to Elicit Fear of Gaining Weight, Body Anxiety and Body-Related Attentional Bias in Patients with Anorexia Nervosa. *J. Clin. Med.* **2020**, *9*, 3210. [CrossRef] [PubMed]
25. Koerner, T.; Haas, V.; Heese, J.; Karacic, M.; Ngo, E.; Correll, C.U.; Voderholzer, U.; Cuntz, U. Outcomes of an Accelerated Inpatient Refeeding Protocol in 103 Extremely Underweight Adults with Anorexia Nervosa at a Specialized Clinic in Prien, Germany. *J. Clin. Med.* **2020**, *9*, 1535. [CrossRef] [PubMed]
26. Truttmann, S.; Philipp, J.; Zeiler, M.; Franta, C.; Wittek, T.; Merl, E.; Schöfbeck, G.; Koubek, D.; Laczkovics, C.; Imgart, H.; et al. Long-Term Efficacy of the Workshop Vs. Online SUCCEAT (Supporting Carers of Children and Adolescents with Eating Disorders) Intervention for Parents: A Quasi-Randomised Feasibility Trial. *J. Clin. Med.* **2020**, *9*, 1912. [CrossRef] [PubMed]
27. Philipp, J.; Truttmann, S.; Zeiler, M.; Franta, C.; Wittek, T.; Schöfbeck, G.; Mitterer, M.; Mairhofer, D.; Zanko, A.; Imgart, H.; et al. Reduction of High Expressed Emotion and Treatment Outcomes in Anorexia Nervosa—Caregivers' and Adolescents' Perspective. *J. Clin. Med.* **2020**, *9*, 2021. [CrossRef]

Publisher's Note: MDPI stays neutral with regard to jurisdictional claims in published maps and institutional affiliations.

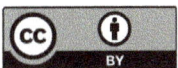

© 2020 by the authors. Licensee MDPI, Basel, Switzerland. This article is an open access article distributed under the terms and conditions of the Creative Commons Attribution (CC BY) license (http://creativecommons.org/licenses/by/4.0/).

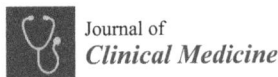

Article

Polygenic Score for Body Mass Index Is Associated with Disordered Eating in a General Population Cohort

Mohamed Abdulkadir [1], Moritz Herle [2,3], Bianca L. De Stavola [2], Christopher Hübel [4,5,6], Diana L. Santos Ferreira [7,8], Ruth J. F. Loos [9], Rachel Bryant-Waugh [10], Cynthia M. Bulik [6,11,12] and Nadia Micali [1,2,13,*]

1. Department of Psychiatry, Faculty of Medicine, University of Geneva, CH–1205 Geneva, Switzerland; mohamed.abdulkadir@unige.ch
2. Great Ormond Street Institute of Child Health, University College London, London WC1N 1EH, UK; moritz.herle.12@ucl.ac.uk (M.H.); b.destavola@ucl.ac.uk (B.L.D.S.)
3. Department of Biostatistics & Health Informatics, Institute of Psychiatry, Psychology & Neuroscience, King's College London, London SE5 8AB, UK
4. Social, Genetic & Developmental Psychiatry Centre, Institute of Psychiatry, Psychology & Neuroscience, King's College London, London SE5 8AF, UK; christopher.1.huebel@kcl.ac.uk
5. UK National Institute for Health Research (NIHR) Biomedical Research Centre, South London and Maudsley Hospital, London SE5 8AF, UK
6. Department of Medical Epidemiology and Biostatistics, Karolinska Institutet, SE-171 77 Stockholm, Sweden; cynthia_bulik@med.unc.edu
7. Medical Research Council Integrative Epidemiology, University of Bristol, Bristol BS8 2BN, UK; diana.santosferreira@bristol.ac.uk
8. Population Health Sciences, Bristol Medical School, University of Bristol, Bristol BS8 2PS, UK
9. The Charles Bronfman Institute for Personalized Medicine, The Mindich Child Health and Development Institute, Icahn School of Medicine at Mount Sinai, New York, NY 10029, USA; ruth.loos@mssm.edu
10. Maudsley Centre for Child and Adolescent Eating Disorders, Michael Rutter Centre for Children and Young People, Maudsley Hospital, London SE5 8AZ, UK; rachel.bryant-waugh@slam.nhs.uk
11. Department of Psychiatry, University of North Carolina at Chapel Hill, Chapel Hill, NC 27599, USA
12. Department of Nutrition, University of North Carolina at Chapel Hill, Chapel Hill, NC 27599, USA
13. Department of Pediatrics, Gynecology and Obstetrics, University of Geneva, CH–1205 Geneva, Switzerland
* Correspondence: n.micali@ucl.ac.uk or nadia.micali@unige.ch; Tel.: +020-7905-2163 or +41-22-372-89-55; Fax: +020-7831-7050 or +41-22-372-24-38

Received: 31 March 2020; Accepted: 18 April 2020; Published: 21 April 2020

Abstract: Background: Disordered eating (DE) is common and is associated with body mass index (BMI). We investigated whether genetic variants for BMI were associated with DE. *Methods*: BMI polygenic scores (PGS) were calculated for participants of the Avon Longitudinal Study of Parents and Children (ALSPAC; N = 8654) and their association with DE tested. Data on DE behaviors (e.g., binge eating and compensatory behaviors) were collected at ages 14, 16, 18 years, and DE cognitions (e.g., body dissatisfaction) at 14 years. Mediation analyses determined whether BMI mediated the association between the BMI-PGS and DE. *Results*: The BMI-PGS was positively associated with fasting (OR = 1.42, 95% CI = 1.25, 1.61), binge eating (OR = 1.28, 95% CI = 1.12, 1.46), purging (OR = 1.20, 95% CI = 1.02, 1.42), body dissatisfaction (Beta = 0.99, 95% CI = 0.77, 1.22), restrained eating (Beta = 0.14, 95% CI = 0.10, 1.17), emotional eating (Beta = 0.21, 95% CI = 0.052, 0.38), and negatively associated with thin ideal internalization (Beta = −0.15, 95% CI = −0.23, −0.07) and external eating (Beta = −0.19, 95% CI = −0.30, −0.09). These associations were mainly mediated by BMI. *Conclusions*: Genetic variants associated with BMI are also associated with DE. This association was mediated through BMI suggesting that weight potentially sits on the pathway from genetic liability to DE.

Keywords: Avon Longitudinal Study of Parents and Children (ALSPAC); body mass index; disordered eating behaviors; disordered eating cognitions; polygenic scores

1. Introduction

Disordered eating (DE) behaviors [1–3], including fasting, binge eating, and related cognitions (such as body dissatisfaction) are widely prevalent in the general population (14–22%) and are considered behavioral and psychological features of a clinical diagnosis of anorexia nervosa (AN), bulimia nervosa (BN), and binge-eating disorder (BED) [1,4–7]. DE typically arises during pre-adolescence and adolescence [1,7,8] and individuals with DE are at greater risk for mood disorders, psychosocial impairment, and suicidal behavior, as well as at elevated risk for developing a full eating disorder [9,10]. Identification of risk factors that may contribute to DE is an active area of inquiry and may offer new prevention and therapeutic interventions as the current treatment strategies for eating disorders (ED) are limited in their efficacy [11,12].

DE and related cognitions are moderate to highly heritable, with estimates from twin studies ranging between 20–85% making it suitable for genetic analyses [13,14]. Polygenic score (PGS) analyses are an effective method that allow for direct testing of whether common genetic variants associated with one trait are also associated with another [15,16]. PGS approaches to understand DE are of interest as they allow interrogation of the shared genetic etiology of two traits that are associated at the phenotypic level, such as DE and body mass index (BMI) [17,18]. Previous research has highlighted that DE and related cognitions are present across the entire weight spectrum, including AN (at one extreme of the weight spectrum) and BED (often at the other extreme of the weight spectrum) [19]. In addition, children who develop an ED have been shown to follow different BMI trajectories prior to diagnosis [20–22]. More specifically, children who go on to develop AN show consistently lower childhood BMI, whereas children who later develop BED show higher premorbid childhood BMIs [20].

It is well established that BMI has a substantial genetic component [23] with the SNP-based heritability ranging between 17–27% [24]. Recent studies have shown a negative genetic correlation between AN and BMI (r_g ~ -0.24) suggesting shared genetic etiology between AN and BMI, whereby genetic variants associated with higher BMI were associated with lower risk for AN [25,26]. However, less is known about the extent to which DE shares genetic etiology with BMI.

The first study to investigate the association between DE and a BMI-PGS found that a BMI-PGS is associated with weight loss behaviors [27]. Nagata et al. reported that the BMI-PGS was associated with a higher odds of weight loss behaviors (e.g., dieting, vomiting) and a lower odds of weight gain behaviors (e.g., eating more or different foods than normal). In addition, Nagata et al. found that the association between the BMI-PGS and weight loss behaviors was mediated by measured BMI; a higher BMI-PGS was associated with a higher measured BMI, which in turn was associated with higher odds of engaging in weight loss behaviors. However, this study [27] investigated the association only in a sample of young adults and evidence is currently lacking in adolescence—a critical period for the development of EDs and DE. Furthermore, this study failed to include pre-morbid BMI (measurement of BMI prior to DE) in the mediation analyses, which complicates establishing potential causal pathways that lead from measured BMI to DE.

In the current study, we investigated whether a BMI-PGS is longitudinally associated with a broad range of DE behaviors and cognitions in a large UK-based population study across adolescence. We hypothesized that the BMI-PGS will be positively correlated with binge eating, emotional eating, and inappropriate compensatory behaviors, such as purging and fasting for weight loss. Based on a previous positive correlation of higher body weight with higher adolescent body dissatisfaction [1] and restrained eating [27,28], we hypothesized that the BMI-PGS will positively correlate with later body dissatisfaction and restrained eating. We also expected a negative association between BMI-PGS and both thin ideal internalization and high external eating—both of which have been found to be negatively correlated with weight or BMI in population-based studies [28,29]. One possible pathway that genetic risk could lead to DE could be through changes in measured BMI which then could lead to increased risk for DE; therefore, we aimed to determine the role of measured BMI as a mediator of these associations. Considering the prospective nature of the data, we also examined developmental differences, determining whether the strength of the association between the BMI-PGS and DE differs across the three time-points during adolescence.

2. Methods and Materials

2.1. Participants

The Avon Longitudinal Study of Parents and Children (ALSPAC) study is an ongoing population-based birth cohort study of 15,454 mothers and their children (that were born between 1 April 1991 and 31 December 1992) residing in the south west of England (UK) [30–33]. From the 15,454 pregnancies, 13,988 were alive at 1 year. At age 7 years this sample was bolstered with an additional 913 children. Participants are assessed at regular intervals using clinical interviews, self-report questionnaires, medical records, and physical examinations. We included children based on three waves of data collection which were at age 14 (wave 14, $N = 10,581$), 16 (wave 16, $N = 9702$), and 18 years (wave 18, $N = 9505$). Further details on ALSPAC are available in previous publications [30,32] and the study website contains details of available data through a fully searchable data dictionary: http://www.bristol.ac.uk/alspac/researchers/our-data/. To avoid potential confounding due to relatedness, one sibling per set of multiple births was randomly selected to guarantee independence of participants ($N = 75$). Furthermore, individuals who were closely related to each other, defined as a phi hat > 0.2 (calculated using PLINK v1.90b), were removed; this meant removal of any duplicates or monozygotic twins, first-degree relatives (i.e., parent-offspring and full siblings), and second-degree relatives (i.e., half-siblings, uncles, aunts, grandparents, and double cousins). The authors assert that all procedures contributing to this work comply with the ethical standards of the relevant national and institutional committees on human experimentation and with the Helsinki Declaration of 1975, as revised in 2008.Ethical approval for the study was obtained from the ALSPAC Ethics and Law Committee and the Local Research Ethics Committees (Bristol and Weston Health Authority: E1808 Children of the Nineties: ALSPAC. 28th November 1989. for details see: http://www.bristol.ac.uk/alspac/researchers/research-ethics/). Informed consent for the use of data collected via questionnaires and clinics was obtained from participants following the recommendations of the ALSPAC Ethics and Law Committee at the time. The main caregiver initially provided consent for child participation and from the age 16 years the offspring themselves have provided informed written consent.

2.2. Measures

2.2.1. Binary Outcomes

Information on fasting, binge eating, and purging, were assessed at ages 14, 16, and 18 years using questions modified from the Youth Risk Behavior Surveillance System questionnaire [34]. For fasting (N age 14 = 4584, N age 16 = 3844, N age 18 = 2586), participants were asked, "During the past year, how often did you fast (not eat for at least a day) to lose weight or avoid gaining weight?" with the response options "Never", "Less than once a month", "1–3 times a month", "Once a week", and "2 or more times a week". This variable was dichotomized as fasting at least once a month in the previous year versus no fasting [8]. For binge eating (N age 14 = 4144, N age 16 = 3336, N age 18 = 1910), participants were asked how often they engaged in overeating (eating a very large amount of food) in the previous year. Participants who answered this question positively were subsequently asked whether they felt out of control during these episodes. We dichotomized the binge eating variable as eating a very large of amount of food at least once a month (with the feeling of loss of control) versus no binge eating. Regarding purging (N age 14 = 4588, N age 16 = 3871, N age 18 = 2582), participants were asked how often they self-induced vomiting or had taken laxatives (or other weight loss medications) to lose weight or avoid weight gain in the previous year; this variable was then dichotomized as purging at least once a month versus no purging.

2.2.2. Continuous Outcomes

All continuous DE outcomes were assessed at age 14 years and included thin ideal internalization, body dissatisfaction, emotional eating, external eating, and restrained eating. Thin ideal internalization ($N = 4496$) was assessed using the Ideal-Body Stereotype Scale-Revised with gender-specific items used to assess different aspects of appearance-ideal internalization for boys (six items) and girls (five items) [8,35,36]. The responses were rated on a five-point Likert scale from "strongly agree" to "strongly disagree" and the items from this scale were summed to obtain a total score; a higher score corresponded with increased internalization of the thin ideal Body dissatisfaction ($N = 4625$) was assessed using the Body Dissatisfaction Scale [36,37]. Participants were asked gender-specific questions rating their satisfaction with nine body parts with responses on a six-point Likert scale ranging from 'extremely satisfied' to 'extremely dissatisfied'. We constructed a continuous score from this scale with a higher score corresponding to higher body dissatisfaction [8,36]. Restrained eating ($N = 4530$), emotional eating ($N = 4345$), and external eating ($N = 3995$) were assessed using a modified version of the Dutch Eating Behavior Questionnaire (DEBQ; [38]). The restrained eating subscale was assessed with two questions, the emotional eating subscale with 14, and the external eating subscale with seven [36,39].

2.2.3. Body Mass Index.

BMI (weight/height^2) was calculated using objectively measured weight and height obtained during a face-to-face assessment at age 11 years ($N = 5902$) [30–32]. Height was measured to the nearest millimeter using a Harpenden Stadiometer (Holtain Ltd., Crymych, UK) and weight was measured using the Tanita Body Fat analyzer (Tanita TBF UK Ltd., Middlesex, UK) to the nearest 50 g. Age- and sex-standardized BMI z-scores (zBMI) were calculated according to UK reference data, indicating the degree to which a child is heavier (>0) or lighter than expected according to his/her age and sex [40].

2.3. Genotyping

Genotype data were available for 9915 children out of the total of 15,247 ALSPAC participants. Participants were genome-wide genotyped on the Illumina HumanHap550 quad chip. Details of the quality control checks are described in the Supplementary Information.

2.4. PGS Calculations

PGS were derived from summary statistics of the Genetic Investigation of Anthropometric Traits (GIANT) consortium, referred to as the discovery cohort [41]. The calculation, application, and evaluation of the PGS was carried out with PRSice (2.1.3 beta; github.com/choishingwan/PRSice/) [42,43]. PRSice relies on PLINK to carry out necessary cleaning steps prior to PGS calculation [42,44]. Strand-ambiguous SNPs were removed prior to the scoring. A total of 1,488,001 SNPs were present in both the discovery and in the target cohort. Clumping was applied to extract independent SNPs according to linkage disequilibrium and p-value: the SNP with the smallest p-value in each 250 kilobase window was retained and all those in linkage disequilibrium ($r^2 > 0.1$) with this SNP were removed. To calculate the PGS, for each participant the sum of the risk alleles was taken and was then weighted by the effect size estimated from the discovery cohort. The PGS were calculated using the high-resolution scoring (PGS calculated across a large number of p-value thresholds) option in PRSice, to identify an optimal p-value threshold at which the PGS is optimally associated with the outcome.

2.5. Statistical Analyses

2.5.1. Sensitivity Analyses (Linkage Disequilibrium Score Regression)

The discovery genome-wide association study (GWAS) from which the BMI-PGS was derived included participants from the UK Biobank [41]. Considering a potential overlap in participants between ALSPAC and the UK Biobank we performed a BMI GWAS with biological sex as a covariate using PLINK in the ALSPAC sample [44]. Subsequently we determined the genetic covariance with the BMI GWAS [41] using linkage disequilibrium score regression (LDSC) v1.0.0. [45].

2.5.2. Regression Analyses

Logistic regressions models were applied for binary outcomes (e.g., fasting at age 14, 16, and 18 years) and linear regression models were used for continuous variables (e.g., thin ideal internalization) with biological sex and the first four ancestry-informative principal components as covariate in all models. We also tested for an interaction between the BMI-PGS and sex and conducted gender stratified analyses.

As confirmatory analyses, we investigated the association between the BMI-PGS and BMI at age 11 and 18 years and the association between the BMI-PGS and the age and sex standardized BMI (i.e., BMI z-scores) measured at age 11 years. We then investigated the association of DE symptoms at age 14 years, except for purging due to its low endorsement and hence exclusion from our analyses (N purging at age 14 years = 74). We repeated the same analyses at age 16 and 18 years for fasting, binge eating, and purging. We report the regression models that explain the largest R^2 or Nagelkerke's pseudo-R^2 at the optimal BMI-PGS p-value threshold. For the binary outcome measures we report the Nagelkerke's pseudo-R^2 on the liability scale [46]. Empirical p-values were calculated through permutation (N = 11,000) that account for multiple testing (i.e., number of p-value thresholds tested) and overfitting [42]. We additionally calculated False Discovery Rate-corrected Q-values adjusting for the number of phenotypes tested [47]. The significance threshold was met if the False Discovery Rate-adjusted Q was <0.05.

2.5.3. Generalized Linear Mixed Models (GLMM)

To understand whether the association of the BMI-PGS with DE differs across the ages (i.e., developmental differences), we used generalized linear mixed models, including BMI-PGS, biological sex, the first four ancestry-informative principal components as fixed effects, and age at self-report as an interaction term. We included random intercepts for each individual in the model, to take into account variance in DE that is due to inter-individual differences. To generate comparable results across the ages, we calculated the PGS at a p-value threshold (P_t) of 1 for each behavioral trait at each age.

2.5.4. Exploratory Causal Mediation Analysis

The association between BMI-PGS and adolescent DE could be explained through childhood BMI prior to assessment of DE. We used sex- and age-adjusted BMI z-scores (zBMI) measured around the age of 11 years (prior to assessment of DE and related cognitions) to capture a possible pathway linking genetic liability measured by the standardized BMI-PGS to DE (Figure S1). We estimated the BMI-PGS effects that are mediated and not mediated by childhood zBMI scores using concepts proposed in modern causal inference; the natural direct and indirect effects [48]. The natural direct effect (also known as the "average direct effect", ADE) measures the expected risk difference of the binary outcome measures (e.g., fasting) had the BMI-PGS been hypothetically set to change by 1 SD from 0 to 1, while at the same time childhood zBMI scores had been set to take their natural value (i.e., the zBMI value that would be experienced had the BMI-PGS been set at the reference value of 0, i.e., under no exposure). For the continuous outcome measures (e.g., thin ideal internalization), the ADE measured as the mean difference of the outcome had the BMI-PGS been set to change by 1 SD while childhood zBMI scores were set to take their natural value under no exposure. The natural indirect effect ("average causal mediated effect", ACME) measures the expected risk difference in binary outcome measures had the BMI-PGS been hypothetically set to take the value 1, while at the same time childhood zBMI scores had been set to take their potential values had BMI-PGS been set to 0 or 1. The ADE was defined in a similar fashion for the continuous outcome measures except that the ACME measured the expected mean difference of the outcome. When summed together, these direct and indirect effects give the total causal effects and therefore are useful measures of the contribution made by a particular pathway to a causal relationship.

We estimated these effects, expressed as risk differences/mean differences, using the R package 'mediation' (version 4.4.6; [49]). Our analyses were controlled for biological sex, and the first four ancestry-informative principal components. Furthermore, we assumed that there were no additional unaccounted confounders nor any intermediate confounders [48].

2.5.5. Missing Data

Considering the longitudinal nature of ALSPAC, study participants tend to drop out as time goes on leading to missing data. In our analyses we carried out complete cases analyses (CCA) and to counter potential bias introduced by carrying out CCA we included relevant confounders (sex), as well as BMI-PGS, both of which are related to missingness in our data [50]. Hence estimates are unbiased under the missing at random (MAR) assumption.

3. Results

3.1. Sample Description

Following quality control of the genetic data, a total of 8654 children with genotyping data and at least one outcome measure were included in the analyses (Table 1). Information regarding age, sex, and ancestry for each timepoint can be found in Table S1. Our sensitivity analyses did not find evidence of sample overlap between our discovery (i.e., BMI GWAS; 25) and target cohort (i.e., ALSPAC) using LDSC, as the intercept from the genetic covariance (0.0068) was less than one standard error (0.0103) from zero, suggesting no sample overlap.

Table 1. Descriptive statistics of disordered eating behaviors and cognitions and BMI of the participants in the Avon Longitudinal Study of Parents and Children [a].

Binary Outcomes	Age Outcome Measured (Years)	Cases			Controls		
		Total N	N (%)	% Female	N		% Female
Fasting [b]	14	4584	300 (3.4%)	83.7%	4284		53.3%
Fasting [b]	16	3844	516 (5.9%)	90.7%	3328		53.8%
Fasting [b]	18	2586	143 (1.6%)	93%	2443		62.1%
Binge eating [b]	14	4144	257 (2.9%)	71.6%	3887		53.4%
Binge eating [b]	16	3336	434 (5.0%)	83.2%	2902		55.3%
Binge eating [b]	18	1910	365 (4.2%)	85.2%	1545		62.2%
Purging [b]	16	3871	237 (2.7%)	92.4%	3634		56.7%
Purging [b]	18	2582	166 (1.9%)	90.9%	2416		62.0%

Continuous Outcomes	Age Outcome Measured (Years)	Total N	Mean	SD	Observed Range (min)	Observed Range (max)
Thin ideal internalization [c]	14	4496	15.33	2.69	5	25
Body dissatisfaction [d]	14	4625	21.85	7.75	9	46.3
Restrained eating [e]	14	4530	0.68	1.13	0	5
Emotional eating [e]	14	4345	5.22	5.53	0	28
External eating [e]	14	3995	8.45	3.34	0	21
Age- and sex-adjusted body mass index (zBMI) [f]	11	4037	0.59	1.13	−3.22	3.78
Total sample size [g]		8654				

SD = standard deviation. [a] Full description of the Avon Longitudinal Study of Parents and Children is described elsewhere; [30–33]. [b] Assessed using questions modified from the Youth Risk Behavior Surveillance System questionnaire [34]. [c] Assessed the Ideal-Body Stereotype Scale-Revised with gender-specific items used to assess different aspects for boys and girls [8,35,36]. [d] Assessed using the Body Dissatisfaction scale [36,37]. [e] As measured by a modified version of the Dutch Eating Behavior Questionnaire [38]. [f] Calculated as weight in kilograms divided by height in meters squared. Height was measured to the nearest millimeter using a Harpenden Stadiometer (Holtain Ltd., Crymych, UK) and weight was measured using the Tanita Body Fat analyzer (Tanita TBF UK Ltd., Middlesex, UK) to the nearest 50 g. zBMI was calculated by standardizing BMI by age and sex. [g] Individuals with at least one outcome measurement (e.g., fasting, binge eating, body dissatisfaction) and available genotyping data.

3.2. PGS Analyses

3.2.1. BMI

In our confirmatory analyses we found that the BMI-PGS was significantly associated with BMI at age 11 years and 18 years and to zBMI measured at age 11 years (Table S2).

3.2.2. DE Behaviors

The BMI-PGS was positively associated with fasting and binge eating at the ages 14, 16, and 18 years and with purging at age 16 years but not at age 18 years (Table 2, Figure 1). There was no significant interaction between the BMI-PGS and sex. When female participants were investigated separately we found similar effect sizes (Table S3). The effect of the best-fit BMI-PGS on fasting was fairly consistent; for one SD increase in the BMI-PGS children were 1.42 (95% CI 1.25, 1.61), 1.29 (95% CI 1.17, 1.42), and 1.26 (95% CI 1.06, 1.51) times more likely to engage in fasting behavior at age 14, 16, and 18 years, respectively. We did not find evidence for a significant interaction between the PGS-BMI and fasting across the three ages indicating that the effect of the BMI-PGS is not age-dependent.

Table 2. Associations of body mass index polygenic score (BMI-PGS) with disordered eating behaviors and cognitions correcting for biological sex in the Avon Longitudinal Study of Parents and Children.

Binary Outcomes	Age Outcome Measured (Years)	Threshold [a]	N SNPs	R^2	OR (95% CI) [b]	Q [c]
Fasting	14	0.085	33,379	0.021	1.42 (1.25, 1.61)	<0.001
Fasting	16	0.17	43,956	0.012	1.29 (1.17, 1.42)	<0.001
Fasting	18	0.1	36,088	0.008	1.26 (1.06, 1.51)	0.045
Binge eating	14	0.014	17,929	0.010	1.28 (1.12, 1.46)	0.003
Binge eating	16	0.0016	9523	0.006	1.20 (1.08, 1.34)	0.006
Binge eating	18	0.0047	12,708	0.008	1.23 (1.09, 1.39)	0.008
Purging	16	0.00025	6115	0.007	1.22 (1.07, 1.41)	0.02
Purging	18	0.033	23,731	0.005	1.20 (1.02, 1.42)	0.10
Continuous Outcomes	Age Outcome Measured (Years)	Threshold [a]	N SNPs	R^2	β (95% CI) [d]	Q [c]
Thin ideal internalization	14	0.5	66,077	0.003	−0.15 (−0.23, −0.07)	0.003
Body dissatisfaction	14	0.0013	9075	0.015	0.99 (0.77, 1.22)	<0.001
Restrained eating	14	0.1	36,088	0.015	0.14 (0.10, 0.17)	<0.001
Emotional eating	14	0.0091	15,467	0.001	0.21 (0.052, 0.38)	0.046
External eating	14	0.0026	10,780	0.003	−0.19 (−0.30, −0.09)	0.003

SNP = single nucleotide polymorphism; R^2, Nagelkerke's Pseudo squared multiple correlation on the liability scale for the binary outcome measures and the squared multiple correlation for the continuous outcomes; OR, odds ratio; CI, confidence interval. [a] The optimal p-value threshold for the inclusion of SNPs in the calculation of the body mass index (BMI) polygenic score (PGS) as determined by PRSice's high-resolution scoring [42]. [b] Odds ratios reflect one standard deviation change in the standardized (to mean zero and standard deviation of one) BMI-PGS. [c] Benjamini & Hochberg False Discovery Rate adjustment for the number of phenotypes tested [47]. [d] Standardized betas reflect one standard deviation increase in the standardized (to mean zero and standard deviation of one) BMI-PGS.

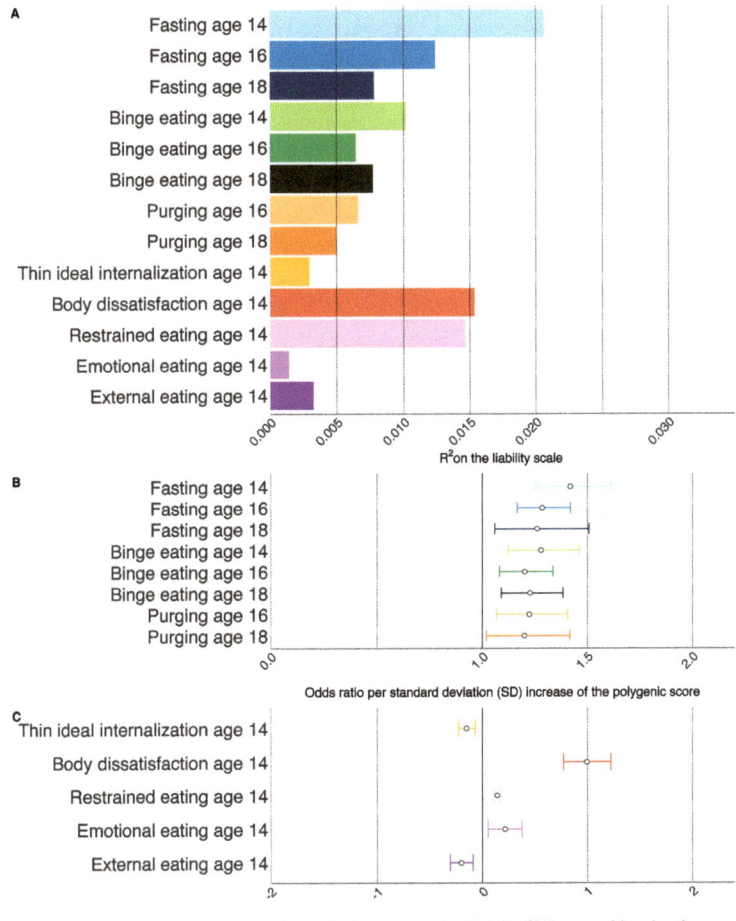

Figure 1. Association between the body mass index polygenic score (BMI-PGS) and disordered eating (DE) behaviors and cognitions in the Avon Longitudinal Study of Parents and Children using generalized linear models [30–33]. Analyses were corrected for biological sex. Age is measured in years. Sample sizes per outcome were fasting (age 14, n cases = 300, n controls = 4284; age 16, n cases = 516, n controls = 3328; age 18, n cases =143, n controls = 2443;), binge eating (age 14, n cases = 257, n controls = 3887; age 16, n cases = 434, n controls = 2902; age 18, n cases =365, n controls = 1545;), and purging (age 16, n cases = 237, n controls = 3634; age 18, n cases= 166, n controls = 2416), thin ideal internalization (n = 4496), body dissatisfaction (n = 4625), restrained eating (n = 4530), emotional eating (n = 4345), external eating (n = 3995). (**A**) Explained variance as measured by Nagelkerke's Pseudo squared multiple correlation (R^2) for the DE phenotypes. All associations were statistically significant (False Discovery Rate-corrected Q-values < 0.05) except for purging at age 18 years. (**B**) Effect size of the association between the standardized BMI-PGS (to mean zero and standard deviation of one) as measured by odds ratios (ORs) and the DE behaviors. The dots represent the point estimates of the ORs for an increase of one standard deviation in the BMI-PGS and the lines represent the 95% confidence interval of the point estimate. (**C**) Effect size of the association between the standardized BMI-PGS (to mean zero and standard deviation of one) as measured by standardized betas and the DE cognitions. The dots represent the point estimates of the standardized betas for an increase of one standard deviation in the BM-PGS and the lines represent the 95% confidence interval of the point estimate.

Children with higher BMI-PGS were also more likely to report binge eating at all three ages with ORs of 1.28 (95% CI 1.12, 1.46), 1.20 (95% CI 1.08, 1.34), and 1.23 (95% CI: 1.09, 1.39), for the ages 14, 16, and 18 years, respectively. Furthermore, the effect of the BMI-PGS on binge eating did not differ across the three ages. Individuals with higher BMI-PGS were 1.22 (95% CI 1.07, 1.41) times more likely to report purging at age 16 years. We did not find an interaction between the BMI-PGS and age at reporting suggesting that the effect of the BMI-PGS did not differ across the reported ages (Table S4).

3.2.3. DE Cognitions

The BMI-PGS was positively correlated with body dissatisfaction and with the DEBQ restrained and emotional eating scale (Table 2). The effect of this association was strongest for body dissatisfaction; children with a higher BMI-PGS (an increase of 1 SD) were more likely to have higher scores on body dissatisfaction at age 14 years ($\beta = 0.99$, 95% CI 0.77, 1.22). This effect was less pronounced for the restrained ($\beta = 0.14$, 95% CI: 0.10, 1.17) and emotional eating ($\beta = 0.21$, 95% CI: 0.05, 0.38) scale of the DEBQ in which a higher BMI-PGS corresponded with lower scores for both behaviors.

In contrast to all other DE outcomes, we found that the BMI-PGS was negatively correlated with thin ideal internalization and with external eating; i.e., individuals with a higher BMI-PGS reported lower scores for thin ideal internalization ($\beta = -0.15$, 95% CI: -0.23, -0.07) and external eating ($\beta = -0.19$, 95% CI: -0.30, -0.09). There was no significant interaction between the BMI-PGS and sex in relation to the DE cognitions. Furthermore, the effect sizes of the association between the BMI-PGS and DE cognitions did not differ (95% confidence intervals overlapped) when female participants were analyzed separately (Table S3).

3.3. Exploratory Causal Mediation Analyses

Causal mediation analyses indicated that the zBMI scores mediated the association between the BMI-PGS and DE except for thin ideal internalization (Table 3). Estimate (β_{ACME}) of the average causal mediation effect ranged between -0.11 (external eating) and 0.93 (body dissatisfaction). For almost all mediation models, one standard deviation (SD) increase in the BMI-PGS corresponded to an increase in zBMI scores at age 11 years, which in turn led to an increased probability of endorsing DE. The exception to this direction of effect was external eating; one standard deviation increase in the BMI-PGS led to an increase in zBMI scores at age 11 years, which corresponded to lower external eating scores at 14 years.

Table 3. Exploratory causal mediation analysis of the association between the disordered eating outcomes and the standardized body mass index polygenic score (BMI-PGS) with the age- and sex-adjusted body mass index z-scores at age 11 years as mediator [a]. p-values for mediation were generated with bootstrapping methods.

Phenotype	Age [b]	Total Effect Estimate β total effect (95% CI)	Total Effect p-Value	Average Direct Effect β ADE (95% CI)	Average Direct Effect p-Value	Average Causal Mediation Effect β ACME (95% CI)	Average Causal Mediation Effect p-Value
Fasting	14	0.022 (0.01, 0.032)	<0.0001	0.011 (0.001, 0.022)	0.038	0.011 (0.007, 0.014)	<0.0001
Fasting	16	0.035 (0.019, 0.051)	<0.0001	0.021 (0.005, 0.037)	0.004	0.014 (0.008, 0.019)	<0.0001
Fasting	18	0.014 (0.002, 0.028)	0.02	0.009 (−0.002, 0.024)	0.146	0.005 (0.001, 0.01)	0.03
Binge eating	14	0.01 (−0.001, 0.02)	0.07	0.004 (−0.007, 0.014)	0.464	0.006 (0.002, 0.01)	<0.0001
Binge eating	16	0.015 (0.001, 0.031)	0.04	−0.001 (−0.015, 0.014)	0.95	0.016 (0.01, 0.022)	<0.0001
Binge eating	18	0.028 (0.006, 0.053)	0.01	0.01 (−0.013, 0.034)	0.348	0.017 (0.009, 0.026)	<0.0001
Purging	16	0.011 (0.002, 0.022)	0.02	0.007 (−0.003, 0.018)	0.168	0.004 (0.001, 0.008)	0.006
Purging	18	0.014 (0.001, 0.03)	0.04	0.004 (−0.008, 0.019)	0.494	0.009 (0.005, 0.014)	<0.0001
Thin ideal internalization	14	−0.133 (−0.245, −0.017)	0.03	−0.118 (−0.228, −0.001)	0.042	−0.015 (−0.055, 0.027)	0.47
Body dissatisfaction	14	1.097 (0.819, 1.378)	<0.0001	0.171 (−0.097, 0.439)	0.218	0.926 (0.798, 1.061)	<0.0001
Restrained eating	14	0.161 (0.819, 0.208)	<0.0001	0.03 (−0.014, 0.072)	0.162	0.13 (0.113, 0.149)	<0.0001
Emotional eating	14	0.129 (−0.071, 0.356)	0.26	0.03 (−0.181, 0.269)	0.804	0.098 (0.023, 0.176)	0.01
External eating	14	−0.195 (−0.335, −0.053)	0.006	−0.087 (−0.228, 0.06)	0.212	−0.108 (−0.162, −0.057)	<0.0001

[a] The BMI-PGS was derived from summary statistics of the genome-wide association study (GWAS) carried out by the Genetic Investigation of Anthropometric Traits (GIANT) consortium [41] and were calculated for participants in the Avon Longitudinal Study of Parents and Children [30–33]. The age- and sex-adjusted BMI (zBMI) at age 11 years was included as a mediator in the causal mediation analyses that was carried out using the R package 'mediation' (version 4.4.6; 32) which is based on concepts proposed in modern causal inference [48]. Prior to the mediation analyses the BMI-PGS was standardized and the analysis was controlled for biological sex. [b] Age was measured in years. [c] Measured using the Dutch Eating Behavior Questionnaire (DEBQ) [38]).

4. Discussion

To our knowledge this is the largest study to date that has investigated whether a BMI-PGS is longitudinally associated with DE in a general population cohort (N = 8654). We demonstrate that genetic factors that underlie BMI are also associated with DE suggesting possible shared genetic etiology between BMI and DE. This association was mainly mediated through measured age- and sex-adjusted BMI (i.e., zBMI at age 11 years). Our results mirror findings from epidemiological studies that report higher BMI to be positively correlated with binge eating, emotional eating, restrained eating, purging, fasting, and body dissatisfaction, and negatively correlated with external eating [28,51–55]. The negative genetic correlation between the BMI-PGS and thin ideal internalization is also consistent with findings for AN, reported to be negatively genetically correlated (r_g = −0.32) with BMI [25,26]. The non-significant association between the BMI-PGS and purging at age 18 years was likely due to the relatively rare endorsement of purging behavior (N = 166) emphasizing the need for larger samples. Furthermore, we did not find evidence for developmental differences; i.e., the strength of the association between the BMI-PGS and DE did not differ across ages.

It is important to emphasize that our study focused on DE as present in a general population cohort, which has important implications in interpreting our findings. Given the high incidence of overweight and obesity [56] in the general population, more individuals than ever could be at risk of developing DE and particularly those with elevated BMI-PGS could be at greater risk. Consistent with our findings, Nagata et al. reported that higher BMI-PGS is positively correlated with weight loss behaviors (e.g., fasting, use of laxatives) in a population cohort [27]. Findings from our group have also previously implicated BMI-related genes in adolescent binge eating in this sample [51]. Taken together, our data and those of others support the notion of a shared genetic etiology between DE and propensity for higher BMI [27,51,57].

Results from our mediation analyses extend previous findings from Reed et al. that reported a causal effect of higher BMI in childhood on increased risk of DE at age 13 years using Mendelian randomization [52]. The importance of BMI in predicting ED has also been highlighted in prospective studies in which BMI trajectories of children who develop an ED during adolescence were found to significantly deviate from children without an eating disorder [20]. We found differences in the estimates of the mediated effect by age- and sex-corrected BMI (zBMI) in the association between the BMI-PGS and DE; suggesting that the effect of actual BMI in late childhood is important for body dissatisfaction, but less for DE behaviors (e.g., purging and fasting for weight loss). As previously shown [1], cognitions such as body dissatisfaction are likely to be influenced by body image distortion and might be more influenced by environmental factors (e.g., comments and teasing about shape and weight). Furthermore, it is important to note that the zBMI scores did not mediate the association between the BMI-PGS and thin ideal internalization. The non-significant mediation for thin ideal internalization might suggest that other pathways apart from prior BMI might account for this association (e.g., environmental factors such as exposure to family or peer factors; [58]). Overall, our findings add to the considerable wealth of literature suggesting an important role for BMI in DE [1,20,25–27,52].

This study benefitted from a large discovery sample (N ~ 789,224) that included participants from the GIANT consortium and the UK Biobank [41,59] and a relatively large target sample (N = 8654). In addition, the availability of a wide range of DE outcomes collected at different time points enriched our analyses. The availability of objectively measured BMI at age 11 years allowed us to investigate the possible role that BMI plays in the association between the BMI-PGS and DE.

Findings from this study should be interpreted in the context of some limitations. Participants were all recruited from the same geographical region in the southwest of England and therefore the results of this study might not be broadly generalizable to other populations. However, the homogeneity of the sample lends itself to genetic analyses as bias from population stratification is expected to be less pronounced [60]. It is important to note that ED symptoms included in this study were derived from self-reports and the questions asked pertained to the previous year, which may have resulted in misclassification and recall bias. However, we emphasize that observational measures on eating behaviors are not feasible in large cohort studies such as ALSPAC. We did not have information on DE behaviors and related cognitions in late childhood; occurrence of these behaviors prior to the measurement of BMI at age 11 years could have biased estimates of our mediation analysis. However, it is likely that prevalence of these behaviors and cognitions would have been very low in late childhood. We also highlight that the focus of our study was on DE as present in the general population and while this information could improve our understanding of threshold ED, caution should be taken when interpreting these results in the context of threshold ED; a proportion of the individuals endorsing DE do not go on to develop an ED. The dichotomizing of categorical behaviors (fasting, binge eating, and purging) might have resulted in grouping less severe cases with more severe cases and in a loss of variance in the outcome which could have weakened our findings. Furthermore, considering the longitudinal nature of the study, participants tend to drop out as time goes on leading to missing data. Attrition (i.e., loss to follow up) in longitudinal studies such as ALSPAC was reported to be associated with higher BMI-PGS [61]. Given what is known about this cohort, we have assumed that the missingness observed in our data was at random, given certain individual characteristics, including the BMI-PGS; for this reason we do not expect substantial bias affecting our complete cases analyses because they included covariates that were related to missingness in our dataset. We acknowledge that some remaining bias might result from selective attrition (i.e., more severe cases dropping out from the study) [50].

The results of our mediation analyses are promising and suggest that joint approaches to the prevention of both obesity and DE might yield better clinical outcomes than those targeting the former or the latter independently [7]. Furthermore, increased awareness amongst pediatricians or general practitioners that children who have overweight or obesity are at increased risk of DE might aid in early screening, detection, and prevention of DE potentially mitigating the development of threshold ED [3]. BMI-PGS can also be used in conjunction with other PGS (e.g., eating disorder PGS) and environmental risk factors in constructing clinical risk prediction models for ED. A robust clinical risk prediction model could for example aid in prediction and guide personalization of treatment, an approach that has shown to be fruitful in many somatic illnesses including coronary artery diseases [62]. However, given the effect sizes observed in this study, the utility of PGS for clinical application for DE is premature.

In conclusion, our results suggest that genetic propensity for higher BMI is associated with DE, and that this association is mediated by actual measured BMI. Our findings add to the consistent epidemiological literature that implicates BMI in DE. The current study has demonstrated that DE and related cognitions need to be understood in a broad context that includes anthropometry as well as behavioral and developmental components. Future research should focus on multifactorial risk and consider the role of environment as well as genetic predisposition to other DE-related traits.

Supplementary Materials: The following are available online at http://www.mdpi.com/2077-0383/9/4/1187/s1, Quality control checks; Figure S1: Directed acyclic graph (DAG) of the causal mediation analyses; Table S1: Age, sex, and ethnicity of the participants in the Avon Longitudinal Study of Parents and Children at all three time points; Table S2: Associations of body mass index polygenic score (BMI-PGS) with BMI in the Avon Longitudinal Study of Parents and Children; Table S3: Effect size of associations of body mass index polygenic score (BMI-PGS) with disordered eating behaviors and cognitions in the total samples and separately for female participants of the Avon Longitudinal Study of Parents and Children; Table S4: Generalized linear mixed models for the association between the body mass index polygenic score (BMI-PGS) and the disordered eating behaviors with age at self-report of the disordered eating as an interaction term [a].

Author Contributions: Conceptualization, B.L.D.S., C.M.B. and N.M.; Data curation, M.H. and N.M.; Formal analysis, M.A., M.H., B.L.D.S. and N.M.; Funding acquisition, N.M. Investigation, M.A., M.H., B.L.D.S. and N.M.; Project administration, N.M.; Supervision, B.L.D.S., R.J.F.L., R.B.-W., C.M.B. and N.M.; Visualization, M.A.; Writing—original draft, M.A., M.H., B.L.D.S. and N.M.; Writing—review & editing, M.A., M.H., B.L.D.S., C.H., D.L.S.F., R.J.F.L., R.B.-W., C.M.B. and N.M. All authors have read and agreed to the published version of the manuscript.

Funding: This research was funded by the UK Medical Research Council and the Medical Research Foundation (MR/R004803/1). The UK Medical Research Council and Wellcome (102215/2/13/2) and the University of Bristol provide core support for ALSPAC. A comprehensive list of grants funding is available on the ALSPAC website (http://www.bristol.ac.uk/alspac/external/documents/grant-acknowledgements.pdf). This research was also funded by the National Institute of Health (MH087786, MH115397) and the National Institute for Health Research (CS/01/2008/014). GWAS data was generated by Sample Logistics and Genotyping Facilities at Wellcome Sanger Institute and LabCorp (Laboratory Corporation of America) using support from 23andMe. This publication is the work of the authors and M.A. will serve as guarantors for the contents of this paper. CMB acknowledges funding from the Swedish Research Council (538-2013-8864) and the National Institute of Mental Health (R01MH120170, R01MH119084). DSF works in a unit that receives funds from the University of Bristol and the UK Medical Research Council (MC_UU_00011/6). The funders were not involved in the design or conduct of the study; collection, management, analysis or interpretation of the data; or preparation, review or approval of the manuscript. M.H. is funded by a fellowship from the Medical Research Council UK (MR/T027843/1).

Acknowledgments: We wish to thank the Genetic Investigation of Anthropometric Traits (GIANT) consortium for providing the summary statistics of the GWAS on BMI. We are also extremely grateful to all the families who took part in the ALSPAC study, the midwives for their help in recruiting them, and the whole ALSPAC team, which includes interviewers, computer and laboratory technicians, clerical workers, research scientists, volunteers, managers, receptionists, and nurses.

Conflicts of Interest: C.B. reports conflict of interest with Shire (grant recipient, Scientific Advisory Board member), Idorsia (consultant), and Pearson (author, royalty recipient). All other authors have indicated they have no conflicts of interest to disclose.

References

1. Micali, N.; De Stavola, B.; Ploubidis, G.; Simonoff, E.; Treasure, J.; Field, A.E. Adolescent eating disorder behaviours and cognitions: Gender-specific effects of child, maternal and family risk factors. *Br. J. Psychiatry* **2015**, *207*, 320–327. [CrossRef] [PubMed]
2. Micali, N.; Horton, N.J.; Crosby, R.D.; Swanson, S.A.; Sonneville, K.R.; Solmi, F.; Calzo, J.P.; Eddy, K.T.; Field, A.E. Eating disorder behaviours amongst adolescents: Investigating classification, persistence and prospective associations with adverse outcomes using latent class models. *Eur. Child Adolesc. Psychiatry* **2017**, *26*, 231–240. [CrossRef] [PubMed]
3. Hayes, J.F.; Fitzsimmons-Craft, E.E.; Karam, A.M.; Jakubiak, J.; Brown, M.L.; Wilfley, D.E. Disordered Eating Attitudes and Behaviors in Youth with Overweight and Obesity: Implications for Treatment. *Curr. Obes. Rep.* **2018**, *7*, 235–246. [CrossRef] [PubMed]
4. Swanson, S.A.; Crow, S.J.; Le Grange, D.; Swendsen, J.; Merikangas, K.R. Prevalence and Correlates of Eating Disorders in Adolescents. *Arch. Gen. Psychiatry* **2011**, *68*, 714–723. [CrossRef]
5. Field, A.E.; Sonneville, K.R.; Micali, N.; Crosby, R.D.; Swanson, S.A.; Laird, N.M.; Treasure, J.; Solmi, F.; Horton, N.J. Prospective Association of Common Eating Disorders and Adverse Outcomes. *Pediatrics* **2012**, *130*, e289–e295. [CrossRef]
6. Solmi, F.; Sonneville, K.R.; Easter, A.; Horton, N.J.; Crosby, R.D.; Treasure, J.; Rodriguez, A.; Jarvelin, M.R.; Field, A.E.; Micali, N. Prevalence of purging at age 16 and associations with negative outcomes among girls in three community-based cohorts. *J. Child Psychol. Psychiatry Allied Discip.* **2015**, *56*, 87–96. [CrossRef]
7. Neumark-Sztainer, D.; Wall, M.; Guo, J.; Story, M.; Haines, J.; Eisenberg, M. Obesity, disordered eating, and eating disorders in a longitudinal study of adolescents: How do dieters fare 5 years later? *J. Am. Diet. Assoc.* **2006**, *106*, 559–568. [CrossRef] [PubMed]
8. Micali, N.; Solmi, F.; Horton, N.J.; Crosby, R.D.; Eddy, K.T.; Calzo, J.P.; Sonneville, K.R.; Swanson, S.A.; Field, A.E. Adolescent Eating Disorders Predict Psychiatric, High-Risk Behaviors and Weight Outcomes in Young Adulthood. *J. Am. Acad. Child Adolesc. Psychiatry* **2015**, *54*, 652–659.e1. [CrossRef]
9. Crow, S.; Eisenberg, M.E.; Story, M.; Neumark-Sztainer, D. Are body dissatisfaction, eating disturbance, and body mass index predictors of suicidal behavior in adolescents? A longitudinal study. *J. Consult. Clin. Psychol.* **2008**, *76*, 887–892. [CrossRef]
10. Chamay-Weber, C.; Narring, F.; Michaud, P.-A. Partial eating disorders among adolescents: A review. *J. Adolesc. Heal.* **2005**, *37*, 416–426. [CrossRef]
11. Berkman, N.; Bulik, C.; Brownley, K.; Lohr, K.; Sedway, J.; Rooks, A.; Gartlehner, G. *Management of Eating Disorders. Evidence Report/Technology Assessment No. 135*; (Prepared by the RTI International-University of North Carolina Evidence-Based Practice Center under Contract No. 290-02-0016.) AHRQ Publication No. 06-E010; Agency for Healthcare Research and Quality: Rockville, MD, USA, 2006.
12. Keel, P.K.; Haedt, A. Evidence-Based Psychosocial Treatments for Eating Problems and Eating Disorders. *J. Clin. Child Adolesc. Psychol.* **2008**, *37*, 39–61. [CrossRef] [PubMed]
13. Culbert, K.M.; Racine, S.E.; Klump, K.L. Research Review: What we have learned about the causes of eating disorders—A synthesis of sociocultural, psychological, and biological research. *J. Child Psychol. Psychiatry* **2015**, *56*, 1141–1164. [CrossRef] [PubMed]

14. Culbert, K.M.; Racine, S.E.; Klump, K.L. The influence of gender and puberty on the heritability of disordered eating symptoms. In *Behavioral neurobiology of eating disorders*; Springer: Berlin/Heidelberg, Germany, 2010; pp. 177–185.
15. Martin, A.R.; Daly, M.J.; Robinson, E.B.; Hyman, S.E.; Neale, B.M. Predicting Polygenic Risk of Psychiatric Disorders. *Biol. Psychiatry* **2019**, *86*, 97–109. [CrossRef] [PubMed]
16. Choi, S.W.; Shin, T.; Mak, H.; Reilly, P.F.O. A guide to performing Polygenic Risk Score analyses. *bioRxiv* **2018**, *5*, 11–13.
17. Tanofsky-Kraff, M.; Yanovski, S.Z.; Wilfley, D.E.; Marmarosh, C.; Morgan, C.M.; Yanovski, J.A. Eating-Disordered Behaviors, Body Fat, and Psychopathology in Overweight and Normal-Weight Children. *J. Consult. Clin. Psychol.* **2004**, *72*, 53–61. [CrossRef] [PubMed]
18. Torstveit, M.K.; Aagedal-Mortensen, K.; Stea, T.H. More than half of high school students report disordered eating: A cross sectional study among Norwegian boys and girls. *PLoS ONE* **2015**, *10*, 1–15. [CrossRef]
19. Flament, M.F.; Henderson, K.; Buchholz, A.; Obeid, N.; Nguyen, H.N.T.; Birmingham, M.; Goldfield, G. Weight Status and DSM-5 Diagnoses of Eating Disorders in Adolescents from the Community. *J. Am. Acad. Child Adolesc. Psychiatry* **2015**, *54*, 403–411.e2. [CrossRef]
20. Yilmaz, Z.; Gottfredson, N.C.; Zerwas, S.C.; Bulik, C.M.; Micali, N. Developmental Premorbid Body Mass Index Trajectories of Adolescents with Eating Disorders in a Longitudinal Population Cohort. *J. Am. Acad. Child Adolesc. Psychiatry* **2019**, *58*, 191–199. [CrossRef]
21. Herle, M.; De Stavola, B.; Hübel, C.; Abdulkadir, M.; Ferreira, D.S.; Loos, R.J.F.; Bryant-Waugh, R.; Bulik, C.M.; Micali, N. A longitudinal study of eating behaviours in childhood and later eating disorder behaviours and diagnoses. *Br. J. Psychiatry* **2019**, 1–7. [CrossRef]
22. Föcker, M.; Bühren, K.; Timmesfeld, N.; Dempfle, A.; Knoll, S.; Schwarte, R.; Egberts, K.M.; Pfeiffer, E.; Fleischhaker, C.; Wewetzer, C.; et al. The relationship between premorbid body weight and weight at referral, at discharge and at 1-year follow-up in anorexia nervosa. *Eur. Child Adolesc. Psychiatry* **2015**, *24*, 537–544. [CrossRef]
23. Albuquerque, D.; Stice, E.; Rodríguez, R.; Licíno, L.-R.; Manco, L.; Nóbrega, C. Current review of genetics of human obesity: From molecular mechanisms to an evolutionary perspective. *Mol. Genet. Genomics* **2015**, *290*, 1191–1221. [CrossRef] [PubMed]
24. Khera, A.V.; Chaffin, M.; Wade, K.H.; Zahid, S.; Brancale, J.; Xia, R.; Distefano, M.; Senol-Cosar, O.; Haas, M.E.; Bick, A.; et al. Polygenic Prediction of Weight and Obesity Trajectories from Birth to Adulthood. *Cell* **2019**, *177*, 587–596.e9. [CrossRef] [PubMed]
25. Watson, H.J.; Yilmaz, Z.; Thornton, L.M.; Hübel, C.; Coleman, J.R.I.I.; Gaspar, H.A.; Bryois, J.; Hinney, A.; Leppä, V.M.; Mattheisen, M.; et al. Genome-wide association study identifies eight risk loci and implicates metabo-psychiatric origins for anorexia nervosa. *Nat. Genet.* **2019**, *51*, 1207–1214. [CrossRef] [PubMed]
26. Duncan, L.; Yilmaz, Z.; Gaspar, H.; Walters, R.; Goldstein, J.; Anttila, V.; Bulik-Sullivan, B.; Ripke, S.; Thornton, L.; Hinney, A.; et al. Significant locus and metabolic genetic correlations revealed in genome-wide association study of anorexia nervosa. *Am. J. Psychiatry* **2017**, *174*, 850–858. [CrossRef]
27. Nagata, J.M.; Braudt, D.B.; Domingue, B.W.; Bibbins-Domingo, K.; Garber, A.K.; Griffiths, S.; Murray, S.B. Genetic risk, body mass index, and weight control behaviors: Unlocking the triad. *Int. J. Eat. Disord.* **2019**, *52*, 825–833. [CrossRef]
28. Snoek, H.M.; Engels, R.C.M.E.; van Strien, T.; Otten, R. Emotional, external and restrained eating behaviour and BMI trajectories in adolescence. *Appetite* **2013**, *67*, 81–87. [CrossRef]
29. Juarascio, A.S.; Forman, E.M.; Timko, C.A.; Herbert, J.D.; Butryn, M.; Lowe, M. Implicit internalization of the thin ideal as a predictor of increases in weight, body dissatisfaction, and disordered eating. *Eat. Behav.* **2011**, *12*, 207–213. [CrossRef]
30. Fraser, A.; Macdonald-wallis, C.; Tilling, K.; Boyd, A.; Golding, J.; Davey smith, G.; Henderson, J.; Macleod, J.; Molloy, L.; Ness, A.; et al. Cohort profile: The avon longitudinal study of parents and children: ALSPAC mothers cohort. *Int. J. Epidemiol.* **2013**, *42*, 97–110. [CrossRef]
31. Golding; Pembrey; Jones; The Alspac Study Team ALSPAC-The Avon Longitudinal Study of Parents and Children. *Paediatr. Perinat. Epidemiol.* **2001**, *15*, 74–87. [CrossRef]
32. Golding, J.; Team, S. The Avon Longitudinal Study of Parents and Children (ALSPAC) – Study design and collaborative opportunities. *Eur. J. Endocrinol.* **2004**, *151* (Suppl. 3), U119–U123. [CrossRef] [PubMed]

33. Boyd, A.; Golding, J.; Macleod, J.; Lawlor, D.A.; Fraser, A.; Henderson, J.; Molloy, L.; Ness, A.; Ring, S.; Smith, G.D. Cohort profile: The 'Children of the 90s'-The index offspring of the avon longitudinal study of parents and children. *Int. J. Epidemiol.* **2013**, *42*, 111–127. [CrossRef] [PubMed]
34. Kann, L.; Warren, C.W.; Harris, W.A.; Collins, J.L.; Williams, B.I.; Ross, J.G.; Kolbe, L.J. Youth Risk Behavior Surveillance-United States, 1995. *J. Sch. Health* **1996**, *66*, 365–377. [CrossRef] [PubMed]
35. Stice, E. Modeling of eating pathology and social reinforcement of the thin-ideal predict onset of bulimic symptoms. *Behav. Res. Ther.* **1998**, *36*, 931–944. [CrossRef]
36. Calzo, J.P.; Austin, S.B.; Micali, N. Sexual orientation disparities in eating disorder symptoms among adolescent boys and girls in the UK. *Eur. Child Adolesc. Psychiatry* **2018**, *27*, 1–8. [CrossRef]
37. Stice, E. A prospective test of the dual-pathway model of bulimic pathology: Mediating effects of dieting and negative affect. *J. Abnorm. Psychol.* **2001**, *110*, 124–135. [CrossRef]
38. van Strien, T.; Frijters, J.E.R.; Bergers, G.P.A.; Defares, P.B. The Dutch Eating Behavior Questionnaire (DEBQ) for assessment of restrained, emotional, and external eating behavior. *Int. J. Eat. Disord.* **1986**, *5*, 295–315. [CrossRef]
39. Schaumberg, K.; Zerwas, S.; Goodman, E.; Yilmaz, Z.; Bulik, C.M.; Micali, N. Anxiety disorder symptoms at age 10 predict eating disorder symptoms and diagnoses in adolescence. *J. Child Psychol. Psychiatry Allied Discip.* **2018**. [CrossRef]
40. Cole, T.J.; Bellizzi, M.; Flegal, K.; Dietz, W. Establishing a standard definition for child overweight and obesity worldwide: International survey. *BMJ* **2000**, *320*, 1240. [CrossRef]
41. Yengo, L.; Sidorenko, J.; Kemper, K.E.; Zheng, Z.; Wood, A.R.; Weedon, M.N.; Frayling, T.M.; Hirschhorn, J.; Yang, J.; Visscher, P.M. Meta-analysis of genome-wide association studies for height and body mass index in ~700000 individuals of European ancestry. *Hum. Mol. Genet.* **2018**, *27*, 3641–3649. [CrossRef]
42. Euesden, J.; Lewis, C.M.; O'Reilly, P.F. PRSice: Polygenic Risk Score software. *Bioinformatics* **2015**, *31*, 1466–1468. [CrossRef]
43. Choi, S.W.; O'Reilly, P.F. PRSice-2: Polygenic Risk Score software for biobank-scale data. *Gigascience* **2019**, *8*, 1–6. [CrossRef] [PubMed]
44. Purcell, S.; Neale, B.; Todd-Brown, K.; Thomas, L.; Ferreira, M.A.R.; Bender, D.; Maller, J.; Sklar, P.; de Bakker, P.I.W.; Daly, M.J.; et al. PLINK: A tool set for whole-genome association and population-based linkage analyses. *Am. J. Hum. Genet.* **2007**, *81*, 559–575. [CrossRef] [PubMed]
45. Bulik-Sullivan, B.; Loh, P.R.; Finucane, H.K.; Ripke, S.; Yang, J.; Patterson, N.; Daly, M.J.; Price, A.L.; Neale, B.M.; Corvin, A.; et al. LD score regression distinguishes confounding from polygenicity in genome-wide association studies. *Nat. Genet.* **2015**, *47*, 291–295. [CrossRef] [PubMed]
46. Lee, S.H.; Goddard, M.E.; Wray, N.R.; Visscher, P.M. A better coefficient of determination for genetic profile analysis. *Genet. Epidemiol.* **2012**, *36*, 214–224. [CrossRef]
47. Benjamini, Y.; Hochberg, Y. Controlling the False Discovery Rate: A Practical and Powerful Approach to Multiple Testing. *J. R. Stat. Soc. Ser. B* **1995**, *57*, 289–300. [CrossRef]
48. VanderWeele, T. *Explanation in Causal Inference: Methods for Mediation and Interaction*; Oxford University Press: Oxford, UK, 2015.
49. Tingley, D.; Yamamoto, T.; Hirose, K.; Keele, L.; Imai, K. mediation: R Package for Causal Mediation Analysis. *J. Stat. Softw.* **2014**, *59*, 1–38. [CrossRef]
50. White, I.R.; Carlin, J.B. Bias and efficiency of multiple imputation compared with complete-case analysis for missing covariate values. *Stat. Med.* **2010**, *29*, 2920–2931. [CrossRef]
51. Micali, N.; Field, A.E.; Treasure, J.L.; Evans, D.M. Are obesity risk genes associated with binge eating in adolescence? *Obesity* **2015**, *23*, 1729–1736. [CrossRef]
52. Reed, Z.E.; Micali, N.; Bulik, C.M.; Davey Smith, G.; Wade, K.H. Assessing the causal role of adiposity on disordered eating in childhood, adolescence, and adulthood: A Mendelian randomization analysis. *Am. J. Clin. Nutr.* **2017**, ajcn154104. [CrossRef]
53. Bucchianeri, M.M.; Arikian, A.J.; Hannan, P.J.; Eisenberg, M.E.; Neumark-Sztainer, D. Body dissatisfaction from adolescence to young adulthood: Findings from a 10-year longitudinal study. *Body Image* **2013**, *10*, 1–7. [CrossRef]
54. Keel, P.K.; Baxter, M.G.; Heatherton, T.F.; Joiner, T.E. A 20-year longitudinal study of body weight, dieting, and eating disorder symptoms. *J. Abnorm. Psychol.* **2007**, *116*, 422–432. [CrossRef] [PubMed]

55. Stice, E.; Gau, J.M.; Rohde, P.; Shaw, H. Risk factors that predict future onset of each DSM–5 eating disorder: Predictive specificity in high-risk adolescent females. *J. Abnorm. Psychol.* **2017**, *126*, 38–51. [CrossRef] [PubMed]
56. Bentham, J.; Di Cesare, M.; Bilano, V.; Bixby, H.; Zhou, B.; Stevens, G.A.; Riley, L.M.; Taddei, C.; Hajifathalian, K.; Lu, Y.; et al. Worldwide trends in body-mass index, underweight, overweight, and obesity from 1975 to 2016: A pooled analysis of 2416 population-based measurement studies in 128·9 million children, adolescents, and adults. *Lancet* **2017**, *390*, 2627–2642.
57. Hinney, A.; Kesselmeier, M.; Jall, S.; Volckmar, A.-L.; Föcker, M.; Antel, J.; Heid, I.M.; Winkler, T.W.; Grant, S.F.A.; Guo, Y.; et al. Evidence for three genetic loci involved in both anorexia nervosa risk and variation of body mass index. *Mol. Psychiatry* **2017**, *22*, 192–201. [CrossRef]
58. Field, A.E.; Javaras, K.M.; Aneja, P.; Kitos, N.; Camargo, C.A.; Taylor, C.B.; Laird, N.M. Family, Peer, and Media Predictors of Becoming Eating Disordered. *Arch. Pediatr. Adolesc. Med.* **2008**, *162*, 574. [CrossRef]
59. Bycroft, C.; Freeman, C.; Petkova, D.; Band, G.; Elliott, L.T.; Sharp, K.; Motyer, A.; Vukcevic, D.; Delaneau, O.; O'Connell, J.; et al. The UK Biobank resource with deep phenotyping and genomic data. *Nature* **2018**, *562*, 203–209. [CrossRef]
60. Hellwege, J.N.; Keaton, J.M.; Giri, A.; Gao, X.; Velez Edwards, D.R.; Edwards, T.L. Population Stratification in Genetic Association Studies. *Curr. Protoc. Hum. Genet.* **2017**, *95*, 1.22.1–1.22.23. [CrossRef]
61. Taylor, A.E.; Jones, H.J.; Sallis, H.; Euesden, J.; Stergiakouli, E.; Davies, N.M.; Zammit, S.; Lawlor, D.A.; Munafò, M.R.; Smith, G.D.; et al. Exploring the association of genetic factors with participation in the Avon Longitudinal Study of Parents and Children. *Int. J. Epidemiol.* **2018**, *47*, 1207–1216. [CrossRef]
62. Lambert, S.A.; Abraham, G.; Inouye, M. Towards clinical utility of polygenic risk scores. *Hum. Mol. Genet.* **2019**, *00*, 1–10. [CrossRef]

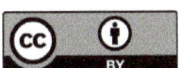

© 2020 by the authors. Licensee MDPI, Basel, Switzerland. This article is an open access article distributed under the terms and conditions of the Creative Commons Attribution (CC BY) license (http://creativecommons.org/licenses/by/4.0/).

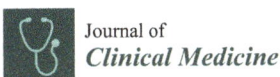

Review

Eating Disorders, Heredity and Environmental Activation: Getting Epigenetic Concepts into Practice

Howard Steiger [1,2,3,*,†] and Linda Booij [3,4,5,*,†]

1. Eating Disorders Continuum, Douglas University Institute, Montreal, Quebec H4H 1R3, Canada
2. Douglas Institute Research Centre, McGill University, Montreal, Quebec H4H 1R3, Canada
3. Department of Psychiatry, McGill University, Montreal, Quebec H3A 1A1, Canada
4. Department of Psychology, Concordia University, Montreal, Quebec H4B 1R6, Canada
5. Sainte-Justine Hospital Research Centre, University of Montreal, Montreal, Quebec H3T 1C5, Canada
* Correspondence: stehow@douglas.mcgill.ca (H.S.); linda.booij@concordia.ca (L.B.)
† Authorship for this paper is shared equally.

Received: 11 March 2020; Accepted: 30 April 2020; Published: 3 May 2020

Abstract: Epigenetic mechanisms are believed to link environmental exposures to alterations in gene expression, and in so doing, to provide a physical substrate for the activation of hereditary potentials by life experiences. In keeping with this idea, accumulating data suggest that epigenetic processes are implicated in eating-disorder (ED) etiology. This paper reviews literature on putative links between epigenetic factors and EDs, and examines ways in which epigenetic programming of gene expression could account for gene-environment interactions acting in the EDs. The paper also presents evidence suggesting that epigenetic processes link malnutrition and life stresses (gestational, perinatal, childhood, and adult) to risk of ED development. Drawing from empirical evidence and clinical experience, we propose that an epigenetically informed understanding of ED etiology can benefit patients, caregivers, and clinicians alike, in the sense that the perspective can reduce judgmental or blameful attitudes on the part of clinicians and caregivers, and increase self-acceptance and optimism about recovery on the part of those affected.

Keywords: epigenetics; anorexia nervosa; bulimia nervosa; eating disorders; DNA methylation; gene-environment interactions

---

1. Introduction

Anorexia nervosa (AN), bulimia nervosa (BN), and related eating disorders (EDs) have traditionally been viewed as "sociocultural creations," or as products of disturbed family environments [1,2]. Not to downplay social and family influences in certain instances of ED, empirical evidence suggests that environmental "impacts" influence ED development by acting upon an environmentally malleable, heritable biology. In this paper, we review evidence for the concept that EDs involve the environmental regulation (through epigenetic processes) of hereditary susceptibilities, and discuss various potential benefits of providing patients, caregivers, and clinicians with a good understanding of a putative causal interplay, in the EDs, between genetic and environmental processes. Our intention with this paper is not to conduct a systematic review on epigenetics in the eating disorders (as such reviews exist elsewhere (e.g., [3,4]), but rather to provide an informed update on the latest findings, along with a discussion of clinical implications. Nonetheless, our review covers important recent articles related to the topic, as identified using PubMED and Google Scholar.

2. What are Eating Disorders (EDs)?

Eating disorders (EDs) are characterized by intense preoccupations with eating, weight, and body image, and such maladaptive eating practices as excessive caloric restraint, binge eating, self-induced vomiting, and compulsive exercise [5]. These disorders are often associated with marked morbidity and mortality [6,7], and high personal and social costs, including lower educational and vocational achievement, decreased quality of life, and social isolation [7–9]. The current version of the Diagnostic and Statistical Manual of Mental Disorders (DSM-5) refers to EDs as "Feeding and Eating Disorders" (FEDs), and recognizes six subtypes: anorexia nervosa (AN), bulimia nervosa (BN), binge eating disorder (BED), avoidant/restrictive food intake disorder (ARFID), rumination disorder (RD), and pica. Two residual diagnoses (other specified feeding or eating disorder and unspecified feeding or eating disorder) capture ED variants that have clinical significance without fulfilling criteria for full-threshold syndromes [5].

AN is defined by restriction of energy intake and persistent avoidance of weight gain, resulting in subnormal body weight. The disorder has two sub-types: AN-restricting type, characterized by restriction of food intake without binging or purging; and AN-binge-eating/purging type, in which individuals regularly engage in binge-eating followed by compensatory behaviors (like self-induced vomiting or misuse of laxatives). People with BN also display recurrent binge-eating and compensatory behaviors, but in the absence of marked weight loss [5]. Individuals with BED, roughly 40% of whom are obese [10], show recurrent binge-eating without compensatory behaviors [5]. Newly introduced in DSM-5, ARFID is characterized by restriction of food intake for reasons unrelated to weight and body image—for instance, compulsive avoidance of foods judged to be impure or unhealthy, or that elicit disgust or aversion [5]. People affected by RD bring already swallowed foods back up and re-chew, whereas pica is a disorder in which people eat non-food items [5]. To date, there are no genetic or epigenetic studies involving ARFID, RD, or pica and, thus, our review does not address these entities.

3. Etiology

EDs are understood to be multiply determined by genetic factors (that shape emotion regulation, reward sensitivity, energy metabolism, appetite, and other variations), environmental triggers (including perinatal insults, developmental stressors, later-life stressors), state-related effects (owing to the nutritional and mental status) and ultimately, social inducements toward intensive caloric restraint [11,12].

3.1. Heredity

Multiple sources of evidence point to the importance of heredity in the EDs. Family aggregation studies have shown that AN and BN are substantially more common in female first-degree relatives of people who themselves have AN or BN (e.g., Strober, et al. [13]), and one study shows that levels of eating and body-image concerns correspond in biological sister pairs, but not in adoptive pairs [14]. Even more convincingly, studies comparing concordance rates for EDs between mono- and dizygotic twin pairs reveal heritability coefficients for AN, BN, and BED ranging from 32% to 76% [15], 28% to 83% [15], and 39% to 45% [15], respectively. Aside from emphasizing unique genetic effects, these studies generally indicate non-shared environmental factors (e.g., a particular stressor experienced by one twin) to be more influential in ED development than are shared environmental factors (e.g., living in the same family environment) [15]. The preceding tends to refute ED formulations that are couched strongly in terms of family dynamics.

3.2. Genetics

There have been various efforts to identify gene variants that may be associated with risk of an ED. Candidate-gene approaches (which examine single gene variants) are generally driven by a theory-based "guess" about which of the tens of thousands of genes may be an important contributor to risk for a disorder—something akin to guessing around which star in the night sky might there be a life-harboring planet. Nonetheless, some findings point to associations between EDs and polymorphisms of genes regulating key neurotransmitters (e.g., serotonin [16]), neuromodulators (e.g., brain-derived neurotropic factor (BDNF) [17]), hormones (e.g., estrogen [18]), or eating behavior (e.g., ghrelin [19]). Despite some leads, the candidate approach has not yielded many replicable findings. Detailed reviews of findings from candidate-gene studies in EDs can be found in several previous reviews (e.g., [3,20]).

Recent technologies support genome-wide association studies (GWASs), which allow for hypothesis-free investigations aimed at uncovering novel genetic markers that reach what is called "genome-wide statistical significance" for association with a phenotype of interest. Given that genome-wide methods test thousands of common human gene variant markers at a time, a strict threshold for significance ($p < 5 \times 10^{-8}$) has been established to correct for chance associations that could occur when conducting large numbers of simultaneous comparisons. The cost of maintaining such stringency, however, is that genome-wide studies require enormous sample sizes.

To date, GWASs in the field have been completed only for AN—although studies examining BN and BED are underway. The earliest published GWASs in AN were underpowered, and hence failed to yield findings of genome-wide significance [21–24]. However, two recently published GWASs, both conducted by the Eating Disorders Work Group of the Psychiatric Genomics Consortium (PGC-ED), have yielded intriguing findings reaching genome-wide significance. The first of these, involving DNA from 3,495 people with AN and 10,982 normal-eater controls, associated a locus on chromosome 12 with AN, at a site linked to type-1 diabetes and autoimmune diseases [25]. In addition, genetic correlations (computed using linkage disequilibrium scores) associated AN with mental-illness phenotypes (e.g., neuroticism) and physical-health phenotypes (rapid glucose and lipid metabolism, low body mass index (BMI)). In other words, in addition to expected psychiatric components, findings characterized AN as having important metabolic and autoimmune components. The autoimmune aspect of these findings, incidentally, corroborates a report from a study in more than 930,000 Swedish hospital records showing that children having a parent with an auto-immune disorder are unusually likely to develop an ED [26].

The second GWAS, involving data from 16,992 people with AN and 55,525 controls [27], identified eight significant genetic loci, and again implicated psychiatric traits (e.g., obsessive-compulsive and major depressive disorders), metabolic traits (e.g., insulin resistance, lipid metabolism) and anthropometric traits (e.g., low BMI, low fat mass). According to these studies, the genetic architecture of AN not only implicates psychiatric traits, but also metabolic factors and particular physical (anthropometric) characteristics.

4. Genes and Environmental Activation

It is an intuitive point that the genetic contribution to many mental-health problems acts only when triggered by the environment—and the preceding is very likely to be true of EDs. As we have already noted, twin data have shown that EDs involve a strong genetic diathesis, but also a contribution from the non-shared environment [15]. In other words, ED development is likely to implicate gene-environment interaction effects. Supporting this point, animal data suggest that genetic susceptibility, in combination with adolescent social stress and caloric restraint can produce a mouse "analog" to AN—mice that let themselves starve [28]. Similarly, clinical data show risk of AN to be increased in genetically disposed individuals when subjected to familial distress [29]. Diverse environmental influences have been postulated to act in AN, including obstetric insults, gestational stress, childhood trauma, familial conflict, adult victimization experiences, social inducement towards caloric restraint, and one's actual nutritional state [30].

Epigenetic Processes

Epigenetic processes influence gene expression (and corresponding phenotypic variations) in the absence of actual DNA sequence changes, and are believed to act in an environmentally responsive fashion [31,32]. Mechanisms involved include DNA methylation/demethylation and hydroxylmethylation, histone acetylation/deacetylation, histone phosphorylation/ dephosphorylation, noncoding RNA and microRNAs, as well as transcriptome actions [32]. The most widely studied of these, DNA methylation, involves the addition of methyl groups to regions of the gene referred to as CpG sites—at which cytocine is followed by guanine [32]. Methylation in certain CpGs can silence or suppress gene expression—in theory, allowing for environmental programming of gene expression [31,32]. Available findings provide compelling evidence of a role of DNA methylation in rendering gene expression responsive to environmental exposures. However, these findings are not without limitations—from both methodological and conceptual standpoints. As a full discussion of such limitations is beyond the scope of this paper, the interested reader is referred to full treatments of such questions presented elsewhere [4,33].

Environments of Concern

The Prenatal Environment

A famous study, capitalizing on a "natural experiment" in malnutrition, showed that Dutch children born to starving mothers (due to a World War II induced food blockade) showed altered physical stature and emotional adjustment and, after six decades, altered DNA methylation in genes regulating growth and metabolism compared to those of their siblings [34]. In a similar vein, studies have linked maternal depression during gestation to altered methylation of the glucocorticoid receptor (NR3C1) gene and altered stress reactivity in the offspring [35]. Likewise, Suarez et al. [36] observed that maternal antenatal depression was associated with an epigenetic marker (lower epigenetic gestational age) associated with mental-health problems in pre-school age boys. Fathers matter, too. Germ cells in the sperm line convey epigenetic information, meaning that fathers can also influence fetal programming in their offspring [37]. There is a now-sizable literature demonstrating that stress in parents of both sexes can impact neurodevelopment in their offspring via epigenetic processes (see [38] for a thorough review). Also of relevance are findings of a recent study associating fathers' periconception BMI with DNA methylation patterns in their children at age 3 and 7 years, independently of mothers' BMI [39].

One of our group's recent studies showed that children of mothers who were exposed to intense, third-trimester gestational distress during very-severe weather conditions—the 1998 Quebec Ice Storm (regarded as Canada's worst natural disaster)—showed more ED symptoms at age $13\frac{1}{2}$ than did children of mothers who had less environmental-stress exposure [40]. Indicating the effect to have likely epigenetic origins, in a separate study, degree of *in utero* stress exposure in the same children was associated with extent of alteration of methylation in genes involved in Type-1 and -2 diabetes mellitus [41]. Interestingly, children who had higher methylation levels at age 13 concurrently had a lower BMI and lower central adiposity [41]. Investigating possible epigenetic effects of maternal EDs upon their offspring, Kazmi and colleagues [42] measured genome-wide methylation of cord blood DNA in 21 babies of women with active AN, 43 with a past AN, and 126 normal-eater controls. Infants of women with AN had lower global methylation levels than did controls. In addition, babies of women who were actively eating-disordered during pregnancy had altered methylation in genes implicated in biosynthesis of cholesterol and neuronal survival, whereas those whose mothers once had AN showed altered methylation in a gene linked to inflammation and immune response.

The Childhood Environment

Although it is uncertain to what extent findings obtained in animal studies inform processes in humans, animal studies have one advantage when studying possible epigenetic effects of early-life stress—as environmental stress exposures can be randomized across animals and experimentally manipulated and controlled in a way that could never be done in studies on developing humans. The preceding allows for differentiation of gene-environment correlations (in which the actor, because of a particular trait, induces an environmental effect) from gene-environment interactions (in which the environment has an action that is fully independent of the actor). There are many demonstrations that animals raised in stressful conditions show altered DNA methylation in systems associated with stress accommodation (e.g., [43–45]. Studies by Roth and colleagues indicate that infant rats exposed to adverse rearing experiences evinced lasting changes in the methylation status of the *BDNF* gene, and corresponding behavioral alterations [45]. Likewise, studies by Meaney and colleagues showed that rat pups receiving low maternal care compared to pups, that received high maternal care had greater hippocampal DNA methylation of the glucocorticoid receptor gene (*NR3C1*) and decreased hippocampal glucocorticoid receptor messenger RNA (mRNA) expression (e.g., [43,46]). In parallel, in a postmortem study, human suicide victims who had experienced childhood abuse have been shown to display higher methylation of the *NR3C1* gene promoter and decreased levels of glucocorticoid receptor mRNA in the hippocampus relative to non-abused suicide victims and controls [44]. Numerous other observations in humans associate early-life stress exposures (such as physical or sexual abuse, deprivation from parental care, or natural disasters), with epigenetic alterations and later behavioral and mental-health outcomes [33,47–51].

Suggesting that comparable effects apply in EDs, we previously found that women with BN who report a history of suicidality have greater methylation of specific CpG sites in the *NR3C1* gene promoter region [52]. We also observed hypermethylation of specific CpG sites in the promoter region of the *BDNF* gene in bulimic women who report a history of childhood sexual or physical abuse [53]. BDNF is thought to play a role in neural plasticity, learning of traumatic memory and binge eating [54]. Furthermore, we reported that women with BN and comorbid borderline personality disorder, who tend to report high levels of childhood adversity, show hypermethylation of the dopamine *DRD2* receptor gene promoter region [55].

The Nutritional Environment

Since EDs profoundly affect nutritional status, an important question is "How do ED-induced nutritional deficits affect the epigenome?" An even more important question may be: "Does nutritional rehabilitation during ED recovery reverse disorder-linked epigenetic alterations?". Central to the preceding questions is that nutrients, such as folate, B12, and choline, influence the functioning of one carbon metabolism—a physiological process crucial for generating methyl-transfer reactions upon which DNA methylation depends [56]. While most of the evidence for the influence of nutrients on DNA methylation comes from animal studies, there is now increasing evidence in humans that dietary intake of folate, choline, and B-vitamins also affect DNA methylation and brain function across the life-cycle [56,57]. Furthermore, numerous studies suggest that peoples' nutritional state can make epigenetically mediated contributions to psychiatric disorders [58]. Our group is presently studying pathways, in people with AN, linking self-reported eating behaviors, plasma levels of nutrients involved in one-carbon metabolism, and DNA methylation levels. At the time of this writing, results are in a preliminary state. However, initial indices suggest that nutritional factors do impinge directly upon DNA methylation levels [59].

5. Findings on DNA Methylation in People with EDs

5.1. Methylation Studies in Candidate Genes

We emphasize from the start that candidate-gene methylation studies are subject to all of the limitations inherent in any candidate study—including problems of power and stability of results. Nonetheless, interpreted judiciously, available studies offer some intriguing indications: Available studies in AN have reported altered methylation of genes regulating expression of alpha-synuclein (involved in neurotransmitter release) [60], dopamine [61] (implicated in mood, impulse-control, reward sensitivity and binge-like eating), oxytocin [62,63] (linked to social attachment), histone deacetylase [64] (broadly influencing gene expression), and leptin [65] (which inhibits hunger). Combining measures of serotonin transporter (*SLC6A4*) gene methylation with resting-state functional connectivity data, Boehm, et al. [66] associated epigenetic variation in the *SLC6A4* gene with neural connectivity in the salience network—an important brain circuit for emotion regulation. Another research group reported that individuals with BN had greater methylation of the atrial natriuretic peptide (ANP) gene promoter (involved in cardiovascular homeostasis) than controls [67]. Similarly, studies noted earlier have documented alterations in the methylation of candidate genes that might, in theory, be relevant to bulimic ED variants—including glucocorticoid receptor [52] and dopamine *DRD2* receptor genes [55]. However, we note that available findings seem to indicate that the epigenetic variations noted may be more pertinent to comorbidity (e.g., suicidality or personality disorders) than to BN itself.

We identified no studies investigating methylation differences between patients with a primary diagnosis of BED and normal-eater controls. However, one study reported that patients who showed concurrent bipolar disorders and binge-eating had hypomethylation of the *SLC1A2* gene (involved in removing glutamate from the synaptic cleft) relative to patients with bipolar disorder who displayed no binge eating [68].

5.2. Global Methylation Level Studies

A handful of recent studies has attempted to quantify global methylation across the whole genome. Such studies allow for the evaluation of hypotheses about global variations in methylation levels, but are "blind" to possibly more meaningful variations in methylation acting at specific genomic loci. Studies of this type have tended to produce inconsistent results, largely (we suspect) because of small samples and a diversity of methods involved. Across available studies comparing participants with AN to those with no ED, we find one reporting no global differences [69], two reporting global hypomethylation in AN [60,70], and one reporting hypermethylation [71].

5.3. Epigenome-Wide Methylation Studies

Superior to either candidate-gene or global methylation measures, genome-wide methylation measures allow for the analysis of site-specific alterations at multiple genomic loci. A first study of this kind, performed by our group, used a high-throughput (Illumina 450K) technology to perform a genome-wide comparison of methylation levels in DNA obtained from leukocytes in 30 women with active AN and 15 normal-weight, normal eaters [71]. False discovery rate corrected comparisons identified differentially methylated CpG probes corresponding to genes associated with histone acetylation, cholesterol storage, lipid transport, and dopamine and glutamate signaling. Findings also linked chronicity of illness to DNA methylation levels at probes that mapped onto genes associated with anxiety, immunity, and central nervous system functioning. An independent study (using the same technology) reported on methylation in 47 females with AN and 100 population-based control females [72]. Intriguingly, two of the differentially methylated genes identified in case-control comparisons—*NR1H3* (involved in lipid metabolism and inflammation) and *TNXB* (associated with connective-tissue disorders)—corresponded to those identified by our group. TNXB encodes an extracellular matrix glycoprotein, absence of which has been associated with Ehlers–Danlos syndrome, a connective tissue disorder characterized by joint hypermobility that is noted to co-occur with AN [73].

Our group subsequently reported on an expanded methylome-wide study, involving enlarged samples of participants with active AN or no ED, and a new sample of individuals in whom AN had remitted for at least one year [74]. Methylation levels in members of the remitted group differed from those in the active group on probes that, among others, isolated genes associated with serotonin and insulin activity, glucose metabolism, and immunity. Intriguingly, the direction of methylation effects in remitted participants tended to be opposite to that seen in individuals with active AN, suggesting that epigenetic alterations in actively ill individuals may be reversible. If so, DNA methylation could serve as a marker of disease staging or therapeutic response. Furthermore, we find it intriguing that altered methylation findings seem to parallel results of the GWASs described earlier [25]—i.e., they also implicate psychiatric, metabolic, and immune functions.

6. Clinical Applications

Traditional etiological models are replete with blameful and pathologizing innuendos concerning roles in ED development of "maladaptive personality traits" in affected individuals and "problematic interaction patterns" in their families. As our review has shown, contemporary conceptualizations refute such notions—promoting instead the point that people do not develop EDs because of "character weaknesses," "stubbornness," "superficial concern with appearance," or "bad parenting" but because they carry real genetic susceptibilities that get "switched on" by a lifetime of environmental exposures. In other words, EDs are understood to result from factors that are far beyond the willful control of those affected. It is our belief that perspectives on ED development that properly accommodate genetic and epigenetic influences improve clinicians' sensitivity to their patients' realities, and help make treatment more palatable and humane.

We take inspiration from several recent efforts to apply gene x environment interaction concepts clinically in the ED area. One recent study showed that an approach to ED psychoeducation that was couched in epigenetic terms (referred to as "malleable biology"), when compared to approaches framed in purely biological or cognitive terms, led to greater recovery optimism and felt self-efficacy on ED patients' part [75]. A recent paper makes a similar point, that when counseling for people affected by EDs places causal responsibility upon interacting genetic and environmental influences, it has potential to relieve blame and to legitimize patients' experiences [76]. One of the co-authors of the paper in question, Jehannine Austin, has been a strong proponent of the application, across a variety of mental-health contexts, of a new "breed" of genetic counseling. She and her colleagues have shown that counseling that informs patients and those close to them about gene-environment interactions helps empower and increase self-efficacy in individuals with mental illness [77]. In one of their studies, patients reported that this style of counseling made them better able to manage their illnesses, and more open to talking about them with family and friends [77]. We have similarly argued that epigenetically informed models improve clinicians' empathy surrounding the ways in which EDs can become entrenched and difficult to overcome [30]. Encouragingly (and a bit paradoxically), formulations of ED development that accommodate neuroscience concepts actually seem to "humanize" the understanding of ED illness and recovery. Arguably, genetically and epigenetically informed models of ED development contribute positively to efforts of clinicians and carers in various ways:

1. They blame affected individuals less. Since the causes of EDs are increasingly understood to involve the activation of real physical susceptibilities by real environmental exposures, it becomes possible to trace with patients the sequence of life events (that may include perinatal insults, childhood adversities, school-related stresses and, invariably, the effects of prolonged caloric restraint) that served to activate inherited susceptibilities toward ED development. Likewise, because they take into account multiple causal factors (and complex interactions among them), informed models do less "finger pointing" at parents and other caregivers. It is never a single event or action (e.g., parents' divorce, or a care-taker's depressive episode) that caused someone's ED.

2. They help promote greater self-acceptance. Clinical experience dictates that a common "symptom" of an ED is shame. People invariably feel stupid to have developed their disorder, weak to not yet have overcome it, and guilty for the distress their disorder causes relatives and friends. When with someone experiencing shame around his/her ED, and speaking from an epigenetically informed understanding, we might often say something like: "You didn't ask to have an ED. At the end of the day, when you fully understand why you developed this disorder, you won't have to feel ashamed. You'll just say, 'I see why I got an ED'". This stance on therapists' part, when sincere, helps promote self-acceptance in people who are prone instead to self-disparagement. Likewise, especially when afflicted by an ED after several rounds of therapy, or decades of suffering, it is natural for affected people to feel inadequate, and perhaps deserving of messages they may have received from uninformed carers or therapists that "you aren't trying hard enough" or "You're choosing to keep your ED". Findings from the epigenetic literature suggest that chronic exposure

to malnutrition and dietary distress amplify psychological tendencies (e.g., compulsivity, anxiety) and metabolic adaptations (e.g., altered lipid metabolism) that help "lock" the ED into place. The difficulty one may experience in recovering from an ED becomes understood, not as an index of character weakness or obstinacy, but of the extent to which biological processes anchor symptoms and behaviors into place.

3. They help patients (and therapists) accept "incremental response." Epigenetic data in AN suggest that there are many disorder-induced alterations in the expression of genes that affect mental status, metabolism, and immune/inflammatory processes—and that such alterations become more pronounced with increasing chronicity of illness (see [71,74]). It is likely that these same factors need to be "reset" before someone affected can take back control. Encouragingly, some findings show that nutritional rehabilitation does help undo problematic changes—but it remains unclear over what span of time such alterations take place.

4. They assign proper importance to nutritional factors. It is clear that malnutrition and dietary distress amplify physical and psychological problems in ED patients, and help lock the disorder into place. Various recent findings suggest that epigenetic processes may contribute to ED entrenchment through nutritionally-induced alterations in gene expression [71,72,74]. An implicit message is that: "Your ED was triggered by too much caloric restraint and, logically, recovery will depend upon re-establishing a healthy nutritional state". Although further research is required to establish parameters, a related concern may help moderate messages aimed at preventing obesity that encourage dietary restraint.

5. They help separate the person affected from his/her illness. "Externalizing the illness" is an explicit operation in family-based treatment approaches [78], and an implicit one in Cognitive Behavioral Therapy [79] and other established ED treatments. Recognizing that one is separate from one's disorder (and the behaviors that it drives) helps affected people overcome shame, and increases empathy on the part of family members, partners, and friends. A genetically/epigenetically informed model implicitly separates individuals from the factors that caused and perpetuate their illnesses—in the sense that the model makes explicit the point that EDs represent the activation of heritable physical susceptibilities by real-life experiences. We often say: "You did not ask to have this disorder. You are responsible for repairing the damage and recovering, but not for what caused the illness in the first place". In a related vein, because of its ego-syntonic nature, people with AN sometimes identify positively with their disorder, or assume it as an identity. We believe that an epigenetically informed perspective helps counteract such tendencies. It helps people affected by the disorder recognize that "you are not 'an anorexic'. Rather, you are someone in whom a vulnerability has been switched on by too much dieting. And the effect is that restricting food intake feels good in a bit the same way that abusing drugs feels good to a person with an addiction."

The following clinical vignette illustrates the potential value of an epigenetically informed stance: Some time ago, we admitted a woman with severe anorexia nervosa onto our inpatient unit. She was bewildered and frightened in the early days of her stay on our unit. A voluntary patient, after only a few days she took essentially the stance: "Thank you, I'm feeling much better and would like to go home." This was not a plan that could be safe for her. As a program invested in practices governed by notions of autonomy support (See [80,81]), we made efforts to avoid involuntary admission. But rational arguments aimed at helping this woman opt to stay voluntarily failed to be convincing, and she became increasingly adamant about returning home. Thankfully, serendipity made involuntary admission unnecessary. This woman spontaneously asked why she felt so bloated after eating, and we explained that this was a symptom of delayed stomach emptying time typical in AN. She replied: "You mean it's not in my head". We replied: "No. It's not in your head; it's in your stomach. There's a real physical cause". We explained further. "And speaking of real physical causes, you know that study on epigenetics in which we asked you to take part? Can we talk about that a bit?" We elaborated on what epigenetics is, how it is a science that promises to explain how genetic tendencies get activated by the environment. How life stresses and too much dieting seem to be among the factors that cause epigenetic changes in AN. After a brief discussion, and after addressing the patient's various questions and confusions, she stated: "That's so interesting". Signs of indignity fell away. She not only consented to take part in the study, but agreed to stay longer on the unit.

Author Contributions: H.S. conceptualized the review. H.S. and L.B. drafted the article. Both authors have read and agreed to the published version of the manuscript. All authors have read and agreed to the published version of the manuscript.

Funding: Authors' research described in this paper was made possible by generous contributions towards research from the Canadian Institutes for Health Research (grants 142717 and 391362), the Douglas Institute Foundation and from Cogir Corporation. L.B. was supported by a salary award from the Fonds de Recherche du Québec-Santé.

Conflicts of Interest: The authors declare no conflicts of interest.

References

1. Gordon, R. *Eating Disorders: Anatomy of a Social Epidemic*, 2nd ed.; Wiley-Blackwell: Hoboken, NJ, USA, 2000.
2. Minuchin, S.; Baker, L.; Rosman, B.L.; Liebman, R.; Milman, L.; Todd, T.C. A conceptual model of psychosomatic illness in children. Family organization and family therapy. *Arch. Gen. Psychiatry* **1975**, *32*, 1031–1038. [CrossRef]
3. Himmerich, H.; Bentley, J.; Kan, C.; Treasure, J. Genetic risk factors for eating disorders: An update and insights into pathophysiology. *Ther. Adv. Psychopharmacol.* **2019**, *9*. [CrossRef]
4. Hubel, C.; Marzi, S.J.; Breen, G.; Bulik, C.M. Epigenetics in eating disorders: A systematic review. *Mol. Psychiatry* **2019**, *24*, 901–915. [CrossRef] [PubMed]
5. American Psychiatric Association. *Diagnostic and Statistical Manual of Mental Disorders*, 5th ed.; American Psychiatric Publishing: Washington, DC, USA, 2013.
6. Arcelus, J.; Mitchell, A.J.; Wales, J.; Nielsen, S. Mortality rates in patients with anorexia nervosa and other eating disorders. A meta-analysis of 36 studies. *Arch. Gen. Psychiatry* **2011**, *68*, 724–731. [CrossRef] [PubMed]
7. Weigel, A.; Konig, H.H.; Gumz, A.; Lowe, B.; Brettschneider, C. Correlates of health related quality of life in anorexia nervosa. *Int. J. Eat. Disord.* **2016**, *49*, 630–634. [CrossRef] [PubMed]
8. Maxwell, M.; Thornton, L.M.; Root, T.L.; Pinheiro, A.P.; Strober, M.; Brandt, H.; Crawford, S.; Crow, S.; Fichter, M.M.; Halmi, K.A.; et al. Life beyond the eating disorder: Education, relationships, and reproduction. *Int. J. Eat. Disord.* **2011**, *44*, 225–232. [CrossRef]
9. Wentz, E.; Gillberg, I.C.; Anckarsater, H.; Gillberg, C.; Rastam, M. Adolescent-onset anorexia nervosa: 18-year outcome. *Br. J. Psychiatry* **2009**, *194*, 168–174. [CrossRef]
10. Kessler, R.C.; Berglund, P.A.; Chiu, W.T.; Deitz, A.C.; Hudson, J.I.; Shahly, V.; Aguilar-Gaxiola, S.; Alonso, J.; Angermeyer, M.C.; Benjet, C.; et al. The prevalence and correlates of binge eating disorder in the World Health Organization World Mental Health Surveys. *Biol. Psychiatry* **2013**, *73*, 904–914. [CrossRef]
11. Steiger, H.; Coelho, J.; Thaler, L.; Van den Eynde, F. Eating disorders. In *Oxford Textbook of Psychopathology*; Blaney, P., Krueger, R., Millon, T., Eds.; Oxford University Press: New York, NY, USA, 2015.
12. Striegel-Moore, R.H.; Bulik, C.M. Risk factors for eating disorders. *Am. Psychol.* **2007**, *62*, 181–198. [CrossRef]
13. Strober, M.; Freeman, R.; Lampert, C.; Diamond, J.; Kaye, W. Controlled family study of anorexia nervosa and bulimia nervosa: Evidence of shared liability and transmission of partial syndromes. *Am. J. Psychiatry* **2000**, *157*, 393–401. [CrossRef]
14. Klump, K.L.; Suisman, J.L.; Burt, S.A.; McGue, M.; Iacono, W.G. Genetic and environmental influences on disordered eating: An adoption study. *J. Abnorm. Psychol.* **2009**, *118*, 797–805. [CrossRef] [PubMed]
15. Wade, T.C.; Bulik, C.M. Genetic Influences on Eating Disorders. In *The Oxford Handbook of Eating Disorders*; Agras, W.S., Robinson, A., Eds.; Oxford University Press: New York, NY, USA, 2018.
16. Calati, R.; De Ronchi, D.; Bellini, M.; Serretti, A. The 5-HTTLPR polymorphism and eating disorders: A meta-analysis. *Int. J. Eat. Disord.* **2011**, *44*, 191–199. [CrossRef] [PubMed]
17. Ceccarini, M.R.; Tasegian, A.; Franzago, M.; Patria, F.F.; Albi, E.; Codini, M.; Conte, C.; Bertelli, M.; Dalla Ragione, L.; Stuppia, L.; et al. 5-HT2AR and BDNF gene variants in eating disorders susceptibility. *Am. J. Med. Genet. B NeuroPsychiatr. Genet.* **2019**, *183*, 155–163. [CrossRef] [PubMed]

18. Nilsson, M.; Naessen, S.; Dahlman, I.; Linden Hirschberg, A.; Gustafsson, J.A.; Dahlman-Wright, K. Association of estrogen receptor beta gene polymorphisms with bulimic disease in women. *Mol. Psychiatry* **2004**, *9*, 28–34. [CrossRef] [PubMed]

19. Muller, T.D.; Tschop, M.H.; Jarick, I.; Ehrlich, S.; Scherag, S.; Herpertz-Dahlmann, B.; Zipfel, S.; Herzog, W.; de Zwaan, M.; Burghardt, R.; et al. Genetic variation of the ghrelin activator gene ghrelin O-acyltransferase (GOAT) is associated with anorexia nervosa. *J. Psychiatr. Res.* **2011**, *45*, 706–711. [CrossRef]

20. Baker, J.H.; Schaumberg, K.; Munn-Chernoff, M.A. Genetics of anorexia nervosa. *Curr. Psychiatry Rep.* **2017**, *19*, 84. [CrossRef]

21. Boraska, V.; Franklin, C.S.; Floyd, J.A.; Thornton, L.M.; Huckins, L.M.; Southam, L.; Rayner, N.W.; Tachmazidou, I.; Klump, K.L.; Treasure, J.; et al. A genome-wide association study of anorexia nervosa. *Mol. Psychiatry* **2014**, *19*, 1085–1094. [CrossRef]

22. Huckins, L.M.; Hatzikotoulas, K.; Southam, L.; Thornton, L.M.; Steinberg, J.; Aguilera-McKay, F.; Treasure, J.; Schmidt, U.; Gunasinghe, C.; Romero, A.; et al. Investigation of common, low-frequency and rare genome-wide variation in anorexia nervosa. *Mol. Psychiatry* **2018**, *23*, 1169–1180. [CrossRef]

23. Wang, K.; Zhang, H.; Bloss, C.S.; Duvvuri, V.; Kaye, W.; Schork, N.J.; Berrettini, W.; Hakonarson, H.; Price Foundation Collaborative, G. A genome-wide association study on common SNPs and rare CNVs in anorexia nervosa. *Mol. Psychiatry* **2011**, *16*, 949–959. [CrossRef]

24. Li, D.; Chang, X.; Connolly, J.J.; Tian, L.; Liu, Y.; Bhoj, E.J.; Robinson, N.; Abrams, D.; Li, Y.R.; Bradfield, J.P.; et al. A genome-wide association study of anorexia nervosa suggests a risk locus implicated in dysregulated leptin signaling. *Sci. Rep.* **2017**, *7*, 3847. [CrossRef]

25. Duncan, L.; Yilmaz, Z.; Gaspar, H.; Walters, R.; Goldstein, J.; Anttila, V.; Bulik-Sullivan, B.; Ripke, S.; Eating Disorders Working Group of the Psychiatric Genomics; Thornton, L.; et al. Significant locus and metabolic genetic correlations revealed in genome-wide association study of anorexia nervosa. *Am. J. Psychiatry* **2017**, *174*, 850–858. [CrossRef] [PubMed]

26. Zerwas, S.; Larsen, J.T.; Petersen, L.; Thornton, L.M.; Quaranta, M.; Koch, S.V.; Pisetsky, D.; Mortensen, P.B.; Bulik, C.M. Eating disorders, autoimmune, and autoinflammatory disease. *Pediatrics* **2017**, *140*. [CrossRef] [PubMed]

27. Watson, H.J.; Yilmaz, Z.; Thornton, L.M.; Hubel, C.; Coleman, J.R.I.; Gaspar, H.A.; Bryois, J.; Hinney, A.; Leppa, V.M.; Mattheisen, M.; et al. Genome-wide association study identifies eight risk loci and implicates metabo-psychiatric origins for anorexia nervosa. *Nat. Genet.* **2019**, *51*, 1207–1214. [CrossRef] [PubMed]

28. Madra, M.; Zeltser, L.M. BDNF-Val66Met variant and adolescent stress interact to promote susceptibility to anorexic behavior in mice. *Transl. Psychiatry* **2016**, *6*, e776. [CrossRef]

29. Karwautz, A.F.; Wagner, G.; Waldherr, K.; Nader, I.W.; Fernandez-Aranda, F.; Estivill, X.; Holliday, J.; Collier, D.A.; Treasure, J.L. Gene-environment interaction in anorexia nervosa: Relevance of non-shared environment and the serotonin transporter gene. *Mol. Psychiatry* **2011**, *16*, 590–592. [CrossRef]

30. Steiger, H.; Thaler, L. Eating disorders, gene-environment interactions and the epigenome: Roles of stress exposures and nutritional status. *Physiol. Behav.* **2016**, *162*, 181–185. [CrossRef]

31. Szyf, M. DNA methylation, behavior and early life adversity. *J. Genet. Genom.* **2013**, *40*, 331–338. [CrossRef]

32. Szyf, M. Epigenetics, a key for unlocking complex CNS disorders? Therapeutic implications. *Eur. Neuropsychopharmacol.* **2015**, *25*, 682–702. [CrossRef]

33. Cecil, C.A.M.; Zhang, Y.; Nolte, T. Childhood maltreatment and DNA methylation: A systematic review. *NeuroSci. BioBehav. Rev.* **2020**, *112*, 392–409. [CrossRef]

34. Tobi, E.W.; Goeman, J.J.; Monajemi, R.; Gu, H.; Putter, H.; Zhang, Y.; Slieker, R.C.; Stok, A.P.; Thijssen, P.E.; Muller, F.; et al. DNA methylation signatures link prenatal famine exposure to growth and metabolism. *Nat. Commun.* **2014**, *5*, 5592. [CrossRef]

35. Nemoda, Z.; Szyf, M. Epigenetic alterations and prenatal maternal depression. *Birth Defects Res.* **2017**, *109*, 888–897. [CrossRef] [PubMed]

36. Suarez, A.; Lahti, J.; Czamara, D.; Lahti-Pulkkinen, M.; Knight, A.K.; Girchenko, P.; Hamalainen, E.; Kajantie, E.; Lipsanen, J.; Laivuori, H.; et al. The epigenetic clock at birth: Associations with maternal antenatal depression and child psychiatric problems. *J. Am. Acad Child. Adolesc. Psychiatry* **2018**, *57*, 321–328. [CrossRef] [PubMed]
37. Marcho, C.; Oluwayiose, O.A.; Pilsner, J.R. The preconception environment and sperm epigenetics. *Andrology* **2020**. [CrossRef] [PubMed]
38. Chan, J.C.; Nugent, B.M.; Bale, T.L. Parental advisory: Maternal and paternal stress can impact offspring neurodevelopment. *Biol. Psychiatry* **2018**, *83*, 886–894. [CrossRef]
39. Noor, N.; Cardenas, A.; Rifas-Shiman, S.L.; Pan, H.; Dreyfuss, J.M.; Oken, E.; Hivert, M.F.; James-Todd, T.; Patti, M.E.; Isganaitis, E. Association of periconception paternal body mass index with persistent changes in DNA methylation of offspring in childhood. *JAMA Netw. Open* **2019**, *2*. [CrossRef]
40. St-Hilaire, A.; Steiger, H.; Liu, A.; Laplante, D.P.; Thaler, L.; Magill, T.; King, S. A prospective study of effects of prenatal maternal stress on later eating-disorder manifestations in affected offspring: Preliminary indications based on the Project Ice Storm cohort. *Int. J. Eat. Disord.* **2015**, *48*, 512–516. [CrossRef]
41. Cao-Lei, L.; Dancause, K.N.; Elgbeili, G.; Massart, R.; Szyf, M.; Liu, A.; Laplante, D.P.; King, S. DNA methylation mediates the impact of exposure to prenatal maternal stress on BMI and central adiposity in children at age 13(1/2) years: Project Ice Storm. *Epigenetics* **2015**, *10*, 749–761. [CrossRef]
42. Kazmi, N.; Gaunt, T.R.; Relton, C.; Micali, N. Maternal eating disorders affect offspring cord blood DNA methylation: A prospective study. *Clin. Epigenet.* **2017**, *9*, 120. [CrossRef]
43. Weaver, I.C.; Cervoni, N.; Champagne, F.A.; D'Alessio, A.C.; Sharma, S.; Seckl, J.R.; Dymov, S.; Szyf, M.; Meaney, M.J. Epigenetic programming by maternal behavior. *Nat. NeuroSci.* **2004**, *7*, 847–854. [CrossRef]
44. McGowan, P.O.; Sasaki, A.; D'Alessio, A.C.; Dymov, S.; Labonte, B.; Szyf, M.; Turecki, G.; Meaney, M.J. Epigenetic regulation of the glucocorticoid receptor in human brain associates with childhood abuse. *Nat. NeuroSci.* **2009**, *12*, 342–348. [CrossRef]
45. Roth, T.L.; Sweatt, J.D. Epigenetic marking of the BDNF gene by early-life adverse experiences. *Horm. Behav.* **2011**, *59*, 315–320. [CrossRef] [PubMed]
46. Suderman, M.; McGowan, P.O.; Sasaki, A.; Huang, T.C.; Hallett, M.T.; Meaney, M.J.; Turecki, G.; Szyf, M. Conserved epigenetic sensitivity to early life experience in the rat and human hippocampus. *Proc. Natl. Acad. Sci. USA* **2012**, *109*, 17266–17272. [CrossRef] [PubMed]
47. Holmes, L., Jr.; Shutman, E.; Chinaka, C.; Deepika, K.; Pelaez, L.; Dabney, K.W. Aberrant epigenomic modulation of glucocorticoid receptor gene (NR3C1) in early life stress and major depressive disorder correlation: Systematic review and quantitative evidence synthesis. *Int. J. Environ. Res. Public Health* **2019**, *16*, 4280. [CrossRef] [PubMed]
48. Jawahar, M.C.; Murgatroyd, C.; Harrison, E.L.; Baune, B.T. Epigenetic alterations following early postnatal stress: A review on novel aetiological mechanisms of common psychiatric disorders. *Clin. Epigenet.* **2015**, *7*, 122. [CrossRef] [PubMed]
49. Park, C.; Rosenblat, J.D.; Brietzke, E.; Pan, Z.; Lee, Y.; Cao, B.; Zuckerman, H.; Kalantarova, A.; McIntyre, R.S. Stress, epigenetics and depression: A systematic review. *NeuroSci. BioBehav. Rev.* **2019**, *102*, 139–152. [CrossRef] [PubMed]
50. Jawaid, A.; Roszkowski, M.; Mansuy, I.M. Transgenerational epigenetics of traumatic stress. *Prog. Mol. Biol. Transl. Sci.* **2018**, *158*, 273–298. [CrossRef]
51. Watkeys, O.J.; Kremerskothen, K.; Quide, Y.; Fullerton, J.M.; Green, M.J. Glucocorticoid receptor gene (NR3C1) DNA methylation in association with trauma, psychopathology, transcript expression, or genotypic variation: A systematic review. *NeuroSci. BioBehav. Rev.* **2018**, *95*, 85–122. [CrossRef]
52. Steiger, H.; Labonte, B.; Groleau, P.; Turecki, G.; Israel, M. Methylation of the glucocorticoid receptor gene promoter in bulimic women: Associations with borderline personality disorder, suicidality, and exposure to childhood abuse. *Int. J. Eat. Disord.* **2013**, *46*, 246–255. [CrossRef]
53. Thaler, L.; Gauvin, L.; Joober, R.; Groleau, P.; de Guzman, R.; Ambalavanan, A.; Israel, M.; Wilson, S.; Steiger, H. Methylation of BDNF in women with bulimic eating syndromes: Associations with childhood abuse and borderline personality disorder. *Prog. Neuropsychopharmacol. Biol. Psychiatry* **2014**, *54*, 43–49. [CrossRef]
54. Notaras, M.; van den Buuse, M. Neurobiology of BDNF in fear memory, sensitivity to stress, and stress-related disorders. *Mol. Psychiatry* **2020**. [CrossRef]

55. Groleau, P.; Joober, R.; Israel, M.; Zeramdini, N.; DeGuzman, R.; Steiger, H. Methylation of the dopamine D2 receptor (DRD2) gene promoter in women with a bulimia-spectrum disorder: Associations with borderline personality disorder and exposure to childhood abuse. *J. Psychiatr. Res.* **2014**, *48*, 121–127. [CrossRef] [PubMed]
56. Amenyah, S.D.; Hughes, C.F.; Ward, M.; Rosborough, S.; Deane, J.; Thursby, S.-J.; Walsh, C.P.; Kok, D.E.; Strain, J.J.; McNulty, H.; et al. Influence of nutrients involved in one-carbon metabolism on DNA methylation in adults—a systematic review and meta-analysis. *Nutr. Rev.* **2020**. [CrossRef] [PubMed]
57. McGarel, C.; Pentieva, K.; Strain, J.J.; McNulty, H. Emerging roles for folate and related B-vitamins in brain health across the lifecycle. *Proc. Nutr. Soc.* **2015**, *74*, 46–55. [CrossRef] [PubMed]
58. Stevens, A.J.; Rucklidge, J.J.; Kennedy, M.A. Epigenetics, nutrition and mental health. Is there a relationship? *Nutr. NeuroSci.* **2018**, *21*, 602–613. [CrossRef]
59. Burdo, J.; Booij, L.; Kahan, E.; McGregor, K.; Greenlaw, K.; Agellon, L.B.; Thaler, L.; Labbe, A.; Israël, M.; Wykes, L.; et al. Association between plasma nutrient levels and methylation of selected genomic probes in women with anorexia nervosa. In Proceedings of the International Conference on Eating Disorders, New York, NY, USA, 15 March 2019.
60. Frieling, H.; Gozner, A.; Romer, K.D.; Lenz, B.; Bonsch, D.; Wilhelm, J.; Hillemacher, T.; de Zwaan, M.; Kornhuber, J.; Bleich, S. Global DNA hypomethylation and DNA hypermethylation of the alpha synuclein promoter in females with anorexia nervosa. *Mol. Psychiatry* **2007**, *12*, 229–230. [CrossRef]
61. Frieling, H.; Römer, K.D.; Scholz, S.; Mittelbach, F.; Wilhelm, J.; De Zwaan, M.; Jacoby, G.E.; Kornhuber, J.; Hillemacher, T.; Bleich, S. Epigenetic dysregulation of dopaminergic genes in eating disorders. *Int. J. Eat. Disord.* **2010**, *43*, 577–583. [CrossRef]
62. Kim, Y.-R.; Kim, J.-H.; Kim, M.J.; Treasure, J. Differential methylation of the oxytocin receptor gene in patients with anorexia nervosa: A pilot study. *PLoS ONE* **2014**, *9*, e88673. [CrossRef]
63. Thaler, L.; Brassard, S.; Booij, L.; Kahan, E.; McGregor, K.; Labbe, A.; Israel, M.; Steiger, H. Methylation of the OXTR gene in women with anorexia nervosa: Relationship to social behavior. *Eur. Eat. Disord. Rev.* **2020**, *28*, 79–86. [CrossRef]
64. Subramanian, S.; Braun, P.R.; Han, S.; Potash, J.B. Investigation of differential HDAC4 methylation patterns in eating disorders. *Psychiatr. Genet.* **2018**, *28*, 12–15. [CrossRef]
65. Neyazi, A.; Buchholz, V.; Burkert, A.; Hillemacher, T.; de Zwaan, M.; Herzog, W.; Jahn, K.; Giel, K.; Herpertz, S.; Buchholz, C.A.; et al. Association of leptin gene DNA methylation with diagnosis and treatment outcome of anorexia nervosa. *Front. Psychiatry* **2019**, *10*, 197. [CrossRef]
66. Boehm, I.; Walton, E.; Alexander, N.; Batury, V.L.; Seidel, M.; Geisler, D.; King, J.A.; Weidner, K.; Roessner, V.; Ehrlich, S. Peripheral serotonin transporter DNA methylation is linked to increased salience network connectivity in females with anorexia nervosa. *J. Psychiatry NeuroSci.* **2019**, *45*, 190016. [CrossRef]
67. Frieling, H.; Bleich, S.; Otten, J.; Romer, K.D.; Kornhuber, J.; de Zwaan, M.; Jacoby, G.E.; Wilhelm, J.; Hillemacher, T. Epigenetic downregulation of atrial natriuretic peptide but not vasopressin mRNA expression in females with eating disorders is related to impulsivity. *Neuropsychopharmacology* **2008**, *33*, 2605–2609. [CrossRef] [PubMed]
68. Jia, Y.F.; Choi, Y.; Ayers-Ringler, J.R.; Biernacka, J.M.; Geske, J.R.; Lindberg, D.R.; McElroy, S.L.; Frye, M.A.; Choi, D.S.; Veldic, M. Differential SLC1A2 promoter methylation in bipolar disorder with or without addiction. *Front. Cell NeuroSci.* **2017**, *11*, 217. [CrossRef] [PubMed]
69. Saffrey, R.; Novakovic, B.; Wade, T.D. Assessing global and gene specific DNA methylation in anorexia nervosa: A pilot study. *Int. J. Eat. Disord.* **2014**, *47*, 206–210. [CrossRef]
70. Tremolizzo, L.; Conti, E.; Bomba, M.; Uccellini, O.; Rossi, M.S.; Marfone, M.; Corbetta, F.; Santarone, M.E.; Raggi, M.E.; Neri, F.; et al. Decreased whole-blood global DNA methylation is related to serum hormones in anorexia nervosa adolescents. *World J. Biol. Psychiatry* **2014**, *15*, 327–333. [CrossRef]
71. Booij, L.; Casey, K.F.; Antunes, J.M.; Szyf, M.; Joober, R.; Israel, M.; Steiger, H. DNA methylation in individuals with anorexia nervosa and in matched normal-eater controls: A genome-wide study. *Int. J. Eat. Disord.* **2015**, *48*, 874–882. [CrossRef]
72. Kesselmeier, M.; Putter, C.; Volckmar, A.L.; Baurecht, H.; Grallert, H.; Illig, T.; Ismail, K.; Ollikainen, M.; Silen, Y.; Keski-Rahkonen, A.; et al. High-throughput DNA methylation analysis in anorexia nervosa confirms TNXB hypermethylation. *World J. Biol. Psychiatry* **2018**, *19*, 187–199. [CrossRef]

73. Lee, M.; Strand, M. Ehlers-Danlos syndrome in a young woman with anorexia nervosa and complex somatic symptoms. *Int. J. Eat. Disord.* **2018**, *51*, 281–284. [CrossRef]
74. Steiger, H.; Booij, L.; Kahan, E.; McGregor, K.; Thaler, L.; Fletcher, E.; Labbe, A.; Joober, R.; Israel, M.; Szyf, M.; et al. A longitudinal, epigenome-wide study of DNA methylation in anorexia nervosa: Results in actively ill, partially weight-restored, long-term remitted and non-eating-disordered women. *J. Psychiatry NeuroSci.* **2019**, *44*, 205–213. [CrossRef]
75. Farrell, N.R.; Lee, A.A.; Deacon, B.J. Biological or psychological? Effects of eating disorder psychoeducation on self-blame and recovery expectations among symptomatic individuals. *Behav. Res. Ther.* **2015**, *74*, 32–37. [CrossRef]
76. Bulik, C.M.; Blake, L.; Austin, J. Genetics of eating disorders: What the clinician needs to know. *Psychiatr. Clin. North. Am.* **2019**, *42*, 59–73. [CrossRef] [PubMed]
77. Semaka, A.; Austin, J. Patient perspectives on the process and outcomes of psychiatric genetic counseling: An "empowering encounter". *J. Genet. Couns* **2019**, *28*, 856–868. [CrossRef] [PubMed]
78. Lock, J.; Le Grange, D. *Treatment Manual for Anorexia Nervosa*, 2nd ed.; Guilford Press: New York, NY, USA, 2012.
79. Fairburn, C.G. *Cognitive Behavior Therapy and Eating Disorders*; Guilford Press: New York, NY, USA, 2008.
80. Steiger, H. Evidence-informed practices in the real-world treatment of people with eating disorders. *Eat. Disord.* **2017**, *25*, 173–181. [CrossRef] [PubMed]
81. Steiger, H.; Sansfacon, J.; Thaler, L.; Leonard, N.; Cottier, D.; Kahan, E.; Fletcher, E.; Rossi, E.; Israel, M.; Gauvin, L. Autonomy support and autonomous motivation in the outpatient treatment of adults with an eating disorder. *Int. J. Eat. Disord.* **2017**, *50*, 1058–1066. [CrossRef]

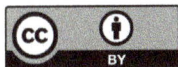

© 2020 by the authors. Licensee MDPI, Basel, Switzerland. This article is an open access article distributed under the terms and conditions of the Creative Commons Attribution (CC BY) license (http://creativecommons.org/licenses/by/4.0/).

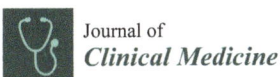

Article

Unexpected Association of Desacyl-Ghrelin with Physical Activity and Chronic Food Restriction: A Translational Study on Anorexia Nervosa

Philibert Duriez [1,2], Lauralee Robichon [1], Roland Dardennes [2], Guillaume Lavoisy [2], Dominique Grouselle [1], Jacques Epelbaum [1,3], Nicolas Ramoz [1], Philip Gorwood [1,2], Virginie Tolle [1,†] and Odile Viltart [1,4,*,†]

1. Institute of Psychiatry and Neuroscience of Paris (IPNP), Université de Paris, INSERM UMR-S 1266, F-75014 Paris, France; p.duriez@ghu-paris.fr (P.D.); lauralee.robichon@sfr.fr (L.R.); dominique.grouselle@inserm.fr (D.G.); jacques.epelbaum@inserm.fr (J.E.); nicolas.ramoz@inserm.fr (N.R.); p.gorwood@ghu-paris.fr (P.G.); virginie.tolle@inserm.fr (V.T.)
2. GHU Paris Psychiatrie et Neurosciences, Hôpital Sainte-Anne, F-75014 Paris, France; r.dardennes@ghu-paris.fr (R.D.); guillaumelavoisy@hotmail.com (G.L.)
3. UMR 7179 CNRS, MNHN, Adaptive mechanism and Evolution (MECADEV), 91800 Brunoy, France
4. Cité scientifique, SN4, Université de Lille, 59491 Villeneuve d'Ascq, France
* Correspondence: odile.viltart@univ-lille.fr
† Both authors contributed equally to this work.

Received: 27 July 2020; Accepted: 22 August 2020; Published: 28 August 2020

Abstract: Anorexia nervosa (AN) is a severe metabopsychiatric disorder characterised by caloric intake restriction and often excessive physical exercise. Our aim is to assess in female AN patients and in a rodent model, the co-evolution of physical activity and potential dysregulation of acyl—(AG) and desacyl—(DAG) ghrelin plasma concentrations during denutrition and weight recovery. AN inpatients were evaluated at inclusion (T0, $n = 29$), half—(T1) and total (T2) weight recovery, and one month after discharge (T3, $n = 13$). C57/Bl6 mice with access to a running wheel, were fed ad libitum or submitted to short—(15 days) or long—(50 days) term quantitative food restriction, followed by refeeding (20 days). In AN patients, AG and DAG rapidly decreased during weight recovery (T0 to T2), AG increased significantly one-month post discharge (T3), but only DAG plasma concentrations at T3 correlated negatively with BMI and positively with physical activity. In mice, AG and DAG both increased during short- and long-term food restriction. After 20 days of ad libitum feeding, DAG was associated to persistence of exercise alteration. The positive association of DAG with physical activity during caloric restriction and after weight recovery questions its role in the adaptation mechanisms to energy deprivation that need to be considered in recovery process in AN.

Keywords: restrictive anorexia nervosa; weight recovery; animal models; acyl-ghrelin; desacyl-ghrelin; physical activity; chronic food restriction

1. Introduction

Anorexia nervosa (AN) is a psychiatric disorder where the severe weight loss due to a reduction on food intake is associated with high levels of physical activity. Indeed, 31% to 80% of AN patients display inappropriate quantity of exercise with respect to their energy resources [1,2]. Hyperactivity has been associated with an increase in the length of hospitalisation stay [3], a poor treatment outcome both interfering with refeeding therapies and increasing the risk of relapse [4]. One out of two patients relapses within a year following inpatient treatment and approximately 20% of patients experience recurrent patterns of remission and relapse or chronic disease [5,6]. The disorder affects predominantly women and girls, with female to male ratios of approximately 10/1 to 15/1 [7]. The etiology of AN is complex, but recent evidences emphasise metabolic and endocrine aspects as key pathophysiological determinants of the disorder [8–12].

Amongst many metabolic and endocrine factors, ghrelin a 28-amino-acid peptide orexigenic gut hormone produced by the X/A-like endocrine cells in the oxyntic glands of the gastric fundus [13–15], is involved in many physiological processes associated with feeding and exercise including the regulation of energy metabolism and appetite [16], the cardiovascular system as autonomic nervous system [17–20], and the modulation of reward and motivation [11,21,22]. Ghrelin has rapidly been considered as a biomarker of AN since its plasma concentrations are significantly increased in AN patients and return to control values after renutrition as also observed in animal models mimicking several symptoms of AN [23–25]. Acylation (on its third serine residue) by ghrelin O-acyl transferase allows acyl-ghrelin (AG) to bind to its receptor, the growth hormone secretagogue receptor (GHSR) type 1a that is widely distributed within the central nervous system [13,26]. Desacyl-ghrelin (DAG) is also present in the blood circulation [27]. Original studies using competition assays showed that DAG accounts for 80–90% of total circulating ghrelin [28]. More recently, using very selective sandwich immunoassays for AG and DAG, DAG accounted for 76% of the total circulating ghrelin (i.e., AG+DAG) [29]. Despite a number of studies reporting a physiological role for DAG, usually opposite to AG [27,30–32], its role remains elusive.

Beside appetite, many clinical and preclinical studies support an association of ghrelin with physical exercise. More particularly, in healthy subjects, acute or short-term exercise duration is associated with a decrease in ghrelin plasma concentrations while chronic physical activity is correlated with increased concentrations of ghrelin [33–35]. Increased ghrelin plasma concentrations are also described in rodents performing chronic treadmill exercise [36]. In pathological situations associated with excessive physical activity such as AN, total ghrelin is positively correlated with physical activity, measured by daily step counts [37]. In the activity-based anorexia (ABA) model, where time-restriction in food access is associated with running activity, mice display excessive daytime physical activity in the context of limited access to food [38,39]. Interestingly, in ABA mice, a single intracerebroventricular injection or chronic peripheral treatment with a GHS-R1a antagonist lead to a significant decrease of daytime activity [38]. Moreover, GHS-R KO mice show a more rapid exhaustion in an endurance exercise as compared to wild-type mice [40]. However, the differential effect or association of AG and DAG with chronic physical activity, in clinical or preclinical studies is controversial, because of the kind of exercise considered (acute, endurance, etc. ...) or the sex of the participants (usually males, in human or rodents). Furthermore, in healthy conditions, only plasma AG concentrations were modulated by exercise [41–43]. Finally, most of the studies that investigated the role of ghrelin in AN have focused on variations in plasma total ghrelin or AG, neglecting the potential involvement of DAG. To our knowledge, longitudinal data are not yet available on AG and DAG levels during a refeeding hospital program and after body weight recovery associated with physical activity. A standardised definition of remission, recovery and relapse is still lacking [44]. We thus hypothesised that in long-term food restriction and in nutritional recovery, AG and DAG plasma concentrations evolve differentially according to the level of physical activity. For this purpose, we first assessed the evolution of plasma concentrations of AG and DAG in ill- and recovered-AN patients, in relation with their physical activity. Then, we used a modified mouse ABA model of chronic quantitative food restriction associated with a voluntary running activity in a wheel, to determine whether AG and DAG plasma concentrations reflect the level of physical activity during the periods of chronic food restriction and nutritional recovery [45,46]. Here, "nutritional recovery" is used to identify patients or rodents that followed a program of refeeding and included weight restoration.

2. Materials and Methods

2.1. Experiment 1. Clinical Investigation

Participants. Twenty-nine female patients suffering from anorexia nervosa (AN) in undernourished state were included in the study (Table 1). Thirteen patients had full weight recovery during intensive in-patient program and were evaluated one-month post discharge. Participants, aged 18–37 years, fulfilled DSM-V criteria for AN (APA, 2013). All patients attended a structured in-patient program in the Eating Disorders Unit of *Clinique des Maladies Mentales et de l'Encéphale* (CMME, Sainte-Anne Hospital, Paris, France) and received behavioural nutritional rehabilitation program with progressive and controlled access to physical activity and were discharged after reaching their target weight and maintaining it for at least 2 weeks. We excluded patients with active malignancies, active inflammatory or infectious diseases, epilepsy, and other psychiatric disorders. Several clinical parameters were recorded at the different time-points. Patients were weighted at every inpatient and follow-up assessment, size was measured and corresponding body mass indexes (BMIs) were calculated. Physical activity was assessed with the self-reported International Physical Activity Questionnaire (IPAQ) [47]. The study protocol was approved by *Comité de Protection des Personnes Ile de France III* (EUDRACT N: 2008-A008 17–48; CPP N Am5355-2-2592). All patients gave written informed consent prior to participation. All data were recorded anonymously.

Table 1. Demographic, anthropometric and socio-economic characteristics of anorexia nervosa in the clinical samples. Data are presented as mean +/− SD. T0: at admission; T1: 50–70% of target BMI reached; T2-T3: weight recovered patients with evaluation one month post discharge; AN: anorexia nervosa; AN-R: anorexia nervosa restrictive type; AN-BP: anorexia nervosa binge-eating/purging type; BMI: body mass index; EDI2: Eating Disorder Inventory version 2.

	T0 (n = 29)		T1 (n = 28)		T2-T3 (n = 13)	
	Mean +/−SD	%	Mean +/−SD	%		%
Age (years)	25.8+/−6.8		26.2 +/−6.44		26+/−7	
AN-Duration (years)	7.4+/−5.4		7.4+/−5.5		8.8+/−6.5	
Age of onset	18.4+/−3.8		18.4 +/−3.9		17.2+/−1.9	
AN Subtype						
AN-R		59%		57%		60%
AN-BP		41%		43%		40%
BMI at inclusion (kg/m^2)	14.6+/−1.3		14.6+/−1.4		14.8+/−1.2	
Partner ship						
Single		79%		78%		69%
In a relationship		21%		22%		31%
Daily psychiatric drugs		62%		62%		62%
EDI-2 at inclusion						
Total	116+/−5		118+/−52		114+/−53.7	
Drive for thinness	11.9+/−7.4		12.2+/−7.3		11.5+/−8.6	
Bulimia	4.9+/−7		5.1+/−7.1		5+/−7.62	
Body dissatisfaction	17+/−6.9		17.1+/−7		17+/−6.7	
Ineffectiveness	16+/−8.9		16.5+/−8.7		15.5+/−9.3	
Perfectionism	7.5+/−4.4		7.3+/−4.4		7.7+/−4.6	
Interpersonal distrust	9.4+/−4.8		9.3+/−4.9		9.4+/−4.5	
Interoceptive awareness	14.7+/−7.3		14.8+/−7.4		14.2+/−5.9	
Maturity fears	8.3+/−6.5		8.6+/−6.4		8.2+/−7.5	
Asceticism	9+/−5.74		9.3+/−5.8		9+/−6.32	
Impulse Regulation	7+/−7.25		7+/−7.3		6+/−7.4	
Social Insecurity	11+/−5.52		10.8+/−5.4		11+/−6.3	

In order to assay hormonal longitudinal variations in different nutritional conditions, blood samplings were performed in undernourished conditions (T0) (5–8 days after the arrival at the Hospital) during the acute phase of the disorder, in the course of the refeeding process (T1: 50–70% target BMI of 20 kg/m^2), after complete weight recovery (T2: 90–100% target BMI) or during the stabilisation process (T3: 1 month following discharge).

Conditions of Blood Sampling, Processing and Storage of Blood. Blood sampling was performed after an overnight fast. Blood was collected on tubes containing 15% EDTA and Aprotinin 250 KIU (tube BD vacutainer EDTA K3 Aprotinin). Blood samples were immediately centrifuged at 4 °C ($1000\times g$ for 15 min). In addition, plasma samples were aliquoted and supplemented with HCl at a final concentration of 0.1 N immediately after collection in order to preserve acylation and frozen at −80 °C.

Acyl—and Desacyl-Ghrelin Immunoassays. Acyl- (AG) and desacyl-ghrelin (DAG) concentrations were assayed in duplicates with selective two-sites sandwich enzyme-immunoassays (EIA) using two different monoclonal antibodies for capture and revelation (human AG and DAG EIA Easy Sampling Elisa kits, Ref A05306 and Ref A05319, respectively, Bertin Bioreagent, Montigny-le-Bretonneaux, France). For AG, the limit of detection is 4 pg/mL. Intra- and inter-assay coefficients of variation are 9 and 16%, respectively. For DAG, the limit of detection is 10 pg/mL. Intra- and inter-assay coefficients of variation are 6 and 16%, respectively.

2.2. Experiment 2. Preclinical Investigation

Animals. Seven-week old C57BL/6J female mice (Charles River Laboratories, L'Arbresle, France) weighing 18.3 ± 0.1 g were housed by cages of two to avoid isolation stress and hypothermia [45]. They were kept in a pathogen-free barrier facility maintained at 22–24 °C with a 12:12-h dark-light cycle (lights on at 07:00 a.m.). During one week of habituation, mice were weighted every day to get acclimatised to handling. Mice within the same cage had a similar initial body weight. They had free access to water and to standard chow diet (3% fat, 16% protein, 60% carbohydrate, 4% fibres, 2.79 kcal/g; Safe A04). All experiments were carried out in accordance with the European Communities Council Directive (86/609/EEC) and approved by the Regional ethical committed of Paris Descartes University France.

Short-Term Food Restriction Protocol. In this first set of experiments, mice were randomised into two experimental groups according to their initial body weight. Mice of the group "ad libitum and wheel" (group ALW, $n = 12$) were placed in a cage equipped with a free running wheel (ActiviWheel Software; Intellibio, Seichamps, France) and had free access to food. In the group "food restriction and wheel" (group FRW, $n = 12$), mice were placed in a cage equipped with a free running wheel and exposed to a 30% quantitative food restriction for three days followed by 50% quantitative food restriction through the end of the protocol. This restriction was calculated every day from the total food consumed by each mouse in the ALW group the previous day, by weighing the whole pellets in the feeder. Food (on pellet per mouse) was distributed directly into the cage every day at 6:30 p.m. Body weight was monitored daily at the same time. In 8 out of the 12 cages, the locomotor activity was assessed daily with a running wheel (diameter: 230 mm; width: 50 mm; 1 revolution = 0.72 m) linked to a computer system that measured interval counts (10 min) per mean wheel revolution (ActiviWheel Software; Intellibio, Seichamps, France). In 4 out of the 6 cages of ALW mice, the physical activity was measured with a manual counter (Sigma Germany BC 9.16 ATS), which indicated total distance, mean speed, and maximum speed in 12-h periods. Manual counters were read twice per day: between 7:30 and 8:00 a.m. to evaluate ALW nocturnal activity and around 6:00 p.m., before the food distribution, for the diurnal activity. The wheel running activity was measured per cage, because ethologically speaking and for the welfare of the animals, we decided to avoid stress isolation and the hypothermia induced by our long-term caloric restriction protocol. The recording of physical activity thus reflected the activity of two mice that usually run two by two in the wheel (personal observation), resulting in 6 ALW and 6 FRW cages. Since we measured each animal body weight daily, we were able to detect changes in feeding or running activity and thus avoided the cage-effect of these analyses. As mentioned, weight loss in a same cage is usually similar (considering the standard deviation) leading us to consider the cage value of physical activity in wheel for each mouse. Data were extracted with an excel macro (Microsoft Office Standard, 2016) to obtain cumulative activity or day/night activity. To establish a link between plasma concentrations of AG and DAG with physical activity, blood samples were collected twice: in the morning (D11) at 9:00 a.m. and before food distribution (at D10) at 5:00 p.m., when the anticipatory food activity was developed in the FRW mice (see results).

Long-Term Food Restriction and Nutritional Recovery Protocols. In the second set of experiments, mice were randomised according to their initial body weight into two experimental groups FRW ($n = 6$) and ALW ($n = 6$) as described above. The experimental protocol was exactly similar to the short-term food restriction, except that we maintained the groups of mice in this protocol for 8 weeks. Body weight was monitored three times a week. The locomotor activity was assessed daily with a running wheel linked to a computer system that measured interval counts (10 min) per mean wheel revolution (ActiviWheel Software; Intellibio, Seichamps, France). After 8 weeks of this protocol, nutritional recovery was achieved by giving ad libitum access to standard diet to all FRW mice while free access to the running wheel was maintained. As mentioned above, the activity was evaluated per cage. Data were extracted with an Excel® macro (Microsoft Office Standard, 2016) to obtain cumulative activity or day/night activity. To evaluate the kinetic of plasma ghrelin concentrations during the refeeding period, two blood samples were withdrawn at 5:00 p.m.: on day 51, one day after the beginning of the refeeding, and on day 70, at sacrifice (after two weeks of nutritional recovery).

Blood Samples Collection. AG and DAG Plasma Assays. Blood samples were collected from the caudal vein with a 1-mL syringe in EDTA coated tubes (1 mg/mL final, Microvette® CB 300 µL, Sarstedt, Germany) containing p-hydroxy-mercuribenzoic acid (PHMB 0.4 mM final), which is a serine protease inhibitor, and kept at 4 °C until processing. At the end of the short- and long-term protocols, mice were deeply anesthetised with an overdose of ketamine (100 mg/kg) and xylazine (20 mg/kg) mix. Blood was collected through cardiac puncture with a 1-mL syringue and transferred into EDTA coated tubes. Samples were rapidly centrifuged ($1000\times g$ for 10 min, 4 °C), to collect plasma (around 80 µL), which was immediately acidified with HCl (0.1 N final) to preserve ghrelin acylation. Plasma aliquots were frozen in dry ice before being stored at −80 °C until they were assayed. Plasma AG and DAG concentrations were evaluated by specific EIA (A05118 for the acylated form and A05117 for the des-acylated form; Bertin Bioreagents, Montigny le Bretonneux, France). All samples were analysed in duplicates. Intra- and inter-assay coefficients of variations were 6.1% and 5.7% for AG and 5.5% and 4.8% for DAG, respectively.

Statistical Analysis. Analysis of normality and equality of variances were tested by Shapiro-Wilk test. Statistical analysis were performed using one-way ANOVA followed by a Fisher *post-hoc* test when the *p* value of the ANOVA was significant ($p < 0.05$) or a non-parametric ANOVA followed by Tukey or Bonferroni post hoc test was used when appropriate, using Statview® software (SAS institute Inc., Cary, NC, USA).

Clinical values are given as mean ±SD. Preclinical values are given as mean ±SEM. For both clinical and preclinical values correlations we used Pearson correlation test if normality is respected (Shapiro-Wilk $p > 0.05$) or Spearman's rank correlation coefficient if not (Shapiro-Wilk $p < 0.05$). We used Jamovi Softare (Version 1.1; R Core Team 2018). The level for significance was established at 5%. We considered a tendency at $0.1 > p > 0.05$. Graphs were generated using GraphPad Prism® 5.01 (Abacus Concepts, Berkeley, CA, USA).

3. Results

3.1. Experiment 1. Clinical Investigation

3.1.1. Longitudinal Evolution of BMI and Physical Activity during Inpatient Weight Recovery and One-Month Post Discharge

At inclusion (T0), 29 female patients were evaluated. Only one patient left the protocol before T1. Thirteen patients out of the 29 were re-evaluated both at T2 (90–100% target BMI) and one-month post-discharge (T3). Our analysis focused on recovery and early modifications of metabolic parameters after discharge (Time T3). We thus considered only patients who succeeded in obtaining "full" weight recovery during treatment in our clinical unit, namely the 13 patients presented in our study. The other patients ($n = 16$) did not fulfil the criteria and left hospital mainly after "partial" weight recovery (about 16 kg/m^2). Table 1 describes the clinical sample.

Between T0 and T2, patients increased their BMI according to the strict clinical protocol with weight therapeutic contract ($U = 51, p < 0.001$) and reduced their physical activity ($U = 53.5, p = 0.002$). The BMI significantly increased between T0 and T2 ($F_{(2-75)} = 186, p < 0.001$; Figure 1A). More specifically, post-hoc analysis revealed a significant increase between T0 and T1 ($p < 0.001$) and between T1 and T2 ($p < 0.001$). Physical activity was permitted after 50% of total expected weight gain, explaining no physical activity reported at T1 (Figure 1B).

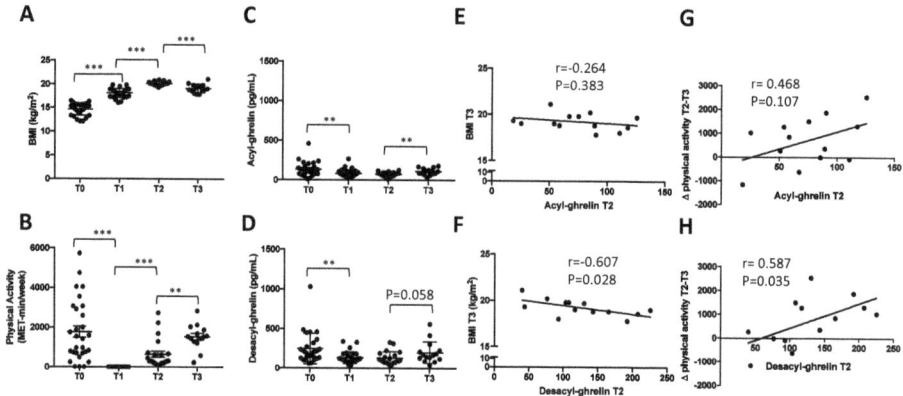

Figure 1. Longitudinal evolution of acyl-ghrelin (AG) and desacyl-ghrelin (DAG) during inpatient weight restoration and one-month post discharge. One-month post hospitalisation (T3), BMI (**A**) and physical activity (**B**) significantly decreased and plasma concentrations of AG (**C**) increased but not DAG (**D**). Plasma concentrations of DAG at the end of hospitalisation (T2) were negatively correlated to BMI one month later (T3,**F**), but not AG (**E**) and positively correlated to the increase of physical activity between the end of hospitalisation and one month later (**H**), but not AG (**G**). Only statistical differences between two consecutive time-points are reported. T0 = 1-week post-admission; T1 = 50–70% of target BMI reached; T2 = discharge BMI (close to target BMI); T3 = 1-month post-discharge visit. BMI: body mass index. MET: metabolic equivalent of task. ** $p < 0.01$; *** $p < 0.001$.

3.1.2. Rapid Decrease of Circulating AG and DAG during Refeeding Period

Both AG and DAG plasma concentrations significantly decreased during weight recovery (respectively $F_{(2-75)} = 7.68, p < 0.001$; $F_{(2-75)} = 6.86, p = 0.002$, Figure 1C,D). More specifically, post-hoc analysis revealed a significant decrease of these two forms of ghrelin between T0 and T1 (AG: $p = 0.006$; DAG: $p = 0.005$), T0 and T2 (AG: $p = 0.003$; DAG: $p = 0.009$) and T1 and T2 (AG: n.s.; DAG: n.s.). The AG/DAG ratio was calculated, and ANOVA analysis did not show any significant effect of time ($F_{(2-75)} = 0.04, p = 0.963$).

3.1.3. Early Increase of Circulating AG but Not DAG One Month after Discharge

One month after discharge (T3), patients BMI globally decreased (20.1 ± 0.09 vs. 19.1 ± 0.24; T2 vs. T3, $U = 51$, $p < 0.001$, Figure 1A). Physical activity was significantly increased (T2 vs. T3, $U = 53.5$, $p = 0.002$, Figure 1B). Plasma concentrations of AG were significantly increased (73.2 ± 30.9 vs. 111 ± 43.6; T2 vs. T3, $U = 79$, $p = 0.011$, Figure 1C), with mean circulating DAG at T3 was 153% of that at T2 ($U = 08$, $p = 0.058$, Figure 1D). The AG/DAG ratio was calculated and no significant difference was noted between T2 vs. T3 ($U = 146$, $p = 0.727$).

3.1.4. Correlations between Circulating DAG after Weight Recovery (T2) and BMI at T3

The correlations are presented in Table 2. At T2, AG and DAG plasma concentrations were not correlated to BMI (respectively: $r = 0.107$, $p = 0.73$; $r = -0.378$, $p = 0.202$). DAG plasma concentrations, but not AG, were positively correlated with physical activity (respectively: rho = -0.609, $p = 0.027$; rho = -0.322, $p = 0.283$). Furthermore, DAG value at T2 was negatively correlated with BMI at T3 ($r = -0.607$, $p = 0.028$, Figure 1F), while it was not the case for the AG value ($r = -0.264$, $p = 0.383$, Figure 1E). Finally, the increase of physical activity between T2 and T3 was significantly correlated to DAG value at T2 ($r = 0.587$, $p = 0.035$ Figure 1H), but not AG value at T2 ($r = 0.468$, $p = 0.107$, Figure 1G).

3.2. Experiment 2. Preclinical Investigation

3.2.1. Short Term Food Restriction Protocol: Link between AG, DAG and Physical Activity

At D0, the body weight was not significantly different between ALW and FRW mice (17.3 ± 0.25 vs. 17.0 ± 0.19 g). At D14, the body weight of FRW mice was significantly decreased (12.92 ± 0.21 g) compared to ALW mice (17.89 ± 0.27; $t = 14.63$, $p < 0.0001$; Figure 2A). Physical activity was evaluated per cage (2 mice per cage). Total 24 h activity was similar between ALW and FRW at D0 ($U = 71$, $p = 0.96$; ALW vs. FRW: 564,302 ± 196,102 vs. 348,602 ± 113,549) and at D14 ($U = 50$, $p = 0.22$; ALW vs. FRW: 1,032,292 ± 308,989 vs. 564,872 ± 183,051). From D8, only FRW mice developed a food anticipatory activity (FAA, $p < 0.01$ FRW vs. ALW; Figure 2B) 4 h 30 before the distribution of food (2:00 p.m. to 6:30 p.m.). From D10 to D14, ANOVA analysis for repeated measures revealed an interaction between group and day/night activity ($F_{(1-160)} = 8.86$, $p = 0.049$). When considering the cumulative activity between D10 and D14, post-hoc analysis indicated that ALW showed the highest activity during the night (day vs. night: 52,178 ± 18,874 cm vs. 4,850,005 ± 1,358,516 cm, $p = 0.008$), and FRW mice did not show any significant differences between day and night activity (day vs. night: 877,885 ± 189,871 cm vs. 1,026,869 ± 189,585 cm, $p = 0.61$) reflecting the FAA.

Plasma ghrelin concentrations were measured when the FAA was clearly developed: before distribution of food for FRW (at 5:00 p.m.) and when mice were fed (at 9:00 a.m.). At 9:00 a.m. AG plasma concentrations in fed mice were not different between ALW and FRW ($p = 0.15$), but were significantly increased only for FRW mice at 5:00 p.m. as compared to ALW mice ($U = 79.5$, $p < 0.0001$, Figure 2C). DAG plasma concentrations were significantly higher in FRW mice both at 9:00 a.m. ($U = 151$, $p = 0.0041$) and at 5:00 p.m. ($U = 32$, $p < 0.0001$) than in ALW mice (Figure 2D). Finally, AG and DAG were significantly increased between morning and afternoon ($p < 0.0001$, Figure 2C,D). The AG/DAG ratio was significantly different between ALW and FRW at 9:00 a.m. (0.22 ± 0.02 vs. 0.13 ± 0.01, $U = 140$, $p = 0.0018$), but not at 5:00 p.m. (0.25 ± 0.04 vs. 0.24 ± 0.03, $U = 250.5$, $p = 0.44$).

The high quantity of physical activity performed by FRW mice during FAA (day 12) was correlated with high plasma concentrations of AG (Figure 2E, rho = 0.661, $p = 0.001$) and DAG (Figure 2F; rho = 0.614, $p = 0.002$).

Table 2. Correlations between BMI, physical activity, AG and DAG plasma concentrations in the clinical samples after weight restoration and one-month post discharge.

	BMI T2	PA T2 [1]	AG T2	DAG T2	BMI T3	PA T3	AG T3	DAG T3 [1]	Δ BMI	Δ PA	Δ AG	Δ DAG
BMI T2	—											
PA T2 [1]	0.007	—										
AG T2	0.107	−0.322	—									
DAG T2	−0.378	**−0.609 ***	0.205	—								
BMI T3	0.533	0.111	−0.264	**−0.607 ***	—							
PA T3	−0.188	0.165	0.159	0.192	−0.038	—						
AG T3	−0.107	0.146	0.369	0.186	−0.510	0.527	—					
DAG T3 [1]	−0.302	0.069	0.346	0.319	−0.494	0.301	0.445	—				
Δ BMI	0.087	0.141	−0.369	−0.511	**0.890 *****	0.050	−0.543	−0.278	—			
Δ PA	−0.121	**−0.664 ***	0.468	**0.587 ***	−0.204	**0.613 ***	0.412	0.159	−0.175	—		
Δ AG	−0.190	0.085	−0.492	0.002	−0.257	0.344	**0.628 ***	0.143	−0.200	−0.006	—	
Δ DAG	−0.222	0.198	0.355	−0.063	−0.101	−0.015	−0.072	**0.791 ****	0.001	−0.113	−0.364	—

T2: after weight restoration (90–100% BMI target); T3: one-month post discharge. BMI: body mass index; PA: physical activity measured by IPAQ; AG: acyl-ghrelin; DAG: desacyl-ghrelin. Δ: delta between T2 and T3. * $p<0.05$; ** $p<0.01$; *** $p<0.001$.
[1] Shapiro-Wilk $p < 0.05$; Spearman's rank correlation coefficient is indicated.

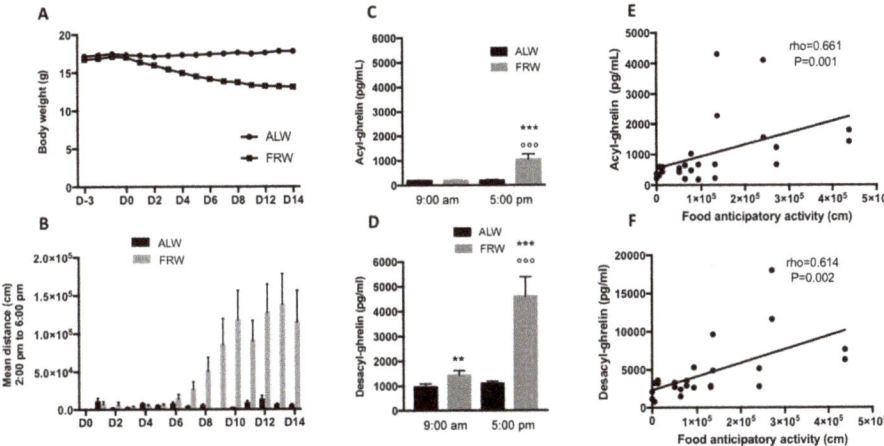

Figure 2. Short-term food restriction protocol. (**A**) Body weight evolution with a significant decrease from D2 to D14 for FRW vs. ALW mice. (**B**) Implementation of the food anticipatory activity (FAA, day activity) in the FRW mice from D6 to D14. (**C**) Mean plasma concentrations of acyl- (AG) and (**D**) desacyl-ghrelin (DAG) sampled at D10 (5:00 p.m.) and D11 (9:00 a.m.). Significant increases of AG and DAG were observed between morning and late afternoon samples only for FRW mice. (**E,F**) Plasma concentrations of AG (**E**) and DAG (**F**) were positively correlated with food anticipatory activity. Data are expressed as mean ± SEM; $n = 24$/group. $^{\circ\circ\circ}$ $p < 0.001$ 9 h vs. 17 h; ** $p < 0.01$, *** $p < 0.001$ ALW vs. FRW. ALW: ad libitum and wheel; FRW: food restriction and wheel.

3.2.2. Long Term Food Restriction Protocol and Refeeding

Fifty days after the beginning of quantitative food restriction for the FRW group, ad libitum food regimen was fully restored. The body weight of the FRW mice was rapidly restored after one day of refeeding (Figure 3A). In 4 days, FRW mice exhibited higher food intake as compared to the ALW group (D1: 213% of ALW food intake, D2: 167%, D3: 147%, Figure 3B).

It was not possible to properly measure physical activity during early refeeding from D51, because of the high binge-eating-like behaviour that interfered with FRW mice daily exercise. However, at D70, when FRW mice body weight was completely restored, activity in running wheels was significantly lower as compared to ALW mice during night-time only ($U = 0$, $p = 0.007$, Figure 3C).

On the first day of the refeeding period (D51), AG and DAG plasma concentrations were significantly decreased in FRW mice compared to ALW mice (respectively $U = 3$, $p = 0.015$; $U = 3$, $p = 0.015$, Figure 3D,E), whereas at D70, no difference was noted between the two groups for AG ($U = 13$, $p = 0.792$, Figure 3F) and DAG ($U = 10$, $p = 0.429$, Figure 3G).

At D70, night and total activities in ALW mice were positively correlated to AG (respectively, rho = 0.887, $p = 0.018$; rho = 0.888, $p = 0.018$), but not DAG. In contrast, total activity in FRW mice was positively correlated to DAG (rho = 0.96, $p = 0.01$) with a tendency only for day activity (rho = 0.820, $p = 0.089$) but not AG (Table 3).

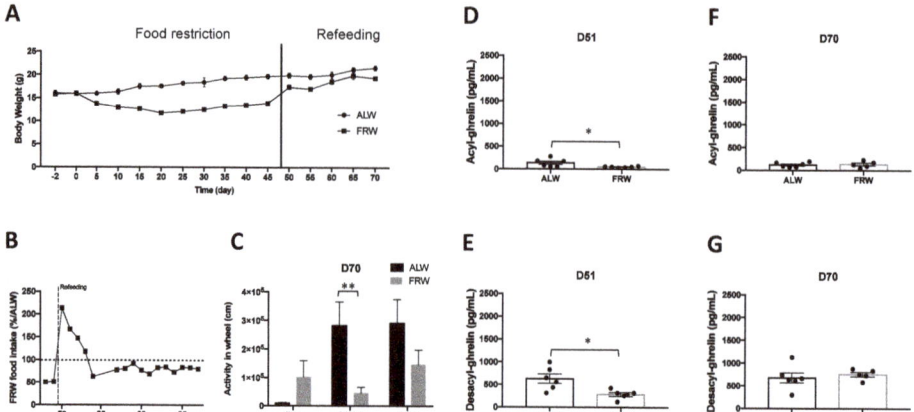

Figure 3. Long-term food restriction protocol and nutritional recovery (refeeding). (**A**) Longitudinal evolution of body weight during long term protocol. (**B**) Evolution of food intake during the refeeding period. (**C**) Total, day and night voluntary exercise in wheel at the end of the refeeding period; FRW mice showed an alteration in the daily distribution of their physical activity. (**D,E**) Acyl- (**D**) and desacyl-ghrelin (**E**) after one day of refeeding (D51). (**F,G**) Acyl- (**F**) and desacyl-ghrelin (**G**) after 20 days of refeeding (D70). Data are expressed as mean ± SEM; n = 6/group. Dotted lines in **B** represent the percentage value corresponding to the food eaten by ALW mice. * $p < 0.05$; ** $p < 0.01$. ALW: ad libitum and wheel; FRW: food restriction and wheel.

Table 3. Correlation between physical activity in wheel (total, day and night) and acyl- and desacyl-ghrelin plasma concentrations, in FRW and ALW mice at D70 (20 days of refeeding). Spearman's rank correlation coefficient is indicated by rho.

		ALW		FRW	
		AG	DAG	AG	DAG
Activity in Wheel	Total	0.887 *	0.609	0.699	0.960 *
	Day	−0.297	−0.407	0.569	0.820
	Night	0.888 *	0.614	0.117	0.049

* $p < 0.05$. Significant values are indicated in bold. AG: acyl-ghrelin; DAG: desacyl-ghrelin; ALW: ad libitum and wheel; FRW: food restriction and wheel.

4. Discussion

In the present study, we aimed to improve our understanding of the link between plasma concentrations of the two isoforms of ghrelin and the level of physical activity in condition of chronic food restriction and during nutritional recovery. In AN patients, under an inpatient therapeutic program, we observed that one month after discharge only plasma DAG concentrations were negatively correlated to BMI and positively to the level of physical activity. In keeping with this observation in AN patients, we also showed in mice that after two weeks of nutritional recovery, plasma DAG concentrations were positively correlated with diurnal physical activity.

In AN, refeeding is accompanied by a significant reduction in plasma ghrelin concentrations [23,48]. To our knowledge, only one study reported a differential evolution of plasma AG and DAG concentrations during nutritional recovery in five women with restrictive-type AN [49]. Plasma DAG concentrations decreased more rapidly than AG in the early stage of hospitalisation and after 8 weeks they remained significantly lower than in ten control subjects [49].

Relapse after hospitalisation is a major clinical challenge, especially within the first year following treatment [44,50]. Thus, the identification of factors influencing recovery is a research priority for AN [51]. During hospitalisation, the therapeutic program followed by our AN patients involves reduction of exercise and physical activity limitations and both quantitative and qualitative food intake modifications. During this period, we observed that plasma concentrations of total ghrelin, AG and DAG decreased rapidly, as previously demonstrated in longitudinal studies [23,49]. The therapeutic program includes a progressive exposure to home after weight recovery and before discharge, with regular home visits. However, the period following weight recovery remains a challenge both for patients and caregivers, most patients losing weight one month after discharge and resuming their physical hyperactivity routine. In the present study plasma AG concentrations increase faster than DAG after return in an ecological environment. More specifically, BMI and DAG are negatively correlated. Recent data showed that physical activity correlated positively with total plasma ghrelin levels in acute state of AN [37]. Here, only DAG plasma concentrations at discharge were associated with increased physical activity one month later. Although the follow-up was too short to conclude about a possible relapse, our data further support that early variations of body weight and physical activity may be influenced by metabolic factors at discharge. Length of hospitalisation and balance between inpatient and intensive outpatient treatment might benefit from objective metabolic biomarkers, such as AG and DAG.

To better decipher the potential interaction between daily physical activity and metabolic alterations, we used a preclinical mouse model of chronic food restriction associated with voluntary physical activity, in which metabolic parameters have been characterised previously following either a short- (2 weeks) or long-term (8 weeks) protocol [45,46]. In the present study, AG and DAG plasma concentrations were assessed at different key stages of the protocol, using selective and sensitive immunoassays [29]. We first assessed such variations in mice submitted to a two-week food restriction that had the ability to run in a wheel. The association between ghrelin and exercise had previously been demonstrated in the "activity-based anorexia" (ABA) model. Indeed during 5 days of ABA protocol, GHRS-R1a antagonism inhibited food anticipatory activity (FAA) in mice [38] and the motivational drive to eat in rats [52]. Moreover, ghrelin knockout mice exhibited a lower FAA in wheel during a time-restricted feeding protocol and acute administration of GHRP-6, a GHSR-1a agonist, was sufficient to enhance the amount of voluntary exercise in ghrelin KO mice [53]. This increase of FAA induced by GHRP-6 is mediated by an increase of dopaminergic activity in the nucleus accumbens [53]. These data are of importance since they emphasise how ghrelin, usually studied for its involvement in the modulation of food intake [54], is essential to initiate voluntary exercise in parallel to feeding behaviour. Here, in our quantitative food-restricted model, we consolidated the data obtained by Mifune et al. in their time-food restricted model [53]. Indeed, only the food-restricted mice that developed the highest FAA displayed the highest plasma concentrations of both AG and DAG. The mechanisms by which animals anticipate feeding remain yet unresolved (see. Mistlberger (1994) for review) [55]. Food anticipatory activity might be induced by both food-inducible oscillators—the precise location into the brain of which remains to be determined [56,57]—and circadian-clocks located in the suprachiasmatic nucleus [58]. LeSauter et al. (2009) suggested that stomach-producing ghrelin cells contain food-entrainable oscillators [59]. They showed that intraperitoneal ghrelin administration in non-deprived mice, but in the absence of food, induced an increase in the locomotor activity while mice lacking ghrelin receptors displayed a significant reduction of FAA. Acylated ghrelin appears to stimulate both the appetitive (anticipatory locomotor behaviour) and the consummatory component (food intake) of feeding behaviour. However, AG does not appear to be necessary for FAA although anticipatory activity rhythms may exhibit a reduced peak level or duration in *ghsr* −/− mice; supporting a modulatory influence of ghrelin rather than a full food-inducible oscillator role [56,60–63]. Although the potential role of DAG as a hormone remains a matter of debate, DAG is suggested to be a signalling molecule that has specific targets, including the brain, with mostly opposite and independent effects to AG on food intake and glucose homeostasis [27,30,64,65]. To our knowledge, a relation between DAG and physical activity anticipatory to feeding had not been previously demonstrated in food-restricted rodents. An elegant study on bird migratory behaviours demonstrated that injections of DAG decrease food intake and increase migratory restlessness [66]. Indeed, ethologic condition of migration associates voluntary exercise to voluntary immediate food renunciation permitting long-term gain for the species [67]. As mentioned by Guisinger et al. (2003) "AN's distinctive symptoms of restricting food, denial of starvation, and hyperactivity are likely to be evolved adaptive mechanisms that facilitated ancestral nomadic foragers leaving depleted environments; genetically susceptible individuals who lose too much weight may trigger these archaic adaptations." [67]. Although highly speculative and lacking enough empirical substantiation, these findings prompted us to determine whether the evolution of AG and DAG in relation with physical activity during and after feeding evolved similarly to establish them as reliable post-remission predictors.

The food restriction protocol was thus extended to 50 days followed by a long-term nutritional recovery protocol. Such a protocol better mimicked the physiological changes that occur during weight recovery in AN patients. In this perspective, our preclinical model may fulfil face validity (phenomenological similarities for the physiological alterations) and predictive validity, criteria that are essential to model pathology [68]. After long-term food restriction, plasma AG and DAG concentrations remained elevated. Then, the prolongation of the protocol impacted the day-night exercise setting out even after 20 days of nutritional recovery, despite the technical necessity of maintaining two mice per cage to limit social stress. Nevertheless, this suggested that after 20 days of nutritional recovery, the voluntary physical activity remained differentially correlated with AG or DAG, in control or food restricted mice respectively. Indeed, DAG positively correlated with exercise performed during the day, only in the FRW group.

The effects of exercise on plasma total or AG plasma ghrelin levels have been investigated in multiple human and rodent studies although the results have been inconsistent, demonstrating either a decrease, increase, or no change [40,69]. Only total and AG concentrations have been measured. To our knowledge, no study described the impact of physical activity on DAG. Here, we benefited from the development of selective and sensitive assays, validated both in humans (personal data) and rodents [29]. Our results converge in both rodents and humans and highlight the importance of the balance between AG and DAG. Indeed on one side, AG is rapidly converted into a DAG because of the rapid action of blood esterases [70]. On the other side, the ghrelin O-acyl transferase (GOAT) that permits the octanoylation of ghrelin (AG) is now considered to be a key regulator in energy metabolism and hedonic feeding [71–73]. DAG has long been considered to be an inactive product of degradation of AG but subsequent data suggest that it is a metabolically active peptide acting through a yet unknown receptor [27]. Mostly, DAG antagonises but sometimes acts synergistically with AG, since it can bind and activate the AG receptor but with a lower affinity in vitro and in vivo [74]. However, DAG does not reach the necessary concentrations in tissues to do so, at least under physiological conditions [27]. Overall, studies in rodents and humans support a role of DAG to decrease body weight, food intake and body fat [75,76]. Indeed, DAG overexpressing mice exhibit a decrease in body weight, food intake, fat pad mass weight accompanied by a modest decrease in linear growth [76]. These physiological changes are attributable to (1) the decrease in gastric emptying and (2) an anorexigenic effect of DAG mediated by a specific activation of hypothalamic neurons [76,77]. In the present FRW model, intraperitoneal injection of DAG increased physical activity [78]. Therefore, we hypothesise an indirect action of DAG on physical activity. Indeed, GOAT activity has been detected in the hypothalamus and pituitary and its hypothalamic expression is nutritionally regulated [73,79]. Thus, increased DAG plasma concentrations during chronic food restriction might indirectly activate GHS-R via a local hypothalamic conversion into AG, leading to an adaptive increase of physical activity [80].

The present clinical data enlightened the potential role of DAG in recovery processes in AN and suggested a potential negative impact of DAG on weight recovery. Such interpretation might be paralleled with data obtained from the mouse model where increased plasma DAG correlated with an unusual physical activity during daytime, since rodents are used to exercise during night-time. This may reflect a sustainable alteration of physiological regulation of feeding-relative behaviours away from a long- period of caloric restriction that can interfere with a proper recovery. DAG has also been implicated in myogenesis and thus may protect the muscle integrity along weight loss [54,81]. Finally, we cannot exclude the role of elevated DAG plasma concentrations in the development of osteopenia and osteoporosis even if DAG effects on bone physiology are currently very limited and contradictory. On one side, DAG stimulates human osteoblasts proliferation in the absence of GHS-R1a [82]. On the other side, mice overexpressing DAG show a moderate decrease in their linear growth suggesting an impairment of the skeletal integrity [76]. Further mechanistic studies will help to decipher how AG and DAG modulate both muscle and bone integrity and functioning.

Translational data might be a prerequisite to stress the mechanisms that support a successful recovery in AN. On one hand, ghrelin agonists induced motivation to exercise through activation of the central reward circuit [53]. Furthermore, central administration of ghrelin enhances exercise through dopamine release in the nucleus accumbens [83]. In AN, an alteration of the reward circuit is now well accepted [11]. Further studies are needed to determine the action of DAG on this brain circuit. On the other hand, several data have linked the body temperature with the level of activity both in mice, in rats and in AN patients [84,85]. Thus, increasing physical activity through a direct or indirect action of AG or DAG could maintain appropriate body temperature in AN.

Limitations and perspectives. There are several limitations to this study. First, the small size of the clinical sample prevents generalisation and calls for replication. Second, we need to be cautious with the interpretation of data related to physical activity measurement in clinical and preclinical experiments. In the clinical sample, we used an internationally valid self-report assessment (IPAQ). Actimetry, heart rate monitoring, and recent progress on portable devices would allow investigating physical activity based on objective measures, which would be more accurate. Indeed, physical activity in AN patients is underestimated by subjective assessment (IPAQ) when compared with objective (Actiheart) measurement [86]. We also confirmed that objective assessment of physical activity could be more informative than subjective ratings, to reflect for example cognitive specificities of anorexia nervosa [87]. As surprising as it may seem, physical activity assessment in AN is so far not well defined, and there is currently no real consensus on how to measure it. In future research, it seems necessary to assess the different aspects of physical exercise conjointly (obligatory exercise, addiction exercise, commitment for exercise, reasons for exercise, isometry...) [88]. Recent studies support the need to investigate more in depth this unsuitable behaviour in a condition of reduced energy supplies [2,89]. Third, the choice to maintain as long as possible two restricted mice in a cage equipped with a wheel to avoid social stress and hypothermia, could limit the measurement of physical activity. However, separate experiments done in metabolic cages (where the ALW and FRW mice were singly housed for 5 to 6 days), validated that singly housed FRW mice exhibited similar FAA after 15 days of protocol (Duriez et al., unpublished data, [45]). For the welfare of the animals and to avoid stress isolation and hypothermia induced by a long-term caloric restriction, mice were maintained as two per cage. The recording of physical activity reflected the activity of two mice that usually run two by two in the wheel (ALW or FRW, personal observation). We also observed that the nutritional recovery was extremely rapid in our animal experiment, with a rapid body weight gain, that is consistent with a faster metabolism observed in rodents than in human. It might be interesting to validate another protocol of slow nutritional refeeding monitored by the investigator. Altogether, this reflects the limitations of animal modelling of psychiatric disorders. The rapid decrease of AG and DAG plasma concentrations, rapid weight gain and binge-eating like behaviour in the first three days of nutritional recovery suggest the persistence of food directed motivation after a long caloric restriction period. However, our conclusion asks the question to compare progressive to rapid weight recovery in mice. Indeed, clinical practice reported in some cases a rapid weight recovery in AN, especially in the case of clinical switch from AN to bulimia nervosa [90,91]. Ghrelin gene variants may also predict crossover rate from restricting-type AN to binge-purging subtype or bulimia nervosa [92]. We need to know whether the changes in AG and DAG during a rapid or a progressive weight recovery associated or not with binge-eating crisis forecast sustainable altered eating behaviour. Finally, weight gain cannot be considered as the unique remission factor. Preclinical models appear then to be crucial tools to decipher long-term metabolic alterations after full weight recovery and despite their limitations, they could permit to test pharmacological options. Shall DAG-signalling be a pharmacological target in AN?

Author Contributions: O.V. was responsible for the study concept and design of animal experiments and R.D., G.L. and J.E. for the study concept and design of the clinical protocol. V.T. was responsible for the design and analyses of biomarkers assays in both experimental and clinical protocols. O.V., P.D. and V.T. wrote the paper. P.D., L.R., V.T. and O.V. performed animal experimentations. D.G. performed immunoassays. P.D., P.G., N.R., L.R., V.T. and O.V. contributed to data analysis and interpretation of findings. R.D., G.L. were in charge of the recruitment of patients and data analysis. All authors have read and agreed to the published version of the manuscript.

Funding: This work was supported by University Paris Descartes Sorbonne Paris Cité, Institut National de la Santé et de la Recherche Médicale (INSERM) (to PG and JE) and Agence Nationale de la Recherche (ANR) JCJC ANR-12-JSV1-0013-01 grant to V.T.

Acknowledgments: We first warmly acknowledge Cécile Bergot and Emilie Grasset (CMME, Ste Anne Hospital) for the care of the patients and their contribution to the clinical study. We are grateful to the staff in the animal experimentation platform at the Institute of Psychiatry and Neurosciences of Paris (IPNP) for the care of the animals and to the PhenoBrain phenotyping for providing a platform for animal experimentation. We are grateful to Bertin Biotechnologies (Montigny-le-Bretonneaux, France) for providing the acyl-ghrelin and desacyl-ghrelin assays.

Conflicts of Interest: The authors declare no conflict of interest.

References

1. Hebebrand, J.; Exner, C.; Hebebrand, K.; Holtkamp, C.; Casper, R.C.; Remschmidt, H.; Herpertz-Dahlmann, B.; Klingenspor, M. Hyperactivity in patients with anorexia nervosa and in semistarved rats: Evidence for a pivotal role of hypoleptinemia. *Physiol. Behav.* **2003**, *79*, 25–37. [CrossRef]
2. Rizk, M.; Mattar, L.; Kern, L.; Berthoz, S.; Duclos, J.; Viltart, O.; Godart, N. Physical Activity in Eating Disorders: A Systematic Review. *Nutrients* **2020**, *12*, 183. [CrossRef]
3. Solenberger, S.E. Exercise and eating disorders: A 3-year inpatient hospital record analysis. *Eat. Behav.* **2001**, *2*, 151–168. [CrossRef]
4. Taranis, L.; Meyer, C. Associations between specific components of compulsive exercise and eating-disordered cognitions and behaviors among young women. *Int. J. Eat. Disord.* **2011**, *44*, 452–458. [CrossRef]
5. Steinhausen, H.-C. The outcome of anorexia nervosa in the 20th century. *Am. J. Psychiatry* **2002**, *159*, 1284–1293. [CrossRef]
6. Strober, M.; Freeman, R.; Morrell, W. The long-term course of severe anorexia nervosa in adolescents: Survival analysis of recovery, relapse, and outcome predictors over 10–15 years in a prospective study. *Int. J. Eat. Disord.* **1997**, *22*, 339–360. [CrossRef]
7. Treasure, J.; Zipfel, S.; Micali, N.; Wade, T.; Stice, E.; Claudino, A.; Schmidt, U.; Frank, G.K.; Bulik, C.M.; Wentz, E. Anorexia nervosa. *Nat. Rev. Dis. Primers* **2015**, *1*, 15074. [CrossRef]
8. Duncan, L.; Yilmaz, Z.; Gaspar, H.; Walters, R.; Goldstein, J.; Anttila, V.; Bulik-Sullivan, B.; Ripke, S.; Eating Disorders Working Group of the Psychiatric Genomics Consortium; Thornton, L.; et al. Significant Locus and Metabolic Genetic Correlations Revealed in Genome-Wide Association Study of Anorexia Nervosa. *Am. J. Psychiatry* **2017**, *174*, 850–858. [CrossRef]
9. Schorr, M.; Miller, K.K. The endocrine manifestations of anorexia nervosa: Mechanisms and management. *Nat. Rev. Endocrinol.* **2017**, *13*, 174–186. [CrossRef]
10. Watson, H.J.; Yilmaz, Z.; Thornton, L.M.; Hübel, C.; Coleman, J.R.I.; Gaspar, H.A.; Bryois, J.; Hinney, A.; Leppä, V.M.; Mattheisen, M.; et al. Genome-wide association study identifies eight risk loci and implicates metabo-psychiatric origins for anorexia nervosa. *Nat. Genet.* **2019**, *51*, 1207–1214. [CrossRef]
11. Duriez, P.; Ramoz, N.; Gorwood, P.; Viltart, O.; Tolle, V. A Metabolic Perspective on Reward Abnormalities in Anorexia Nervosa. *Trends Endocrinol. Metab.* **2019**, *30*, 915–928. [CrossRef] [PubMed]
12. Viltart, O.; Duriez, P.; Tolle, V. Metabolic and neuroendocrine adaptations to undernutrition in anorexia nervosa: From a clinical to a basic research point of view. *Horm. Mol. Biol. Clin. Investig.* **2018**, *36*. [CrossRef] [PubMed]
13. Kojima, M.; Hosoda, H.; Date, Y.; Nakazato, M.; Matsuo, H.; Kangawa, K. Ghrelin is a growth-hormone-releasing acylated peptide from stomach. *Nature* **1999**, *402*, 656–660. [CrossRef] [PubMed]

14. Date, Y.; Kojima, M.; Hosoda, H.; Sawaguchi, A.; Mondal, M.S.; Suganuma, T.; Matsukura, S.; Kangawa, K.; Nakazato, M. Ghrelin, a novel growth hormone-releasing acylated peptide, is synthesized in a distinct endocrine cell type in the gastrointestinal tracts of rats and humans. *Endocrinology* **2000**, *141*, 4255–4261. [CrossRef] [PubMed]
15. Müller, T.D.; Nogueiras, R.; Andermann, M.L.; Andrews, Z.B.; Anker, S.D.; Argente, J.; Batterham, R.L.; Benoit, S.C.; Bowers, C.Y.; Broglio, F.; et al. Ghrelin. *Mol. Metab.* **2015**, *4*, 437–460. [CrossRef]
16. De Vriese, C.; Perret, J.; Delporte, C. Focus on the short- and long-term effects of ghrelin on energy homeostasis. *Nutrition* **2010**, *26*, 579–584. [CrossRef]
17. Pradhan, G.; Samson, S.L.; Sun, Y. Ghrelin: Much more than a hunger hormone. *Curr. Opin. Clin. Nutr. Metab. Care* **2013**, *16*, 619–624. [CrossRef]
18. Tajiri, Y. Ghrelin and exercise: A possible virtuous circle. *Diabetol. Int.* **2017**, *8*, 347–349. [CrossRef]
19. Tokudome, T.; Otani, K.; Miyazato, M.; Kangawa, K. Ghrelin and the heart. *Peptides* **2019**, *111*, 42–46. [CrossRef]
20. Camargo-Silva, G.; Turones, L.C.; da Cruz, K.R.; Gomes, K.P.; Mendonça, M.M.; Nunes, A.; de Jesus, I.G.; Colugnati, D.B.; Pansani, A.P.; Pobbe, R.L.H.; et al. Ghrelin potentiates cardiac reactivity to stress by modulating sympathetic control and beta-adrenergic response. *Life Sci.* **2018**, *196*, 84–92. [CrossRef]
21. Perello, M.; Dickson, S.L. Ghrelin signalling on food reward: A salient link between the gut and the mesolimbic system. *J. Neuroendocrinol.* **2015**, *27*, 424–434. [CrossRef] [PubMed]
22. Bake, T.; Edvardsson, C.E.; Cummings, C.J.; Dickson, S.L. Ghrelin's effects on food motivation in rats are not limited to palatable foods. *J. Neuroendocrinol.* **2018**, e12665. [CrossRef]
23. Tolle, V.; Kadem, M.; Bluet-Pajot, M.-T.; Frere, D.; Foulon, C.; Bossu, C.; Dardennes, R.; Mounier, C.; Zizzari, P.; Lang, F.; et al. Balance in ghrelin and leptin plasma levels in anorexia nervosa patients and constitutionally thin women. *J. Clin. Endocrinol. Metab.* **2003**, *88*, 109–116. [CrossRef] [PubMed]
24. Pardo, M.; Roca-Rivada, A.; Al-Massadi, O.; Seoane, L.M.; Camiña, J.P.; Casanueva, F.F. Peripheral leptin and ghrelin receptors are regulated in a tissue-specific manner in activity-based anorexia. *Peptides* **2010**, *31*, 1912–1919. [CrossRef]
25. Méquinion, M.; Chauveau, C.; Viltart, O. The use of animal models to decipher physiological and neurobiological alterations of anorexia nervosa patients. *Front. Endocrinol. (Lausanne)* **2015**, *6*, 68. [CrossRef] [PubMed]
26. Zigman, J.M.; Jones, J.E.; Lee, C.E.; Saper, C.B.; Elmquist, J.K. Expression of ghrelin receptor mRNA in the rat and the mouse brain. *J. Comp. Neurol.* **2006**, *494*, 528–548. [CrossRef]
27. Delhanty, P.J.; Neggers, S.J.; van der Lely, A.J. Des-acyl ghrelin: A metabolically active peptide. *Endocr. Dev.* **2013**, *25*, 112–121. [CrossRef]
28. Hosoda, H.; Kojima, M.; Matsuo, H.; Kangawa, K. Ghrelin and des-acyl ghrelin: Two major forms of rat ghrelin peptide in gastrointestinal tissue. *Biochem. Biophys. Res. Commun.* **2000**, *279*, 909–913. [CrossRef]
29. Hassouna, R.; Grouselle, D.; Chiappetta, G.; Lipecka, J.; Fiquet, O.; Tomasetto, C.; Vinh, J.; Epelbaum, J.; Tolle, V. Combination of Selective Immunoassays and Mass Spectrometry to Characterize Preproghrelin-Derived Peptides in Mouse Tissues. *Front. Neurosci.* **2017**, *11*, 211. [CrossRef]
30. Stevanovic, D.M.; Grefhorst, A.; Themmen, A.P.N.; Popovic, V.; Holstege, J.; Haasdijk, E.; Trajkovic, V.; van der Lely, A.-J.; Delhanty, P.J.D. Unacylated ghrelin suppresses ghrelin-induced neuronal activity in the hypothalamus and brainstem of male rats [corrected]. *PLoS ONE* **2014**, *9*, e98180. [CrossRef]
31. Allas, S.; Caixàs, A.; Poitou, C.; Coupaye, M.; Thuilleaux, D.; Lorenzini, F.; Diene, G.; Crinò, A.; Illouz, F.; Grugni, G.; et al. AZP-531, an unacylated ghrelin analog, improves food-related behavior in patients with Prader-Willi syndrome: A randomized placebo-controlled trial. *PLoS ONE* **2018**, *13*, e0190849. [CrossRef] [PubMed]
32. Beauloye, V.; Diene, G.; Kuppens, R.; Zech, F.; Winandy, C.; Molinas, C.; Faye, S.; Kieffer, I.; Beckers, D.; Nergårdh, R.; et al. High unacylated ghrelin levels support the concept of anorexia in infants with prader-willi syndrome. *Orphanet J. Rare Dis.* **2016**, *11*, 56. [CrossRef] [PubMed]
33. King, J.A.; Deighton, K.; Broom, D.R.; Wasse, L.K.; Douglas, J.A.; Burns, S.F.; Cordery, P.A.; Petherick, E.S.; Batterham, R.L.; Goltz, F.R.; et al. Individual Variation in Hunger, Energy Intake, and Ghrelin Responses to Acute Exercise. *Med. Sci. Sports Exerc.* **2017**, *49*, 1219–1228. [CrossRef]

34. Dundar, A.; Kocahan, S.; Sahin, L. Associations of apelin, leptin, irisin, ghrelin, insulin, glucose levels, and lipid parameters with physical activity during eight weeks of regular exercise training. *Arch. Physiol. Biochem.* **2019**, 1–5. [CrossRef] [PubMed]
35. Sartorio, A.; Morpurgo, P.; Cappiello, V.; Agosti, F.; Marazzi, N.; Giordani, C.; Rigamonti, A.E.; Muller, E.E.; Spada, A. Exercise-induced effects on growth hormone levels are associated with ghrelin changes only in presence of prolonged exercise bouts in male athletes. *J. Sports Med. Phys. Fit.* **2008**, *48*, 97–101.
36. Fathi, R.; Ghanbari-Niaki, A.; Kraemer, R.R.; Talebi-Garakani, E.; Saghebjoo, M. The effect of exercise intensity on plasma and tissue acyl ghrelin concentrations in fasted rats. *Regul. Pept.* **2010**, *165*, 133–137. [CrossRef]
37. Hofmann, T.; Elbelt, U.; Haas, V.; Ahnis, A.; Klapp, B.F.; Rose, M.; Stengel, A. Plasma kisspeptin and ghrelin levels are independently correlated with physical activity in patients with anorexia nervosa. *Appetite* **2017**, *108*, 141–150. [CrossRef]
38. Verhagen, L.A.W.; Egecioglu, E.; Luijendijk, M.C.M.; Hillebrand, J.J.G.; Adan, R.A.H.; Dickson, S.L. Acute and chronic suppression of the central ghrelin signaling system reveals a role in food anticipatory activity. *Eur. Neuropsychopharmacol.* **2011**, *21*, 384–392. [CrossRef]
39. Wu, H.; van Kuyck, K.; Tambuyzer, T.; Luyten, L.; Aerts, J.-M.; Nuttin, B. Rethinking food anticipatory activity in the activity-based anorexia rat model. *Sci. Rep.* **2014**, *4*, 3929. [CrossRef]
40. Mani, B.K.; Castorena, C.M.; Osborne-Lawrence, S.; Vijayaraghavan, P.; Metzger, N.P.; Elmquist, J.K.; Zigman, J.M. Ghrelin mediates exercise endurance and the feeding response post-exercise. *Mol. Metab.* **2018**, *9*, 114–130. [CrossRef]
41. Mackelvie, K.J.; Meneilly, G.S.; Elahi, D.; Wong, A.C.K.; Barr, S.I.; Chanoine, J.-P. Regulation of appetite in lean and obese adolescents after exercise: Role of acylated and desacyl ghrelin. *J. Clin. Endocrinol. Metab.* **2007**, *92*, 648–654. [CrossRef] [PubMed]
42. Shiiya, T.; Ueno, H.; Toshinai, K.; Kawagoe, T.; Naito, S.; Tobina, T.; Nishida, Y.; Shindo, M.; Kangawa, K.; Tanaka, H.; et al. Significant lowering of plasma ghrelin but not des-acyl ghrelin in response to acute exercise in men. *Endocr. J.* **2011**, *58*, 335–342. [CrossRef] [PubMed]
43. Tiryaki-Sonmez, G.; Ozen, S.; Bugdayci, G.; Karli, U.; Ozen, G.; Cogalgil, S.; Schoenfeld, B.; Sozbir, K.; Aydin, K. Effect of exercise on appetite-regulating hormones in overweight women. *Biol. Sport* **2013**, *30*, 75–80. [CrossRef]
44. Khalsa, S.S.; Portnoff, L.C.; McCurdy-McKinnon, D.; Feusner, J.D. What happens after treatment? A systematic review of relapse, remission, and recovery in anorexia nervosa. *J. Eat. Disord.* **2017**, *5*, 20. [CrossRef] [PubMed]
45. Méquinion, M.; Caron, E.; Zgheib, S.; Stievenard, A.; Zizzari, P.; Tolle, V.; Cortet, B.; Lucas, S.; Prévot, V.; Chauveau, C.; et al. Physical activity: Benefit or weakness in metabolic adaptations in a mouse model of chronic food restriction? *Am. J. Physiol. Endocrinol. Metab.* **2015**, *308*, E241–E255. [CrossRef]
46. Duriez, P.; Eddarkaoui, S.; Blum, D.; Dickson, S.L.; Gorwood, P.; Tolle, V.; Viltart, O. Does physical activity associated with chronic food restriction alleviate anxiety like behaviour, in female mice? *Horm. Behav.* **2020**, *124*, 104807. [CrossRef]
47. Craig, C.L.; Marshall, A.L.; Sjöström, M.; Bauman, A.E.; Booth, M.L.; Ainsworth, B.E.; Pratt, M.; Ekelund, U.; Yngve, A.; Sallis, J.F.; et al. International physical activity questionnaire: 12-country reliability and validity. *Med. Sci. Sports Exerc.* **2003**, *35*, 1381–1395. [CrossRef]
48. Otto, B.; Cuntz, U.; Fruehauf, E.; Wawarta, R.; Folwaczny, C.; Riepl, R.L.; Heiman, M.L.; Lehnert, P.; Fichter, M.; Tschöp, M. Weight gain decreases elevated plasma ghrelin concentrations of patients with anorexia nervosa. *Eur. J. Endocrinol.* **2001**, *145*, 669–673. [CrossRef]
49. Koyama, K.-I.; Yasuhara, D.; Nakahara, T.; Harada, T.; Uehara, M.; Ushikai, M.; Asakawa, A.; Inui, A. Changes in acyl ghrelin, des-acyl ghrelin, and ratio of acyl ghrelin to total ghrelin with short-term refeeding in female inpatients with restricting-type anorexia nervosa. *Horm. Metab. Res.* **2010**, *42*, 595–598. [CrossRef]
50. Keel, P.K.; Dorer, D.J.; Franko, D.L.; Jackson, S.C.; Herzog, D.B. Postremission predictors of relapse in women with eating disorders. *Am. J. Psychiatry* **2005**, *162*, 2263–2268. [CrossRef]
51. Van Furth, E.F.; van der Meer, A.; Cowan, K. Top 10 research priorities for eating disorders. *Lancet Psychiatry* **2016**, *3*, 706–707. [CrossRef]

52. Merkestein, M.; Brans, M.A.D.; Luijendijk, M.C.M.; de Jong, J.W.; Egecioglu, E.; Dickson, S.L.; Adan, R.A.H. Ghrelin mediates anticipation to a palatable meal in rats. *Obesity (Silver Spring)* **2012**, *20*, 963–971. [CrossRef] [PubMed]
53. Mifune, H.; Tajiri, Y.; Sakai, Y.; Kawahara, Y.; Hara, K.; Sato, T.; Nishi, Y.; Nishi, A.; Mitsuzono, R.; Kakuma, T.; et al. Voluntary exercise is motivated by ghrelin, possibly related to the central reward circuit. *J. Endocrinol.* **2020**, *244*, 123–132. [CrossRef] [PubMed]
54. Yanagi, S.; Sato, T.; Kangawa, K.; Nakazato, M. The Homeostatic Force of Ghrelin. *Cell Metab.* **2018**, *27*, 786–804. [CrossRef]
55. Mistlberger, R.E. Circadian food-anticipatory activity: Formal models and physiological mechanisms. *Neurosci. Biobehav. Rev.* **1994**, *18*, 171–195. [CrossRef]
56. Mistlberger, R.E. Neurobiology of food anticipatory circadian rhythms. *Physiol. Behav.* **2011**, *104*, 535–545. [CrossRef]
57. Chen, Y.; Lin, Y.-C.; Zimmerman, C.A.; Essner, R.A.; Knight, Z.A. Hunger neurons drive feeding through a sustained, positive reinforcement signal. *Elife* **2016**, *5*. [CrossRef]
58. Challet, E. Circadian clocks, food intake, and metabolism. *Prog. Mol. Biol. Transl. Sci.* **2013**, *119*, 105–135. [CrossRef]
59. LeSauter, J.; Hoque, N.; Weintraub, M.; Pfaff, D.W.; Silver, R. Stomach ghrelin-secreting cells as food-entrainable circadian clocks. *Proc. Natl. Acad. Sci. USA* **2009**, *106*, 13582–13587. [CrossRef]
60. Blum, I.D.; Patterson, Z.; Khazall, R.; Lamont, E.W.; Sleeman, M.W.; Horvath, T.L.; Abizaid, A. Reduced anticipatory locomotor responses to scheduled meals in ghrelin receptor deficient mice. *Neuroscience* **2009**, *164*, 351–359. [CrossRef]
61. Gunapala, K.M.; Gallardo, C.M.; Hsu, C.T.; Steele, A.D. Single gene deletions of orexin, leptin, neuropeptide Y, and ghrelin do not appreciably alter food anticipatory activity in mice. *PLoS ONE* **2011**, *6*, e18377. [CrossRef] [PubMed]
62. Patton, D.F.; Katsuyama, A.M.; Pavlovski, I.; Michalik, M.; Patterson, Z.; Parfyonov, M.; Smit, A.N.; Marchant, E.G.; Chung, S.H.; Chung, J.; et al. Circadian mechanisms of food anticipatory rhythms in rats fed once or twice daily: Clock gene and endocrine correlates. *PLoS ONE* **2014**, *9*, e112451. [CrossRef] [PubMed]
63. Dailey, M.J.; Stingl, K.C.; Moran, T.H. Disassociation between preprandial gut peptide release and food-anticipatory activity. *Endocrinology* **2012**, *153*, 132–142. [CrossRef] [PubMed]
64. Toshinai, K.; Yamaguchi, H.; Sun, Y.; Smith, R.G.; Yamanaka, A.; Sakurai, T.; Date, Y.; Mondal, M.S.; Shimbara, T.; Kawagoe, T.; et al. Des-acyl ghrelin induces food intake by a mechanism independent of the growth hormone secretagogue receptor. *Endocrinology* **2006**, *147*, 2306–2314. [CrossRef] [PubMed]
65. Delhanty, P.J.D.; Neggers, S.J.; van der Lely, A.J. Should we consider des-acyl ghrelin as a separate hormone and if so, what does it do? *Front. Horm. Res.* **2014**, *42*, 163–174. [CrossRef]
66. Goymann, W.; Lupi, S.; Kaiya, H.; Cardinale, M.; Fusani, L. Ghrelin affects stopover decisions and food intake in a long-distance migrant. *Proc. Natl. Acad. Sci. USA* **2017**. [CrossRef]
67. Guisinger, S. Adapted to flee famine: Adding an evolutionary perspective on anorexia nervosa. *Psychol. Rev.* **2003**, *110*, 745–761. [CrossRef]
68. Willner, P. Validation criteria for animal models of human mental disorders: Learned helplessness as a paradigm case. *Prog. Neuropsychopharmacol. Biol. Psychiatry* **1986**, *10*, 677–690. [CrossRef]
69. Holliday, A.; Blannin, A. Appetite, food intake and gut hormone responses to intense aerobic exercise of different duration. *J. Endocrinol.* **2017**, *235*, 193–205. [CrossRef]
70. Hosoda, H.; Doi, K.; Nagaya, N.; Okumura, H.; Nakagawa, E.; Enomoto, M.; Ono, F.; Kangawa, K. Optimum collection and storage conditions for ghrelin measurements: Octanoyl modification of ghrelin is rapidly hydrolyzed to desacyl ghrelin in blood samples. *Clin. Chem.* **2004**, *50*, 1077–1080. [CrossRef]
71. Yang, J.; Brown, M.S.; Liang, G.; Grishin, N.V.; Goldstein, J.L. Identification of the acyltransferase that octanoylates ghrelin, an appetite-stimulating peptide hormone. *Cell* **2008**, *132*, 387–396. [CrossRef] [PubMed]
72. Davis, J.F.; Perello, M.; Choi, D.L.; Magrisso, I.J.; Kirchner, H.; Pfluger, P.T.; Tschoep, M.; Zigman, J.M.; Benoit, S.C. GOAT induced ghrelin acylation regulates hedonic feeding. *Horm. Behav.* **2012**, *62*, 598–604. [CrossRef] [PubMed]

73. Kirchner, H.; Gutierrez, J.A.; Solenberg, P.J.; Pfluger, P.T.; Czyzyk, T.A.; Willency, J.A.; Schurmann, A.; Joost, H.G.; Jandacek, R.; Hale, J.E.; et al. GOAT links dietary lipids with the endocrine control of energy balance. *Nat. Med.* **2009**, *15*, 741–745. [CrossRef]
74. Heppner, K.M.; Piechowski, C.L.; Müller, A.; Ottaway, N.; Sisley, S.; Smiley, D.L.; Habegger, K.M.; Pfluger, P.T.; Dimarchi, R.; Biebermann, H.; et al. Both acyl and des-acyl ghrelin regulate adiposity and glucose metabolism via central nervous system ghrelin receptors. *Diabetes* **2014**, *63*, 122–131. [CrossRef] [PubMed]
75. Delhanty, P.J.D.; Neggers, S.J.; van der Lely, A.J. Mechanisms in endocrinology: Ghrelin: The differences between acyl- and des-acyl ghrelin. *Eur. J. Endocrinol.* **2012**, *167*, 601–608. [CrossRef] [PubMed]
76. Asakawa, A.; Inui, A.; Fujimiya, M.; Sakamaki, R.; Shinfuku, N.; Ueta, Y.; Meguid, M.M.; Kasuga, M. Stomach regulates energy balance via acylated ghrelin and desacyl ghrelin. *Gut* **2005**, *54*, 18–24. [CrossRef]
77. Asakawa, A.; Ataka, K.; Fujino, K.; Chen, C.-Y.; Kato, I.; Fujimiya, M.; Inui, A. Ghrelin family of peptides and gut motility. *J. Gastroenterol. Hepatol.* **2011**, *26* (Suppl. 3), 73–74. [CrossRef]
78. Robichon, L.; Adda, S.; Tolle, V.; Viltart, O. Deacyl-ghrelin: A potential role on the food anticipatory activity in a mouse model of chronic food restriction? *Eur. Neuropsychopharmacol.* **2019**, *29*, S189–S190. [CrossRef]
79. Gahete, M.D.; Córdoba-Chacón, J.; Salvatori, R.; Castaño, J.P.; Kineman, R.D.; Luque, R.M. Metabolic regulation of ghrelin O-acyl transferase (GOAT) expression in the mouse hypothalamus, pituitary, and stomach. *Mol. Cell. Endocrinol.* **2010**, *317*, 154–160. [CrossRef]
80. Hopkins, A.L.; Nelson, T.A.S.; Guschina, I.A.; Parsons, L.C.; Lewis, C.L.; Brown, R.C.; Christian, H.C.; Davies, J.S.; Wells, T. Unacylated ghrelin promotes adipogenesis in rodent bone marrow via ghrelin O-acyl transferase and GHS-R1a activity: Evidence for target cell-induced acylation. *Sci. Rep.* **2017**, *7*, 45541. [CrossRef]
81. Gortan Cappellari, G.; Zanetti, M.; Semolic, A.; Vinci, P.; Ruozi, G.; Falcione, A.; Filigheddu, N.; Guarnieri, G.; Graziani, A.; Giacca, M.; et al. Unacylated Ghrelin Reduces Skeletal Muscle Reactive Oxygen Species Generation and Inflammation and Prevents High-Fat Diet-Induced Hyperglycemia and Whole-Body Insulin Resistance in Rodents. *Diabetes* **2016**, *65*, 874–886. [CrossRef]
82. Delhanty, P.J.D.; van der Eerden, B.C.J.; van der Velde, M.; Gauna, C.; Pols, H.A.P.; Jahr, H.; Chiba, H.; van der Lely, A.J.; van Leeuwen, J.P.T.M. Ghrelin and unacylated ghrelin stimulate human osteoblast growth via mitogen-activated protein kinase (MAPK)/phosphoinositide 3-kinase (PI3K) pathways in the absence of GHS-R1a. *J. Endocrinol.* **2006**, *188*, 37–47. [CrossRef] [PubMed]
83. Jerlhag, E.; Egecioglu, E.; Dickson, S.L.; Douhan, A.; Svensson, L.; Engel, J.A. Ghrelin administration into tegmental areas stimulates locomotor activity and increases extracellular concentration of dopamine in the nucleus accumbens. *Addict. Biol.* **2007**, *12*, 6–16. [CrossRef]
84. Carrera, O.; Adan, R.A.H.; Gutierrez, E.; Danner, U.N.; Hoek, H.W.; van Elburg, A.A.; Kas, M.J.H. Hyperactivity in anorexia nervosa: Warming up not just burning-off calories. *PLoS ONE* **2012**, *7*, e41851. [CrossRef] [PubMed]
85. Inoue, Y.; Nakahara, K.; Maruyama, K.; Suzuki, Y.; Hayashi, Y.; Kangawa, K.; Murakami, N. Central and peripheral des-acyl ghrelin regulates body temperature in rats. *Biochem. Biophys. Res. Commun.* **2013**, *430*, 278–283. [CrossRef] [PubMed]
86. Alberti, M.; Galvani, C.; El Ghoch, M.; Capelli, C.; Lanza, M.; Calugi, S.; Dalle Grave, R. Assessment of physical activity in anorexia nervosa and treatment outcome. *Med. Sci. Sports Exerc.* **2013**, *45*, 1643–1648. [CrossRef]
87. Di Lodovico, L.; Gorwood, P. The relationship between moderate to vigorous physical activity and cognitive rigidity in anorexia nervosa. *Psychiatry Res.* **2020**, *284*, 112703. [CrossRef]
88. Rizk, M.; Lalanne, C.; Berthoz, S.; Kern, L.; EVHAN Group; Godart, N. Problematic Exercise in Anorexia Nervosa: Testing Potential Risk Factors against Different Definitions. *PLoS ONE* **2015**, *10*, e0143352. [CrossRef] [PubMed]
89. Meyer, C.; Taranis, L.; Touyz, S. Excessive exercise in the eating disorders: A need for less activity from patients and more from researchers. *Eur. Eat. Disord. Rev.* **2008**, *16*, 81–83. [CrossRef]
90. Eddy, K.T.; Dorer, D.J.; Franko, D.L.; Tahilani, K.; Thompson-Brenner, H.; Herzog, D.B. Diagnostic crossover in anorexia nervosa and bulimia nervosa: Implications for DSM-V. *Am. J. Psychiatry* **2008**, *165*, 245–250. [CrossRef]

91. Schaumberg, K.; Jangmo, A.; Thornton, L.M.; Birgegård, A.; Almqvist, C.; Norring, C.; Larsson, H.; Bulik, C.M. Patterns of diagnostic transition in eating disorders: A longitudinal population study in Sweden. *Psychol. Med.* **2019**, *49*, 819–827. [CrossRef] [PubMed]
92. Ando, T.; Komaki, G.; Nishimura, H.; Naruo, T.; Okabe, K.; Kawai, K.; Takii, M.; Oka, T.; Kodama, N.; Nakamoto, C.; et al. A ghrelin gene variant may predict crossover rate from restricting-type anorexia nervosa to other phenotypes of eating disorders: A retrospective survival analysis. *Psychiatr. Genet.* **2010**, *20*, 153–159. [CrossRef] [PubMed]

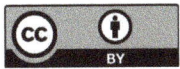

© 2020 by the authors. Licensee MDPI, Basel, Switzerland. This article is an open access article distributed under the terms and conditions of the Creative Commons Attribution (CC BY) license (http://creativecommons.org/licenses/by/4.0/).

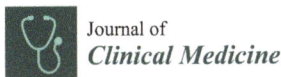

Article

Assessment of Physical Activity Patterns in Adolescent Patients with Anorexia Nervosa and Their Effect on Weight Gain

Miriam Kemmer [1], Christoph U. Correll [1,2,3], Tobias Hofmann [4], Andreas Stengel [4,5], Julia Grosser [1] and Verena Haas [1,*]

[1] Department of Child and Adolescent Psychiatry, Charité-Universitätsmedizin Berlin, Corporate Member of Freie Universität Berlin, Humboldt-Universität zu Berlin, and Berlin Institute of Health, 13353 Berlin, Germany; miriam.kemmer@charite.de (M.K.); CCorrell@northwell.edu (C.U.C.); julia.grosser@charite.de (J.G.)
[2] Donald and Barbara Zucker School of Medicine at Hofstra/Northwell, Hempstead, NY 11549, USA
[3] Department of Psychiatry, The Zucker Hillside Hospital, Glen Oaks, NY 11004, USA
[4] Center for Internal Medicine and Dermatology, Department for Psychosomatic Medicine, Charité-Universitätsmedizin Berlin, Corporate Member of Freie Universität Berlin, Humboldt-Universität zu Berlin, and Berlin Institute of Health Berlin, 12200 Berlin, Germany; tobias.hofmann@charite.de (T.H.); Andreas.Stengel@med.uni-tuebingen.de (A.S.)
[5] Department of Psychosomatic Medicine and Psychotherapy, Medical University Hospital Tübingen, 72076 Tübingen, Germany
* Correspondence: verena.haas@charite.de; Tel.: +49-30-450-566-399

Received: 29 January 2020; Accepted: 4 March 2020; Published: 7 March 2020

Abstract: (1) Background: Altered physical activity (PA) affects weight recovery in anorexia nervosa (AN) patients. The study aimed to objectively characterize PA patterns and their effect on weight trajectory in adolescent AN patients. (2) Methods: PA was assessed in 47 patients on admission to inpatient treatment, in $n = 25$ of these patients again 4 weeks after discharge (follow-up, FU), as well as in 20 adolescent healthy controls using the Sense Wear™ armband. The following PA categories were defined by metabolic equivalent (MET) ranges: sedentary behavior (SB), light (LPA), moderate (MPA), vigorous (VPA), and high-level PA (HLPA= MPA + VPA). (3) Results: LPA on admission was significantly higher in AN patients than in controls (103 vs. 55 min/d, $p < 0.001$), and LPA in AN decreased over time to 90 min/d ($p = 0.006$). Patients with higher admission LPA ($n = 12$) still had elevated LPA at FU ($p = 0.003$). High admission LPA was associated with a higher inpatient BMI percentage gain (ΔBMI%; 18.2% ± 10.0% vs. 12.0% ± 9.7%, $p = 0.037$) but with a loss of ΔBMI% at FU (−2.3% ± 3.6% vs. 0.8% ± 3.6%, $p = 0.045$). HLPA at baseline was associated with a lower inpatient ΔBMI% ($p = 0.045$). (4) Conclusion: Elevated LPA in AN patients decreased after inpatient treatment, and PA patterns had an impact on weight trajectory.

Keywords: anorexia nervosa; physical activity; accelerometry; weight gain

1. Introduction

Anorexia nervosa (AN) is characterized by the restriction of energy intake, low body weight, fear of weight gain, and distorted body image [1]. Increased physical activity (PA) has been observed in 31–80% of patients suffering from AN [2], yet varying definitions and terminology, such as hyperactivity [3], excessive activity, and problematic exercise [4], are used in the literature to describe this phenomenon. These definitions include different types of PA, ranging from light PA, such as standing and walking, to high-level PA, such as running or biking. Due to the lack of a common definition, the AN-specific PA patterns as well as the effect of these PA patterns on the illness course are difficult to discern [4].

Additionally, when assessing PA in AN patients, there is a discrepancy between self-reported and objectively measured PA; patients tend to both either over- or underestimate their PA [5–7]. Despite the high clinical relevance of objectively measured PA in AN patients, considering its impact on weight recovery [8,9], few studies have objectively assessed PA in AN patients.

In the present study, the terms high-level PA and light PA will be used to distinguish between high and low intensity PA. In previous studies, average total PA did not vary between AN patients and healthy controls [5,10], but high-level PA was both higher [11] and lower [12] than in healthy controls. Several studies demonstrated increased light PA in AN patients, such as more time on feet during daytime [8], more time spent in PA intensities of between 1.8 and 3 metabolic equivalents (METs) [12], and more time 'fidgeting' compared to healthy controls [8,13]. However, varying definitions for fidgeting have been used, such as changes in body position while seated per time unit, and average acceleration from both feet in meters/second^2/minute. There is high interpersonal variation in PA patterns among AN patients [11,12]. Longitudinal PA assessment indicated a link between pre-hospital exercise behavior and objectively measured total PA at the time of admission [14]. The findings on long-term patterns of the PA behavior of AN patients during and after treatment are controversial, as some studies state that total PA increased during weight restoration [8,15], while in others total PA decreased [16]. After discharge from inpatient treatment, both light PA and high-level PA remained constant [16], and, overall, PA did not vary between recovered AN patients and healthy controls [17]. Little data exist on how objectively measured PA affects weight trajectory. One study found no association between light PA (<3 METs) and BMI trajectory in adult AN patients [18], while others found that BMI trajectories were associated with time on feet when weight restored [8], the number of steps per day, the time spent in light PA (1.8–3.0 METs) [12], and the time spent in high-level PA (3–6 METs) [12,19]. In an outpatient setting, higher levels of total PA were associated with higher BMI values [20]. While this finding is somewhat counterintuitive, i.e., more PA that may have been driven by the desire to lose weight did not reduce BMI, it also highlights the bidirectional interdependence of BMI and PA, as it is also possible that a higher BMI reflects a healthier state that can result in higher and healthy activity.

Prior studies in an inpatient setting have shown that even under PA restricted inpatient conditions, there is a high variance in regards to PA amongst AN patients [11,12,16]. In one study, steps ranged from 2479 to 31,876 per day [12]. This variance is observable even when PA is specifically restricted as part of the treatment program [16]. Our study aims to better characterize these PA patterns and to assess their impact on weight trajectory in order to identify subgroups of patients at risk for a poorer treatment outcome. Identifying these patients at the beginning of treatment may allow for future studies to explore new approaches to treatment tailored to the needs of patients with specific types of hyperactivity.

We propose that PA levels impact weight trajectory, while not all physical activity levels will have the same impact on the weight recovery of patients. Based on our prior research [12], we hypothesize that high light physical activity will correlate with a poorer weight trajectory while increased high level physical activity will not have this same impact. We also propose that physical activity patterns are closely linked to the phenotype of AN; therefore, PA patterns will vary between adolescent AN patients and healthy controls. To pursue these aims, the following hypotheses were tested:

- Similar to adults, inpatient adolescent AN patients spend more time in light PA than age-matched healthy controls, while moderate PA and vigorous PA will be lower in AN patients.
- Within AN patients, different subgroups exist with respect to PA patterns (i.e., increased light PA or high-level PA defined as moderate PA + vigorous PA), and this PA pattern is an individual trait that remains constant over time, irrespective of therapy.
- More time spent in light PA, but not in high-level PA, on admission is a significant risk factor for lower inpatient weight gain and greater weight loss between discharge and outpatient follow-up.

2. Experimental Section

2.1. Study Populations

Adolescent female patients (age 12–18 years) hospitalized between 2014–2018 in the Department of Child and Adolescent Psychiatry, Psychosomatic Medicine and Psychotherapy at Charité-Universitätsmedizin Berlin were enrolled in this study. The inclusion criteria were: AN diagnosis (restricting, purging, and atypical subtype) according to International Statistical Classification of Diseases and Related Health Problems, 10th Revision (ICD-10). Patients diagnosed with a condition in addition to AN, which might significantly affect PA behavior (e.g., half-sided paralysis) were excluded. During the inpatient stay aimed at medical stabilization and weight recovery, all patients received psychotherapy, nutrition counselling, and body-oriented therapy. According to current German guidelines, target weight for discharge was set at the 25th BMI percentile, with an expected rate of weekly weight gain between 500 and 1000 g/week. PA was limited as part of the treatment program. Patients under the 3rd BMI percentile were given strict resting hours, one hour of sitting still after each mealtime and half an hour after each in-between meal. Resting times may have been prolonged based on individual treatment decisions. PA was limited to a 15-min walk a day and a one-hour yoga class per week focusing on relaxation techniques. Patients over the 3rd percentile were allowed to attend hospital school on an hourly basis. There was no mandatory bed rest, no one-on-one surveillance of patients, and patients were able to move freely in the ward. Patients over the 15th percentile were not given specific resting times and were able to attend a physical therapy group once a week. Additionally, patients who were clinically stable had the possibility to be granted a two-day leave. Patients were given dietary plans at the beginning of the program that they were instructed to adhere to, and mealtimes were supervised by clinical staff. On average, patients were given a plan of 1860 kilocalories (kcal) per day (range: 800–2600 kcal). The daily intake was increased by 200 kcal/ week in order to enable the targeted weight gain of 500g/week. Once patients achieved this weight gain, the meal plan was adjusted accordingly. In the patients participating in the study, no feeding tubes were used during the treatment. By the end of treatment program patients were free to make their own decisions about meals and did not have a specific dietary plan. Instead, patients were encouraged to stabilize their weight by making healthy choices about their food intake based on the nutritional training they had received during the treatment program. Information about illness duration, medication, admission weight and height, comorbidities, and length of stay was obtained from medical records.

We also recruited sex- and age-matched healthy controls between 2017–2018. The Sick, Control, One stone (14 lbs./6.5 kg.), Fat, Food (SCOFF) questionnaire was used in the screening process to identify and exclude all possible participants that exhibited early signs of altered eating behavior and/or negative body perception linked to body weight. Further exclusion criteria for healthy controls were any other physical or psychiatric diseases with a significant impact on PA behavior.

In total, 106 patients were approached about participating in the study, and 56 agreed to participate. Four patients were excluded retrospectively from analysis, because they were male, 5 datasets were excluded due to being incomplete. Forty-seven patient data sets were included in this analysis.

Forty-five possible participants for the control group responded to our informational online pamphlet. All of them received the screening questionnaire and 35 returned screening questionnaires to the study office. Of the healthy participants who completed the screening, 11 were excluded as part of the screening process. Twenty-five girls participated in the study assessment and in total 20 data sets were complete and included in the data analysis.

All participants and their legal guardians (if patients were <18 years old) provided written informed consent before participating in this study. The study was approved by the institutional ethics committee of the Charité-Universitätsmedizin Berlin (Identification code: EA2/034/14; date of approval 06/24/2014) and is in accordance with the Declaration of Helsinki on 'Ethical Principles for Medical Research Involving Human Subjects'.

2.2. Anthropometry

Height and weight were measured in undergarments and empty-stomached during morning weigh-ins (7–8 a.m.) for patients at admission/discharge, and during the afternoon at follow-up, and similarly for healthy controls using a digital scale (KERN, MCB, Berlin, Germany) and a stadiometer (Sicca 2016, Hamburg, Germany).

2.3. Physical Activity Assessment

The SenseWear™ Pro3 Armband was used to assess PA. The SenseWear™ Pro3 is a two-axis accelerometer that also measures skin temperature, galvanic skin response and heat flux in order to calculate PA. It has been previously used in several studies to assess PA objectively both in controlled and free-range settings [21–23]. PA was assessed for three consecutive days, with recordings always taking place on Friday to Sunday, at the first study assessment and at outpatient follow-up. The same patients were given the SenseWear™ Pro3 within an average of 21 days of admission (first study assessment) and at the post-discharge outpatient follow-up visit, as described before [24], in order to assess longitudinal changes in activity; at both time points, patients were asked to wear the SenseWear™ Pro3 device on their dominant arm continuously for three consecutive days (data admissible if worn >20, 5 h on at least two out of the three days), except when showering, bathing, or swimming. As part of the inpatient treatment program, PA was limited; meanwhile, during post-discharge follow-up, PA was unrestricted. Healthy controls were given the SenseWear™ Pro3 Armband on one occasion on the day of their assessment and were instructed to wear the device for three consecutive days (Friday to Sunday) continuously except when showering, bathing, or swimming. PA was unrestricted in the control group.

In accordance with previous work [12,19], we defined PA intensity levels as follows:

- Sedentary behavior: ≥ 1.1 to ≤ 1.8 METs
- Light-intensity PA: > 1.8 and < 3 METs
- Moderate-intensity PA: ≥ 3 to < 6 METs
- Vigorous-intensity PA: ≥ 6 METs

For the purpose of this paper, the category very light PA used previously was renamed as sedentary behavior, as new research suggests that 1.1–1.8 METs are more in line with this terminology [25]. The following activities are associated with each category. Sedentary behavior (SB) includes behavior such as lying down, watching television, eating, sitting, reading, and standing. LPA includes light physical work, walking slowly (less than 2.0 miles per hour), household errands and activities of daily life such as getting ready for bed. MPA involves activities such as descending stairs, walking for pleasure, dance practice, low impact aerobics, and bicycling (less than 10 miles per hour). Vigorous PA (VPA) includes running (<15 min/mile), competitive football or dance and high intensity cycling [26].

2.4. Statistical Analysis

A p-value of 0.05 was set as the significance threshold. All variables were tested two-sided. Analyses were conducted using R version 3.5.3 (2019-03-11). Comparing high vs. low physical activity was limited to AN patients and was calculated via median split. Descriptive statistics were selected according to scale level as absolute and relative frequencies for categories, median, the 25th/75th percentile, and extreme values for ordinal data, and the mean, standard deviation, and extreme values for normally distributed continuous measures. Group comparisons were performed using Fisher's exact test, the Wilcoxon rank sum test, and a t-test, accordingly. Correlations between measures were computed using the Spearman rank correlation. Range-based variability was calculated using the Siegel-Tukey test for equality in variability with adjustments for the median.

3. Results

3.1. Characterization of the Study Population

Within the study population of 47 patients, 25 patients (53%) were diagnosed with restrictive, 11 (23%) with purging, and 11 (23%) with atypical AN. Twenty-eight patients (60%) had their first inpatient admission, and, for the remaining patients, the number of prior inpatient therapies varied from 1 to 4. The mean illness duration was 11 months, ranging from 6.2–16.8 months. Thirty patients (64%) had comorbidities, including major depression ($n = 9$; 19%), borderline personality disorder ($n = 3$; 6%), anxiety disorders ($n = 5$; 11%), and obsessive-compulsive disorder ($n = 5$; 11%). Only eight patients (17%) received psychopharmacological medications, i.e., stimulating antidepressants ($n = 4$; 9%) and antipsychotics ($n = 2$; 4%). Three patients received oral contraceptives (6%). None of the healthy controls took any psychopharmacological medication, and 4 participants (20%) took oral contraceptives. The time between admission and first study assessment was on average 21 (2–50) days, and during this time, the patients' weight had increased by 0.9 ± 1.1 (−2.6–3.5) kilogram (kg). Table 1 shows the clinical characteristics and PA parameters of the AN patients on admission compared to healthy controls. The number of steps was significantly lower in AN patients ($p = 0.048$), but there was no between-group difference in the range of steps. AN patients spent significantly more time in light PA ($p < 0.001$) and less in moderate PA ($p = 0.009$) than healthy controls.

Table 1. General characteristics and physical activity parameters of patients with AN at first study assessment compared to healthy controls.

Participant Characteristics and PA	AN Total ($n = 47$)	Healthy Controls ($n = 20$)	p-Value
Age, years	15.70 (14.68/16.64) (12.44–17.85)	15.02 (13.59/15.84) (12.07–17.86)	0.139
Height, centimeters	164.3 ± 6.4 (150.2–183.0)	165.1 ± 7.1 (153.0–178.0)	0.672
Weight, kilograms	42.2 ± 6.0 (31.3–58.2)	57.3 ± 9.4 (38.8–70.8)	<0.001
BMI, kilogram/meter^2	15.60 ± 1.78 (12.80–20.40)	20.96 ± 2.88 (16.00–27.60)	<0.001
BMI, percentile	4.6 ± 9.9 (0.0–43.0)	51.8 ± 25.5 (7.0–93.0)	<0.001
Steps	8430 (6522/10398) (2026–26439)	11390 (8261/13680) (4427–23139)	0.048
Sedentary behavior (min) (≥ 1.1 to ≤ 1.8 METs)	705 (624/765) (189–868)	647 (557/732) (386–853)	0.118
Light PA (min) (>1.8 and <3 METs)	105 (73/204) (41–530)	55 (42/88) (14–303)	<0.001
Moderate PA (min) (≥ 3 to <6 METs)	77.0 (44.3/114.2) (3.0–268.0)	121.5 (82.3/188.2) (25.0–302.0)	0.009
Vigorous PA (min) (≥ 6 METs)	2.0 (0.0/10.2) (0.0–212.0)	2.0 (0.4/15.8) (0.0–55.0)	0.697

Values are means ± SDs (range) (first quartile/ third quartile). AN, anorexia nervosa; BMI, body mass index; MET, metabolic equivalent of task; PA, physical activity.

3.2. General Parameters and Physical Activity of AN Patients and Healthy Controls

The median length of stay for all patients was 17.0 weeks (range: 9.0 to 28.4 weeks), with a weight change from admission to discharge from 42.2 ± 6.0 to 48.1 ± 4.8 kg (total weight gain: 5.96 ± 3.62 kg; rate of weight gain: 391 ± 245 g/week). Of the 47 patients, 25 (53%) returned for outpatient follow-up, 36 days (range: 27–119 days) after discharge. This subgroup had a body weight increase from 41.9 ± 4.4 kg to 48.9 ± 3.1 kg during hospitalization that lasted 17.0 (9.0 to 28.4) weeks, which translates into an increase of 6.98 ± 3.45 kg and a rate of weight gain of 445 ± 241 g/week. Compared to the patients who returned, the patients not returning for a follow-up visit had similar admission BMI and PA parameters, but were significantly younger ($p = 0.006$). On average, weight between discharge and follow-up remained constant at 48.3 ± 3.8 kg ($p = 0.102$; range: −3.8 to +3.4). However, at follow-up, body weight and BMI of the AN patients remained significantly lower than in healthy controls ($p < 0.001$).

Clinical characteristics and PA of the patient subgroup returning for their follow-up in comparison with healthy controls are shown in Table 2. At the first study assessment, AN patients had significantly lower body weight ($p < 0.001$), BMI ($p < 0.001$), and BMI percentile ($p < 0.001$), and spent significantly more time in light PA than healthy controls ($p < 0.001$). At outpatient follow-up, AN patients were significantly older ($p < 0.001$), had a significantly lower body weight ($p < 0.001$), BMI ($p < 0.001$), BMI percentile ($p < 0.001$), and spent more time in light PA ($p = 0.039$) and vigorous PA ($p = 0.006$) than healthy controls. From admission to follow-up, AN patients gained significant weight ($p < 0.001$), BMI ($p < 0.001$) and BMI percentile ($p < 0.001$), had higher number of daily steps ($p = 0.037$), and spent significantly less time in light PA ($p = 0.008$) and more time in vigorous PA ($p < 0.001$).

Table 2. General characteristics and PA parameters for AN patients at first study assessment, AN patients at outpatient follow-up and healthy controls [°].

Participant Characteristics and PA	AN (First Study Assessment) (n = 25)	AN (Follow-Up) (n = 25)	Healthy Controls (n = 20)
Age, years	16.49 (15.08/17.38) (12.44–17.85)	16.90 (15.49/17.82) [b] (12.88–18.20)	15.02 (13.59/15.84) [2] (12.07–17.86)
Height, centimeters	165.4 ± 5.5 (156.3–183.0)	164.9 ± 5.1 [a] (156.6–181.3)	165.1 ± 7.1 (153.0–178.0)
Weight, kilograms	41.9 ± 4.4 (35.3–53.0)	48.3 ± 3.8 [b] (41.1–56.6)	57.3 ± 9.4 [II 2] (38.8–70.8)
BMI, kilogram/meter^2	15.34 ±1.72 (12.80–20.40)	17.87 ± 1.56 [b] (14.50–21.80)	20.96 ± 2.88 [II 2] (16.00–27.60)
BMI, percentile	2.8 ± 8.9 (0.0–43.0)	13.2 ± 13.7 [b] (0.0–61.0)	51.8 ± 25.5 [II 2] (7.0–93.0)
Steps	7821 (5948/9296) (2753–23923)	10475 (8612/14975) [a] (646–23273)	11390 (8261/13680) (4427–23139)
Sedentary behavior (min) (≥1.1 to ≤ 1.8 METs)	712 (634/760) (483–868)	681 (636/747) (499–848)	647 (557/732) (386–853)
Light PA (min) (>1.8 and < 3 METs)	103.0 (89.7/155.7) (41.0–293.0)	90.0 (64.0/117.7) [a] (49.0–162.0)	55.0 (41.8/88.1) [II 2] (14.0–303.0)
Moderate PA (min) (≥3 to < 6 METs)	73.0 (35.7/108.7) (22.0–268.0)	96.0 (73.0/132.3) (3.0–275.0)	121.5 (82.3/188.2) (25.0–302.0)
Vigorous PA (min) (≥6 METs)	1.0 (0.0/3.3) (0.0–23.0)	13.0 (5.0/33.3) [b] (0.0–116.0)	2.0 (0.4/15.8) [1] (0.0–55.0)

[°] The values are means ± SDs (range) (first quartile/ third quartile). AN, anorexia nervosa; BMI, body mass index; MET, metabolic equivalent of task; PA, physical activity; AN (first study assessment) vs. AN (follow-up): [a], $p < 0.05$; [b], $p < 0.01$; AN (first study assessment) vs. healthy controls: [II], $p < 0.01$; AN (follow-up) vs. healthy controls: [1], $p < 0.05$; [2], $p < 0.01$.

3.3. Light PA in AN Patients Over Time

As shown in Figure 1, total time spent in light PA in AN patients decreased significantly between the first study assessment and follow-up ($p = 0.008$). Nevertheless, at follow-up a significant difference between low light PA and high light PA patients remained, as high light PA patients continued to show higher levels of light PA at follow-up ($p = 0.003$). When analyzing the subgroups separately, the decrease in light PA over time was only significant in the group with high baseline light PA ($n = 12$, $p < 0.001$), and not in the low light PA group ($n = 13$, $p = 0.147$).

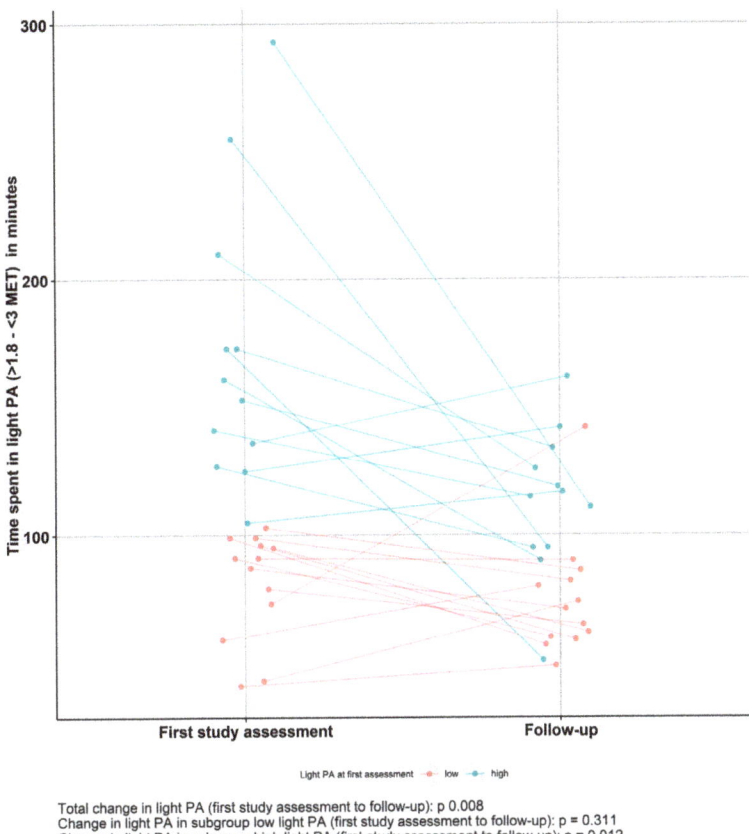

Total change in light PA (first study assessment to follow-up): p 0.008
Change in light PA in subgroup low light PA (first study assessment to follow-up): p = 0.311
Change in light PA in subgroup high light PA (first study assessment to follow-up): p = 0.012
Difference in light PA between subgroups (low and high light PA) at first study assessment: p < 0.001
Difference in light PA between subgroups (low and high light PA) at follow-up: p = 0.003

Figure 1. Light physical activity (PA) patterns in anorexia nervosa (AN) patients over time grouped by median split based on light PA at first study assessment (low light PA, $n = 13$; high light PA, $n = 12$).

3.4. Impact of light PA/ High-Level PA at Admission on Weight Trajectory

Compared to patients with low baseline light PA ($n = 13$), those with high baseline light PA ($n = 12$) showed a significantly higher inpatient BMI percentage increase, but less significant outpatient BMI percentage improvement (Table 3). Although the average time spent in high-level PA was short, increased high-level PA had a negative impact on inpatient BMI percentage change, as patients with higher baseline levels of high-level PA ($n = 11$) had significantly lower inpatient BMI percentage change than those with lower baseline levels of high-level PA ($n = 14$). Nevertheless, there were no differences in BMI percentage change in the outpatient setting (Table 3).

Table 3. Impact of light PA and high-level PA in anorexia nervosa patients at admission on BMI trajectory (BMI percentage change) from admission to discharge and from discharge to outpatient follow-up.

Weight Trajectory in PA Subgroups	Low Light PA (n = 13)	High Light PA (n = 12)	p-value	Low HLPA (n = 14)	High HLPA (n = 11)	p-value
Inpatient BMI percentage change (admission to discharge)	12.0 ± 9.7 (−3.6–33.6)	18.2 ± 10.0 (−0.5–38.6)	0.037	21.3 ± 9.7 (7.7–38.6)	13.43 ± 8.50 (−0.52–25.83)	0.045
Outpatient BMI percentage change (discharge to follow-up)	0.80 ± 3.61 (−3.70–9.42)	−2.28 ± 3.63 (−7.59–4.49)	0.045	−0.91 ± 3.90 (−6.25–9.42)	−0.38 ± 4.02 (−7.59–5.96)	0.740

Values are means ± SDs (range) (first quartile/ third quartile); unit = %; BMI, body mass index; HLPA, high level physical activity; PA, physical activity.

3.5. Characteristics of Patients Grouped by Low/High Levels of Light PA and Longitudinal Impact of Time Spent in Light PA

Comparing the two subgroups of patients (low light PA, n = 23; high light PA, n = 24) at admission, there were no differences with regards to AN subtype, comorbidities, medication, the presence of amenorrhea, hormonal contraception, age, and duration of illness (Ref. Table A1). The two subgroups presented a similar duration of inpatient stay and height. However, patients with high levels of light PA did have a significantly lower weight ($p = 0.015$), BMI ($p < 0.001$), and BMI percentile ($p = 0.026$) than low light PA patients. This difference was still present at discharge, where high light PA AN patients continued to present a significantly lower weight ($p < 0.001$), BMI ($p < 0.001$), and BMI percentile ($p = 0.018$). There was no significant difference in the BMI change between the first study assessment and discharge, or in daily steps. High light PA AN patients spent less time in sedentary behavior than low light PA AN patients ($p < 0.001$), but had similar levels of moderate PA and vigorous PA.

At outpatient follow-up, there was no significant difference with regards to age and height between the two subgroups. High light PA AN had significantly lower weight ($p = 0.003$) and BMI percentile ($p = 0.042$); but there was no significant difference in the BMI. High light PA AN patients had a lower BMI percentage change between discharge and outpatient follow-up ($p = 0.045$). There was no significant difference in daily steps and sedentary behavior. High light PA AN patients continued to present significantly higher light PA values ($p = 0.003$). Moderate PA was comparable and high light PA AN patients presented lower amounts of vigorous PA ($p = 0.034$).

The time spent in light PA at first study assessment showed a significant association with BMI at admission ($p = 0.041$), while time spent in light PA at admission and the BMI at outpatient follow-up were only associated trend-level significance ($p = 0.059$) (Figure 2).

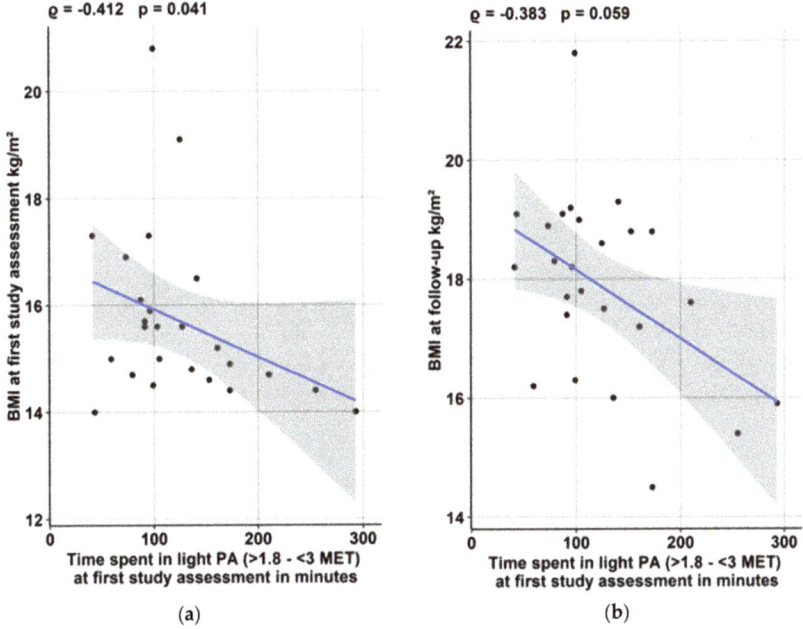

Figure 2. Impact of time spent in light physical activity (PA) at first study assessment (**a**) on admission BMI and (**b**) BMI at outpatient follow-up.

4. Discussion

Objectively assessing PA patterns in adolescent AN patients compared to healthy controls and their impact on the weight trajectories of AN patients yielded following results: (1) There was no difference in sedentary behavior, AN inpatients exhibited more light PA, less moderate PA, and similar vigorous PA compared to healthy controls; (2) The time spent in light PA by AN patients decreased between admission and outpatient follow-up, but patients who had spent relatively more time in light PA on admission continued to do so at outpatient follow-up; (3) The decrease in light PA over time was only significant in the subgroup with high baseline light PA; (4) Contrary to our hypothesis, high baseline light PA was associated with a higher inpatient BMI percentage change, but as expected, with a poorer outpatient BMI percentage change; (5) High-level PA had a negative impact on inpatient but not on outpatient BMI percentage change.

4.1. Comparison of Activity Patterns Between AN Patients and Healthy Controls

Consistent with our previous study in adult AN inpatients [19], adolescent AN patients in the present study spent significantly more time in light PA than healthy, age-matched controls. High light PA was not mirrored by a high daily step count, pointing out the importance of a detailed PA assessment using intensity categories. In the literature, "fidgeting" assessed using a shoe-based monitor was higher in AN inpatients [13] than in controls and was similar when assessed using the Intelligent Device for Energy Expenditure and Activity (IDEEA™) accelerometer [8]. A comparison of data is difficult due to inconsistent definitions of light PA and different PA dimensions being assessed with varying devices. 'Fidgeting' in the second study may be more similar to sedentary behavior in the present study, which was similar between the two groups. For high-level PA, controversial results have been reported. In the present study, AN patients spent less time in moderate PA, and similar time in vigorous PA. A previous study using the Actiwatch™ (AW7) in a day hospital setting found similar amounts of high-level PA in AN and control subjects (no distinction was made between moderate PA and vigorous PA) [27], while a study using the SenseWear™ Armband in inpatient adolescent and adult AN patients reported higher high-level PA than in controls (3–6 METs, which corresponds to the category of moderate PA in the present study) [11]. The different amounts of high-level PA may be a result of different treatment programs and varying approaches to PA restriction. No information about the handling of PA during treatment was given in the cited studies. Furthermore, a variation in PA behavior patterns within the different control groups and different recruitment locations may have impacted the results.

4.2. Longitudinal Development of Light PA in AN Patients

The current study assessed light PA longitudinally at the beginning of inpatient treatment and at outpatient follow-up. While on average, light PA decreased over time, there were two characteristic subgroups: patients grouped in either high or low light PA at the first study assessment continued to exhibit these same PA patterns at follow-up. These findings lead to the question as to whether time spent in high or low light PA is an individual trait, which persists over time, regardless of therapy and setting, or whether the time needed to normalize varies and takes up more than a median of 36.0 days. Casper et al. proposed a dysregulation of PA called 'restless activation' as a phenotype of AN and hypothesized that it may be linked to improved self-esteem and wellbeing [28]. In rodent models, PA has been linked to dopamine and endocannabinoid signaling networks that suggest an addictive property [29]. Similar findings using MRI imagining in AN patients have linked altered neurological responses in the reward system to excessive exercise [30]. We are only aware of one comparable study, which reported a trend for increased time spent on feet between low-weight and weight restored AN patients, while 'fidgeting' did not vary when using the IDEEA™ [8]. The varying age of the study populations (adolescent and adult patients vs. only adolescents in the present study), the different admission BMIs (16.1 ± 1.0 vs. 15.6 ± 1.8 in the current study), and the different measurement instruments may have impacted PA behaviors and readings.

4.3. Impact of PA Patterns on Weight Trajectory

Contrary to our hypothesis, increased time spent in light PA was linked to a higher inpatient BMI percentage change. Previous studies on the impact of light PA on inpatient weight trajectory have yielded mixed findings. In an exploratory, non-linear model based on 50 adult AN patients, time spent in light PA was a potential predictor for poor BMI increase during inpatient treatment [19]. In adolescent and adult AN patients, time spent in light PA was inversely linked to BMI at discharge, while there was no significant relationship to BMI percentage change [19]. No association between 'fidgeting', assessed with a shoe-based accelerometer, and weight gain was found in a group of 11 adolescent and adult AN patients [13]. Age differences may have led to different results, as in healthy participants, PA behaviors vary between adolescents and adults. Healthy adolescents are more active and spent more time in high-level PA than adults [31,32]. Additionally, some of these previous studies were small. In the present study, the group of patients with high light PA had a significantly lower BMI at admission; a higher BMI increase in this group may have been caused the program's discharge weight target at the 25th BMI percentile requiring more weight gain in this group in order to be discharged. There also might be a link between increased LPA and muscle gain as it has been shown that LPA can improve muscle strength [33], which may contribute to the increased BMI percentage change within the high LPA group. The present study found a statistical trend ($p = 0.059$) for an inverse association between high light PA at admission and inpatient BMI gain, as well as a significant inverse association with BMI percentile at follow-up. Therefore, the assessment of PA patterns at admission might hold the potential to identify patients at risk of poor weight gain. The time spent on feet in 61 AN patients at the assessment point weight, but not at low weight, was linked to a poorer weight trajectory at the 12 month follow-up [8]. Heterogeneous results may thus be caused either by different time points of PA assessment during treatment or by different follow-up durations. Consistent with our previous study [19], high-level PA was inversely associated with inpatient BMI change. Conversely, in a group of 88 AN patients in a day hospital setting, high-level PA assessed using an Actiwatch™ (AW7) was directly associated with achieving BMI > 18.5 and with decreased AN-specific cognitions and reduced binge/purge behavior [27]. Different settings (inpatient vs. day hospital treatment) may have impacted the patients' ability to exercise at higher intensities and the impact high-level PA had on the weight trajectory.

When assessing the impact of PA patterns on weigh status in healthy adolescents, two trends can be observed: high levels of high-level PA (HLPA) are associated with a lower BMI and a lower body fat mass. Additionally, more time in sedentary behavior is linked to a higher BMI and higher body fat [34–36]. These trends are also replicable when analyzing only healthy female participants [37,38]. Further sedentary behavior in both gender-mixed groups and female-only groups was also linked to a higher BMI increase in the long run [39,40]. However, in a sample of female secondary school students, there was no correlation between being underweight and PA patterns (both SB and HLPA) [41].

4.4. Limitations

The limitations of this study first include the prolonged and variable times between the admission and the first study assessment, and between discharge and the follow-up assessment. Second, a high drop-out ($n = 22$) may have reduced the generalizability of the findings, yet comparable studies had both similar ($n = 26$) [8] and lower ($n = 3$) [16] drop-outs. Third, there was a significant age difference between the patients at follow-up and the healthy controls. Fourth, the validity of the SenseWear™ Pro 3 Armand has not been assessed for PA parameters in underweight AN patients; thus, the validity of the obtained data is unknown. Fifth different cutoff points for PA are used in the literature. We used a definition for sedentary behavior (very low PA) with a cutoff point at 1.8 METs [42] to establish compatibility with our previous work [12,19], but a new definition proposed a cutoff point at 1.5 METs [25]. Therefore, the actual activities associated with sedentary behavior in this study may not fully represent all aspects of sedentary behavior. Sixth, it is unknown if wearing a SenseWear™ Armand affects PA behavior. Seventh, no data about the caloric intake of patients after discharge were obtained. Finally, potential differences in PA based on socioeconomic status were not assessed. However, despite these limitations, this is one of the first studies to assess the longitudinal development of light PA and its impact on weight trajectories in adolescent AN patients.

5. Conclusions

In summary, PA patterns vary between AN patients and healthy controls and impact weight trajectories in AN patients. Our study aims to raise awareness of the different types of hyperactivity and their impact on the weight development of AN patients. Our research may provide a foundation for future research into the benefit of objectively measured PA patterns in AN patients and may allow for a better understanding of PA as a disease maintaining factor as well as the identification of high risk patients at the beginning of treatment. This could enable research into new treatment interventions that are tailored to the different PA subgroups of patients, such as high light PA patients. An early intervention that focuses on reducing light PA hyperactivity from the beginning of the treatment program on may positively impact short- and long-term weight development. Our study shows that the detailed assessment of PA patterns, rather than general PA parameters, such as steps or activity counts, provides valuable insight into PA behavior of AN patients.

Author Contributions: Conceptualization, V.H., T.H., A.S.; Methodology, V.H., T.H., A.S.; Formal analysis and investigation, M.K.; Resources, Swiss Anorexia Nervosa Foundation (Project Number 23-13); Data curation, J.G., M.K.; writing-original draft preparation, M.K.; writing-review and editing, V.H., C.U.C., T.H. and A.S.; visualization, M.K.; supervision, V.H., C.U.C.; project administration, V.H.; funding acquisition, V.H. All authors have read and agreed to the published version of the manuscript.

Funding: This work was supported by funding of the Swiss Anorexia Nervosa Foundation (Project Number 23-13). We acknowledge support from the German Research Foundation (DFG) and the Open Access Publication Funds of Charité-Universitätsmedizin Berlin. The sponsors had no role in design, conduct or data interpretation of the study.

Acknowledgments: We thank Andreas Busjahn for assistance with biostatistical analysis and Nathalie Engelhaus for support with data assessment of healthy controls.

Conflicts of Interest: Correll has been a consultant and/or advisor to or has received honoraria from: Alkermes, Allergan, Angelini, Boehringer-Ingelheim, Gedeon Richter, Gerson Lehrman Group, Indivior, IntraCellular Therapies, Janssen/J&J, LB Pharma, Lundbeck, MedAvante-ProPhase, Medscape, Merck, Neurocrine, Noven, Otsuka, Pfizer, Recordati, Rovi, Servier, Sumitomo Dainippon, Sunovion, Supernus, Takeda, and Teva. He has provided expert testimony for Bristol-Myers Squibb, Janssen, and Otsuka. He served on a Data Safety Monitoring Board for Boehringer-Ingelheim, Lundbeck, Rovi, Supernus, and Teva. He received royalties from UpToDate and grant support from Janssen and Takeda. He is also a shareholder of LB Pharma. The other authors declared no conflicts of interest.

Appendix A

Table A1. General characteristics and PA parameters of AN patients at admission, first study assessment and discharge grouped by a low/high level of light PA (median split).

Participant Characteristics and PA	Low Light PA ($n = 23$)	High Light PA ($n = 24$)	p-value
Duration of illness, months	12.0 (7.3/15.8) (3.0–64.0)	9.0 (4.0/17.6) (1.0–56.0)	0.176
Admission age, y	15.82 (14.87/16.64) (13.78–17.85)	15.11 (13.89/16.70) (12.44–17.82)	0.250
Admission height, cm	166.7 ± 6.4 (159.0–183.0)	164.1 ± 4.3 (156.3–170.0)	0.253
Admission weight, kg	43.9 ± 4.1 (39.6–53.0)	39.8 ± 3.8 (35.3–46.5)	0.015
Admission BMI, kg/m^2	15.84 ± 1.73 (13.90–20.40)	14.80 ± 1.61 (12.80–19.10)	0.135
Admission BMI percentile (%)	4.1 ± 11.7 (0.0–43.0)	1.33 ± 4.31 (0.00–15.00)	0.443
Steps	8586 (7136/9735) (2753–24536)	7870 (6159/12179) (2026–26439)	0.882
Sedentary behavior (min) (≥ 1.1 to ≤ 1.8 METs)	730 (698/789) (581–856)	646 (497/715) (189–868)	<0.001
Light PA (min) (>1.8 and <3 METs)	73.0 (54.3/93.5) (41.0–103.0)	192 (146/273) (105–530)	<0.001
Moderate PA (min) (≥ 3 to <6 METs)	73.0 (46.5/103.5) (22.0–268.0)	89.5 (39.3/120.8) (3.0–241.0)	0.663
Vigorous PA (min) (≥ 6 METs)	2.0 (1.0/10.0) (0.0–54.0)	1.5 (0.0/8.9) (0.0–212.0)	0.729
Time between admission and discharge, days	95.0 (74.8/118.8) (47.0–225.0)	121.0 (88.8/135.6) (41.0–171.0)	0.097
Discharge weight, kg	51.4 ± 3.3 (45.3–61.1)	45.0 ± 3.9 (36.6–52.5)	<0.001
Discharge BMI, kg/m^2	18.38 ± 0.96 (16.50–20.50)	17.31 ± 1.15 (15.50–19.40)	<0.001
Discharge BMI percentile (%)	18.4 ± 11.1 (0.0–45.0)	11.4 ± 8.4 (0.0–36.0)	0.018
BMI change from first study assessment to discharge kg/m^2	1.85 ± 1.41 (−0.70–4.70)	2.60 ± 1.36 (−0.10–5.40)	0.072
BMI percentile change from first study assessment to discharge (%)	12.0 ± 9.7 (−3.6–33.6)	18.2 ± 10.0 (−0.5–38.6)	0.037

Values are means ± SDs (range) (first quartile/ third quartile). AN, anorexia nervosa; BMI, body mass index; METs, metabolic equivalents; PA, physical activity.

References

1. Association, American Psychiatric. *Diagnostic and Statistical Manual of Mental Disorders: Dsm-5*; Amer Psychiatric Pub Incorporated: Washington, DC, USA, 2013.
2. Solenberger, S.E. Exercise and eating disorders: A 3-year inpatient hospital record analysis. *Eat. Behav.* **2001**, *2*, 151–168. [CrossRef]
3. Achamrah, N.; Coeffier, M.; Dechelotte, P. Physical activity in patients with anorexia nervosa. *Nutr. Rev.* **2016**, *74*, 301–311. [CrossRef] [PubMed]
4. Rizk, M.; Lalanne, C.; Berthoz, S.; Kern, L.; Godart, N. Problematic Exercise in Anorexia Nervosa: Testing Potential Risk Factors against Different Definitions. *PLoS ONE* **2015**, *10*, e0143352. [CrossRef] [PubMed]
5. Keyes, A.; Woerwag-Mehta, S.; Bartholdy, S.; Koskina, A.; Middleton, B.; Connan, F.; Webster, P.; Schmidt, U.; Campbell, I.C. Physical activity and the drive to exercise in anorexia nervosa. *Int. J. Eat. Disord.* **2015**, *48*, 46–54. [CrossRef] [PubMed]
6. Alberti, M.; Galvani, C.; Capelli, C.; Lanza, M.; El Ghoch, M.; Calugi, S.; Dalle Grave, R. Physical fitness before and after weight restoration in anorexia nervosa. *J. Sports Med. Phys. Fit.* **2013**, *53*, 396–402.
7. Bratland-Sanda, S.; Sundgot-Borgen, J.; Ro, O.; Rosenvinge, J.H.; Hoffart, A.; Martinsen, E.W. "I'm not physically active - I only go for walks": Physical activity in patients with longstanding eating disorders. *Int. J. Eat. Disord.* **2010**, *43*, 88–92. [CrossRef]
8. Gianini, L.M.; Klein, D.A.; Call, C.; Walsh, B.T.; Wang, Y.; Wu, P.; Attia, E. Physical activity and post-treatment weight trajectory in anorexia nervosa. *Int. J. Eat. Disord.* **2016**, *49*, 482–489. [CrossRef]
9. Gummer, R.; Giel, K.E.; Schag, K.; Resmark, G.; Junne, F.P.; Becker, S.; Zipfel, S.; Teufel, M. High Levels of Physical Activity in Anorexia Nervosa: A Systematic Review. *Eur. Eat. Disord. Rev.* **2015**, *23*, 333–344. [CrossRef]
10. Hechler, T.; Rieger, E.; Touyz, S.; Beumont, P.; Plasqui, G.; Westerterp, K. Physical activity and body composition in outpatients recovering from anorexia nervosa and healthy controls. *Adapt. Phys. Act. Q.* **2008**, *25*, 159–173. [CrossRef]
11. El Ghoch, M.; Calugi, S.; Pellegrini, M.; Milanese, C.; Busacchi, M.; Battistini, N.C.; Bernabe, J.; Dalle Grave, R. Measured physical activity in anorexia nervosa: Features and treatment outcome. *Int. J. Eat. Disord.* **2013**, *46*, 709–712. [CrossRef]
12. Lehmann, C.S.; Hofmann, T.; Elbelt, U.; Rose, M.; Correll, C.U.; Stengel, A.; Haas, V. The Role of Objectively Measured, Altered Physical Activity Patterns for Body Mass Index Change during Inpatient Treatment in Female Patients with Anorexia Nervosa. *J. Clin. Med.* **2018**, *7*, 289. [CrossRef] [PubMed]
13. Belak, L.; Gianini, L.; Klein, D.A.; Sazonov, E.; Keegan, K.; Neustadt, E.; Walsh, B.T.; Attia, E. Measurement of fidgeting in patients with anorexia nervosa using a novel shoe-based monitor. *Eat. Behav.* **2017**, *24*, 45–48. [CrossRef] [PubMed]
14. Klein, D.A.; Mayer, L.E.; Schebendach, J.E.; Walsh, B.T. Physical activity and cortisol in anorexia nervosa. *Psychoneuroendocrinology* **2007**, *32*, 539–547. [CrossRef] [PubMed]
15. Bratland-Sanda, S.; Sundgot-Borgen, J.; Ro, O.; Rosenvinge, J.H.; Hoffart, A.; Martinsen, E.W. Physical activity and exercise dependence during inpatient treatment of longstanding eating disorders: An exploratory study of excessive and non-excessive exercisers. *Int. J. Eat. Disord.* **2010**, *43*, 266–273. [CrossRef]
16. Kostrzewa, E.; van Elburg, A.A.; Sanders, N.; Sternheim, L.; Adan, R.A.; Kas, M.J. Longitudinal changes in the physical activity of adolescents with anorexia nervosa and their influence on body composition and leptin serum levels after recovery. *PLoS ONE* **2013**, *8*, e78251. [CrossRef]
17. Dellava, J.E.; Hamer, R.M.; Kanodia, A.; Reyes-Rodriguez, M.L.; Bulik, C.M. Diet and physical activity in women recovered from anorexia nervosa: A pilot study. *Int. J. Eat. Disord.* **2011**, *44*, 376–382. [CrossRef]
18. El Ghoch, M.; Calugi, S.; Pellegrini, M.; Chignola, E.; Dalle Grave, R. Physical activity, body weight, and resumption of menses in anorexia nervosa. *Psychiatry Res.* **2016**, *246*, 507–511. [CrossRef]
19. Großer, J.; Hofmann, T.; Stengel, A.; Zeeck, A.; Winter, S.; Correll, C.H. *Psychological and Nutritional Correlates of Objectively Assessed Physical Activity in Patients with Anorexia Nervosa, Submitted*; German Association for Psychiatry, Psychotherapy and Psychosomatics Congress: Berlin, Germany, 12 January 2018.
20. Bouten, C.V.; van Marken Lichtenbelt, W.D.; Westerterp, K.R. Body mass index and daily physical activity in anorexia nervosa. *Med. Sci. Sports Exerc.* **1996**, *28*, 967–973. [CrossRef]

21. Calabro, M.A.; Lee, J.M.; Saint-Maurice, P.F.; Yoo, H.; Welk, G.J. Validity of physical activity monitors for assessing lower intensity activity in adults. *Int. J. Behav. Nutr. Phys. Act.* **2014**, *11*, 119. [CrossRef]
22. van Hoye, K.; Mortelmans, P.; Lefevre, J. Validation of the SenseWear Pro3 Armband using an incremental exercise test. *J Strength Cond. Res.* **2014**, *28*, 2806–2814. [CrossRef]
23. Johannsen, D.L.; Calabro, M.A.; Stewart, J.; Franke, W.; Rood, J.C.; Welk, G.J. Accuracy of armband monitors for measuring daily energy expenditure in healthy adults. *Med. Sci. Sports Exerc.* **2010**, *42*, 2134–2140. [CrossRef] [PubMed]
24. Stengel, A.; Haas, V.; Elbelt, U.; Correll, C.U.; Rose, M.; Hofmann, T. Leptin and Physical Activity in Adult Patients with Anorexia Nervosa: Failure to Demonstrate a Simple Linear Association. *Nutrients* **2017**, *9*, 1210. [CrossRef] [PubMed]
25. Tremblay, M.S.; Aubert, S.; Barnes, J.D.; Saunders, T.J.; Carson, V.; Latimer-Cheung, A.E.; Chastin, S.F.M.; Altenburg, T.M.; Chinapaw, M.J.M. Sedentary Behavior Research Network (SBRN)—Terminology Consensus Project process and outcome. *Int. J. Behav. Nutr. Phys. Act.* **2017**, *14*, 75. [CrossRef] [PubMed]
26. Ainsworth, B.E.; Haskell, W.L.; Herrmann, S.D.; Meckes, N.; Bassett, D.R.J.; Tudor-Locke, C.; Greer, J.L.; Vezina, J.; Whitt-Glover, M.C.; Leon, A.S. 2011 Compendium of Physical Activities: A second update of codes and MET values. *Med. Sci. Sports Exerc.* **2011**, *43*, 1575–1581. [CrossRef]
27. Sauchelli, S.; Arcelus, J.; Sanchez, I.; Riesco, N.; Jimenez-Murcia, S.; Granero, R.; Gunnard, K.; Banos, R.; Botella, C.; de la Torre, R.; et al. Physical activity in anorexia nervosa: How relevant is it to therapy response? *Eur. Psychiatry J. Assoc. Eur. Psychiatr.* **2015**, *30*, 924–931. [CrossRef]
28. Casper, R.C. Not the Function of Eating, but Spontaneous Activity and Energy Expenditure, Reflected in "Restlessness" and a "Drive for Activity" Appear to Be Dysregulated in Anorexia Nervosa: Treatment Implications. *Front. Psychol.* **2018**, *9*, 2303. [CrossRef]
29. Garland, T.J.; Schutz, H.; Chappell, M.A.; Keeney, B.K.; Meek, T.H.; Copes, L.E.; Acosta, W.; Drenowatz, C.; Maciel, R.C.; van Dijk, G.; et al. The biological control of voluntary exercise, spontaneous physical activity and daily energy expenditure in relation to obesity: Human and rodent perspectives. *J. Exp. Biol.* **2011**, *214*, 206–229. [CrossRef]
30. Kullmann, S.; Giel, K.E.; Hu, X.; Bischoff, S.C.; Teufel, M.; Thiel, A.; Zipfel, S.; Preissl, H. Impaired inhibitory control in anorexia nervosa elicited by physical activity stimuli. *Soc. Cogn. Affect Neurosci.* **2014**, *9*, 917–923. [CrossRef]
31. Gordon-Larsen, P.; Nelson, M.C.; Popkin, B.M. Longitudinal physical activity and sedentary behavior trends: Adolescence to adulthood. *Am. J. Prev. Med.* **2004**, *27*, 277–283. [CrossRef]
32. Nelson, M.C.; Gordon-Larsen, P.; Adair, L.S.; Popkin, B.M. Adolescent physical activity and sedentary behavior: Patterning and long-term maintenance. *Am. J. Prev. Med.* **2005**, *28*, 259–266. [CrossRef]
33. Chantler, I.; Szabo, C.P.; Green, K. Muscular strength changes in hospitalized anorexic patients after an eight week resistance training program. *Int. J. Sports Med.* **2006**, *27*, 660–665. [CrossRef] [PubMed]
34. Werneck, A.O.; Silva, E.C.A.; Bueno, M.R.O.; Vignadelli, L.Z.; Oyeyemi, A.L.; Romanzini, C.L.P.; Ronque, E.R.V.; Romanzini, M. Association(s) Between Objectively Measured Sedentary Behavior Patterns and Obesity Among Brazilian Adolescents. *Pediatric Exerc. Sci.* **2019**, *31*, 37–41. [CrossRef] [PubMed]
35. Augustin, N.H.; Mattocks, C.; Cooper, A.R.; Ness, A.R.; Faraway, J.J. Modelling fat mass as a function of weekly physical activity profiles measured by actigraph accelerometers. *Physiol. Meas.* **2012**, *33*, 1831–1839. [CrossRef] [PubMed]
36. Machado-Rodrigues, A.M.; Coelho-e-Silva, M.J.; Mota, J.; Padez, C.; Ronque, E.; Cumming, S.P.; Malina, R.M. Cardiorespiratory fitness, weight status and objectively measured sedentary behaviour and physical activity in rural and urban Portuguese adolescents. *J. Child Health Care Prof. Work. Child. Hosp. Community* **2012**, *16*, 166–177. [CrossRef] [PubMed]
37. Allender, S.; Kremer, P.; de Silva-Sanigorski, A.; Lacy, K.; Millar, L.; Mathews, L.; Malakellis, M.; Swinburn, B. Associations between activity-related behaviours and standardized BMI among Australian adolescents. *J. Sci. Med. Sport* **2011**, *14*, 512–521. [CrossRef] [PubMed]
38. Jones, M.A.; Skidmore, P.M.; Stoner, L.; Harrex, H.; Saeedi, P.; Black, K.; Barone Gibbs, B. Associations of accelerometer-measured sedentary time, sedentary bouts, and physical activity with adiposity and fitness in children. *J. Sports Sci.* **2020**, *38*, 114–120. [CrossRef]

39. Altenburg, T.M.; Singh, A.S.; van Mechelen, W.; Brug, J.; Chinapaw, M.J. Direction of the association between body fatness and self-reported screen time in Dutch adolescents. *Int. J. Behav. Nutr. Phys. Act.* **2012**, *9*, 4. [CrossRef]
40. Hands, B.P.; Chivers, P.T.; Parker, H.E.; Beilin, L.; Kendall, G.; Larkin, D. The associations between physical activity, screen time and weight from 6 to 14 yrs: The Raine Study. *J. Sci. Med. Sport* **2011**, *14*, 397–403. [CrossRef]
41. Kantanista, A.; Osinski, W. Underweight in 14 to 16 year-old girls and boys: Prevalence and associations with physical activity and sedentary activities. *Ann. Agric. Environ. Med. Aaem* **2014**, *21*, 114–119.
42. Ainsworth, B.E.; Haskell, W.L.; Whitt, M.C.; Irwin, M.L.; Swartz, A.M.; Strath, S.J.; O'Brien, W.L.; Bassett, D.R.J.; Schmitz, K.H.; Emplaincourt, P.O.; et al. Compendium of physical activities: An update of activity codes and MET intensities. *Med. Sci. Sports Exerc.* **2000**, *32*, S498–S504. [CrossRef]

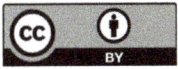

© 2020 by the authors. Licensee MDPI, Basel, Switzerland. This article is an open access article distributed under the terms and conditions of the Creative Commons Attribution (CC BY) license (http://creativecommons.org/licenses/by/4.0/).

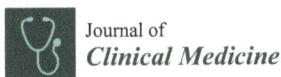

Article

Somatotype Components as Useful Predictors of Disordered Eating Attitudes in Young Female Ballet Dance Students

José Ramón Alvero-Cruz [1,2,3,*], Verónica Parent Mathias [1] and Jerónimo C. García-Romero [1,2]

[1] Department of Human Physiology, Histology, Pathological Anatomy and Physical Education and Sport, University of Málaga-Andalucía Tech, 29071 Málaga, Spain; veronicaparent@hotmail.com (V.P.M.); jeronimo@uma.es (J.C.G.-R.)
[2] The Biomedical Research Institute of Málaga (IBIMA), 29010 Málaga, Spain
[3] Edificio López de Peñalver, Campus de Teatinos, Universidad de Málaga, 29071 Málaga, Spain
* Correspondence: alvero@uma.es

Received: 18 May 2020; Accepted: 25 June 2020; Published: 27 June 2020

Abstract: The current study used receiver operating characteristic (ROC) curve analysis to examine the accuracy of somatotype components in correctly classifying disordered eating attitudes (DEA) in female dance students. Participants were a sample of 81 female dancers distributed in two groups: beginner training (BT; age (mean ± SD) = 10.09 ± 1.2 years, n = 32) and advanced training (AT; age = 15.37 ± 2.1 years, n = 49). For evaluation of DEA, the Eating Attitudes Test- 26 (EAT-26) questionnaire was used. We defined an EAT-26 score ≥20 as positive for DEA. Somatotype components were calculated using the Heath-Carter anthropometric method. The risk of presenting DEA was 28.1% (n = 9) in the BT group and 6.1% (n = 3) in the AT group. In the BT group, mesomorphy demonstrated moderate–high accuracy in predicting DEA (area under the curve (AUC) = 0.82, 95% confidence interval (CI): 0.64–0.93). The optimal cut-off of 6.34 yielded a sensitivity of 0.77 and a specificity of 0.95. Ectomorphy showed moderate accuracy in predicting DEA (AUC = 0.768, 95% CI: 0.58–0.89). The optimal cut-off of 2.41 yielded a sensitivity of 0.78 and a specificity of 0.78. In the AT group, none of the components demonstrated accuracy in predicting DEA. Somatotype components were good predictors of disordered eating attitudes in the younger dance student group (beginner training). Further research is needed to identify the determinants of these differences between the two groups.

Keywords: dance students; disordered eating attitudes; Eating Attitudes Test-26 (EAT-26); mesomorphy; ectomorphy; Receiver Operating Characteristics (ROC) curve analysis

1. Introduction

Eating disorders (EDs) are mental disorders defined by abnormal eating habits that negatively affect a person's physical or mental health. Anorexia nervosa, one of the main EDs, has two distinct symptoms: low body weight (body mass index (BMI) less than 17.5 kg/m^2 or less than 85% of the expected weight for height, age and sex) and body image disturbance. Bulimia nervosa is defined by three criteria: recurrent binge eating, recurrent compensatory behavior, and preoccupation with one's body weight or shape. Others EDs include avoidant/restrictive food intake disorder, pica, regurgitation disorders, and other specified feeding and eating disorder [1]. In most EDs, the association with depression and anxiety states and substance abuse is common [1,2].

The influence of cultural and social factors on the development of EDs and their manifestations have been investigated from multiple perspectives [3]. The reasons for these rates of EDs have been centered on elements including personality factors and traits such as perfectionism and low self-esteem.

Epigenetic reasons are currently found in the etiology of EDs, with evidence suggesting that epigenetic processes link malnutrition and life stresses (gestational, perinatal, childhood, and adult) to the risk of developing EDs [4]. In dancers, it is well known that they spend countless hours practicing in front of mirrors where their bodies are closely examined by themselves and others. In addition, high levels of perfectionism concerning dance and a specific body shape, combined with the socio-cultural pressures for thinness inherent in the dance profession and expectations of high performance, produce the ideal social climate for the development of EDs [5,6].

Similarly, the Tripartite Influence Model, which is an etiological model of body image disturbance and eating disorders, proposes that social agents, such as family, friends, and the media, promote ideals of appearance that emphasize a slim ideal for women and a lean, muscular ideal for men [7]. EDs today are a health problem in Western countries [8], and their incidence and prevalence are increasing. The prevalence of EDs in female athletes appears to be high when competitive weight is important [9]. This prevalence is higher in athletes (18%) compared to non-athletes (5%) [10], and is also higher in female athletes (20%) than in non-athletes (5%) [11]. The highest prevalence of EDs is found in aesthetic sports, as well as in sports where athletes are classified by body weight (45%) compared to other sports (12%) [11]. Similar to the trend in the prevalence of Eds, athletes in lean sports exhibit more disordered eating behaviors than those in non-lean sports [12]. Female dancers, in particular, show high levels of perfectionism and when in highly competitive environments, such as dance companies or professional conservatories, may present a higher risk for developing an ED [13,14]. EDs are characterized by chronicity and relapses of disordered eating behavior in which the attitudes of adolescent girls towards body weight, as well as their perception of body shape, are frequently altered.

Numerous efforts have been made to develop instruments to improve the predictive value in the diagnostic screening of these diseases and various tests have been developed (EAT, Children's Eating Attitudes Test (ChEAT), Eating Disorders Examination-Questionnaire (EDE-Q), Sick, Control, One, Fat, Food (SCOFF), Eating Disorder Inventory (EDI), etc.). Of all these questionnaires, the Eating Attitudes Test (EAT) has been the most extensively used because of its reliability and reproducibility in the detection of EDs in the general population [15]; it has also been widely used in sports and dance [16–19]. EDs are complex and have an impact on both the physical and social–emotional health of adolescents as well as young adults [20]. EDs such as anorexia nervosa and bulimia, have well-established effects on body composition, such as decreased fat mass, fat-free mass, and total body water [21], as well as decreased bone mineral density [22].

The somatotype is defined as the quantification of the present shape and composition of the human body. It is expressed as a three-number rating representing the endomorphy, mesomorphy, and ectomorphy components, respectively, always in the same order. Endomorphy is the relative fatness; mesomorphy is the relative musculoskeletal robustness; and ectomorphy is the relative linearity or slenderness of a physique. The Heath-Carter method uses various anthropometric measurements including weight, height, upper arm circumference, maximal calf circumference, femur and humerus breadths, and triceps, subscapular, supraspinal, and medial calf skinfolds [23]. Somatotype determination is useful in the characterization of body shape in contemporary dance and sports dance [24], but the relationship between anthropometric somatotype components and EDs has been rarely studied [25]. Mesomorphy, the second component of the anthropometric somatotype [23], reflects the development of skeleton and muscle tissues. Studies have found associations between body shape and muscularity and an increase in eating problems [26]. The rationale for studying the somatotype components and their association with DEA is that this measurement is a reflection of body shape based on the three components: endomorphy (fatness), mesomorphy (robustness), and ectomorphy (slenderness). In addition, body dissatisfaction seems to be a determining factor for risk behavior for EDs [2,26].

The present study therefore aimed to establish the accuracy of somatotype components using receiver operating characteristic (ROC) curve analysis to assess disordered eating attitudes (DEA) in a group of dance students engaged in beginner and advanced dance training.

2. Methods

This cross-sectional and correlational study conducted in 2017 was approved by the Research Ethics Committee of the University of Málaga, Spain (EMEFYDE 2016–011 report) and carried out according to the principles of the Declaration of Helsinki.

2.1. Participants

A total of 81 female students between the ages of 8 and 21 years participated in this study. All were enrolled in the Professional Conservatory of Granada, Spain, in courses from beginner training (BT) through advanced training (AT). The students in the AT group were distributed into four dance specialties: Flamenco, Spanish, Classical, and Contemporary. Participation in the study was voluntary, and prior to its initiation, written informed consent was obtained from the participants or the legal guardians of those under 18 years of age. The exclusion criteria were the inability to perform some of the anthropometric measurements, incorrectly completing the EAT-26, and male gender.

2.2. Eating Behavior

Eating behavior was assessed with the EAT-26, which is a self-administered questionnaire used worldwide. It has been validated for assessing symptoms, concerns, and attitudes associated with abnormal eating behavior. The EAT-26 consists of 26 items forming three scales: dieting (related to the avoidance of fattening foods and the preoccupation with being thinner), bulimia and food preoccupation (involving items reflecting thoughts about food and those indicating bulimia), and oral control (associated with the self-control of eating and the perceived pressure from others to gain weight). A total score equal to or greater than 20 on the questionnaire is indicative of disordered eating behavior [15]. The EAT-26 has been validated for the Spanish population [16,27,28].

2.3. Anthropometric Assessment

All anthropometric measurements were conducted after a 12-h fast. Weight was measured on a SECA 813 electronic scale (SECA, Hamburg, Germany) accurate to 0.1 kg., and stretch stature was measured using a wall-mounted SECA 216 stadiometer (SECA, Hamburg, Germany) accurate to 0.1 cm. Skinfolds were measured at the following sites: triceps, subscapular, supraspinal, and medial calf with a Holtain skinfold caliper (Holtain, Crymych, UK) accurate to 0.2 mm, computing the means for subsequent calculations. Girths were measured at the following sites: flexed and tensed arm and calf with a Lufkin W606PM anthropometric tape (Apex Tool Group, Lufkin, México) accurate to 0.1 cm. Biepicondylar humerus and Bicondylar femur breadths were measured with a Holtain sliding caliper (Holtain, Crymych, UK) accurate to 0.1 cm. BMI was calculated as weight in kilograms divided by height in meters squared. Anthropometric measurements were performed following standardized techniques adopted by the International Society for the Advancement of Kinanthropometry [29]. The technical error of measurement of the Level 3 anthropometrist was less than 3% for skinfolds and less than 1% for the rest of the anthropometric measurements.

2.4. Anthropometric Somatotype

Anthropometric somatotypes were determined according to the Heath-Carter method [23] by the following equations:

$$\text{Endomorphy} = -0.7182 + 0.1451 (X) - 0.00068 (X^2) + 0.0000014 (X^3) \text{ where } X = \text{sum of triceps, subscapular and supraspinal skinfolds) multiplied by (170.18/height in cm).} \tag{1}$$

This is called height-corrected endomorphy and is the preferred method for calculating endomorphy.

$$\text{Mesomorphy} = 0.858 \times \text{humerus breadth} + 0.601 \times \text{femur breadth} + 0.188 \times \text{corrected arm girth} + 0.161 \times \text{corrected calf girth} - 0.131 \times \text{height} + 4.5 \tag{2}$$

Three different equations are used to calculate ectomorphy according to the height–weight ratio (HWR). If the HWR is greater than or equal to 40.75, then ectomorphy = 0.732 HWR − 28.58. If HWR is less than 40.75 but greater than 38.25, then ectomorphy = 0.463 HWR − 17.63. If HWR is equal to or less than 38.25, then ectomorphy = 0.1.

2.5. Statistical Analysis

Normality was analyzed using the Shapiro-Wilk test. The descriptive characteristics of the group variables were expressed as mean ± standard deviation. Comparisons between groups were performed using a Mann-Whitney U or one-way ANOVA test when appropriate. Associations between EAT-26 subscale scores and somatotype components were assessed by Spearman's rank correlation coefficient (rho) for the two groups separately. The following criteria were adopted to interpret the magnitude of the correlations: $r \leq 0.1$ = trivial; $0.1 < r \leq 0.3$ = small; $0.3 < r \leq 0.5$ = moderate; $0. < r \leq 0.7$ = large; $0.7 < r \leq 0.9$ = very large; and $r > 0.9$ = almost perfect [30]. Cronbach's alpha was performed for investigating the internal consistency of the subscales and the total score of the EAT-26 questionnaire. Test–retest reliability was assessed by intraclass correlation coefficient (ICC). The effect size was calculated using Rosenthal's R-test and the power (1-β) to analyze the type II error by G*Power [31].

ROC curve analysis was used to test the performance of the somatotype components in predicting disordered eating status and to identify a cut-off score. The ROC curve is a graphical representation of a measure's sensitivity plotted against its false positive rate (i.e., 1-specificity). The area under the curve (AUC) summarizes a test's overall accuracy, or ability to distinguish cases from non-cases, based on the average value of sensitivity for all possible values of specificity. AUC values are defined as non-informative (≤0.50), less accurate (0.51 to 0.70), moderately accurate (0.71 to 0.90), highly accurate (0.91 to 0.99), or perfect (1.0) [32]. The likelihood ratios were calculated for each somatotype component. Binary logistic regression was used to evaluate the association between independent variables (somatotype components) and risk behaviors for DEA. The level of significance was set at $p < 0.05$. The statistical analysis was performed on MedCalc Statistical Software version 19.3.1 (MedCalc Software bvba, Ostend, Belgium).

3. Results

The risk of presenting DEA was 28.1% ($n = 9$) in the BT group and 6.1% ($n = 3$) in the AT group. Table 1 shows the comparative data of the study groups. Regarding the anthropometric variables; significant differences were found in age, weight, height, and BMI (all $p = 0.000001$). Similarly, differences were seen in both endomorphy ($p = 0.003$) and mesomorphy ($p = 0.04$). The psychometric assessment of the EAT-26 subscales showed differences between the groups only in bulimia ($p = 0.004$), although the values of the diet subscale and the total score were higher in the BT group (Table 1).

The internal consistency of the EAT-26 was assessed with Cronbach's alpha. The results revealed satisfactory levels for the subsample ($n = 25$). Cronbach's alpha for the total EAT-26 score, bulimia, oral control, and dieting were 0.87, 0.915, 0.89, and 0.906, respectively. The subsample of 25 participants completed the retest after 3-week intervals. Test–retest reliability was good (ICC = 0.864, $p < 0.001$). A Mann–Whitney U test showed no significant differences between the test and re-test scores for the total EAT-26 score ($p = 0.467$).

Bivariate correlations in the beginner training group: bulimia correlated inversely with age (rho = −0.37, $p = 0.035$) and height (rho = −0.465, $p = 0.007$); oral control correlated with mesomorphy (rho = 0.46. $p = 0.007$); bulimia correlated inversely with height (rho = −0.39. $p= 0.027$) and directly with mesomorphy (rho = 0.40, $p = 0.021$); and the total score correlated inversely with height (rho = −0.45, $p = 0.0089$) and directly with mesomorphy (rho = 0.40, $p= 0.02$) (Table 2).

Table 1. Descriptive data for anthropometrics and the Eating Attitudes Test-26 (EAT-26) subscales of the study groups.

Variables	Beginner Training (n = 32)		Advanced Training (n = 49)		p-Value	Effect Size	Statistical Power
	Mean	SD	Mean	SD		r	1-β
Age (years)	10.09	1.23	15.37	2.11	<0.0001	0.84	0.99
Weight (kg)	34.93	3.63	52.28	5.79	<0.0001	0.87	0.99
Height (m)	1.40	0.07	1.59	0.08	<0.0001	0.79	0.99
BMI (kg/m^2)	18.00	1.89	20.69	1.96	<0.0001	0.57	0.99
Endomorphy	3.85	1.23	3.19	0.64	0.003	0.32	0.81
Mesomorphy	5.64	0.95	5.17	1.04	0.041	0.23	0.51
Ectomorphy	2.77	1.27	2.62	1.29	0.60	0.09	0.08
Bulimia	0.94	1.50	0.16	0.55	0.004	0.33	0.83
Oral control	3.44	4.06	3.10	3.05	0.66	0.05	0.07
Dieting	6.72	7.35	4.22	5.21	0.21	0.19	0.38
Total score	11.09	11.58	7.49	8.01	0.46	0.18	0.33

Table 2. Spearman's rank correlation coefficient between body composition variables, somatotype components and the EAT-26 subscales in the Beginner Training group.

	Bulimia	Oral Control	Dieting	Total Score	Age	Weight	Height	BMI	Endo	Meso
Oral control	0.786 **									
Dieting	0.667 **	0.60 **								
Total Score	0.772 **	0.821 **	0.936 **							
Age	−0.37 *	−0.243	−0.158	−0.218						
Weight	−0.132	−0.212	−0.093	−0.17	0.54 **					
Height	−0.46 **	−0.48 **	−0.39 *	−0.45 **	0.81 **	0.528 **				
BMI	0.193	0.197	0.204	0.184	−0.169	0.537 **	−0.37 *			
Endo	0.254	0.206	0.116	0.121	−0.56 **	0.058	−0.65 **	0.63 **		
Meso	0.422 *	0.466 **	0.405 *	0.438 *	−0.166	0.32	−0.43 **	0.82 **	0.49 **	
Ecto	−0.319	−0.338	−0.27	−0.294	0.415 *	−0.291	0.62 **	−0.94 **	−0.73 **	−0.8 **

BMI: body mass index. Endo: endomorphy. Meso: mesomorphy. Ecto: ectomorphy. * $p < 0.05$. ** $p < 0.001$.

Bivariate correlations in the advanced training group: bulimia did not correlate with body composition variables or somatotype components ($p > 0.05$); oral control correlated directly with age (rho = 0.28, $p = 0.047$) and BMI (rho = 0.29, $p = 0.04$); the mesomorphic component correlated inversely with height (rho = −0.75, $p < 0.0001$) and directly with BMI (rho = 0.62, $p < 0.0001$); ectomorphy also correlated directly with diet (rho = 0.34, $p = 0.016$) and height (rho = 0.69, $p < 0.001$); and the total EAT-26 score did not correlate with any of the body composition variables or somatotype components ($p > 0.05$) (Table 3).

Analysis of ROC Curves

Ectomorphy showed moderate accuracy for the diagnosis of DEA (AUC: 0.768, $p = 0.0158$), and mesomorphy showed moderately high accuracy (AUC: 0.82, $p = 0.0003$) in the BT group. Endomorphy in the BT group and all three components for the AT group indicated low accuracy ($p > 0.05$), (Figure 1 and Table 4).

Table 3. Spearman's rank correlation coefficients between body composition variables, somatotype components, and the EAT-26 subscales in the Advanced Training group.

	Bulimia	Oral Control	Dieting	Total Score	Age	Weight	Height	BMI	Endo	Meso
Oral control	0.469 **									
Dieting	0.489 **	0.141								
Total Score	0.482 *	0.828 **	0.616 **							
Age	0.23	0.284 *	−0.093	0.127						
Weight	0.237	0.35 *	−0.035	0.214	0.803 **					
Height	0.187	0.066	0.258	0.219	0.414 **	0.594 **				
BMI	0.103	0.294 *	−0.277	−0.011	0.474 **	0.51 **	−0.322 *			
Endo	−0.016	0.066	−0.107	−0.021	−0.165	−0.213	−0.57 **	0.431 **		
Meso	−0.09	0.102	−0.281	−0.112	−0.022	−0.146	−0.76 **	0.629 **	0.544 **	
Ecto	0.026	−0.177	0.342 *	0.119	−0.127	−0.118	0.692 **	−0.88 **	−0.59 **	−0.80 **

BMI, body mass index; Endo, endomorphy; Meso, mesomorphy; Ecto, ectomorphy. * $p < 0.05$. ** $p < 0.001$.

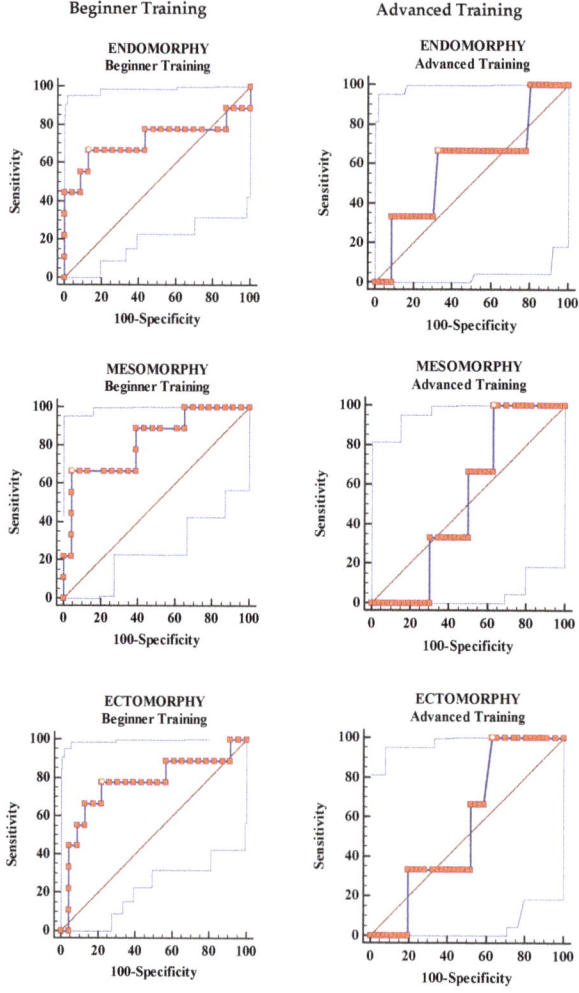

Figure 1. Receiver Operating Characteristics (ROC) curve analysis showing the area under the curve for the prediction of disordered eating attitudes using the Eating Attitudes Test-26 (EAT-26) total score.

Table 4. Characteristics of the ROC curves for somatotype components in the beginner training and advanced training groups.

	Beginner Training			Advanced Training		
	Endo	Meso	Ecto	Endo	Meso	Ecto
Area under the curve	0.72	0.82	0.768	0.601	0.522	0.558
Standard error	0.135	0.089	0.111	0.212	0.114	0.139
95% CI	0.53 to 0.86	0.64 to 0.93	0.58 to 0.89	0.45 to 0.74	0.37 to 0.66	0.41 to 0.70
z statistic	1.631	3.61	2.41	0.477	0.191	0.418
p-value	0.1030	0.003	0.0158	0.633	0.8483	0.6758
Youden's J index	0.5362	0.6232	0.564	0.3406	0.3696	0.3696

ROC, receiver operating characteristic; Endo, endomorphy; Meso, mesomorphy; Ecto, ectomorphy; CI, confidence interval.

The BT group had moderate specificity values for ectomorphy (78.6%) and high values for mesomorphy (95.6%) and endomorphy (87%). Sensitivity values were low and moderate, respectively. In this group, of note is the cut-off point of 6.34 for mesomorphy with a very high positive likelihood ratio value of (15.33). In the AT group, sensitivity values were moderate for endomorphy (67%) and highest for mesomorphy and ectomorphy (both 100%) (Table 5).

Table 5. Sensitivity. specificity and likelihood ratios of somatotype components in the beginner and advanced training groups.

Somatotype Component	Training	Cut-Off	Sens	95% CI	Spec	95% CI	+LR	95% CI	−LR	95% CI
Endomorphy	BT	>4.36	66.67	29.9–92.5	86.96	66.4–97.2	5.11	1.6–16.2	0.38	0.2–1.0
	AT	≤2.88	66.67	9.4–99.2	67.39	52.0–80.5	2.04	0.8–5.0	0.49	0.10–2.5
Mesomorphy	BT	>6.34	66.67	29.9–92.5	95.65	78.1–99.9	15.33	2.1–110	0.35	0.1–0.9
	AT	≤5.72	100	29.2–100.0	36.96	23.2–52.5	1.59	1.3–2.0	0	
Ectomorphy	BT	≤2.41	77.78	40.0–97.2	78.6	56.3–92.5	3.58	1.5–8.4	0.28	0.08–1.0
	AT	>1.76	100	29.2–100.0	36.96	23.2–52.5	1.59	1.3–2.0	0	

BT, beginner training; AT, advanced training; Sens, sensitivity; CI, confidence interval; Spec, specificity; +LR, positive likelihood ratio; −LR, negative likelihood ratio.

A logistic regression analysis was performed to examine independent associations between somatotype components and the probability of DEA (Table 6). The model provided a good fit for all three components in the BT group, particularly the mesomorphic component. However, in the AT group, none of the components achieved a significant fit.

Table 6. Associations between somatotype components and eating disorders.

Group	Variable	OR	95% CI	Overall Model Fit		Hosmer & Lemeshow	
				X^2	p-Value	X^2	p-Value
BT	Endo	2.44	1.1608 to 5.1493	6.878	0.0087	7.3902	0.5966
	Meso	7.14	1.7214 to 29.672	12.47	0.0004	11.0945	0.2693
	Ecto	0.42	0.2041 to 0.8972	6.22	0.0126	9.5698	0.3864
AT	Endo		Not retained in the model				
	Meso		Not retained in the model				
	Ecto		Not retained in the model				

BT, beginner training; AT, advanced training; Endo, endomorphy; Meso, mesomorphy; Ecto, ectomorphy; OR, odds ratio; CI, confidence interval; X^2, chi-squared.

4. Discussion

This study addresses the diagnostic accuracy of somatotype components (endomorphy, mesomorphy, and ectomorphy) to discriminate DEA in two groups of female dance students. The results show important significant differences and indicate that the ectomorphic and mesomorphic components in the BT group (younger students) can discriminate DEA with moderate and high accuracy, respectively; however, none of the somatotype components can do this in the AT group.

The emerging importance of somatotype components in predicting DEA in young female dance students is poorly reflected in the literature. Only one recent study showed that women who support attitudes and/or behaviors aimed at achieving the female muscle ideal may be susceptible to experiencing symptoms of DEA and negative emotional states, such as depression, stress, and anxiety [33].

The differences in the somatotype component associations between the study groups can be explained by the following reasons: the shorter height in the BT group increased mesomorphy scores, and although no significant differences in mesomorphy scores were found between groups, the levels were slightly higher in the BT group. In other words, the musculoskeletal structure was proportionally larger, and therefore a negative body image could have been internalized [34]. This also occurred with ectomorphy, since higher weight in relation to shorter height resulted in a lower ectomorphy value.

Similar results were found by Bartsch et al. who associate bulimia episodes with heavier somatotypes, such as pycnomorphic and metromorphic (similar to Heath and Carter's endomorphic and mesomorphic components) [25]. In the present study, we also observed a relationship between the bulimia subscale and mesomorphy, but this was only in the BT group. It should be noted that all the subscales of the EAT-26 as well as the total score had a significant direct association with the mesomorphic component. The substantial increase in DEA in Western societies may be associated with sociocultural pressures to maintain a slim body shape as well as with the combined influence of perfectionism and learning [5]. This condition becomes more pronounced in aesthetic activities such as dance [35].

Investigating the nature and distribution of DEA in dance students is important for several reasons. First, these studies can provide information about the extent of DEA and weight control in female dancers. Second, on a broader level, many dancers face specific pressures to control their weight and body shape, and this enables us to explore the association between this type of pressure and the development of disordered eating attitudes and behaviors [36].

Although no reference was made to the prevalence of bulimia, anorexia nervosa, or non-specific disorders, due both to this not being an aim of the study and to the limited sample size, the prevalence of these disorders was higher in the BT group, comprising younger students, similar to results published by other authors. In the BT group, this prevalence was around 26% and in the AT group it was 6% [37].

In a study by Fortes et al. that sought to establish the extent to which anthropometric variables can explain body dissatisfaction and eating behavior disturbances in teenage boys and girls, the findings showed that body dissatisfaction was modulated by body fat percentage ($R^2 = 0.18$), but this modulation was low. This was also low for its interaction with BMI ($R^2 = 0.18$). The interaction between eating behavior disturbances and body fat percentage and between body fat percentage and BMI were both ($R^2 = 0.03$) [38]. In contrast, Jáuregui et al. found that although there were correlations between BMI and EAT-40 scores, this did not result in an increased risk of developing an DEA [6]. These associations between BMI and the EAT-26 subscales were not confirmed in either of our study groups. The study by Toro et al. also found no significant inverse correlations between BMI and EAT-26 in dance students aged 14.4 years [39].

Another study in women found associations between BMI and DEA, and when these were mediated by a degree of body dissatisfaction, the associations disappeared [40]. This could explain the different associations between BMI and EAT-26 scores in our study, noting an association between BMI and oral control in the AT group, which implies greater self-control over food intake. In young people, being female, overweight, depressed, and having a high BMI are associated with DEA [41]. The results of a study of athletes competing in weight categories (taekwondo and judo) demonstrated that eating patterns and good dietary management decrease the likelihood of developing an DEA, which appears to be a good strategy [42].

Rouzitalab et al. analyzed a group of physical education students between the ages of 18 and 25 years. They found that EAT-26 had low but significant correlations with body weight and waist circumference in women, indicating these variables as good markers associated with an increase in

DEA [43]. In our study, no correlations were found between weight or BMI and the total score in the AT group, and none of these correlations were found in the BT group.

Several studies are available showing values for the subscales and total score on the EAT-26 in dance students of various ages, with no major differences found between these scores. These studies were performed in ballet dancers between the ages of 11 and 19, the same as those of our study. All the subscale scores in all the studies are higher in dieting than in oral control and bulimia [3,16,44,45].

Female gender, excess weight, living in urban areas, a distorted perception of weight, and body dissatisfaction were factors associated with DEA, suggesting that multiple factors contributed to the development of DEA [46,47]. The highest odds ratios were attributed to factors such as distorted perception of weight and body shape dissatisfaction [42,43]. In a study of 15- to 18-year-olds, the analysis showed significant negative associations between the total EAT-26 score and perceived physical appearance (rho = −0.290, $p < 0.001$) [37]. These data do not agree with those obtained in our study regarding correlations, although the EAT-26 score is very similar. However, for their assessment these differences should be compared with other determinants such as anxiety, stress, dissatisfaction, or body image and with other psychometric instruments that could explain those differences.

The results of this study can be used for prevention and early detection of DEA among young female dance students. Educational programs addressing adolescent eating behaviors should be developed. Future training programs on the significance of somatotype variations with growth, physical activity, and nutrition may be useful in preventing DEA.

5. Limitations

Several limitations of this study should be mentioned including the cross-sectional design, which limits the interpretation of causality. In addition, there was only one study stage, with no clinical interview performed to diagnose DEA. The EAT-26 was used as a screening tool only as the use of a questionnaire alone is not sufficient to diagnose DEA. Another limitation was that our study had a relatively small sample and only female students were included, although the statistical power was acceptable.

6. Conclusions

The ROC curve analysis showed that the mesomorphy and ectomorphy components for the BT group had a high and moderate discriminatory power for classifying DEA. This study allows the identification of a population at risk of DEA, such as young female dance students. We believe that the results found in the group comprising the youngest dancers should serve as an alert for greater control in the onset of DEA.

Author Contributions: Conceptualization, J.R.A.-C.; Data curation, J.R.A.-C. and V.P.M.; Formal analysis, J.R.A.-C., V.P.M., and J.C.G.-R.; Funding acquisition, J.R.A.-C.; Investigation, J.R.A.-C.; Methodology, J.R.A.-C., V.P.M., and J.C.G.-R.; Resources, J.R.A.-C.; Supervision, J.R.A.-C. and J.C.G.-R.; Writing–review and editing, J.R.A.-C., V.P.M., and J.C.G.-R. All authors have read and agreed to the published version of the manuscript.

Funding: This research received no external funding.

Acknowledgments: This study was supported by IBIMA (The Biomedical Research Institute of Málaga). We would like to thank to dance students and their parents for their voluntary participation in this study. We also thank Maria Repice for her help with the English version of the text and Manuel Jiménez for his statistical advice.

Conflicts of Interest: The authors declare that there are no conflicts of interest.

References

1. American Psychiatric Association American Psychiatric Association. *Diagnostic and Statistical Manual of Mental Disorders*, 5th ed.; American Psychiatric Publishing: Gloucester, UK, 2013; ISBN 9780890425541.
2. Treasure, J.; Duarte, T.A.; Schmidt, U. Eating disorders. *Lancet* **2020**, *395*, 899–911. [CrossRef]

3. Toro, J.; Gomez-Peresmitré, G.; Sentis, J.; Vallés, A.; Casulà, V.; Castro, J.; Pineda, G.; Leon, R.; Platas, S.; Rodriguez, R. Eating disorders and body image in Spanish and Mexican female adolescents. *Soc. Psychiatry Psychiatr. Epidemiol.* **2006**, *41*, 556–565. [CrossRef]
4. Steiger, H.; Booij, L. Eating disorders, heredity and environmental activation: Getting epigenetic concepts into practice. *J. Clin. Med.* **2020**, *9*, e1332. [CrossRef] [PubMed]
5. Penniment, K.J.; Egan, S.J. Perfectionism and learning experiences in dance class as risk factors for eating disorders in dancers. *Eur. Eat. Disord. Rev.* **2012**, *20*, 13–22. [CrossRef] [PubMed]
6. Jáuregui-Lobera, I.; Bolaños-Rios, P.; Valero-Blanco, E.; Ortega-de-la-Torre, A. Eating attitudes, body image and risk for eating disorders in a group of Spanish dancers. *Nutr. Hosp.* **2016**, *33*, 1213–1221.
7. Tylka, T.L. Refinement of the tripartite influence model for men: Dual body image pathways to body change behaviors. *Body Image* **2011**, *8*, 199–207. [CrossRef]
8. Uher, R.; Rutter, M. Classification of feeding and eating disorders: Review of evidence and proposals for ICD-11. *World Psychiatry* **2012**, *11*, 80–92. [CrossRef]
9. Joy, E.; Kussman, A.; Nattiv, A. 2016 update on eating disorders in athletes: A comprehensive narrative review with a focus on clinical assessment and management. *Br. J. Sports Med.* **2016**, *50*, 154–162. [CrossRef]
10. Martinsen, M.; Sundgot-Borgen, J. Higher prevalence of eating disorders among adolescent elite athletes than controls. *Med. Sci. Sports Exerc.* **2013**, *45*, 1188–1197. [CrossRef] [PubMed]
11. Sundgot-Borgen, J.; Torstveit, M.K. Prevalence of eating disorders in elite athletes is higher than in the general population. *Clin. J. Sport Med.* **2004**, *14*, 25–32. [CrossRef]
12. Glazer, J.L. Eating disorders among male athletes. *Curr. Sports Med. Rep.* **2008**, *7*, 332–337. [CrossRef]
13. Goodwin, H.; Arcelus, J.; Geach, N.; Meyer, C. Perfectionism and eating psychopathology among dancers: The role of high standards and self-criticism. *Eur. Eat. Disord. Rev.* **2014**, *22*, 346–351. [CrossRef] [PubMed]
14. Abraham, S. Characteristics of eating disorders among young ballet dancers. *Psychopathology* **1996**, *29*, 223–229. [CrossRef] [PubMed]
15. Garner, D.M.; Bohr, Y.; Garfinkel, P.E. The eating attitudes test: Psychometric features and clinical correlates. *Psychol. Med.* **1982**, *12*, 871–878. [CrossRef] [PubMed]
16. Arcelus, J.; Witcomb, G.L.; Mitchell, A. Prevalence of eating disorders amongst dancers: A systemic review and meta-analysis. *Eur. Eat. Disord. Rev.* **2014**, *22*, 92–101. [CrossRef]
17. Sepúlveda, A.R.; Compte, E.J.; Faya, M.; Villaseñor, A.; Gutierrez, S.; Andrés, P.; Graell, M. Spanish validation of the Eating Disorder Examination Questionnaire for Adolescents (EDE-Q-A): Confirmatory factor analyses among a clinical sample. *Eat. Disord.* **2019**, *27*, 565–576. [CrossRef]
18. Rivas, T.; Bersabé, R.; Jimenez, M.; Berrocal, C. The eating attitudes test (EAT-26): Reliability and validity in Spanish female samples. *Span. J. Psychol.* **2010**, *13*, 1044–1056. [CrossRef]
19. Peláez-Fernández, M.A.; Ruiz-Lázaro, P.M.; Labrador, F.J.; Raich, R.M. Validation of the Eating Attitudes Test as a screening instrument for eating disorders in general population. *Med. Clin.* **2014**, *20*, 153–155. [CrossRef]
20. Neumark-Sztainer, D.; Wall, M.; Larson, N.I.; Eisenberg, M.E.; Loth, K. Dieting and disordered eating behaviors from adolescence to young adulthood: Findings from a 10-year longitudinal study. *J. Am. Diet. Assoc.* **2011**, *111*, 1004–1011. [CrossRef]
21. Hübel, C.; Yılmaz, Z.; Schaumberg, K.E.; Breithaupt, L.; Hunjan, A.; Horne, E.; García-González, J.; O'Reilly, P.F.; Bulik, C.M.; Breen, G. Body composition in anorexia nervosa: Meta-analysis and meta-regression of cross-sectional and longitudinal studies. *Int. J. Eat. Disord.* **2019**, *52*, 1205–1223. [CrossRef]
22. Robinson, L.; Micali, N.; Misra, M. Eating disorders and bone metabolism in women. *Curr. Opin. Pediatr.* **2017**, *29*, 488–492. [CrossRef]
23. Heath, B.H.; Carter, J.E.L. A modified somatotype method. *Am. J. Phys. Anthropol.* **1967**, *27*, 57–74. [CrossRef] [PubMed]
24. Liiv, H.; Wyon, M.A.; Jürimäe, T.; Saar, M.; Mäestu, J.; Jürimäe, J. Anthropometry, somatotypes, and aerobic power in ballet, contemporary dance, and DanceSport. *Med. Probl. Perform. Art.* **2013**, *28*, 207–211. [CrossRef] [PubMed]
25. Bartsch, A.J.; Brümmerhoff, A.; Greil, H.; Neumärker, K.J. Shall the anthropometry of physique cast new light on the diagnoses and treatment of eating disorders? *Eur. Child Adolesc. Psychiatry* **2003**, *12*, i54. [CrossRef] [PubMed]
26. Hoffmann, S.; Warschburger, P. Weight, shape, and muscularity concerns in male and female adolescents: Predictors of change and influences on eating concern. *Int. J. Eat. Disord.* **2017**, *50*, 139–147. [CrossRef]

27. De Irala, J.; Cano-Prous, A.; Lahortiga-Ramos, F.; Gual-García, P.; Martínez-González, M.A.; Cervera-Enguix, S. Validation of the Eating Attitudes Test (EAT) as a screening tool in the general population. *Med. Clin.* **2008**, *12*, 487–491. [CrossRef]
28. Castro, J.; Toro, J.; Salamero, M.; Guimerá, E. The eating attitudes test: Validation of the Spanish version. *Evaluación Psicológica* **1991**, *7*, 175–190.
29. Marfell-Jones, M.; Olds, L. *International Standards for Anthropometric Assessment*; International Society for the Advancement of Kinanthropometry: Potchefstroom, South Africa, 2006.
30. Hinkle, D.; Wiersma, W.; Jurs, S. *Applied Statistics for the Behavioural Sciences*, 5th ed.; Houghton Mifflin: Boston, MA, USA, 2003; ISBN 978-0618124053.
31. Faul, F.; Erdfelder, E.; Lang, A.G.; Buchner, A. G*Power 3: A flexible statistical power analysis program for the social, behavioral, and biomedical sciences. *Behav. Res. Methods* **2007**, *39*, 175–191. [CrossRef]
32. Zweig, M.H.; Campbell, G. Receiver-operating characteristic (ROC) plots: A fundamental evaluation tool in clinical medicine. *Clin. Chem.* **1993**, *39*, 561–577. [CrossRef]
33. Cunningham, M.L.; Szabo, M.; Kambanis, P.E.; Murray, S.B.; Thomas, J.J.; Eddy, K.T.; Franko, D.L.; Griffiths, S. Negative psychological correlates of the pursuit of muscularity among women. *Int. J. Eat. Disord.* **2019**, *52*, 1326–1331. [CrossRef]
34. Douglas, V.J.; Kwan, M.Y.; Minnich, A.M.; Gordon, K.H. The interaction of sociocultural attitudes and gender on disordered eating. *J. Clin. Psychol.* **2019**, *75*, 2140–2146. [CrossRef]
35. Ringham, R.; Klump, K.; Kaye, W.; Stone, D.; Libman, S.; Stowe, S.; Marcus, M. Eating disorder symptomatology among ballet dancers. *Int. J. Eat. Disord.* **2006**, *39*, 503–508. [CrossRef] [PubMed]
36. Byrne, S.; McLean, N. Eating disorders in athletes: A review of the literature. *J. Sci. Med. Sport* **2001**, *4*, 145–159. [CrossRef]
37. Costarelli, V.; Antonopoulou, K.; Mavrovounioti, C. Psychosocial characteristics in relation to disordered eating attitudes in Greek adolescents. *Eur. Eat. Disord. Rev.* **2011**, *19*, 322–330. [CrossRef] [PubMed]
38. Fortes, L.D.S.; Almeida, S.D.S.; Ferreira, M.E.C. Impacto de variáveis antropométricas sobre a insatisfação corporal e o comportamento alimentar em jovens atletas. *J. Bras. Psiquiatr.* **2012**, *61*, 235–241. [CrossRef]
39. Toro, J.; Guerrero, M.; Sentis, J.; Castro, J.; Puértolas, C. Eating disorders in Ballet dancing students: Problems and risk factors. *Eur. Eat. Disord. Rev.* **2009**, *17*, 40–49. [CrossRef] [PubMed]
40. Jones, C.L.; Fowle, J.L.; Ilyumzhinova, R.; Berona, J.; Mbayiwa, K.; Goldschmidt, A.B.; Bodell, L.P.; Stepp, S.D.; Hipwell, A.E.; Keenan, K.E. The relationship between body mass index, body dissatisfaction, and eating pathology in sexual minority women. *Int. J. Eat. Disord.* **2019**, *53*, 730–734. [CrossRef]
41. Dooley-Hash, S.; Banker, J.D.; Walton, M.A.; Ginsburg, Y.; Cunningham, R.M. The prevalence and correlates of eating disorders among emergency department patients aged 14–20 years. *Int. J. Eat. Disord.* **2012**, *45*, 883–890. [CrossRef]
42. Rodriguez, A.M.; Salar, N.V.; Carretero, C.M.; Gimeno, E.C.; Collado, E.R. Eating disorders and diet management in contact sports; EAT-26 questionnaire does not seem appropriate to evaluate eating disorders in sports. *Nutr. Hosp.* **2015**, *32*, 1708–1714.
43. Rouzitalab, T.; Gargari, B.P.; Amirsasan, R.; Jafarabadi, M.A.; Naeimi, A.F.; Sanoobar, M. The relationship of disordered eating attitudes with body composition and anthropometric indices in physical education students. *Iran. Red Crescent Med. J.* **2015**, *17*, e20727. [CrossRef] [PubMed]
44. Dotti, A.; Fioravanti, M.; Balotta, M.; Tozzi, F.; Cannella, C.; Lazzari, R. Eating behavior of ballet dancers. *Eat. Weight Disord.* **2002**, *71*, 60–67. [CrossRef]
45. Hayakawa, N.; Tanaka, S.; Hirata, N.; Ogino, S.; Ozaki, N. A battery of self-screening instruments and self-reported body frame could not detect eating disorders among college students. *BMC Res. Notes* **2019**, *12*, 613. [CrossRef] [PubMed]

46. Al-Kloub, M.I.; Al-Khawaldeh, O.A.; ALBashtawy, M.; Batiha, A.M.; Al-Haliq, M. Disordered eating in Jordanian adolescents. *Int. J. Nurs. Pract.* **2019**, *25*, e12694. [CrossRef] [PubMed]
47. Fortes, L.D.S.; Cipriani, F.M.; Ferreira, M.E.C. Risk behaviors for eating disorder: Factors associated in adolescent students. *Trends Psychiatry Psychother.* **2013**, *35*, 279–286. [CrossRef] [PubMed]

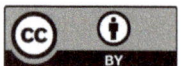

© 2020 by the authors. Licensee MDPI, Basel, Switzerland. This article is an open access article distributed under the terms and conditions of the Creative Commons Attribution (CC BY) license (http://creativecommons.org/licenses/by/4.0/).

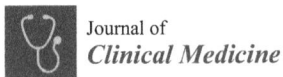

Article

Prevalence and Associated Factors of Nocturnal Eating Behavior and Sleep-Related Eating Disorder-Like Behavior in Japanese Young Adults: Results of an Internet Survey Using Munich Parasomnia Screening

Kentaro Matsui [1,2,3,4], Yoko Komada [5], Katsuji Nishimura [2], Kenichi Kuriyama [4] and Yuichi Inoue [1,6,*]

1. Japan Somnology Center, Neuropsychiatric Research Institute, Tokyo 1510053, Japan; matsui.kentaro@ncnp.go.jp
2. Department of Psychiatry, Tokyo Women's Medical University, Tokyo 1628666, Japan; nishimura.katsuji@twmu.ac.jp
3. Clinical Laboratory, National Institute of Mental Health, National Center of Neurology and Psychiatry, Tokyo 1878551, Japan
4. Department of Sleep-Wake Disorders, National Institute of Mental Health, National Center of Neurology and Psychiatry, Tokyo 1878551, Japan; kenichik@ncnp.go.jp
5. Liberal Arts, Meiji Pharmaceutical University, Tokyo 2048588, Japan; yoko.komada@gmail.com
6. Department of Somnology, Tokyo Medical University, Tokyo 1608402, Japan
* Correspondence: inoue@somnology.com; Tel.: +81-3-6300-5401

Received: 25 March 2020; Accepted: 21 April 2020; Published: 24 April 2020

Abstract: Nocturnal (night) eating syndrome and sleep-related eating disorder have common characteristics, but are considered to differ in their level of consciousness during eating behavior and recallability. To date, there have been no large population-based studies determining their similarities and differences. We conducted a cross-sectional web-based survey for Japanese young adults aged 19–25 years to identify factors associated with nocturnal eating behavior and sleep-related eating disorder-like behavior using Munich Parasomnia Screening and logistic regression. Of the 3347 participants, 160 (4.8%) reported experiencing nocturnal eating behavior and 73 (2.2%) reported experiencing sleep-related eating disorder-like behavior. Smoking ($p < 0.05$), use of hypnotic medications ($p < 0.01$), and previous and/or current sleepwalking ($p < 0.001$) were associated with both nocturnal eating behavior and sleep-related eating disorder-like behavior. A delayed sleep-wake schedule ($p < 0.05$) and sleep disturbance ($p < 0.01$) were associated with nocturnal eating behavior but not with sleep-related eating disorder-like behavior. Both nocturnal eating behavior and sleep-related eating disorder-like behavior had features consistent with eating disorders or parasomnias. Nocturnal eating behavior but not sleep-related eating disorder-like behavior was characterized by a sleep-awake phase delay, perhaps representing an underlying pathophysiology of nocturnal eating syndrome.

Keywords: nocturnal eating syndrome; sleep-related eating disorder; eating disorder; parasomnia; delayed sleep-wake phase; MUPS

1. Introduction

Nocturnal (night) eating syndrome (NES) is characterized by recurrent episodes of eating after the evening meal or after awakening from sleep [1,2]. NES has been described as "other specified feeding or eating disorder" in the Diagnostic and Statistical Manual of Mental Disorders, Fifth Edition [1], but its criteria are relatively unclear. Therefore, the diagnostic criteria proposed by Allison and colleagues [2] have been also used. Similar eating behaviors, but with total amnesia or partial unawareness of eating or drinking, are seen in sleep-related eating disorder (SRED) [3–5]. SRED can be distinguished from NES by its unconscious eating behavior and its inability to recall, which was emphasized in the diagnostic criteria for SRED in the International Classification of Sleep Disorders, Third Edition (ICSD-3) [6]. However, since NES and SRED share several features, the distinction between the two is still controversial [7,8]. NES has been considered an eating disorder with evening hyperphagia, eating episodes occurring upon awakening during the night and resultant morning anorexia [9,10]; the pathology of NES is believed to be a delayed circadian pattern of food intake [11,12]. SRED is classified as parasomnia in the ICSD-3 [6] and characterized by eating while "half-awake, half-asleep" or "asleep" [4,6]. SRED patients often experience sleepwalking [3,4], which is rare in NES patients [13]. To date, no large population-based studies have been conducted on NES and SRED [8], and only a few studies have addressed their similarities and differences in clinical characteristics and pathophysiology [7,13].

Munich Parasomnia Screening (MUPS) is a self-assessment questionnaire consisting of 21 items and is used to evaluate parasomnias and sleep-related movement disorders, including NES and SRED [14]. The questionnaire covers past history and current frequency of abnormal nighttime behaviors and their sensitivity and specificity [14]. Our group previously translated and validated a Japanese version of MUPS [15]. With this questionnaire, we conducted an internet survey for Japanese young adults from the general population and estimated the prevalence of NES and SRED in this cohort. We then analyzed factors related to nocturnal eating behavior and SRED-like behavior in this population to determine similarities and differences in these two disorders.

2. Experimental Section

The present study was conducted as part of a comprehensive research project on the influence of sleep schedule on daytime functioning and depression among young adults [16,17]. This cross-sectional web-based questionnaire for Japanese individuals aged 19–25 years was conducted in February 2012. At that time, ICSD-3 [6] had not been published. The participants were already registered as members of the established internet survey company's research panel and resided throughout Japan. The study protocol was approved by the ethics committee of the Neuropsychiatric Research Institute, Tokyo, Japan (no. 64/2011). Informed consent was obtained from all participants via the survey website.

The questionnaire included demographic information: sex, age, body mass index, residential status (living alone or with family), smoking status, and alcohol consumption. Sleep habits were evaluated as sleep duration (obtained from the Pittsburgh Sleep Quality Index [PSQI], described below), weekday bedtime, and weekday wake-up time. The questionnaire also included the Japanese version of the PSQI for assessing sleep disturbances [18,19], the Japanese version of MUPS for identifying the lifetime incidence of sleepwalking (i.e., walking or sitting up while still asleep), and current episodes of nocturnal eating behavior (i.e., waking again after falling asleep to eat) and SRED-like behavior (i.e., while asleep, eating something or preparing a meal that contains unusual or inedible ingredients, such as a combination of ice cream and cheese or dishwashing detergent instead of butter) [14,15].

Of 3904 participants who accessed the survey website, 3613 responded to the questionnaire. Participants who did not complete the questionnaire ($n = 219$) or who provided invalid answers ($n = 47$) were excluded. The responses of the remaining 3347 participants (92.6%) were included in the analyses of the present study (Figure 1).

To investigate factors associated with nocturnal eating behavior and SRED-like behavior [14,15]), we conducted logistic regression analyses for age, sex, body mass index, living alone, hypnotic medication use (three or more times per week) [18,19]), smoking status, alcohol consumption, previous and/or current sleepwalking [14,15]), typical sleep duration (categorized; see below), sleep-wake schedule (delayed/not delayed; phase delay was defined using the midpoint between sleep onset and sleep offset; 4:00 AM [20]), and subjective sleep quality (categorized; see below). Typical sleep duration and sleep-wake schedule were derived from the PSQI [18,19]. Body mass index was categorized as < 25 kg/m², 25–29 kg/m², and ≥ 30 kg/m² [21]. Typical sleep duration was categorized as < 6 and ≥ 6 hours [22,23]. PSQI scores were grouped as < 6 and ≥ 6 points [18,19]. All variables were examined initially with univariate models, and multivariate logistic regression was conducted for all variables that were significantly correlated in univariate models to determine the main correlates controlling for confounding factors. Wald statistics were used to test the significance of odds ratios (ORs) calculated from the regression analysis. SPSS version 22 (IBM SPSS, Armonk, NY, USA) was used for analysis. Statistical significance was set at $p < 0.05$.

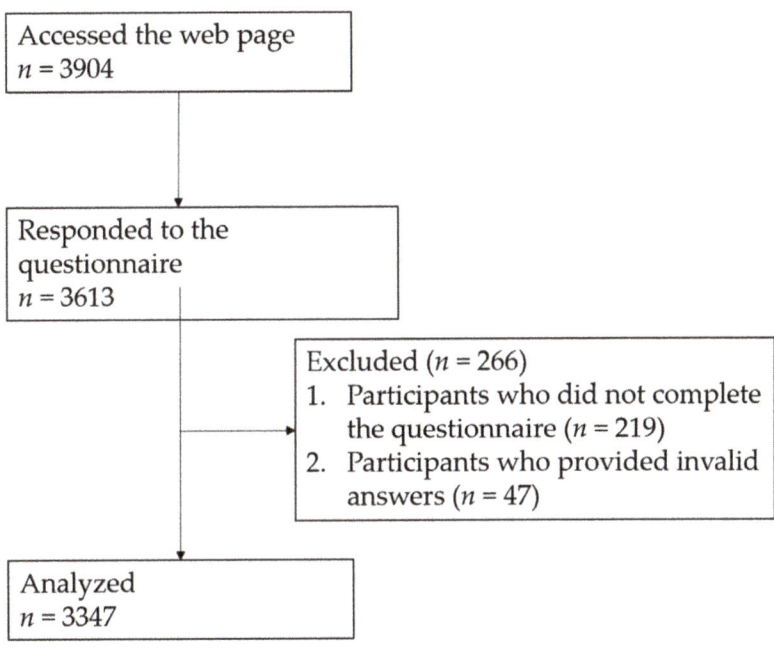

Figure 1. Subject flow diagram.

3. Results

Among the 3347 participants, 160 (4.8%) reported nocturnal eating behavior and 73 (2.2%) reported SRED-like behavior one or more times per year. Nocturnal eating behavior and SRED-like behavior were concomitant in 45 participants, but 72% of participants reporting nocturnal eating behavior and 38% of participants reporting SRED-like behavior did not overlap. Table 1 lists the characteristics of study participants.

Eight factors were significantly associated with nocturnal eating behavior in univariate logistic regression analyses: female sex, body mass index ≥ 30 kg/m², current smoking, use of hypnotic medication, previous and/or current sleepwalking, sleeping < 6 hours, delayed sleep-wake schedule, and higher PSQI scores (≥ 6 points). In the multiple logistic regression model, female sex, current smoking, use of hypnotic medication, previous and/or current sleepwalking, delayed sleep-wake schedule, and higher PSQI scores (≥ 6 points) were associated (Table 2).

Table 1. Characteristics of study participants.

Characteristic	Total (n = 3347)	Nocturnal Eating Behavior (n = 160)	Sleep-Related Eating Disorder-Like Behavior (n = 73)
Age, mean (SD), year	22.9 (1.8)	22.9 (1.8)	22.8 (1.7)
Sex (percent male)	45.3	36.3	46.6
Body mass index, mean (SD), kg/m^2	21.1 (3.6)	21.5 (4.4)	22.2 (4.4)
Current smoker (%)	10.5	20.0	21.9
Regular alcohol consumption (%)	35.1	34.4	47.9
Living alone (%)	34.1	35.0	35.6
Use of hypnotic medication (three or more times per week) (%)	2.8	13.1	12.3
Previous and/or current sleepwalking (%)	8.5	35.0	71.2
Typical sleep duration, mean (SD), hours	6.8 (1.4)	6.9 (1.6)	7.0 (1.7)
Midpoint on weekdays, mean (SD), time	4:22 (1:40)	4:41 (1:51)	4:17 (1:33)
Pittsburgh Sleep Quality Index score, mean (SD), points	5.5 (2.7)	7.6 (3.1)	7.2 (3.3)

Nocturnal eating behavior and sleep-related eating disorder-like behavior were defined as occurring at least once per year. SD, standard deviation.

Table 2. Factors associated with nocturnal eating behavior one or more times per year.

Predictor		Univariate Relative Risk (95% Confidence Interval) [1]	p	Multivariate Relative Risk (95% Confidence Interval) [1]	p
Age (years)	3347		n.s.		n.s.
Sex					
Male	1517				
Female	1830	1.485 (1.068–2.065)	<0.05	1.560 (1.103–2.206)	<0.05
Body mass index (kg/m^2)					
<25	3016				
25–29	247		n.s.		n.s.
≥30	84	2.484 (1.219–5.062)	<0.05		n.s.
Living alone					
No	2204				
Yes	1143		n.s.		n.s.
Current smoker					
No	2995				
Yes	352	2.240 (1.495–3.356)	<0.001	1.980 (1.286–3.047)	<0.01
Regular alcohol consumption					
No	2172				
Yes	1175		n.s.		n.s.
Use of hypnotic medication (three or more times per week)					
No	3253				
Yes	94	6.445 (3.854–10.778)	<0.001	4.054 (2.306–7.129)	<0.001
Previous and/or current sleepwalking					
No	3062				
Yes	285	6.955 (4.894–9.886)	<0.001	6.249 (4.335–9.009)	<0.001
Typical sleep duration (hours)					
≥6	2723				
<6	624	1.539 (1.067–2.219)	<0.05		n.s.
Sleep-wake schedule [2]					
Not delayed	1438				
Delayed	1909	1.507 (1.078–2.107)	<0.05	1.478 (1.042–2.096)	<0.05
Pittsburgh Sleep Quality Index score (points)					
<6	1827				
≥6	1520	2.690 (1.915–3.779)	<0.001	1.871 (1.304–2.684)	<0.01

[1] Relative risks approximated to odds ratios. [2] Phase delay was defined using 4:00 AM as the midpoint. n.s., not significant.

Five factors were associated with SRED-like behavior in univariate logistic regression analyses: body mass index of 25–29 kg/m², current smoking, regular alcohol consumption, previous and/or current sleepwalking, and higher PSQI scores (≥ 6 points). In the multiple logistic regression model, current smoking, use of hypnotic medication, and previous and/or current sleepwalking were associated (Table 3).

Table 3. Factors associated with sleep-related eating disorder-like behavior one or more times per year.

Predictor		Univariate Relative Risk (95% Confidence Interval) [1]	p	Multivariate Relative Risk (95% Confidence interval) [1]	p
Age (years)	3347		n.s.		n.s.
Sex					
Male	1517				
Female	1830		n.s.		n.s.
Body mass index (kg/m²)					
<25	3016				
25–29	247	2.115 (1.068–4.188)	<0.05		n.s.
≥30	84		n.s.		n.s.
Living alone					
No	2204				
Yes	1143		n.s.		n.s.
Current smoker					
No	2995				
Yes	352	2.454 (1.394–4.322)	<0.01	1.998 (1.072–3.724)	<0.05
Regular alcohol consumption					
No	2172				
Yes	1175	1.724 (1.083–2.744)	<0.05		n.s.
Use of hypnotic medication (three or more times per week)					
No	3253				
Yes	94	5.276 (2.542–10.951)	<0.001	3.750 (1.606–8.755)	<0.01
Previous and/or current sleepwalking					
No	3062				
Yes	285	32.318 (19.137–54.576)	<0.001	30.113 (17.764–51.044)	<0.001
Typical sleep duration (hours)					
≥6	2723				
<6	624		n.s.		n.s.
Sleep-wake schedule [2]					
Not delayed	1438				
Delayed	1909		n.s.		n.s.
Pittsburgh Sleep Quality Index (points)					
<6	1827				
≥6	1520	1.848 (1.151–2.969)	<0.05		n.s.

[1] Relative risks approximated to odds ratios. [2] Phase delay was defined using 4:00 AM as the midpoint. n.s., not significant.

4. Discussion

Thus far, sleepwalking has been considered rare in NES subjects [13]. However, we found a relatively strong association between sleepwalking and nocturnal eating behavior, although it was not as strong as the association with SRED-like behavior. This may be attributable to nocturnal eating behavior in the present study being defined as eating behavior after falling asleep or to the overlap reported by some participants between the two conditions. Of note, in this study, both nocturnal eating behavior and SRED-like behavior were associated with the use of hypnotic medication, with relatively high odds ratios. Multiple studies have reported SRED induced by hypnotic medication [24–28], but the evidence for hypnotic medication-induced NES is scarce [29]. but both benzodiazepines and Z-drugs can cause behavioral disinhibition [30,31], which may underlie the association between the use of hypnotic medication and nocturnal eating behavior. In addition, we found that nocturnal eating behavior but not SRED-like behavior was correlated with higher PSQI scores. Although the causal relationship is unclear, an association between insomnia and NES [7,10,32,33] should be considered.

Current smoking was also associated with both nocturnal eating behavior and SRED-like behavior. Smoking is common in eating disorders [34], and especially in bulimia and/or binge eating rather than anorexia [35–37]. Interestingly, NES has been reported to be more frequent in populations with bulimia and/or binge eating disorder rather than anorexia [38]. Thus, nocturnal eating behavior and binge eating may possibly be related to the pathology of addiction, including smoking. As for SRED, several cases in which smoking cessation resulted in SRED have been reported [5,39]. In addition, sleep-related smoking concomitant with NES and/or SRED has been reported [40]. Although Yahia and colleagues did not find a relationship between smoking and NES [32], smoking, as an addiction, may offer an opportunity for studying the pathology of NES and SRED.

Nocturnal eating behavior was associated in our study with the female sex. Just as eating disorders typically affect females [41–43], NES has been reported to be more common in females [10]. However, in both NES and SRED, sex differences in the prevalence are still controversial [5,33,44–50]; some studies have reported that NES was more common in males [44,45]. Thus, our findings should be confirmed in larger studies.

This is the first epidemiological study to indicate a relationship between a delay in the sleep-wake rhythm and nocturnal eating behavior. One study in mice suggested that feeding behavior affects the sleep-wake rhythm via the dopaminergic system [51]. It is still unclear whether delayed eating rhythm results in a delay in the sleep-wake rhythm or vice versa. However, nocturnal secretion of melatonin has been reported to decrease in NES [9]. Moreover, some preliminary studies have suggested that therapeutic interventions that act to consolidate the circadian rhythm, such as bright light therapy [52] and treatment with agomelatine [53,54], are effective for NES. Although these circadian-focused treatments require validation, the findings of the present study indicate that a delay in the sleep-wake rhythm possibly underlies the pathophysiology of NES.

This study has some limitations. First, the study was based on self-rating without face-to-face interviews. A further very important limiting factor is that the MUPS [14] had been developed before the publication of the ICSD-3 [6], and does not include "partial or complete loss of conscious awareness during the eating episode". However, nocturnal eating behavior and SRED-like behavior, which were expressed as "nocturnal eating" and "sleep related eating" in MUPS, respectively, were clearly distinguished by the presence/absence of consciousness [14]. This implication emphasizes the significance of focusing on the differences between nocturnal eating behavior and SRED-like behavior in this study. As this study was an analysis of self-reported data, there is a possibility that we underestimated the prevalence of subjects with SRED-like behavior who could not recall eating behavior at night. In contrast, we may have overestimated the prevalence since we required only one incident over the preceding year. Therefore, the present study should be considered preliminary in assessing the pathophysiology of NES and SRED. The second limitation is a possible sampling bias. Generally, internet users have been reported to experience more sleep problems or shorter sleep durations [55,56]. Third, this study did not confirm any questionnaires or severity scales specific to NES for affected subjects classified only by MUPs. Lastly, we identified the use of hypnotic medication in the survey [18,19], but did not record the type or amount. Similarly, the lack of information on the quantity of alcohol consumed and number of cigarettes smoked is also a limitation.

5. Conclusions

The present study using MUPS suggested that a considerable number of Japanese young adults may have NES, SRED, or both. Factors associated with both nocturnal eating behavior and SRED-like behavior were smoking, sleepwalking, and use of hypnotic medication. Nocturnal eating behavior but not SRED-like behavior was associated with a delayed sleep-wake schedule and sleep disturbances, as well as with the female sex. Confirmation of the reproducibility of these findings and prospective research that includes face-to-face interviews are warranted.

Author Contributions: Conceptualization, Y.K. and Y.I.; investigation, Y.K.; data curation, K.M. and Y.K.; formal analysis, K.M. and Y.I.; supervision, K.N. and K.K.; validation, K.N. and K.K.; original draft writing, K.M.; review and editing, Y.K. and Y.I. All authors have read and agreed to the published version of the manuscript.

Funding: This work was supported by JSPS KAKENHI (grant number JP22700781) from the Ministry of Education, Culture, Sports, Science and Technology.

Acknowledgments: We thank Dean Meyer, ELS from Edanz Group (www.edanzediting.com/ac) for editing a draft of this manuscript.

Conflicts of Interest: The authors declare no conflict of interest. The funder had no role in the design of the study; in the collection, analyses, or interpretation of data; in the writing of the manuscript, or in the decision to publish the results.

References

1. American Psychiatric Association. *Diagnostic and Statistical Manual of Mental Disorders (DSM-5)*, 5th ed.; American Psychiatric Pub: Washington, DC, USA, 2013.
2. Allison, K.C.; Lundgren, J.D.; O'Reardon, J.P.; Geliebter, A.; Gluck, M.E.; Vinai, P.; Mitchell, J.E.; Schenck, C.H.; Howell, M.J.; Crow, S.J.; et al. Proposed diagnostic criteria for night eating syndrome. *Int. J. Eat. Disord.* **2010**, *43*, 241–247. [CrossRef] [PubMed]
3. Schenck, C.H.; Mahowald, M.W. Review of nocturnal sleep-related eating disorders. *Int. J. Eat. Disord.* **1994**, *15*, 343–356. [CrossRef] [PubMed]
4. Winkelman, J.W. Clinical and polysomnographic features of sleep-related eating disorder. *J. Clin. Psychiatry* **1998**, *59*, 14–19. [CrossRef] [PubMed]
5. Schenck, C.H.; Hurwitz, T.D.; O'Connor, K.A.; Mahowald, M.W. Additional Categories of Sleep-Related Eating Disorders and the Current Status of Treatment. *Sleep* **1993**, *16*, 457–466. [CrossRef] [PubMed]
6. American Academy of Sleep Medicine. *International Classification of Sleep Disorders (ICSD-3)*, 3rd ed.; American Academy of Sleep Medicine: Darien, IL, USA, 2014.
7. Vinai, P.; Ferri, R.; Ferini-Strambi, L.; Cardetti, S.; Anelli, M.; Vallauri, P.; Ferrato, N.; Zucconi, M.; Carpegna, G.; Manconi, M. Defining the borders between Sleep-Related Eating Disorder and Night Eating Syndrome. *Sleep Med.* **2012**, *13*, 686–690. [CrossRef] [PubMed]
8. Inoue, Y. Sleep-related eating disorder and its associated conditions. *Psychiatry Clin. Neurosci.* **2015**, *69*, 309–320. [CrossRef]
9. Birketvedt, G.S.; Florholmen, J.; Sundsfjord, J.; Østerud, B.; Dinges, D.; Bilker, W.; Stunkard, A. Behavioral and neuroendocrine characteristics of the night-eating syndrome. *JAMA* **1999**, *282*, 657–663. [CrossRef]
10. Stunkard, A.J.; Grace, W.J.; Wolff, H.G. The night-eating syndrome; a pattern of food intake among certain obese patients. *Am. J. Med.* **1955**, *19*, 78–86. [CrossRef]
11. Boston, R.C.; Moate, P.; Allison, K.C.; Lundgren, J.D.; Stunkard, A.J. Modeling circadian rhythms of food intake by means of parametric deconvolution: Results from studies of the night eating syndrome. *Am. J. Clin. Nutr.* **2008**, *87*, 1672–1677. [CrossRef]
12. Goel, N.; Stunkard, A.J.; Rogers, N.; Van Dongen, H.P.; Allison, K.C.; O'Reardon, J.P.; Ahima, R.S.; Cummings, D.E.; Heo, M.; Dinges, D.F. Circadian rhythm profiles in women with night eating syndrome. *J. Boil. Rhythm.* **2009**, *24*, 85–94. [CrossRef]
13. Vetrugno, R.; Manconi, M.; Ferini-Strambi, L.; Provini, F.; Plazzi, G.; Montagna, P. Nocturnal eating: Sleep-related eating disorder or night eating syndrome? A videopolysomnographic study. *Sleep* **2006**, *29*, 949–954. [CrossRef] [PubMed]
14. Fulda, S.; Hornyak, M.; Muller, K.; Černý, L.; Beitinger, P.A.; Wetter, T.C. Development and validation of the Munich Parasomnia Screening (MUPS). *Somnologie Schlafforsch. Schlafmed.* **2008**, *12*, 56–65. [CrossRef]
15. Komada, Y.; Breugelmans, R.; Fulda, S.; Nakano, S.; Watanabe, A.; Noda, C.; Nishida, S.; Inoue, Y. Japanese version of the Munich Parasomnia Screening: Translation and linguistic validation of a screening instrument for parasomnias and nocturnal behaviors. *Neuropsychiatr. Dis. Treat.* **2015**, *11*, 2953–2958. [CrossRef] [PubMed]

16. Morita, Y.; Sasai-Sakuma, T.; Asaoka, S.; Inoue, Y. The impact of a delayed sleep-wake schedule on depression is greater in women-A web-based cross-sectional study in Japanese young adults. *Chrono Int.* **2015**, *32*, 952–958.
17. Asaoka, S.; Komada, Y.; Aritake, S.; Morita, Y.; Fukuda, K.; Inoue, Y. Effect of delayed sleep phase during university life on the daytime functioning in work life after graduation. *Sleep Med.* **2014**, *15*, 1155–1158. [CrossRef] [PubMed]
18. Buysse, D.J.; Reynolds, C.F.; Monk, T.H.; Berman, S.R.; Kupfer, D.J. The Pittsburgh sleep quality index: A new instrument for psychiatric practice and research. *Psychiatry Res. Neuroimaging* **1989**, *28*, 193–213. [CrossRef]
19. Doi, Y.; Minowa, M.; Uchiyama, M.; Okawa, M.; Kim, K.; Shibui, K.; Kamei, Y. Psychometric assessment of subjective sleep quality using the Japanese version of the Pittsburgh Sleep Quality Index (PSQI-J) in psychiatric disordered and control subjects. *Psychiatry Res. Neuroimaging* **2000**, *97*, 165–172. [CrossRef]
20. Simonelli, G.; Dudley, K.A.; Weng, J.; Gallo, L.C.; Perreira, K.; Shah, N.A.; Alcantara, C.; Zee, P.C.; Ramos, A.R.; Llabre, M.M.; et al. Neighborhood Factors as Predictors of Poor Sleep in the Sueño Ancillary Study of the Hispanic Community Health Study/Study of Latinos (HCHS/SOL). *Sleep* **2016**, *40*, 025.
21. Milano, W.; De Rosa, M.; Milano, L.; Capasso, A. Night eating syndrome: An overview. *J. Pharm. Pharmacol.* **2011**, *64*, 2–10. [CrossRef]
22. Petrov, M.E.; Howard, G.; Grandner, M.A.; Kleindorfer, D.; Molano, J.R.; Howard, V.J. Sleep duration and risk of incident stroke by age, sex, and race. *Neurol.* **2018**, *91*, 1702–1709. [CrossRef]
23. Kaneita, Y.; Ohida, T.; Uchiyama, M.; Takemura, S.; Kawahara, K.; Yokoyama, E.; Miyake, T.; Harano, S.; Suzuki, K.; Fujita, T. The relationship between depression and sleep disturbances: A Japanese nationwide general population survey. *J. Clin. Psychiatry* **2006**, *67*, 196–203. [CrossRef] [PubMed]
24. Molina, S.M.; Joshi, K.G. A Case of Zaleplon-Induced Amnestic Sleep-Related Eating Disorder. *J. Clin. Psychiatry* **2010**, *71*, 210–211. [CrossRef] [PubMed]
25. Najjar, M. Zolpidem and Amnestic Sleep Related Eating Disorder. *J. Clin. Sleep Med.* **2007**, *3*, 637–638. [CrossRef] [PubMed]
26. Nzwalo, H.; Ferreira, L.; Peralta, R.; Bentes, C. Sleep-related eating disorder secondary to zolpidem. *BMJ Case Rep.* **2013**, *2013*. [CrossRef] [PubMed]
27. Park, Y.M.; Shin, H.W. Zolpidem Induced Sleep-related Eating and Complex Behaviors in a Patient with Obstructive Sleep Apnea and Restless Legs Syndrome. *Clin. Psychopharmacol. Neurosci.* **2016**, *14*, 299–301. [CrossRef] [PubMed]
28. Yun, C.H.; Ji, K.H. Zolpidem-induced sleep-related eating disorder. *J. Neurol. Sci.* **2010**, *288*, 200–201. [CrossRef]
29. Kim, H.K.; Kwon, J.T.; Baek, J.; Park, D.S.; Yang, K.I. Zolpidem-Induced Compulsive Evening Eating Behavior. *Clin. Neuropharmacol.* **2013**, *36*, 173–174. [CrossRef]
30. Paton, C. Benzodiazepines and disinhibition: A review. *Psychiatr. Bull.* **2002**, *26*, 460–462. [CrossRef]
31. Olson, L.G. Hypnotic hazards: Adverse effects of zolpidem and other z-drugs. *Aust. Prescr.* **2008**, *31*, 146–149. [CrossRef]
32. Yahia, N.; Brown, C.; Potter, S.; Szymanski, H.; Smith, K.; Pringle, L.; Herman, C.P.; Uribe, M.; Fu, Z.; Chung, M.; et al. Night eating syndrome and its association with weight status, physical activity, eating habits, smoking status, and sleep patterns among college students. *Eat. Weight. Disord. Stud. Anorexia Bulim. Obes.* **2017**, *22*, 421–433. [CrossRef]
33. Ceru-Bjork, C.; Andersson, I.; Rossner, S. Night eating and nocturnal eating-two different or similar syndromes among obese patients? *J. Int. Assoc. Study Obes.* **2001**, *25*, 365–372. [CrossRef] [PubMed]
34. Wiseman, C.V.; Turco, R.M.; Sunday, S.R.; Halmi, K.A. Smoking and body image concerns in adolescent girls. *Int. J. Eat. Disord.* **1998**, *24*, 429–433. [CrossRef]
35. Bulik, C.M.; Epstein, L.H.; McKee, M.; Kaye, W. Drug use in women with bulimia and anorexia nervosa. *NIDA Res. Monogr.* **1990**, *105*, 462–463. [CrossRef]
36. Haug, N.A.; Heinberg, L.J.; Guarda, A.S. Cigarette smoking and its relationship to other substance use among eating disordered inpatients. *Eat. Weight. Disord. Stud. Anorexia, Bulim. Obes.* **2001**, *6*, 130–139. [CrossRef] [PubMed]
37. Anzengruber, D.; Klump, K.L.; Thornton, L.; Brandt, H.; Crawford, S.; Fichter, M.; Halmi, K.A.; Johnson, C.; Kaplan, A.; LaVia, M.; et al. Smoking in eating disorders. *Eat. Behav.* **2006**, *7*, 291–299. [CrossRef] [PubMed]

38. Tu, C.Y.; Tseng, M.C.M.; Chang, C.H. Night eating syndrome in patients with eating disorders: Is night eating syndrome distinct from bulimia nervosa? *J. Formos. Med Assoc.* **2019**, *118*, 1038–1046. [CrossRef]
39. Varghese, R.; De Castro, J.R.; Liendo, C.; Schenck, C.H. Two Cases of Sleep-Related Eating Disorder Responding Promptly to Low-Dose Sertraline Therapy. *J. Clin. Sleep Med.* **2018**, *14*, 1805–1808. [CrossRef]
40. Provini, F.; Vetrugno, R.; Montagna, P. Sleep-related smoking syndrome. *Sleep Med.* **2008**, *9*, 903–905. [CrossRef]
41. Striegel-Moore, R.H.; Bulik, C.M.; Weissman, R.S. Risk factors for eating disorders. *Am. Psychol.* **2007**, *62*, 181–198. [CrossRef]
42. Hoek, H.W. Incidence, prevalence and mortality of anorexia nervosa and other eating disorders. *Curr. Opin. Psychiatry* **2006**, *19*, 389–394. [CrossRef]
43. Hudson, J.I.; Hiripi, E.; Pope, H.G.; Kessler, R.C. The prevalence and correlates of eating disorders in the National Comorbidity Survey Replication. *Boil. Psychiatry* **2006**, *61*, 348–358. [CrossRef] [PubMed]
44. Aronoff, N.J.; Geliebter, A.; Zammit, G. Gender and Body Mass Index as Related to the Night-Eating Syndrome in Obese Outpatients. *J. Am. Diet. Assoc.* **2001**, *101*, 102–104. [CrossRef]
45. Tholin, S.; Lindroos, A.; Tynelius, P.; Åkerstedt, T.; Stunkard, A.J.; Bulik, C.M.; Rasmussen, F. Prevalence of Night Eating in Obese and Nonobese Twins. *Obes.* **2009**, *17*, 1050–1055. [CrossRef] [PubMed]
46. Striegel-Moore, R.H.; Franko, D.L.; Thompson, D.; Affenito, S.; Kraemer, H.C.; Weissman, R.S. Night Eating: Prevalence and Demographic Correlates*. *Obes.* **2006**, *14*, 139–147. [CrossRef]
47. Grilo, C.M.; Masheb, R.M. Night-time eating in men and women with binge eating disorder. *Behav. Res. Ther.* **2004**, *42*, 397–407. [CrossRef]
48. Winkelman, J.W. Efficacy and tolerability of open-label topiramate in the treatment of sleep-related eating disorder: A retrospective case series. *J. Clin. Psychiatry* **2006**, *67*, 1729–1734. [CrossRef]
49. Schenck, C.H.; Hurwitz, T.D.; Bundlie, S.R.; Mahowald, M.W. Sleep-Related Eating Disorders: Polysomnographic Correlates of a Heterogeneous Syndrome Distinct from Daytime Eating Disorders. *Sleep* **1991**, *14*, 419–431. [CrossRef]
50. O'Reardon, J.P.; Ringel, B.L.; Dinges, D.F.; Allison, K.C.; Rogers, N.; Martino, N.S.; Stunkard, A.J. Circadian Eating and Sleeping Patterns in the Night Eating Syndrome. *Obes. Res.* **2004**, *12*, 1789–1796. [CrossRef]
51. Mendoza, J.; Clesse, D.; Pévet, P.; Challet, E. Food-reward signalling in the suprachiasmatic clock. *J. Neurochem.* **2010**, *112*, 1489–1499. [CrossRef]
52. McCune, A.M.; Lundgren, J.D. Bright light therapy for the treatment of night eating syndrome: A pilot study. *Psychiatry Res. Neuroimaging* **2015**, *229*, 577–579. [CrossRef]
53. Milano, W.; De Rosa, M.; Milano, L.; Capasso, A. Agomelatine Efficacy in the Night Eating Syndrome. *Case Rep. Med.* **2013**, *2013*, 1–5. [CrossRef] [PubMed]
54. Milano, W.; De Rosa, M.; Milano, L.; Riccio, A.; Sanseverino, B.; Capasso, A. Successful Treatment with Agomelatine in NES: A Series of Five Cases. *Open Neurol. J.* **2013**, *7*, 32–37. [CrossRef] [PubMed]
55. Cain, N.; Gradisar, M. Electronic media use and sleep in school-aged children and adolescents: A review. *Sleep Med.* **2010**, *11*, 735–742. [CrossRef] [PubMed]
56. Do, Y.K.; Shin, E.; Bautista, M.A.; Foo, K. The associations between self-reported sleep duration and adolescent health outcomes: What is the role of time spent on Internet use? *Sleep Med.* **2013**, *14*, 195–200. [CrossRef] [PubMed]

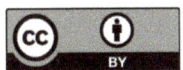

© 2020 by the authors. Licensee MDPI, Basel, Switzerland. This article is an open access article distributed under the terms and conditions of the Creative Commons Attribution (CC BY) license (http://creativecommons.org/licenses/by/4.0/).

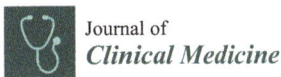

Article

Temperament and Character Traits of Female Eating Disorder Patients with(out) Non-Suicidal Self-Injury

Tinne Buelens [1,*], Koen Luyckx [1,2], Margaux Verschueren [1], Katrien Schoevaerts [3], Eva Dierckx [3,4], Lies Depestele [1,3] and Laurence Claes [1,5]

1   Faculty of Psychology and Educational Sciences, KU Leuven, 3000 Leuven, Belgium; koen.luyckx@kuleuven.be (K.L.); margaux.verschueren@kuleuven.be (M.V.); lies.depestele@azt.broedersvanliefde.be (L.D.); laurence.claes@kuleuven.be (L.C.)
2   UNIBS, University of the Free State, 9300 Bloemfontein, South Africa
3   Psychiatric Hospital Alexianen Zorggroep Tienen, 3300 Tienen, Belgium; katrien.schoevaerts@azt.broedersvanliefde.be (K.S.); eva.dierckx@vub.be (E.D.)
4   Department of Psychology and Educational Sciences, Vrije Universiteit Brussel, 1050 Elsene, Belgium
5   Faculty of Medicine and Health Sciences, Universiteit Antwerpen, 2610 Wilrijk, Belgium
*   Correspondence: tinne.buelens@kuleuven.be; Tel.: +32-163-77-506

Received: 30 March 2020; Accepted: 21 April 2020; Published: 22 April 2020

Abstract: Eating disorder (ED) patients show alarmingly high prevalence rates of Non-Suicidal Self-Injury (NSSI). Adolescents seem to be particularly at risk, as EDs and NSSI both have their onset in mid-adolescence. It has been suggested that personality could be a transdiagnostic mechanism underlying both EDs and NSSI. However, little attention has been given to adolescent clinical samples compared to adult and/or community samples. Therefore, the current study investigated the role of personality in a sample of 189 female inpatients with an ED (M = 15.93, SD = 0.98). Our results confirmed the high prevalence of NSSI in EDs, specifically in patients with bingeing/purging behaviours (ED-BP). Temperamental differences were found between ED-BP and the restrictive ED subtype (ED-R). Namely, ED-BP patients showed more harm avoidance and less self-directedness compared to ED-R. Temperamental differences were found in NSSI as well, regardless of ED subtype: ED patients who had engaged in NSSI during their lifetime reported less self-directedness and more harm avoidance. Interestingly, only ED patients who recently engaged in NSSI showed less novelty seeking. These temperamental profiles should be recognised as key mechanisms in the treatment of adolescent ED patients with and without NSSI.

Keywords: non-suicidal self-injury; temperament; eating disorder; adolescence

1. Introduction

Non-Suicidal Self-Injury (NSSI) is defined as any socially unaccepted behaviour through which individuals deliberately and directly injure their own body [1]. NSSI can serve a wide variety of functions to the individual, but the most common self-reported function is to regulate negative emotions [2]. Typical methods of engaging in NSSI are cutting, scratching, burning, or bruising one's own skin [3]. NSSI is strongly associated with internal distress, rejection by peers, rumination, and psychopathology in general, both internalising and externalising symptoms [4–6]. Adolescents seem to be most vulnerable, as NSSI onset peaks in mid-adolescence, around the ages of 14 and 15 [7]. The vulnerability of adolescents is also reflected in NSSI prevalence rates; epidemiological research consistently indicates that as many as 17% of adolescents in non-clinical samples have engaged in NSSI at least once [8–10]. Prevalence rates rise even higher in clinical samples, with young patients with an eating disorder being particularly at risk as up to 60% of this adolescent population engages in NSSI throughout their lifetime [11–14].

Eating disorder (ED) symptomatology, just like NSSI, can be considered a dysfunctional coping strategy to regulate negative affect [15,16]. Both in NSSI and EDs, the body is often perceived as negative and can become the target of emotional dysregulation [17]. EDs include Bulimia Nervosa (BN), characterised by recurrent binge-eating and compensatory behaviours (e.g., purging), and Anorexia Nervosa (AN), characterised by an irrational fear of gaining weight and restricting food intake. By definition, BN patients are at a healthy weight or slightly overweight, whereas AN patients are underweight [18]. However, some underweight patients do show bulimia-like symptoms, such as binge eating and purging. Consequently, AN is further divided into two subtypes: the binge-eating/purging subtype (AN-BP) and the restrictive subtype (AN-R).

A 2007 review [16] reported that AN-BP patients were most likely to engage in self-harming behaviour, with prevalence rates between 27.8% and 68.1% for this subtype. AN-R patients showed the lowest occurrence with prevalence rates between 13.6% and 42.1%. BN patients were in between the two AN subtypes, with self-harm prevalence rates ranging from 26% to 55.2%. However, this review investigated self-harm, which typically includes suicidal behaviour, in contrast to NSSI, which explicitly excludes suicidal thoughts and behaviours. Yet, several other studies have affirmed that AN-BP patients are engaging more frequently in NSSI compared to AN-R patients [19–21]. For instance, in a sample of 226 female ED patients, the lifetime prevalence of NSSI was significantly higher in AN-BP patients compared to AN-R patients [22]. Some uncertainty remains, however, as a handful of studies did not find any significant differences between AN-BP and AN-R [16,23]. Furthermore, research is lacking regarding the NSSI methods that are used by subtypes of ED patients. To the best of our knowledge, only four studies investigated differences in NSSI methods by subtypes of ED patients. Three of these studies did not find any significant difference [19,24,25], whereas one study by Claes et al. [26] reported that cutting was more common in female ED patients with binge/purge behaviour (AN-BP, BN) as compared to those with restrictive behaviour.

To improve understanding regarding the interplay between EDs and NSSI, researchers have been looking for transdiagnostic mechanisms. It has been suggested that personality could be such a transdiagnostic mechanism, underlying both EDs and NSSI [20,27,28]. According to the psychobiological theory of Cloninger et al. [29,30], there are seven dimensions of personality: four genetically determined temperamental dimensions and three learned character dimensions. Novelty seeking (NS) is the first temperamental dimension and refers to curiosity, impulsivity, enthusiasm regarding new experiences, and rash decision-making. Second, harm avoidance (HA) is characterised by shyness, fearfulness and inhibition in social situations. For example, one HA item reads: "When I have to meet a group of strangers, I am more shy than most people" [31]. Moreover, HA is characterised by excessive worrying, insecurity, and pessimism, even in situations where others would not worry or fear. Third, reward dependence (RD) describes seeking out social approval and support, openness to others, and a tendency to respond to signals of reward. Fourth, persistence (PS) refers to a competitive spirit, being inclined towards perfectionism, and showing perseverance in spite of repeated setbacks, frustration, or fatigue. Self-directedness (SD), the first of three character dimensions, is the strong desire to achieve a set of goals and values and the ability to regulate and adapt one's own behaviour to reach these goals. Cloninger described SD as "willpower" [32], more recent literature linked SD to effortful control [33]. Second, cooperativeness (CO) concerns empathy, tolerance, agreeableness, and identification with others. Low CO is associated with a wide range of personality disorders [30]. Third and finally, self-transcendence (ST) involves spirituality and the idea of a transcendental union with nature and the universe.

Several studies used Cloninger's model to trace temperament and character dimensions in psychopathology. For instance, adolescents engaging in NSSI, both patients and non-clinical controls, are characterised by high novelty seeking and low persistence [20,34–36]. High NS and low PS both indicate high impulsivity, which could partially explain why those who engage in NSSI struggle with resisting the urge to self-injure [37]. Nock and Prinstein [38] corroborated the impulsive nature of NSSI and found that many individuals contemplated the act of self-injury for less than five minutes before committing it. High NS and impulsivity are linked to low self-directedness, which is also part of the personality profile of NSSI [39,40]. Those with low SD are more likely to experience emotion regulation difficulties and end up losing executive functions when they encounter a negative affect [40]. These individuals tend to have lower emotional clarity and are less likely to accept their own emotions [41]. The lack of adaptive emotion regulation strategies might push individuals with low SD towards NSSI once they are confronted with an overwhelming negative affect [42]. Contributing to these emotion regulation difficulties are the high harm avoidance levels in the personality profile of NSSI [34]. According to Cloninger, the combination of high NS and high HA results in an approach-avoidance conflict that can cause further affective instability [29]. Results are less clear regarding levels of cooperativeness in those engaging in NSSI: the scores seem to be dependent on the absence or presence of suicidal thoughts and behaviours (STBs) [43]. Specifically, female adolescents who engaged in self-injury and experienced STBs showed higher CO scores compared to those without STBs [43]. So far, no associations have been found between reward dependence and NSSI [34,36].

The temperament and character dimensions of EDs are similar to those of NSSI in terms of self-directedness and harm avoidance. Namely, like NSSI, all ED types are characterised by high harm avoidance [44–47] and low self-directedness when compared to healthy controls [44,45,47]. Within ED subtypes, it was found that individuals with bingeing and purging behaviour (i.e., AN-BP and BN patients) reached even lower SD levels compared to those restricting their food intake (i.e., AN-R patients [46]). Similar to those engaging in NSSI, individuals with bingeing and purging behaviour show high novelty seeking [44–47] and low persistence [44,46,47]. Thus, the tendency for impulsivity and excitableness is common in both NSSI and binge/purge EDs. However, those with restrictive eating behaviour show the exact opposite pattern: low novelty seeking and high persistence. This combination of characteristics is associated with perfectionism, obsessiveness, and rigidity, which may maintain restrictive, calculated eating behaviour [44–47]. In contrast to NSSI, low cooperativeness is generally found in all ED types [44–47]. Finally, although high reward dependence was hypothesised to be a core characteristic of EDs [48], no associations have been found between reward dependence and ED [49,50].

The vast majority of research on EDs and NSSI has been conducted in adult and/or community samples [9,21]. However, the onset of EDs and NSSI occurs during adolescence and prevalence rates peak during these teenage years, particularly so in clinical samples [7,12,13]. Furthermore, little attention has been given to temperament and character traits in adolescent ED patients, be it with or without NSSI, even though previous research has suggested temperament to be a potential transdiagnostic mechanism in EDs and NSSI [20,28]. Therefore, the current study will investigate temperament and character traits in a large sample of young patients diagnosed with an ED and with(out) NSSI. Our first aim is to investigate the frequency and methods of lifetime and recent NSSI across ED subtypes in this sample. Based on previous literature, we expect higher frequencies of lifetime and recent NSSI in ED patients of the bingeing/purging subtype, compared to the restrictive subtype [19–21]. Research is lacking regarding NSSI methods, which leaves us unable to make strong hypotheses on frequencies of NSSI methods across ED subtypes. As a second aim, we will examine temperament and character dimensions in the adolescent ED patients with and without NSSI. Based on the literature summarised above, we hypothesise both ED types to show high harm avoidance, low self-directedness and low cooperativeness. Furthermore, we hypothesise a combination of high novelty seeking and low persistence in patients with a bingeing/purging ED and the opposite combination, low novelty seeking and high persistence, in patients with a restrictive ED [44–47]. If patients are engaging in NSSI, we hypothesise those individuals to be characterised by high novelty seeking, low persistence, low self-directedness, and high harm avoidance [20,34–36].

2. Materials and Methods

2.1. Procedure and Participants.

Between 2011 and 2018, data was collected in female patients who were hospitalised at a specialised inpatient eating disorder ward in Belgium. Shortly after admission, all patients were invited to participate in the study. Those willing to participate provided written informed consent and completed a series of online questionnaires. All patients under 18 years old provided additional parental consent. The procedure of the current study was approved by both the ethical committee of the psychiatric hospital as well as the ethical committee of the faculty of Psychology and Educational Sciences of the first author to use the data retrospectively for research purposes.

The present study included only minor patients who filled out the Eating Disorder Evaluation Scale [51], the Self-Injury Questionnaire-Treatment Related (SIQ-TR [52]) and the brief Dutch version of Cloninger's Temperament and Character Inventory (VTCI [31]). In total, our sample consisted of 189 female patients with an ED, with a mean age of 15.93 years (SD = 0.98, range 14–17 years).

ED diagnoses, as specified in the DSM-5, were diagnosed by means of an interview conducted by experienced psychiatrists or psychologists and further validated with the Eating Disorder Evaluation Scale [51]. AN-R diagnosis was assigned to 87 participants (46%, M_{adjBMI} = 71.91, SD = 7.32), while 56 participants (29.6%, M_{adjBMI} = 74.32, SD = 6.28) were diagnosed with AN-BP, and 46 (24.3%, M_{adjBMI} = 94.67, SD = 8.16) were diagnosed with BN. Subsequently, data of patients with binge-eating/purging behaviours (AN-BP and BN) were merged, given that these patients show similar temperamental profiles [47]. Thus, we performed our analyses on a group of restrictive ED patients (ED-R; n = 87, 46%, M_{age} = 15.91, SD = 0.97) and a group of patients with binge-eating/purging behaviours (ED-BP; n = 102, 54%, M_{age} = 15.95, SD = 0.99), with no significant age difference between them ($F(1, 187)$ = 0.090, ns). Additionally, we used the 13-item depression subscale of the Symptom Checklist-90 (SCL-90-D, [53]) to further describe our sample. Patients with recent NSSI presented with significantly higher depression scores compared to patients without recent NSSI ($F(1, 188)$ = 13.957, p < 0.000, η_p^2 = 0.070). Similarly, patients with lifetime NSSI presented with significantly higher depression scores compared to patients without lifetime NSSI ($F(1, 188)$ = 9.983, p = 0.002, η_p^2 = 0.051). ED-BP patients reported significantly higher depression scores compared to ED-R patients when lifetime NSSI was included ($F(1, 188)$ = 4.094, p = 0.044, η_p^2 = 0.022), but not when recent NSSI was included in the analysis ($F(1, 188)$ = 2.265, p = 0.134, η_p^2 = 0.012). There was no significant interaction between ED subtype and lifetime/recent NSSI in the prediction of mean depression scores.

2.2. Adjusted Body Mass Index (BMI).

We calculated BMI as weight/height^2 using the weight and height measures provided by the adolescents. Subsequently, we compared the BMI to representative values of adolescent girls in Belgium [54] and computed the adjusted BMI as [(BMI/Percentile 50 of BMI for age and gender) × 100]. The adjusted BMI results in a more accurate determination of the weight status of underaged adolescents and was therefore used throughout this study. In the current sample, 75.1% of the participating patients were underweight (n = 142, adjusted BMI ≤ 85) and 24.9% had a normal weight (n = 47, 85 < adjusted BMI < 120).

2.3. Non-Suicidal Self-Injury

NSSI was assessed using the Self-Injury Questionnaire-Treatment Related (SIQ-TR [55]), a self-report questionnaire that has been proven valid and reliable in female ED patient populations [52]. Patients responded to five yes/no items regarding the absence or presence of scratching, bruising, cutting, burning, and biting oneself. For each self-injurious behaviour, they were asked to complete a number of multiple-choice questions regarding the last time they engaged in that behaviour, how often it happened in certain timeframes, whether they experienced any pain during the behaviour, and which thoughts and feelings preceded and followed the NSSI. Based on these responses, recent NSSI (i.e., any form of NSSI within the last month) and lifetime NSSI (i.e., any form of NSSI throughout their life) were calculated. The Kuder–Richardson reliability coefficient for lifetime NSSI and recent NSSI was 0.673 and 0.489, respectively.

2.4. Temperament

The brief Dutch version of Cloninger's Temperament and Character Inventory (VTCI [31]) was administered to assess Cloninger's seven temperament scales; novelty seeking (NS), harm avoidance (HA), reward dependence (RD), persistence (PS), self-directedness (SD), cooperativeness (CO), and self-transcendence (ST) [29], [56]. Each of the seven scales contains 15 yes/no items, resulting in a total of 105 items. The VTCI was found to be a reliable and valid instrument in adolescent patient populations [57]. In the present study, Cronbach's alphas for these seven scales were, respectively, 0.702, 0.763, 0.609, 0.685, 0.806, 0.750, and 0.764.

2.5. Statistical Analyses

To analyse the frequency of the different lifetime/recent NSSI behaviours, descriptive statistics were calculated. The associations between the presence/absence of lifetime/recent NSSI and ED subtype (ED-R, ED-BP), were investigated with cross-tabulations and the Chi-square test statistic. Finally, to investigate temperamental differences between ED-R/ED-BP patients with and without lifetime/recent NSSI we performed two separate MANOVAs, both with the VTCI temperament scales as dependent variables and the ED subtype (ED-R, ED-BP) as an independent variable. In the first MANOVA, we included lifetime NSSI as an additional independent variable. In the second MANOVA, we included recent NSSI as an additional independent variable. In both MANOVAs, the interaction between ED and NSSI was included as the third and final independent variable. Partial eta squared (η^2) was used as a measure of effect size.

3. Results

3.1. Frequency of Lifetime and Recent NSSI

Overall, 59.8% of the patients ($n = 113$) engaged in at least one act of NSSI during their lifetime whereas 40.2% ($n = 76$) had never engaged in NSSI. The frequency of the reported lifetime NSSI behaviours, when ED-BP and ED-R were examined together, was distributed as follows: cutting (41.8%, $n = 79$), scratching (39.7%, $n = 75$), bruising (27%, $n = 51$), biting (16.9%, $n = 32$), and burning (7.9%, $n = 15$). Table 1 shows the number of different NSSI behaviours (NSSI versatility score) reported by the two ED subtypes. Patients with ED-R reported an average of 2.03 different lifetime NSSI behaviours (SD = 1.13), which was not significantly different from the average of 2.32 different lifetime NSSI behaviours (SD = 1.11) as reported by patients with ED-BP ($F(1, 112) = 1.741, p = 0.190$, partial $\eta^2 = 0.015$). However, on the level of individual NSSI behaviours, patients with ED-BP reported significantly more lifetime scratching, bruising, cutting, burning, and biting behaviours compared to patients with ED-R (see Table 2).

With respect to recent NSSI, 41.3% of patients ($n = 78$) reported at least one act of NSSI during the last week or the last month. The frequency of the recent NSSI behaviours, when ED-BP and ED-R were examined together, was distributed as follows: 25.4% ($n = 48$) reported scratching, 19.6% ($n = 37$) cutting, 12.7% ($n = 24$) bruising, 7.4% ($n = 14$) biting, and 2.6% ($n = 5$) burning oneself during the last week or month. The number of days one engaged in each of the five NSSI behaviours can be found in Supplementary Table S1. Patients with ED-R reported an average of 1.41 different recent NSSI behaviours (SD = 0.73), which was not significantly different from the average of 1.73 different recent NSSI behaviours (SD = 0.80) reported by patients with ED-BP ($F(1, 77) = 2.706, p = 0.104$, partial $\eta^2 = 0.034$, see Table 1). However, on the level of individual NSSI behaviours, patients with ED-BP reported significantly more recent scratching, bruising, cutting, and burning behaviours compared to ED-R patients (see Table 2).

Table 1. The number of different lifetime and recent NSSI behaviours ED-R and ED-BP engaged in.

	Lifetime NSSI n = 113				Recent NSSI n = 78			
	ED-R n = 36		ED-BP n = 77		ED-R n = 22		ED-BP n = 56	
	% [a]	n	% [a]	n	% [a]	n	% [a]	n
1 behaviour	38.9%	14	28.6%	22	68.2%	15	44.6%	25
2 behaviours	36.1%	13	29.9%	23	27.3%	6	41.1%	23
3 behaviours	13.9%	5	23.4%	18	0%	0	10.7%	6
4 behaviours	5.6%	2	16.9%	13	4.5%	1	3.6%	2
5 behaviours	5.6%	2	1.3%	1	0%	0	0%	0

Note. [a] Percentages of NSSI behaviours within ED category; NSSI = Non-Suicidal Self-Injury; ED-R = eating disorder of the restrictive type; ED-BP = eating disorder of the bingeing/purging type.

Table 2. Presence and absence of five NSSI behaviours in two ED subtypes.

	ED-R n = 87				ED-BP n = 102				
	Present		Absent		Present		Absent		
	% [a]	n	% [a]	n	% [a]	n	% [a]	n	$X^2_{(1)}$
Lifetime									
Scratch	28.7%	25	71.3%	62	49.0%	50	51.0%	52	8.071 **
Cut	24.1%	21	75.9%	66	56.9%	58	43.1%	44	20.669 ***
Bruise	17.2%	15	82.8%	72	35.3%	36	64.7%	66	7.766 **
Bite	10.3%	9	89.7%	78	22.5%	23	77.5%	79	4.972 *
Burn	3.4%	3	96.6%	84	11.8%	12	88.2%	90	4.444 *
Recent									
Scratch	12.6%	11	87.4%	76	36.3%	37	63.7%	65	13.838 ***
Cut	11.5%	10	88.5%	77	26.5%	27	73.5%	75	6.689 **
Bruise	4.6%	4	95.4%	83	19.6%	20	80.4%	82	9.542 **
Bite	6.9%	6	93.1%	81	7.8%	8	92.2%	94	0.061
Burn	0%	0	100%	87	4.9%	5	95.1%	97	4.381 *

Note. * $p < 0.05$, ** $p < 0.01$, *** $p < .001$; ED-R = Eating Disorder, Restrictive Subtype; ED-BP = Eating Disorder, Binge Eating/Purging Subtype, NSSI = Non-Suicidal Self-Injury. [a] Percentages of absent/present NSSI behaviour within each ED subtype.

The Pearson correlation coefficients between recent/lifetime NSSI and each of the seven temperament and character dimensions can be found in Table 3.

Table 3. Correlation coefficients between study variables.

	Lifetime NSSI	Recent NSSI	NS	HA	RD	PS	SD	CO
Recent NSSI	0.687 ***							
NS	−0.016	−0.118						
HA	0.205 **	0.252 ***	−0.370 ***					
RD	−0.098	−0.065	0.118	−0.203 **				
PS	−0.049	0.084	−0.345 ***	−0.024	0.121			
SD	−0.225 **	−0.204 **	0.108	−0.488 ***	0.130	0.089		
CO	0.043	0.103	−0.242 **	0.026	−0.214 **	−0.232 **	−0.213 **	
ST	0.093	0.087	0.089	−0.060	0.102	−0.095	−0.185 *	−0.071

Note. * $p < .05$, ** $p < .01$, *** $p < .001$; Significant correlation coefficients are marked in bold; NS = Novelty Seeking, HA = Harm Avoidance, RD = Reward Dependence, PS = Persistence, SD = Self-Directedness, CO = Cooperativeness, ST = Self-Transcendence.

3.2. Temperamental Differences between R/BP Patients with(out) Recent NSSI

With temperamental dimensions as the dependent variables, we included ED type, recent NSSI, and the ED × NSSI interaction as the three independent variables in our first MANOVA. Our results showed a main effect of ED subtype, indicating that there was a significant overall difference in temperamental dimensions, based on ED subtype (Wilks' Lambda = 0.903, $F(7, 179)$ = 2.733, p = 0.01, partial η^2 = 0.097). As reported in Table 4, the univariate results further clarified that ED-BP patients reported significantly more novelty seeking and less persistence compared to ED-R patients. Second, our results showed a main effect of recent NSSI, indicating a significant overall difference in temperamental dimensions based on presence or absence of recent NSSI (Wilks' Lambda = 0.88, $F(7, 179)$ = 3.478, p = 0.002, partial η^2 = 0.12). Namely, the univariate results in Table 4 show how those engaging in recent NSSI reported significantly less novelty seeking, more harm avoidance, and less self-directedness. Finally, there was no significant interaction between ED subtype and recent NSSI (Wilks' Lambda = 0.985, $F(7, 179)$ = 0.392, p = 0.906, partial η^2 = 0.015) in the prediction of temperamental differences. To control for age, we conducted an additional MANCOVA with temperamental dimensions as the dependent variables, ED subtype, recent NSSI and the ED × NSSI interaction as independent variables, and age as a control variable. Age did not reach significance: Wilks' Lambda = 0.974, $F(7, 179)$ = 0.682, p = 0.687, partial η^2 = 0.026 and all other results remained the same (i.e., main effect of ED subtype, main effect of recent NSSI, no interaction effect of ED subtype × NSSI).

Table 4. Means and standard deviations of the z-scores of the brief Dutch version of Cloninger's Temperament and Character Inventory for ED-R/BP patients with(out) recent NSSI (last week/last month).

	Main Effect ED Subtype					Main Effect Absence/Presence of $NSSI_R$				
	ED-R $n = 87$		ED-BP $n = 102$			$NSSI_R = 0$ $n = 111$		$NSSI_R = 1$ $n = 78$		
	M	SD	M	SD	$F(1, 185)$	M	SD	M	SD	$F(1, 185)$
NS	−0.25	(0.91)	0.24	(1.04)	18.47 ***	0.11	(1.02)	−0.13	(0.98)	9.04 **
HA	−0.00	(0.96)	−0.00	(1.02)	1.54	−0.21	(1.03)	0.29	(0.85)	14.23 ***
RD	0.02	(1.04)	−0.01	(0.95)	0.02	0.06	(1.07)	−0.07	(0.86)	0.78
PS	0.14	(.78)	−0.12	(1.15)	4.45 *	−0.07	(1.04)	0.10	(0.95)	2.94
SD	0.09	(1.12)	−0.11	(0.90)	0.03	0.16	(1.11)	−0.26	(0.78)	7.70 **
CO	0.07	(1.09)	−0.07	(0.92)	1.76	−0.09	(1.06)	0.12	(0.91)	2.75
ST	−0.12	(1.01)	0.08	(1.01)	1.08	−0.08	(0.93)	0.09	(1.11)	0.57

Note. * $p < 0.05$, ** $p < 0.01$, *** $p < 0.001$; ED-R = Eating Disorder, Restrictive Subtype; ED-BP = Eating Disorder, Binge Eating/Purging Subtype, $NSSI_R$ = Recent Non-Suicidal Self-Injury; NS = Novelty Seeking, HA = Harm Avoidance, RD = Reward Dependence, PS = Persistence, SD = Self-Directedness, CO = Cooperativeness, ST = Self-Transcendence.

3.3. Temperamental Differences between R/BP Patients with(out) Lifetime NSSI

In a second MANOVA, we substituted recent NSSI for lifetime NSSI while the other variables remained the same as in the first MANOVA. Thus, temperamental dimensions remained included as the dependent variables, and ED subtype, recent NSSI, and the ED × NSSI interaction term were included as the three independent variables. First, the main effect of ED subtype did not reach significance (Wilks' Lambda = 0.93, $F(7, 179)$ = 1.89, p = 0.073, partial η^2 = 0.069). This lack of significance could potentially be ascribed to a statistical artefact. Specifically, by substituting one independent variable with another, the degrees of freedom and the level of explained variance might deviate slightly, which can result in a different main effect. For completeness, we did still include the univariate level in Table 5. Second, our results showed a main effect of NSSI, indicating a significant overall difference in temperamental dimensions based on the presence or absence of lifetime NSSI (Wilks' Lambda = 0.921, $F(7, 179)$ = 2.198, p = 0.036, partial η^2 = 0.079). As described in Table 5, the univariate results clarified that those who engaged in lifetime NSSI reported significantly more harm avoidance and less self-directedness compared to those without lifetime NSSI. Contrasting our findings with recent NSSI, there was no significant difference in the level of novelty seeking between those with and without lifetime NSSI. Finally, the results did not show a significant interaction between ED subtype and lifetime NSSI (Wilks' Lambda = 0.98, $F(7, 179) = 0.49$, $p = 0.838$, partial $\eta^2 = 0.019$), indicating that the association between temperament and NSSI is similar in both ED subtypes. To control for age, we conducted an additional MANCOVA with temperamental dimensions as the dependent variables, ED subtype, lifetime NSSI and the ED × NSSI interaction as independent variables, and age as a control variable. Age did not reach significance: Wilks' Lambda = 0.974, $F(7, 179) = 0.667$, $p = 0.700$, partial $\eta^2 = 0.026$ and all other results remained the same (i.e., main effect of ED subtype, main effect of lifetime NSSI, no interaction effect of ED subtype × NSSI).

Table 5. Means and standard deviations of the z-scores of the brief Dutch version of Cloninger's Temperament and Character Inventory for ED-R/BP patients with(out) lifetime NSSI.

	Main Effect ED Subtype					Main Effect Absence/Presence of NSSI$_L$				
	ED-R n = 87		ED-BP n = 102			NSSI$_L$ = 0 n = 76		NSSI$_L$ = 1 n = 113		
	M	SD	M	SD	F(1, 185)1	M	SD	M	SD	F(1, 185)
NS	−0.25	(0.91)	0.24	(1.04)	12.68 ***	0.03	(0.99)	0.00	(1.03)	2.16
HA	0.00	(0.96)	0.00	(1.02)	0.97	−0.25	(0.97)	0.16	(0.98)	9.19 **
RD	0.02	(1.04)	−0.01	(0.95)	0.07	0.12	(1.01)	−0.07	(0.97)	1.82
PS	0.14	(0.78)	−0.12	(115)	1.87	0.06	(0.87)	−0.04	(1.09)	0.02
SD	0.09	(1.12)	−0.11	(0.90)	0.20	0.26	(1.16)	−0.20	(0.84)	7.82 **
CO	0.08	(1.08)	−0.08	(0.92)	1.92	−0.06	(1.05)	0.03	(0.98)	1.06
ST	−0.12	(1.01)	0.08	(1.01)	0.63	−0.12	(0.93)	0.07	(1.06)	0.82

Note. ** $p < 0.01$, *** $p < 0.001$; ED-R = Eating Disorder, Restrictive Subtype; ED-BP = Eating Disorder, Binge Eating/Purging Subtype, NSSI$_L$ = Lifetime Non-Suicidal Self-Injury; NS = Novelty Seeking, HA = Harm Avoidance, RD = Reward Dependence, PS = Persistence, SD = Self-Directedness, CO = Cooperativeness, ST = Self-Transcendence.

4. Discussion

The prevalence rates of NSSI in patients with any ED are alarmingly high. Both EDs and NSSI are driven by certain temperamental vulnerabilities, which, in their turn, increase the risk for later personality disorders [58,59]. To improve intervention of EDs and NSSI and prevention of later personality disorders, it is crucial to develop a thorough understanding of transdiagnostic temperamental vulnerabilities in adolescents. The vast majority of research on temperamental dimensions in EDs and NSSI has been conducted in adult samples [9,21]. Therefore, the current study examined temperament and character dimensions in a sample of adolescent ED patients with and without NSSI.

As a first aim, the present study investigated the prevalence of NSSI as well as the methods used to engage in NSSI. Our results confirmed the alarmingly high prevalence rates of NSSI previously found in young ED patients [16]. Namely, 60% of the current sample reported lifetime NSSI (i.e., having ever engaged in NSSI) and 40% of the sample reported recent NSSI (i.e., having engaged in NSSI in the past month). Thus, as this information was collected shortly after admission to an inpatient treatment facility, the latter indicates that 40% of the adolescents engaged in NSSI right before and/or during their ED treatment at the hospital ward. Interestingly, previous phenomenological qualitative research described how, during treatment, individuals with an ED experienced a loss of control when they were pressured to eat [60]. To lose control in one domain, be it due to treatment or due to pressure by parents or peers, often requires compensation in another domain [61]. Indeed, the participants in the phenomenological study reported how NSSI functioned as a means of control over anorectic thoughts and overwhelming emotions when they felt pressured to eat [60]. Future systematic research could investigate whether the high prevalence rates of NSSI found in the current study could be due to patients attempting to regain a sense of control.

Our results confirmed cutting and scratching to be the most common forms of NSSI, with, respectively, 42% and 40% of ED patients having engaged in these behaviours [16]. Moreover, each of the five assessed NSSI behaviours was significantly more common in patients of the ED-BP subtype, compared to the ED-R subtype. This ED-R/ED-BP distinction remained unchanged whether lifetime NSSI behaviours or recent NSSI behaviours were assessed. These findings align with previous research, which indicated that ED patients with bingeing/purging symptomatology engaged more often in NSSI overall [19–21]. Only for "biting oneself in the last month" the difference between ED-R and ED-BP did not reach significance, possibly due to the very low prevalence rate of "biting oneself" in both groups. Previously, research was lacking in how the specific NSSI behaviours compared between ED subtypes. With only four previous studies available, our results innovate by providing evidence for higher lifetime prevalence of cutting, scratching, bruising, biting, and burning in ED-BP compared to ED-R patients.

In search of a transdiagnostic mechanism in the ED–NSSI interplay, the current study investigated temperament and character dimensions as a second aim. First, our results showed significant differences in temperament and character based on ED subtype. Namely, patients with ED-BP showed significantly more novelty seeking and less persistence compared to patients with ED-R. Thus, the ED-BP patients had a greater tendency to seek out new, exciting experiences, possibly making impulsive decisions while doing so (high novelty seeking). Additionally, they were less likely than the ED-R patients to persevere and overcome setbacks or frustration, but rather felt frustrated or overwhelmed (low persistence). The differences between ED-BP and ED-R patients as found in the present study are consistent with ED literature [62–65]. Furthermore, both high novelty seeking and low persistence indicate impulse dysregulation, which previous research indeed attributed to bingeing and purging behaviours in ED patients [38]. Importantly, because NSSI too is characterised by high novelty seeking and low persistence [20,34–36], this temperamental profile might function as a transdiagnostic mechanism explaining the high comorbidity between NSSI and ED-BP specifically.

Second, our results showed significant differences in temperament and character based on the presence or absence of NSSI, regardless of the ED subtype. Specifically, ED patients with recent and/or lifetime NSSI reported less self-directedness and more harm avoidance compared to patients who were not engaging in NSSI. Thus, ED patients engaging in NSSI experience less control over their own emotions, they struggle to regulate themselves to set and reach goals (low self-directedness). They lack emotion regulation skills in comparison to adolescent ED patients who do not engage in NSSI. Moreover, NSSI in ED patients was associated with high harm avoidance, which indicates shyness and anxiety in social situations as well as excessive worrying and insecurity regarding interactions with others. These findings align with previous research indicating that emotion dysregulation and an increased amount of negative thoughts and feelings are common in those engaging in NSSI [5,61,66]. Specifically in ED patient populations, high harm avoidance can be related to self-punishment and rumination for those who self-injure. Patients with an ED who additionally engage in NSSI tend to be more concerned about meeting expectations of themselves and others, compared to patients with and ED who do not engage in NSSI [67]. In a qualitative study, ED patients in treatment facilities described how they would use NSSI to punish themselves when they failed to meet their own standards or felt that they had disappointed healthcare workers [60]. In conclusion, the temperamental profile of low self-directedness and high harm avoidance characterises patients with any ED who engage in NSSI.

Interestingly, when studying temperament in ED patients with recent NSSI, one more dimension besides low self-directedness and high harm avoidance showed up as significantly different in those with and without recent NSSI, regardless of ED subtype. Namely, ED patients engaging in recent NSSI reported significantly less novelty seeking. This stands for less curiosity and less impulsivity in those with recent NSSI, as they were less likely to seek out or be interested in new experiences, compared to ED patients without recent NSSI. Previous research, however, typically reported high levels of novelty seeking in adolescent patients engaging in NSSI [20,34–36]. Remarkably, these studies generally assessed lifetime, rather than recent, NSSI. A tentative suggestion as to why we found low novelty seeking in those with recent NSSI, could be the comorbidity of NSSI with depression at the time of assessment.

Depression is typified by high harm avoidance and low self-directedness and, importantly, low novelty seeking; a lack of interest, enthusiasm, and curiosity in one's surroundings [68]. At the time of assessment, those engaging in recent NSSI might have presented with more outspoken depressive symptoms, resulting in lower levels of novelty seeking compared to those without recent NSSI. Previous studies have indeed shown that at NSSI onset, impulsivity and high novelty seeking are common [34,69]. When individuals first start engaging in NSSI, often by experimenting once or twice with a certain method of self-injury, they are more likely to be looking for sensation or a new experience. Consequently, studies investigating lifetime NSSI report high novelty seeking [20,34–36]. However, research on various addictive behaviours suggested that, once the behaviour goes beyond mere experimenting and becomes a coping strategy in response to psychiatric distress, the impulsive, sensation-seeking function loses ground [70]. Rather, the emotion regulation function might become more salient as those with severe, persistent addiction(s) and comorbid psychopathology report engaging in the behaviour to avoid and regulate overwhelming negative affect [70]. Although future research should assess if this parallel with research on addiction is justified, our results on NSSI in ED patients do suggest a similar pattern. Namely, ED patients who present at a treatment facility with recent NSSI show temperamental and character dimensions resembling depression: low self-directedness, high harm avoidance, and, contrasting previous research, low novelty seeking.

The results of the current study support the focus on emotion and impulse dysregulation in evidence-based treatment of NSSI in ED patients. For instance, Dialectical Behavioural Therapy [71] and the Cutting Down treatment programme [72] have been proven effective in this specific patient population. High levels of harm avoidance could be related to serotonergic dysfunction [73] and could, therefore, be targeted by pharmacological treatments, for instance by the use of SSRI to focus on binge eating and self-harm in depressed ED patients [73]. Low levels of self-directedness could be treated by executive function training (e.g., by means of the "Playmancer" computer game [74]).

Although the present study contributes to the understanding of temperament ED patients with and without NSSI, our research is not without limitations. First, our findings are based solely on adolescent self-report questionnaires. Collecting self-report data from a single piece of information could result in reporting bias [75]. However, while we could have assessed peers, parents, or teachers about NSSI and its correlates, research has shown that people do not always observe internalising behaviours accurately in others [76], making NSSI and temperament often difficult to assess by other informants. Additionally, NSSI is often secretive [77] and people close to the adolescent who engages in NSSI, such as parents, are often unaware of the presence or severity of the NSSI [78]. Future research could embrace a multi-method approach and include structured or semi-structured interviews with the adolescents and/or use behavioural measures. Second, because the present study sample solely consists of adolescent girls in an eating disorder treatment facility, we cannot generalise the reported findings to male populations, younger or older individuals, or those receiving ambulatory care. Third, our conclusions are restricted by the cross-sectional nature of our study. As the field moves forward, longitudinal studies will be necessary to examine the developmental course and directionality of effects of temperament in ED patients with and without NSSI.

Supplementary Materials: The following are available online at http://www.mdpi.com/2077-0383/9/4/1207/s1, Table S1: Number of days individuals engaged in five NSSI behaviours in the last month.

Author Contributions: Conceptualisation, K.L., K.S., L.D. and L.C.; data curation, E.D.; formal analysis, T.B. and L.C.; funding acquisition, K.L. and L.C.; investigation, K.S., E.D. and L.D.; methodology, K.L. and L.C.; project administration, T.B., K.L., M.V., K.S., E.D., L.D. and L.C.; resources, K.L. and L.C.; software, E.D.; supervision, K.L. and L.C.; validation, T.B., K.L., M.V., K.S., E.D., L.D. and L.C.; writing—original draft, T.B. and L.C.; writing—review and editing, T.B., K.L., M.V., L.D. and L.C. All authors have read and agreed to the published version of the manuscript.

Funding: This research was funded by Fonds Wetenschappelijk Onderzoek (FWO, Belgium; grant number G062117N).

Conflicts of Interest: The authors declare no conflicts of interests. The funders had no role in the design of the study, in the collection, analyses, or interpretation of data; in the writing of the manuscript, or in the decision to publish the results.

References

1. Favazza, A.R. Nonsuicidal self-injury: Definition and classification. In *Understanding Nonsuicidal Self-Injury: Origins, Assessment, and Treatment*; American Psychological Association (APA): Washington, DC, USA, 2009; pp. 9–18.
2. Nock, M.K.; Cha, C. Psychological models of non-suicidal self-injury. In *Understanding Nonsuicidal Self-Injury: Origins, Assessment, and Treatment*; American Psychological Association (APA): Washington, DC, USA, 2009.
3. Nock, M.K. Why Do People Hurt Themselves? *Curr. Dir. Psychol. Sci.* **2009**, *18*, 78–83. [CrossRef]
4. Wilkinson, P.O.; Qiu, T.; Neufeld, S.; Jones, P.M.; Goodyer, I.M. Sporadic and recurrent non-suicidal self-injury before age 14 and incident onset of psychiatric disorders by 17 years: Prospective cohort study. *Br. J. Psychiatry* **2018**, *212*, 222–226. [CrossRef] [PubMed]
5. Buelens, T.; Luyckx, K.; Gandhi, A.; Kiekens, G.; Claes, L. Non-Suicidal Self-Injury in Adolescence: Longitudinal Associations with Psychological Distress and Rumination. *J. Abnorm. Child Psychol.* **2019**, *47*, 1569–1581. [CrossRef] [PubMed]
6. Crouch, W.; Wright, J. Deliberate Self-Harm at an Adolescent Unit: A Qualitative Investigation. *Clin. Child Psychol. Psychiatry* **2004**, *9*, 185–204. [CrossRef]
7. Gandhi, A.; Luyckx, K.; Baetens, I.; Kiekens, G.; Sleuwaegen, E.; Berens, A.; Maitra, S.; Claes, L. Age of onset of non-suicidal self-injury in Dutch-speaking adolescents and emerging adults: An event history analysis of pooled data. *Compr. Psychiatry* **2018**, *80*, 170–178. [CrossRef]
8. Muehlenkamp, J.J.; Claes, L.; Havertape, L.; Plener, P.L. International prevalence of adolescent non-suicidal self-injury and deliberate self-harm. *Child Adolesc. Psychiatry Ment. Health* **2012**, *6*, 10. [CrossRef]
9. Swannell, S.; Martin, G.; Page, A.N.; Hasking, P.; John, N.J.S. Prevalence of Nonsuicidal Self-Injury in Nonclinical Samples: Systematic Review, Meta-Analysis and Meta-Regression. *Suicide Life-Threat. Behav.* **2014**, *44*, 273–303. [CrossRef]
10. Buelens, T.; Luyckx, K.; Kiekens, G.; Gandhi, A.; Muehlenkamp, J.J.; Claes, L. Investigating the DSM-5 criteria for non-suicidal self-injury disorder in a community sample of adolescents. *J. Affect. Disord.* **2019**, *260*, 314–322. [CrossRef]
11. Muehlenkamp, J.J.; Claes, L.; Smits, D.; Peat, C.M.; Vandereycken, W. Non-suicidal self-injury in eating disordered patients: A test of a conceptual model. *Psychiatry Res.* **2011**, *188*, 102–108. [CrossRef]
12. Volpe, U.; Tortorella, A.; Manchia, M.; Monteleone, A.M.; Albert, U.; Monteleone, P. Eating disorders: What age at onset? *Psychiatry Research* **2016**, *238*, 225–227. [CrossRef]
13. Kostro, K.; Lerman, J.B.; Attia, E. The current status of suicide and self-injury in eating disorders: A narrative review. *J. Eat. Disord.* **2014**, *2*, 19. [CrossRef]
14. Peebles, R.; Wilson, J.L.; Lock, J.D. Self-Injury in Adolescents With Eating Disorders: Correlates and Provider Bias. *J. Adolesc. Health* **2010**, *48*, 310–313. [CrossRef] [PubMed]
15. Claes, L.; Luyckx, K.; Bijttebier, P.; Turner, B.J.; Ghandi, A.; Smets, J.; Norré, J.; Van Assche, L.; Verheyen, E.; Goris, Y.; et al. Non-Suicidal Self-Injury in Patients with Eating Disorder: Associations with Identity Formation Above and Beyond Anxiety and Depression. *Eur. Eat. Disord. Rev.* **2014**, *23*, 119–125. [CrossRef] [PubMed]
16. Svirko, E.; Hawton, K. Self-Injurious Behavior and Eating Disorders: The Extent and Nature of the Association. *Suicide Life-Threat. Behav.* **2007**, *37*, 409–421. [CrossRef] [PubMed]
17. Sansone, R.A.; Sansone, L.A. Personality Disorders as Risk Factors for Eating Disorders. *Nutr. Clin. Pract.* **2010**, *25*, 116–121. [CrossRef] [PubMed]
18. McElroy, S.L.; Frye, M.A.; Hellemann, G.; Altshuler, L.; Leverich, G.S.; Suppes, T.; Keck, P.E.; Nolen, W.A.; Kupka, R.; Post, R.M. Prevalence and correlates of eating disorders in 875 patients with bipolar disorder. *J. Affect. Disord.* **2011**, *128*, 191–198. [CrossRef]

19. Favaro, A.; Santonastaso, P. Self-injurious behaviour in anorexia nervosa. *J. Nerv. Ment. Dis.* **2000**, *188*, 537–543. [CrossRef]
20. Davico, C.; Amianto, F.; Gaiotti, F.; Lasorsa, C.; Peloso, A.; Bosia, C.; Vesco, S.; Arletti, L.; Reale, L.; Vitiello, B. Clinical and personality characteristics of adolescents with anorexia nervosa with or without non-suicidal self-injurious behavior. *Compr. Psychiatry* **2019**, *94*, 152115. [CrossRef]
21. Bühren, K.; Schwarte, R.; Fluck, F.; Timmesfeld, N.; Krei, M.; Egberts, K.; Pfeiffer, E.; Fleischhaker, C.; Wewetzer, C.; Herpertz-Dahlmann, B. Comorbid Psychiatric Disorders in Female Adolescents with First-Onset Anorexia Nervosa. *Eur. Eat. Disord. Rev.* **2013**, *22*, 39–44. [CrossRef]
22. Perez, S.; Marco, J.H.; Cañabate, M. Non-suicidal self-injury in patients with eating disorders: Prevalence, forms, functions, and body image correlates. *Compr. Psychiatry* **2018**, *84*, 32–38. [CrossRef]
23. Claes, L.; Vandereycken, W.; Vertommen, H. Personality traits in eating disordered patients with and without self-injurious behaviours. *J. Personal. Disord.* **2004**, *18*, 399–404. [CrossRef]
24. Favaro, A.; Santonastaso, P. Different types of self-injurious behavior in bulimia nervosa. *Compr. Psychiatry* **1999**, *40*, 57–60. [CrossRef]
25. Claes, L.; Vandereycken, W.; Vertommen, H. Eating-disordered patients with and without self-injurious behaviours: A comparison of psychopathological features. *Eur. Eat. Disord. Rev.* **2003**, *11*, 379–396. [CrossRef]
26. Claes, L.; Vandereycken, W.; Vertommen, H. Self-injurious behaviors in eating-disordered patients. *Eat. Behav.* **2001**, *2*, 263–272. [CrossRef]
27. Baetens, I.; Claes, L.; Willem, L.; Muehlenkamp, J.; Bijttebier, P. The relationship between non-suicidal self-injury and temperament in male and female adolescents based on child- and parent-report. *Pers. Individ. Differ.* **2011**, *50*, 527–530. [CrossRef]
28. Claes, L.; Norré, J.; Van Assche, L.; Bijttebier, P. Non-suicidal self-injury (functions) in eating disorders: Associations with reactive and regulative temperament. *Personal. Individ. Differ.* **2014**, *57*, 65–69. [CrossRef]
29. Cloninger, C.R.; Przybeck, T.R.; Svrakic, D.M.; Wetzel, R.D. *The Temperament and Character Inventory (TCI): A Guide to Its Development and Use*; Center for Psychobiology of Personality: St. Louis, MI, USA, 1994.
30. De Fruyt, F.; Van De Wiele, L.; Van Heeringen, C. Cloninger's Psychobiological Model of Temperament and Character and the Five-Factor Model of Personality. *Personal. Individ. Differ.* **2000**, *29*, 441–452. [CrossRef]
31. Duijsens, I.J.; Spinhoven, P. *Handleiding Van De Nederlandse Verkorte Temperament En Karakter Vragenlijst*; Datec: Leiderdorp, The Netherlands, 2001.
32. Cloninger, C.R.; Svrakic, D.M.; Przybeck, T.R. A Psychobiological Model of Temperament and Character. *Arch. Gen. Psychiatry* **1993**, *50*, 975. [CrossRef]
33. Evans, D.E.; Rothbart, M.K. Developing a model for adult temperament. *J. Res. Personal.* **2007**, *41*, 868–888. [CrossRef]
34. Tschan, T.; Peter-Ruf, C.; Schmid, M.; In-Albon, T. Temperament and character traits in female adolescents with nonsuicidal self-injury disorder with and without comorbid borderline personality disorder. *Child Adolesc. Psychiatry Ment. Health* **2017**, *11*, 4. [CrossRef]
35. Joyce, P.R.; Light, K.J.; Rowe, S.; Cloninger, C.R.; Kennedy, M.A. Self-Mutilation and Suicide Attempts: Relationships to Bipolar Disorder, Borderline Personality Disorder, Temperament and Character. *Aust. N. Z. J. Psychiatry* **2010**, *44*, 250–257. [CrossRef] [PubMed]
36. Hefti, S.; In-Albon, T.; Schmeck, K.; Schmid, M. Temperaments- und Charaktereigenschaften und selbstverletzendes Verhalten bei Jugendlichen. *Nervenheilkd* **2013**, *32*, 45–53. [CrossRef]
37. Bresin, K.; Carter, D.L.; Gordon, K.H. The relationship between trait impulsivity, negative affective states, and urge for nonsuicidal self-injury: A daily diary study. *Psychiatry Res.* **2013**, *205*, 227–231. [CrossRef] [PubMed]
38. Nock, M.K.; Prinstein, M.J. Contextual Features and Behavioral Functions of Self-Mutilation Among Adolescents. *J. Abnorm. Psychol.* **2005**, *114*, 140–146. [CrossRef] [PubMed]
39. Doran, N.; McChargue, D.; Cohen, L. Impulsivity and the reinforcing value of cigarette smoking. *Addict. Behav.* **2007**, *32*, 90–98. [CrossRef]
40. Lüdtke, J.; Weizenegger, B.; Rauber, R.; Contin, B.; In-Albon, T.; Schmid, M. The influence of personality traits and emotional and behavioral problems on repetitive nonsuicidal self-injury in a school sample. *Compr. Psychiatry* **2017**, *74*, 214–223. [CrossRef]

41. Wolz, I.; Agüera, Z.; Granero, R.; Jiménez-Murcia, S.; Gratz, K.L.; Menchón, J.M.; Fernández-Aranda, F. Emotion regulation in disordered eating: Psychometric properties of the Difficulties in Emotion Regulation Scale among Spanish adults and its interrelations with personality and clinical severity. *Front. Psychol.* **2015**, *6*. [CrossRef]
42. Andover, M.S.; Morris, B.W. Expanding and Clarifying the Role of Emotion Regulation in Nonsuicidal Self-Injury. *Can. J. Psychiatry* **2014**, *59*, 569–575. [CrossRef]
43. Ohmann, S.; Schuch, B.; König, M.; Blaas, S.; Fliri, C.; Popow, C. Self-Injurious Behavior in Adolescent Girls. *Psychopathol.* **2008**, *41*, 226–235. [CrossRef]
44. Fassino, S.; Abbate-Daga, G.; Amianto, F.; Leombruni, P.; Boggio, S.; Rovera, G.G. Temperament and character profile of eating disorders: A controlled study with the Temperament and Character Inventory. *Int. J. Eat. Disord.* **2002**, *32*, 412–425. [CrossRef]
45. Fassino, S.; Abbate-Daga, G.; Pierò, A.; Leombruni, P.; Rovera, G.G. Anger and personality in eating disorders. *J. Psychosom. Res.* **2001**, *51*, 757–764. [CrossRef] [PubMed]
46. Klump, K.L.; Bulik, C.M.; Pollice, C.; A Halmi, K.; Fichter, M.; Berrettini, W.H.; Devlin, B.; Strober, M.; Kaplan, A.; Woodside, D.B.; et al. Temperament and Character in Women with Anorexia Nervosa. *J. Nerv. Ment. Dis.* **2000**, *188*, 559–567. [CrossRef] [PubMed]
47. Cassin, S.E.; Von Ranson, K.M. Personality and eating disorders: A decade in review. *Clin. Psychol. Rev.* **2005**, *25*, 895–916. [CrossRef] [PubMed]
48. Strober, M. Disorders of the self in anorexia nervosa: An organismic-developmental perspective. In *Psychodynamic Theory and Treatment of Anorexia Nervosa and Bulimia*; Guildford Press: New York, NY, USA, 1992; pp. 354–373.
49. Brewerton, T.D.; Hand, L.D.; Bishop, E.R. The tridimensional personality questionnaire in eating disorder patients. *Int. J. Eat. Disord.* **1993**, *14*, 213–218. [CrossRef] [PubMed]
50. Bulik, C.M.; Sullivan, P.F.; Fear, J.L.; Pickering, A. Outcome of anorexia nervosa: Eating attitudes, personality, and parental bonding. *Int. J. Eat. Disord.* **2000**, *28*, 139–147. [PubMed]
51. Vandereycken, W. The eating disorder evaluation scale (EDES). *Eat. Disord.* **1993**, *1*, 115–122. [CrossRef]
52. Claes, L.; Vandereycken, W. The Self-Injury Questionnaire-Treatment Related (SIQ-TR): Construction, reliability, and validity in a sample of female eating disorder patients. In *Psychological Tests*; Goldfarb, M., Ed.; Nova Science: New York, NY, USA, 2007.
53. Jorgenson, J. Symptom Checklist-90-Revised. *Encycl. Personal. Individ. Differ.* **2017**, 1–4. [CrossRef]
54. Roelants, M.; Hauspie, R. Groeicurven 2-20 jaar, Vlaanderen 2004 [Growth Charts 2–20 Years, Flanders 2004]. 2004. Available online: http://www.vub.ac.be/groeicurven (accessed on 11 March 2020).
55. Claes, L.; Vandereycken, W. The Self-Injury Questionnaire-Treatment Related. In *Psychological Tests and Testing Research Trends*; Goldfarb, P.M., Ed.; Nova Science: New York, NY, USA, 2007; pp. 111–139.
56. Svrakic, D.M.; Whitehead, C.; Przybeck, T.R.; Cloninger, C.R. Differential Diagnosis of Personality Disorders by the Seven-Factor Model of Temperament and Character. *Arch. Gen. Psychiatry* **1993**, *50*, 991. [CrossRef]
57. Duijsens, I.J.; Spinhoven, P.; Verschuur, M.; Eurelings-Bontekoe, E.H.M. De ontwikkeling van de nederlandse verkorte temperament en karakter vragenlijst (TCI-105). *Ned. Tijdschr. Psychol.* **1999**, *54*, 276–283.
58. Cloninger, C.R. A practical way to diagnosis personality disorder: A proposal. *J. Personal. Disord.* **2000**, *14*, 99–108. [CrossRef]
59. Mervielde, I.; De Clercq, B.; De Fruyt, F.; Van Leeuwen, K. Temperament, Personality, and Developmental Psychopathology as Childhood Antecedents of Personality Disorders. *J. Personal. Disord.* **2005**, *19*, 171–201. [CrossRef] [PubMed]
60. Verschueren, S.; Berends, T.; Kool-Goudzwaard, N.; Van Huigenbosch, E.; Gamel, C.; Dingemans, A.; Van Elburg, A.; Van Meijel, B. Patients With Anorexia Nervosa Who Self-Injure: A Phenomenological Study. *Perspect. Psychiatr. Care* **2014**, *51*, 63–70. [CrossRef] [PubMed]
61. Muehlenkamp, J.J.; Engel, S.G.; Wadeson, A.; Crosby, R.D.; Wonderlich, S.A.; Simonich, H.; Mitchell, J.E. Emotional states preceding and following acts of non-suicidal self-injury in bulimia nervosa patients. *Behav. Res. Ther.* **2008**, *47*, 83–87. [CrossRef] [PubMed]
62. Claes, L.; Vandereycken, W. Is There a Link between Traumatic Experiences and Self-Injurious Behaviors in Eating-Disordered Patients? *Eat. Disord.* **2007**, *15*, 305–315. [CrossRef] [PubMed]

63. DeJong, H.; Oldershaw, A.; Sternheim, L.; Samarawickrema, N.; Kenyon, M.; Broadbent, H.; Lavender, A.; Startup, H.; Treasure, J.; Schmidt, U. Quality of life in anorexia nervosa, bulimia nervosa and eating disorder not-otherwise-specified. *J. Eat. Disord.* **2013**, *1*, 43. [CrossRef]
64. Sanci, L.; Coffey, C.; Olsson, C.; Reid, S.; Carlin, J.; Patton, G. Childhood Sexual Abuse and Eating Disorders in Females. *Arch. Pediatr. Adolesc. Med.* **2008**, *162*, 261. [CrossRef]
65. Vanderlinden, J.; Schoevaerts, K.; Simons, A.; Eede, U.V.D.; Bruffaerts, R.; Serra, R.; Van Roie, E.; Vervaet, M.; Janssens, N.; Vrieze, E. Sociodemographic and clinical characteristics of eating disorder patients treated in the specialized residential settings in Belgium. *Eat. Weight. Disord.—Stud. Anorexia, Bulim. Obes.* **2020**, 1–7. [CrossRef]
66. Klonsky, E.D.; Victor, S.; Saffer, B.Y. Nonsuicidal self-injury: What we know, and what we need to know. *Can. J. Psychiatry* **2014**, *59*, 565–568. [CrossRef]
67. Claes, L.; Soenens, B.; Vansteenkiste, M.; Vandereycken, W. The Scars of the Inner Critic: Perfectionism and Nonsuicidal Self-Injury in Eating Disorders. *Eur. Eat. Disord. Rev.* **2011**, *20*, 196–202. [CrossRef]
68. Bijttebier, P.; Beck, I.; Claes, L.; Vandereycken, W. Gray's Reinforcement Sensitivity Theory as a framework for research on personality–psychopathology associations. *Clin. Psychol. Rev.* **2009**, *29*, 421–430. [CrossRef]
69. Riley, E.N.; Combs, J.L.; Jordan, C.E.; Smith, G.T. Negative Urgency and Lack of Perseverance: Identification of Differential Pathways of Onset and Maintenance Risk in the Longitudinal Prediction of Nonsuicidal Self-Injury. *Behav. Ther.* **2015**, *46*, 439–448. [CrossRef] [PubMed]
70. Brand, M.; Wegmann, E.; Stark, R.; Müller, A.; Wölfling, K.; Robbins, T.W.; Potenza, M.N. The Interaction of Person-Affect-Cognition-Execution (I-PACE) model for addictive behaviors: Update, generalization to addictive behaviors beyond internet-use disorders, and specification of the process character of addictive behaviors. *Neurosci. Biobehav. Rev.* **2019**, *104*, 1–10. [CrossRef] [PubMed]
71. Linehan, M.M. *Skills Training Manual for Treating Borderline Personality Disorder*; Guildford Press: New York, NY, USA, 1993.
72. Taylor, L. *Cutting Down: A CBT Workbook for Treating Young People who Self-Harm*; Informa UK Limited: Colchester, UK, 2015.
73. Claes, L.; Muehlenkamp, J.J. Non-suicidal self-injury and eating disorders: Dimensions of self-harm. In *Non-Suicidal Self-Injury in Eating Disorders*; Claes, L., Muehlenkamp, J.J., Eds.; Springer: Berlin/Heidelberg, Germany, 2014; pp. 3–18.
74. Giner-Bartolomé, C.; Fagundo, A.B.; Sanchez, I.; Jiménez-Murcia, S.; Santamaría, J.J.; Ladouceur, R.; Menchón, J.M.; Fernández-Aranda, F. Can an intervention based on a serious videogame prior to cognitive behavioral therapy be helpful in bulimia nervosa? A clinical case study. *Front. Psychol.* **2015**, *6*, 1–9. [CrossRef] [PubMed]
75. Podsakoff, P.M.; MacKenzie, S.B.; Lee, J.-Y.; Podsakoff, N.P. Common method biases in behavioral research: A critical review of the literature and recommended remedies. *J. Appl. Psychol.* **2003**, *88*, 879–903. [CrossRef]
76. Achenbach, T.M.; Mcconaughy, S.H.; Howell, C.T. Child/adolescent behavioral and emotional problems: Implications of cross-informant correlations for situational specificity. *Psychol. Bull.* **1987**, *101*, 213–232. [CrossRef]
77. Baetens, I.; Claes, L.; Muehlenkamp, J.; Grietens, H.; Onghena, P. Non-Suicidal and Suicidal Self-Injurious Behavior among Flemish Adolescents: A Web-Survey. *Arch. Suicide Res.* **2011**, *15*, 56–67. [CrossRef]
78. Baetens, I.; Claes, L.; Onghena, P.; Grietens, H.; Van Leeuwen, K.; Pieters, C.; Wiersema, J.R.; Griffith, J.W. The effects of nonsuicidal self-injury on parenting behaviors: A longitudinal analyses of the perspective of the parent. *Child Adolesc. Psychiatry Ment. Health* **2015**, *9*, 24. [CrossRef]

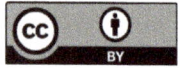

© 2020 by the authors. Licensee MDPI, Basel, Switzerland. This article is an open access article distributed under the terms and conditions of the Creative Commons Attribution (CC BY) license (http://creativecommons.org/licenses/by/4.0/).

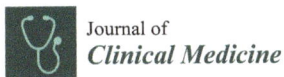

Article

Cortical Complexity in Anorexia Nervosa: A Fractal Dimension Analysis

Enrico Collantoni [1,*], Christopher R. Madan [2], Paolo Meneguzzo [1], Iolanna Chiappini [1], Elena Tenconi [1,3], Renzo Manara [1] and Angela Favaro [1,3]

1. Department of Neurosciences, University of Padua, Via Giustiniani, 2-35128 Padova, Italy; meneguzzo.p@gmail.com (P.M.); iolanna.chiappini@gmail.com (I.C.); elena.tenconi@unipd.it (E.T.); renzo.manara@unipd.it (R.M.); angela.favaro@unipd.it (A.F.)
2. School of Psychology, University of Nottingham, Nottingham NG7 2QL, UK; Christopher.Madan@nottingham.ac.uk
3. Padua Neuroscience Center, University of Padua, 35128 Padova, Italy
* Correspondence: enrico.collantoni@unipd.it; Tel.: +39-0-498-218-175

Received: 18 February 2020; Accepted: 17 March 2020; Published: 19 March 2020

Abstract: Fractal Dimension (FD) has shown to be a promising means to describe the morphology of cortical structures across different neurologic and psychiatric conditions, displaying a good sensitivity in capturing atrophy processes. In this study, we aimed at exploring the morphology of cortical areas by means of FD in 58 female patients with Anorexia Nervosa (AN) (38 currently underweight and 20 fully recovered) and 38 healthy controls (HC). All participants underwent high-resolution MRI. Surface extraction was completed using FreeSurfer, FD was computed using the calcFD toolbox. The whole cortex mean FD value was lower in acute AN patients compared to HC ($p < 0.001$). Recovered AN patients did not show differences in the global FD when compared to HC. However, some brain areas showed higher FD in patients than controls, while others showed the opposite pattern. Parietal regions showed lower FD in both AN groups. In acute AN patients, the FD correlated with age ($p < 0.001$), body mass index ($p = 0.019$) and duration of illness ($p = 0.011$). FD seems to represent a feasible method to explore cortical complexity in patients with AN since it demonstrated to be sensitive to the effects of both severity and duration of malnutrition.

Keywords: eating disorders; anorexia nervosa; malnutrition; neuroimaging; fractal dimension; cortical complexity

1. Introduction

Anorexia Nervosa (AN) is a severe psychiatric disorder with a typical onset during adolescence [1], characterized by severe and prolonged alterations of energy intake and high levels of mortality. Although there is a notable interest in understanding the effects of starvation on the brain, a full characterization of brain changes in patients with AN is still at its first stages [2]. The onset of AN typically occurs when neurodevelopment is still ongoing [3] and it is possible that the effects of malnutrition have a different impact in brain areas that are in a sensitive period of growth at the time of AN onset [4]. Moreover, evidence suggests that prenatal and perinatal factors are involved in the pathogenesis of AN and, for this reason, it is not easy to distinguish the structural brain alterations preceding the AN onset from the ones that might be a consequence of the disorder.

Most studies to date employed a Voxel-Based Morphometry approach and found a globally reduced GM volume, but inconsistent results emerged in the identification of specific regional changes in AN [2]. In addition, only few studies found a significant correlation with body weight or amount of weight loss, and almost none with age of onset or duration of illness [5]. The use of a Surface-Based Morphometry approach did not result in more consistent findings. In fact, while some studies reported a correlation between cortical thickness and BMI, others failed in evidencing a relationship between these two parameters [6–9]. Generally, a reduction of cortical thickness is described in different studies, but the extent of the reduction varies from almost the whole cortex to about a quarter or one third [6,9].

Other surface-based methods, such as the local gyrification index and cortical folding, have been employed to describe brain cortical changes in patients with AN [10–12]. Both measures displayed significant alterations in acute patients, but the interpretation of these findings is not clear, since gyrification tends to develop early in childhood and its alteration is usually attributed to prenatal or very early insults [13].

A novel way to quantify and analyze the cortex from a morphological and structural point of view has been offered by fractal geometry [14], which is specifically designed for the analysis of complex structural and morphological patterns [15]. The application of fractal geometry to neuroscience is consistent with the evidence, already highlighted by the increasing application of complex network science to neuroimaging data, that the central nervous system is organized in nested and hierarchical organization patterns that need to balance both regularity and randomness [16]. This multi-level structural organization of the brain seems to be well-described by fractal geometry, which is based on the concept of "self-similarity" [17]. Since the fractal properties of the cerebral cortex arise secondarily to folding [18], structural MRI studies used fractal dimension to quantify the morphological complexity of the cortex and its convolutional properties both in clinical and non-clinical samples [19–22].

Two types of fractal dimension can be considered, depending on whether the volume of the gray matter is included in the computation. Incorporating the volume of the gray matter into the computation ensures that changes in cortical thickness are directly integrated within the fractal dimension estimation. Thus, interestingly, fractal dimension appears to co-vary with both cortical thickness and gyrification [22]. Furthermore, it also appears to demonstrate a great sensitivity to detect cortical atrophy and to describe age-related effects [15,23]. Prior studies have suggested that FD may provide distinct information from the ones that are provided by conventional cortical structural indices such as gyrification, cortical thickness and sulcal morphology, and evidenced the presence of global and regional FD alterations in different psychiatric disorders such as ADHD, schizophrenia, bipolar and obsessive-compulsive disorders [20,21,24–27]. The use of FD to identify unique characteristics of cortical morphology could be particularly useful in the evaluation of AN, since this disorder has been shown to be characterized by complex (and not entirely determined) patterns of brain morphological alterations. Consistently with this, the first study investigating FD in AN [28] highlighted different patterns of absolute mean curvature and FD alterations in acute AN patients when compared to healthy subjects. More specifically, this research evidenced the presence of a higher FD in the left precentral gyrus as well as a trend toward a lower FD in frontal and occipital areas in patients with AN [28].

In the present study, we used a surface-based approach to explore the use of FD to describe cortical complexity in patients with AN. We hypothesize a reduction of cortical complexity in acute underweight patients and an improvement of this feature after remission.

2. Methods

Fifty-eight patients with AN (38 with acute AN and 20 in full remission) and 38 HC were included in the study. The sample included was the same as in a previous study [29]. Mean age of the patients was 26.1 years (SD = 7.2) ranging from 15.5 to 40.5 years old. Patients with AN were recruited from the Padova Hospital Eating Disorders Unit. AN was defined according to DSM-5 criteria. All patients fulfilling the inclusion criteria who were in treatment or referred to the Unit while the study was being carried out were asked to participate. A sample of HC similar to the patient group in age, ethnicity, educational level and hand lateralization was recruited from the same geographical area.

Patients who recovered from AN had full AN in their lifetime but have been asymptomatic for at least 6 months prior to the time of scanning [mean remission time: 38.5 months (SD = 33.2); range = 6–96 months]. The main clinical characteristics of the sample are reported in Table 1. Exclusion criteria for the recovered group were bingeing, food restriction, excessive exercise, amenorrhea, fasting and purging in the last 6 months. In the year following the study, none of the recovered patients relapsed. Moreover, recovered patients were within the normal weight range at the time of the scan (BMI ≥ 18.5). Exclusion criteria for all subjects were male gender, history of head trauma or injury with loss of consciousness, history of any serious neurological or medical illness, active use of systemic steroids, pregnancy, active suicidality or major depression, history of substance/alcohol abuse or dependence, bipolar disorder or schizophrenia spectrum disorder, moderate mental impairment (IQ < 60) or learning disabilities, use of medications other than antidepressants and known contraindications to conventional MRI. For healthy women, additional exclusion criteria were a history of any psychiatric disorder and the presence of first-degree relatives with an eating disorder.

At the time of recruitment, some individuals were excluded from the study: five AN patients were under antipsychotic medication and/or reported severe comorbidity; one AN patient and one healthy subject reported a previous head trauma; one AN patient, three recovered AN and two healthy subjects were not available to undergo MRI scanning when scheduled. The final sample comprised of 96 women (38 with AN, 20 recovered from AN and 38 HC). No further subject was excluded due to problems with scan acquisition, gross brain alterations or motion artifacts.

Ethical permission was obtained from the ethics committee of the Padova Hospital on 10 June 2008 (ID 1598P). After completely describing the study to the subjects, written informed consent was obtained.

Table 1. Socio-demographic and clinical characteristics of the sample.

	AN (n = 38)		AN-REC (n = 20)		HC (n = 38)		AN vs. HC	AN-REC. vs. HC
	Mean	SD	Mean	SD	Mean	SD	Z (p)	Z (p)
Age (years)	26.1	7.2	26.3	7.0	25.2	6.7	0.38 (0.701)	0.44 (0.659)
Baseline BMI (kg/m^2)	16.0	1.8	19.6	1.6	21.6	3.0	7.42 (0.000)	3.09 (0.002)
Lowest BMI (kg/m^2)	14.0	1.8	15.7	1.4	19.8	2.5	7.17 (0.000)	5.35 (0.000)
Weight loss (kg)	7.1	2.8	5.2	3.1	3.4	1.7	-	-
Age of onset (years)	18.3	5.0	17.7	3.2	-	-	-	-
Duration of illness (months)	78.6	81.2	45.7	65.0	-	-	-	-
Duration of recovery (months)			45.4	47.0	-	-	-	-
Edinburgh laterality index	57.1	37.5	60.0	35.2	55.0	42.0	0.52 (0.603)	0.32 (0.749)
Education (years)	14.2	2.2	14.1	2.6	15.4	2.3	2.63 (0.009)	1.94 (0.053)
Drive to thinness	9.9	6.1	-	-	2.3	4.2	5.492 (0.000)	-
Depression	1.4	0.8	-	-	0.7	0.6	3.844 (0.000)	-
Trait anxiety	56.6	9.7	-	-	39.3	9.6	5.883 (0.000)	-
Cortex volume (mm^3)	440,936	38,526	456,932	36,916	458,753	31,225	9.55 (0.003)	0.07 (0.80)
Gyrification Index	2.85	0.09	2.90	0.09	2.90	0.11	2.09 (0.04)	0.08 (0.93)
Surface area (mm^2)	160,640	13,527	157,348	9381	165,082	12,113	2.20 (0.142)	6.11 (0.017)
Cortical Thickness (mm)	2.49	0.12	2.51	0.11	2.48	0.12	0.52 (0.14)	1.05 (0.30)

GLM, including Total Intracranial Volume as a covariate of no interest; BMI = body mass index Clinical assessment and Follow-up.

A diagnostic interview according to the Eating Disorders Section of the Structured Clinical Interview for DSM-5 [30] was performed in all subjects. A semi-structured interview was also used to collect socio-demographic and clinical variables [29,31]. Depressive and obsessive-compulsive symptoms were assessed by means of the Hopkins Symptoms Checklist [32]. Eating psychopathology was assessed by the Eating Disorders Inventory [33]. The Edinburgh Handedness Inventory [34] was also administered.

All subjects were recruited at the Eating Disorder Unit of the Hospital of Padova, fulfilled the diagnosis for AN according to DSM-IV criteria and were medically stable at the time of scanning. AN diagnosis was established by experienced senior consultants. Different diagnostic subtypes were observed at the time of scanning: 32 AN patients (84%) were restrictive, six AN patients were of the binge-eating/purging subtype and seven patients who were restrictive at the time of the present study reported previous recurrent binge eating and/or purging. Fourteen AN patients and four recovered women were under treatment with antidepressant drugs at the time the study was conducted (acute AN: one case mirtazapine, two paroxetine, two escitalopram, one fluoxetine, eight sertraline; recovered AN: four sertraline).

2.1. MRI Data Acquisition

Data were collected on a Philips Achieva 1.5 Tesla MRI scanner equipped with an eight-channel standard quadrature head coil equipped for echo-planar imaging. A high-resolution three-dimensional (3D) T1-weighted anatomical image was also acquired, in a gradient-echo sequence (repetition-time = 20 s, echo time = 3.78 ms, flip angle = 20°, 160 sagittal slices, acquisition voxel size = $1 \times 0.66 \times 0.66$ mm, field of view 21–22 cm).

2.2. Data Processing and Statistics

Data processing was performed using the FreeSurfer package (Martinos Center for Biomedical Imaging, Massachusetts General Hospital, Boston) version 5.3.0 [35]. The preprocessing was carried out according to the standard description using the following steps: skull-stripping and intensity correction, gray matter–white matter boundary determination for each cortical hemisphere using tissue intensity and neighborhood constraints, and finally, tessellation of the resulting surface boundary to generate multiple vertices across the whole brain before inflating.

Surface reconstruction and segmentation were inspected, and minor manual intervention was performed according to FreeSurfer guidelines. After cortical reconstruction, the cortex was parcellated based on individual gyral and sulcal structures [36]. Cortical thickness and local gyrification index were calculated as described in our previous work [10].

A freely available MATLAB toolbox, calcFD [15] (http://cmadan.github.io/calcFD/), was used to compute the fractal dimension of the cortical ribbon and of parcellated regions of the cortex. The toolbox uses intermediate files generated as part of the standard FreeSurfer analysis pipeline to perform the calculation. Fractal dimension has been shown to be more robust to alignment variability [37] and head motion [38]. We calculated FD of the cortical ribbon (i.e., FD of the filled volume) [15] using the dilation algorithm implemented in the calcFD toolbox and box sizes of 1, 2, and 4. Figure 1 illustrates the fractal dimension calculation for a representative parcellated cortical surface Correlation was performed using Spearmen's ρ (rho), while group comparisons were performed by means of GLM with age and hand-lateralization as covariates of no interest when appropriate. Given that FD values in the different areas of the brain cannot be considered as independent, in order to control for multiple tests, we adjusted for the False Discovery Rate (FDR) [39].

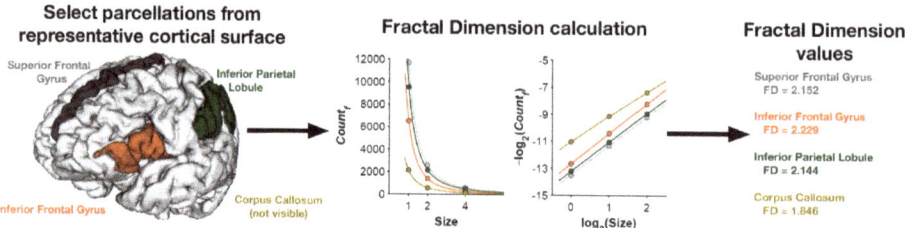

Figure 1. Illustration of the fractal dimension calculation. Individual parcellated regions (or the entire cortical ribbon) are isolated. For each region, the number of voxels at each respective box size is across different spatial resolutions, adjusting for alignment of the 'boxes' to the structure using the dilation algorithm. The counts and box sizes are then log-log transformed and the slope calculated. The slope in log-log space is taken as the fractal dimension of the region.

3. Results

Table 2 shows the average FD values of the three groups in the whole brain and in the frontal, parietal, temporal and occipital lobes.

Table 2. Cortical structures FD differences analysis between AN, REC-AN, and HC groups.

	AN	AN-REC	HC	AN vs. HC	AN-REC vs. HC
	Mean (SD)	Mean (SD)	Mean (SD)	F* (p)	F* (p)
Whole Brain (Cortical Ribbon)	2.49 (0.02)	2.52 (0.02)	2.51 (0.01)	**16.36 (0.000)**	0.32 (0.573)
Frontal Lobe	2.43 (0.02)	2.44 (0.02)	2.44 (0.01)	**13.07 (0.001)**	0.05 (0.829)
Parietal Lobe	2.30 (0.02)	2.32 (0.02)	2.32 (0.01)	**19.75 (0.000)**	0.72 (0.400)
Temporal Lobe	2.34 (0.02)	2.36 (0.01)	2.35 (0.01)	5.40 (0.023)	3.46 (0.068)
Occipital Lobe	2.30 (0.02)	2.32 (0.02)	2.32 (0.01)	**15.31 (0.000)**	0.55 (0.462)
Left Superior Parietal Lobule	2.13 (0.06)	2.16 (0.03)	2.19 (0.04)	**26.956 (0.000)**	**8.711 (0.005)**
Right Superior Parietal Lobule	2.11 (0.06)	2.13 (0.04)	2.16 (0.03)	**23.580 (0.000)**	**9.600 (0.003)**
Left Postcentral Gyrus	2.06 (0.06)	2.07 (0.04)	2.10 (0.04)	**9.851 (0.002)**	5.689 (0.021)
Right Intraparietal Sulcus	2.11 (0.05)	2.12 (0.04)	2.15 (0.03)	**18.715 (0.000)**	**8.170 (0.006)**
Left Parieto-Occipital Sulcus	2.13 (0.04)	2.13 (0.04)	2.16 (0.02)	**12.640 (0.001)**	**10.339 (0.002)**
Right Parieto-Occipital Sulcus	2.15 (0.04)	2.16 (0.04)	2.18 (0.03)	**17.123 (0.000)**	**7.250 (0.009)**

* F (GLM with age and hand lateralization as covariates of no interest; degrees of freedom = 3), p threshold determined based on FDR < 0.025. Significant effects are highlighted in **bold**.

Since the fractal dimension is not sensitive to smaller structures [37,40], we combined small regions with nearby anatomical regions for regions that were insufficient in size. Figure 2 illustrates the area of the original Destrieux parcellations as well as the combined regions. Figure 2 also shows the average surface area for each cortical region and the relationship between area and FD, similar to previous work [37]. As shown in the figure, relatively larger regions have a weak relationship between size and FD, allowing for the shape-related properties of FD to be sensitive to potential group differences (all FD values are included in Tables S1 and S2). Figure 3C shows these regions on the inflated cortical surface for the combined regions.

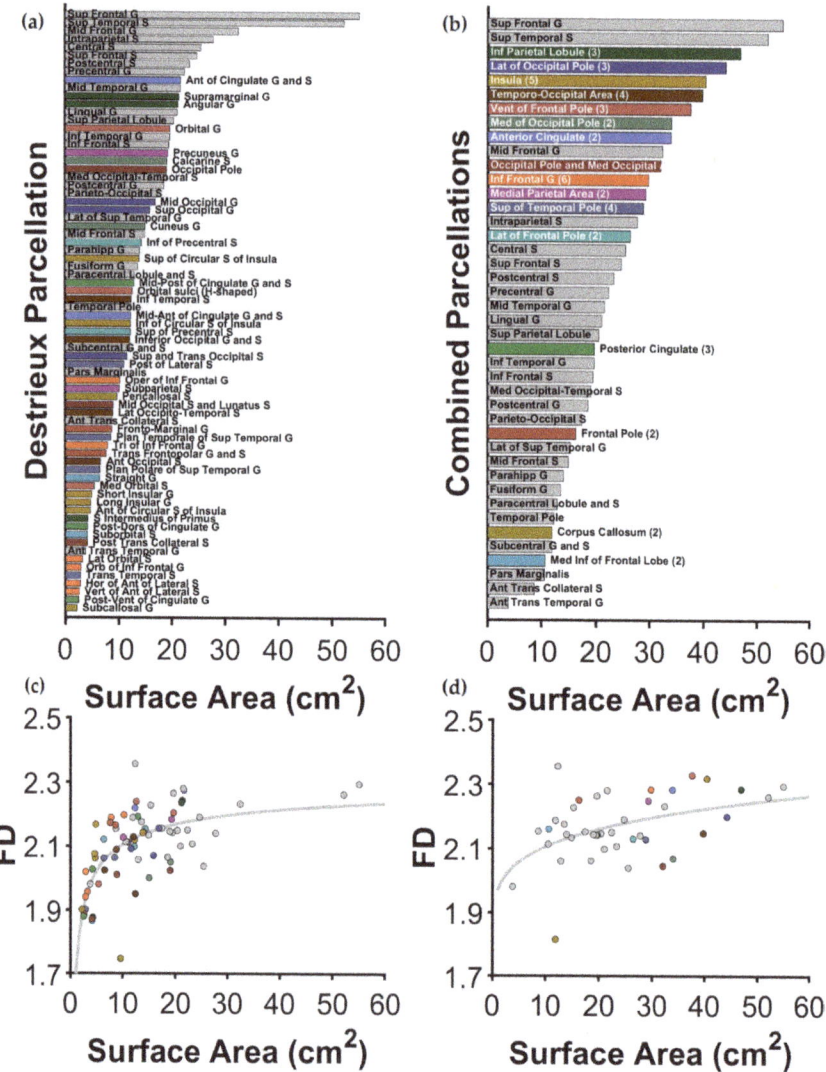

Figure 2. Mean surface area for all parcellation regions using the Destrieux atlas. Figures (**a,c**) show the surface area for parcellations in the original Destrieux atlas; Figures (**b,d**) show areas for combined regions—where the original regions were considered too small for reliable FD calculations. Regions maintained (not combined) in all plots are shown in gray. Regions that were combined to form larger regions are shown in distinct colors, matched between the panels and in Figure 3C. For Figure (**b**), after each combined region's name, the number of Destrieux regions combined is included in parentheses. Figures (**c,d**) show the relationship between surface area and FD (across all participants), showing that FD becomes increasingly distinct from size for larger regions and that the combined regions increased this property. As above, Figure c corresponds to the original Destrieux atlas, whereas figure d uses the recombined regions.

Patients with acute AN displayed significantly lower FD values in comparison to HC in 22 of the considered cortical areas, as shown in Figure 3A. In both hemispheres, the mean FD value of the cortical ribbon was significantly lower in in inferior frontal, middle frontal, superior frontal, postcentral and superior temporal (lateral aspect) gyri, in paracentral, superior parietal and inferior parietal lobules, in superior frontal, intraparietal, parieto-occipital, postcentral and marginal branch of the cingulate sulci, in the lateral aspect of occipital and frontal poles and in a medial parietal area encompassing the precuneus and the subparietal sulcus. In the left hemisphere only, we additionally found significantly decreased FD values in the precentral gyrus, in the superior aspect of the temporal pole and in a temporal-occipital area encompassing the anterior occipital sulcus, the inferior temporal sulcus, the lateral occipito-temporal sulcus and the inferior occipital gyrus. In the right hemisphere, we found decreased FD values in the medial occipital-temporal sulcus. (FD values are reported in Table S1 in the Supplementary Materials). No differences in FD values were observed in patients of the restricting type in comparison to those of the binge-eating/purging type (F (3, 34) = 0.005, p = 0.946 for total FD), nor in those who were taking antidepressants in comparison to those who did not (F (3, 34) = 0.478, p = 0.494, for total FD).

Recovered AN patients did not show differences in the global and lobar FD when compared to HC. The mean FD value of the cortical ribbon was significantly higher in the AN-REC group when compared to HC in the left superior temporal sulcus and in the left subcentral gyrus and sulcus as shown in Figure 3B (FD values are reported in Table S1). Some areas showed reduced FD in both acute and recovered AN patients in comparison to healthy women: the left and right superior parietal lobule, the left postcentral gyrus, the right intraparietal sulcus and the left and right parieto-occipital sulcus.

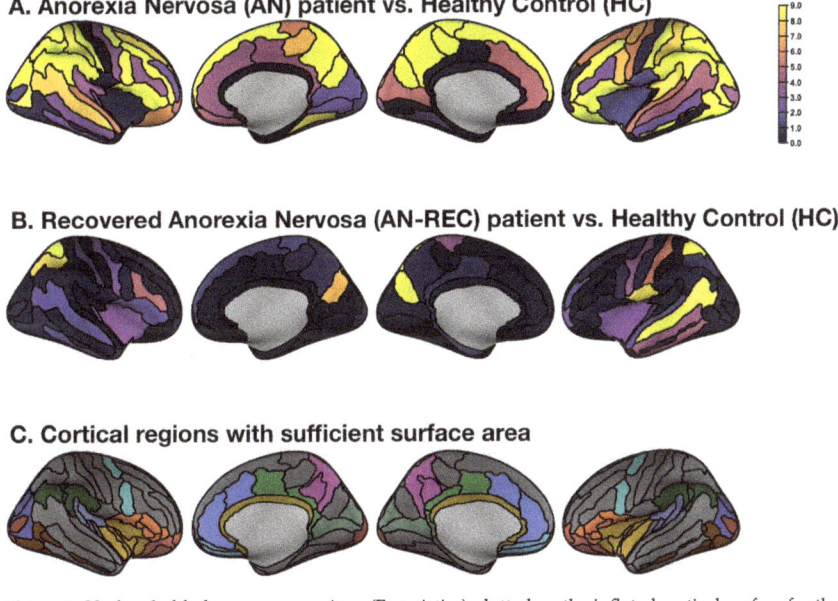

Figure 3. Unthresholded group comparison (F-statistics) plotted on the inflated cortical surface for the combined regions. (**A**) Regional F-statistics comparing Anorexia Nervosa (AN) patients and Healthy Controls (HC). (**B**) Regional F-statistics comparing recovered Anorexia Nervosa (AN-REC) patients with Healthy Controls (HC). (**C**) All cortical regions were included in the analysis. Regions shown in color were recombined with respect to the original Destrieux atlas to yield sufficiently large surfaces areas; colors match the labels and areas shown in Figure 2.

As expected, FD values were significantly negatively correlated with age in all three groups (Table 3) (compare with [15,38,40]). However, the decline of FD along with age tended to be stronger in the acute AN patients than in the other two groups, especially for the frontal and parietal lobes (Figure 4). In all three groups, no differences were observed in left-handed or mixed-handed (Edinburgh scores between −70 to +70) individuals in comparison to right-handed ones. Table 3 shows the correlations (Spearman's ρ [rho] rank correlation) between FD values and clinical variables in the three groups. Significant positive correlations emerged between whole-brain FD and BMI in acute AN, but not in the recovered group (see also [38] for a normative comparison). The FD value was also significantly negatively correlated with the duration of illness in the acute AN group. A significant negative correlation between the age of onset of the disorder and FD emerged in the recovered group. In this last group, the duration of the recovered status showed a negative nonsignificant correlation with FD (rho = −0.386, p = 0.093).

The whole-brain FD positively correlates with the volume of the cortex in all the three groups and with overall local gyrification index in HC, but not in the two AN groups.

Table 3. Correlation between whole-brain (cortical ribbon) FD and clinical variables within each group.

	AN (n = 38) Rho (p)	AN-REC (n = 20) Rho (p)	Healthy Controls (n = 38) Rho (p)
	Whole-brain FD		
Age	−0.608 (0.000) *	−0.617 (0.004) *	−0.527 (0.001) *
Body mass index (BMI)	0.380 (0.019) *	−0.351 (0.130)	−0.209 (0.207)
Duration of illness	−0.406 (0.011) *	−0.111 (0.642)	
Age of AN onset	−0.265 (0.108)	−0.586 (0.007) *	
Cortical volume	0.638 (0.000) *	0.537 (0.015) *	0.496 (0.002) *
Cortical gyrification	0.258 (0.118)	0.376 (0.102)	0.514 (0.001) *
Cortical thickness	0.000 (0.998)	0.65 (0.787)	0.025 (0.883)

FD: Fractal Dimension; Spearman's $ρ(rho)$; * FDR < 0.025.

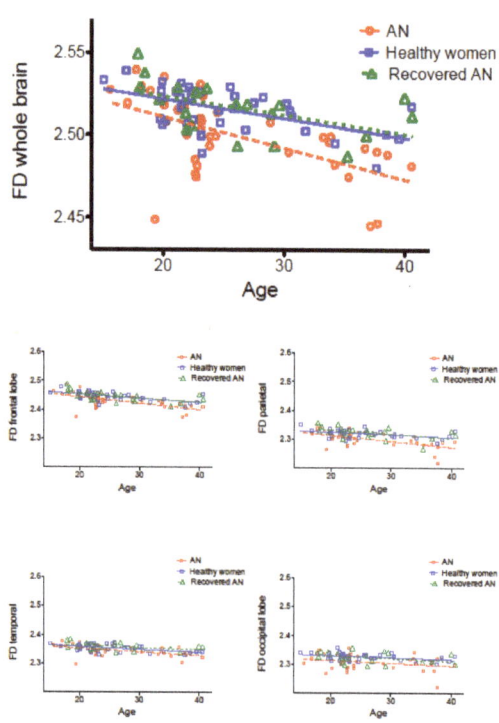

Figure 4. Correlations between whole-brain (cortical ribbon) and lobar FD and age in the three groups.

4. Discussion

In this paper, we explored the morphological complexity of cortical and subcortical brain structures by means of FD and investigated the relationship between FD with clinical variables. Our results showed the presence of a globally reduced cortical FD in patients with acute AN, while patients who recovered from the disorder did not show alterations in global FD values. This observation, together with the correlation between FD and BMI in the acute AN group, allowed us to hypothesize that a global reduction in cortical complexity may be an effect of malnutrition that can be recovered along with weight recovery. FD has been described in the literature as a sensitive measure to describe cortical atrophy and the effects of aging [15,22,23] and our data show that it also seems to describe the complex patterns of cortical morphology that are secondary to the effects of malnutrition in AN. The cortical structural modifications in AN are likely to depend on many factors, such as malnutrition, dehydration and endocrinological factors, but they could also reflect the alterations of neurodevelopmental trajectories that are hypothesized to precede the onset of the disorder [3]. The hypothesized developmental origin of AN [41] and the effects of its onset in critical developmental phases make it important to consider the relationship between any cortical alterations, the duration of the disorder and the patient's age and age of onset in the evaluation of structural MRI findings. Our results indicated that both the patient's age and the duration of the disorder correlate inversely with FD, suggesting an impact of AN on the reduction of cortical complexity. Since cortical complexity, measured by FD, is likely to reduce from adolescence to adulthood as a result of the cortical modeling mechanisms that physiologically occur with aging [42], we hypothesize an impact of the disorder in accelerating this process.

The observed correlation between FD and gyrification in HC, but not in patients with AN, suggests a sensitivity of FD to the effect of malnutrition. A direct correlation between FD and gyrification has been emphasized by previous studies in healthy as well as in neurological populations, indicating the sensitivity of FD in capturing the role of cortical folding in determining cortical complexity [15,22]. Gyrification appears to be largely determined during the earlier neurodevelopmental phases [13] and alterations in this structural parameter have been already pointed out by previous studies on AN patients [10,12]. The absence of a correlation between these two parameters in AN suggests that, in this group, FD could probably be more susceptible than gyrification to the prolonged effects of malnutrition.

From a regional analysis of cortical areas, we identified an FD reduction in various parietal regions that are crucial for the integration of body-image perception abilities both in acute and in recovered AN patients. These results suggest that these areas may be particularly susceptible to disorder-specific alterations and require to be specifically investigated by further research. Except for these regions, in the recovered group we identified some areas that showed no statistically significant differences in cortical complexity, while others showed a higher FD than HC. These findings could reflect reshaping processes induced by re-nutrition, therefore supporting the role of FD in describing how nutritional processes can influence the brain morphology. It is not clear why in the recovered patients the values of FD displayed different patterns in different brain regions. The negative trend we observed between FD and duration of recovery in this group might indicate that after an initial increase of cortical complexity following weight recovery—which probably implies the occurrence of reparative processes—FD tends to decrease towards average values. It is possible that this process occurs with different trajectories in different areas of the brain. In addition, since we observed a negative correlation between FD and age of onset in the recovered group, it seems that these reparative processes are more evident in patients with an earlier age of onset.

The present study has several strengths, as well as important limitations. It explores cortical complexity in AN by means of FD, a novel parameter that has been demonstrated to have a good sensitivity to cortical atrophy and age-related brain differences. The evaluation of cortical morphology with FD allows widening the horizons of surface-based cortical analysis, by integrating the information given by cortical thickness and gyrification with novel and non-redundant data. Furthermore, the correlation between FD alterations and the duration of illness is a new and interesting finding about MRI surface-based analysis in AN, hinting at the potentialities of this morphological index in capturing the effects of prolonged starvation on the cortical structure. A limitation of this study is represented by its cross-sectional design. In fact, longitudinal data could be particularly useful to understand how cortical complexity varies with the clinical course of the disorder and with weight recovery. Another limitation can be found in the absence of male patients in the sample. Any inference about alterations in cortical complexity in male patients with AN cannot be made and would be an interesting topic to explore in future studies.

In conclusion, the present study evidences that FD should be considered particularly useful to investigate the morpho-structural properties of brain cortex in AN, since it demonstrated to be suitable for identifying the negative effects of different clinical variables on cortical structure and giving non-redundant information with respect to other surface-based indexes.

Supplementary Materials: The following are available online at http://www.mdpi.com/2077-0383/9/3/833/s1, Table S1: FD differences analysis for combined cortical regions, comparing the AN, REC-AN and HC groups, Table S2: FD differences analysis for all cortical regions of the Destrieux atlas, comparing the AN, REC-AN and HC groups.

Author Contributions: Conceptualization, E.C. and A.F.; methodology, E.C., C.R.M. and A.F.; formal analysis, E.C., C.R.M., A.F.; data curation, E.C., A.F., R.M., I.C., E.T. and P.M.; writing—original draft preparation, E.C.; writing—review and editing, C.R.M., P.M., A.F. All authors have read and agreed to the published version of the manuscript

Conflicts of Interest: The authors declare no conflict of interest.

References

1. Favaro, A.; Caregaro, L.; Tenconi, E.; Bosello, R.; Santonastaso, P. Time trends in age at onset of anorexia nervosa and bulimia nervosa. *J. Clin. Psychiatry* **2009**, *70*, 1715–1721. [CrossRef]
2. Seitz, J.; Bühren, K.; Von Polier, G.G.; Heussen, N.; Herpertz-Dahlmann, B.; Konrad, K. Morphological Changes in the Brain of Acutely Ill and Weight-Recovered Patients with Anorexia Nervosa a Meta-Analysis and Qualitative Review. *J. Child Adolesc. Psychiatry Psychother.* **2014**, *42*, 7–18.
3. Connan, F.; Campbell, I.C.; Katzman, M.; Lightman, S.L.; Treasure, J. A neurodevelopmental model for anorexia nervosa. *Physiol. Behav.* **2003**, *79*, 13–24. [CrossRef]
4. Andersen, S.L. Trajectories of brain development: Point of vulnerability or window of opportunity? *Neurosci. Biobehav. Rev.* **2003**, *27*, 3–18. [CrossRef]
5. Seitz, J.; Herpertz-Dahlmann, B.; Konrad, K. Brain morphological changes in adolescent and adult patients with anorexia nervosa. *J. Neural Transm.* **2016**, *123*, 949–959. [CrossRef] [PubMed]
6. Bernardoni, F.; King, J.A.; Geisler, D.; Stein, E.; Jaite, C.; Nätsch, D.; Tam, F.I.; Boehm, I.; Seidel, M.; Roessner, V.; et al. Weight restoration therapy rapidly reverses cortical thinning in anorexia nervosa: A longitudinal study. *Neuroimage* **2016**, *130*, 214–222. [CrossRef] [PubMed]
7. Lavagnino, L.; Amianto, F.; Mwangi, B.; D'Agata, F.; Spalatro, A.; Zunta Soares, G.B.; Daga, G.A.; Mortara, P.; Fassino, S.; Soares, J.C. The relationship between cortical thickness and body mass index differs between women with anorexia nervosa and healthy controls. *Psychiatry Res. Neuroimaging* **2016**, *248*, 105–109. [CrossRef]
8. Collantoni, E.; Meneguzzo, P.; Tenconi, E.; Manara, R.; Favaro, A. Small-world properties of brain morphological characteristics in Anorexia Nervosa. *PLoS ONE* **2019**, *14*, e0216154. [CrossRef] [PubMed]
9. Fuglset, T.S.; Endestad, T.; Hilland, E.; Bang, L.; Tamnes, C.K.; Landrø, N.I.; Rø, Ø. Brain volumes and regional cortical thickness in young females with anorexia nervosa. *BMC Psychiatry* **2016**, *16*, 404. [CrossRef] [PubMed]
10. Favaro, A.; Tenconi, E.; Degortes, D.; Manara, R.; Santonastaso, P. Gyrification brain abnormalities as predictors of outcome in anorexia nervosa. *Hum. Brain Mapp.* **2015**, *36*, 5113–5122. [CrossRef] [PubMed]
11. Schultz, C.C.; Wagner, G.; de la Cruz, F.; Berger, S.; Reichenbach, J.R.; Sauer, H.; Bär, K.J. Evidence for alterations of cortical folding in anorexia nervosa. *Eur. Arch. Psychiatry Clin. Neurosci.* **2017**, *267*, 41–49. [CrossRef] [PubMed]
12. Bernardoni, F.; King, J.A.; Geisler, D.; Birkenstock, J.; Tam, F.I.; Weidner, K.; Roessner, V.; White, T.; Ehrlich, S. Nutritional status affects cortical folding: Lessons learned from anorexia nervosa. *Biol. Psychiatry* **2018**, *84*, 692–701. [CrossRef] [PubMed]

13. White, T.; Su, S.; Schmidt, M.; Kao, C.Y.; Sapiro, G. The development of gyrification in childhood and adolescence. *Brain Cogn.* **2010**, *72*, 36–45. [CrossRef] [PubMed]
14. Kiselev, V.G.; Hahn, K.R.; Auer, D.P. Is the brain cortex a fractal? *Neuroimage* **2003**, *20*, 1765–1774. [CrossRef]
15. Madan, C.R.; Kensinger, E.A. Cortical complexity as a measure of age-related brain atrophy. *Neuroimage* **2016**, *134*, 617–629. [CrossRef]
16. Di Ieva, A. *The Fractal Geometry of the Brain: An Overview*; Springer: New York, NY, USA, 2016; ISBN 9781493939954.
17. Mandelbrot, B. How long is the coast of Britain? Statistical self-similarity and fractional dimension. *Science* **1967**, *156*, 636–638. [CrossRef]
18. Hofman, M.A. The fractal geometry of convoluted brains. *J. Hirnforsch.* **1991**, *32*, 103–111.
19. Cook, M.J.; Free, S.L.; Manford, M.R.A.; Fish, D.R.; Shorvon, S.D.; Stevens, J.M. Fractal Description of Cerebral Cortical Patterns in Frontal Lobe Epilepsy. *Eur. Neurol.* **1995**, *35*, 327–335. [CrossRef]
20. Nenadic, I.; Yotter, R.A.; Sauer, H.; Gaser, C. Cortical surface complexity in frontal and temporal areas varies across subgroups of schizophrenia. *Hum. Brain Mapp.* **2014**, *35*, 1691–1699. [CrossRef]
21. Sandu, A.-L.; Rasmussen, I.-A.; Lundervold, A.; Kreuder, F.; Neckelmann, G.; Hugdahl, K.; Specht, K. Fractal dimension analysis of MR images reveals grey matter structure irregularities in schizophrenia. *Comput. Med. Imaging Graph.* **2008**, *32*, 150–158. [CrossRef]
22. King, R.D.; Brown, B.; Hwang, M.; Jeon, T.; George, A.T. Fractal dimension analysis of the cortical ribbon in mild Alzheimer's disease. *Neuroimage* **2010**, *53*, 471–479. [CrossRef] [PubMed]
23. Madan, C.R.; Kensinger, E.A. Age-related differences in the structural complexity of subcortical and ventricular structures. *Neurobiol. Aging* **2017**, *50*, 87–95. [CrossRef] [PubMed]
24. Ha, T.H.; Yoon, U.; Lee, K.J.; Shin, Y.W.; Lee, J.-M.; Kim, I.Y.; Ha, K.S.; Kim, S.I.; Kwon, J.S. Fractal dimension of cerebral cortical surface in schizophrenia and obsessive–compulsive disorder. *Neurosci. Lett.* **2005**, *384*, 172–176. [CrossRef] [PubMed]
25. Li, X.; Jiang, J.; Zhu, W.; Yu, C.; Sui, M.; Wang, Y.; Jiang, T. Asymmetry of prefrontal cortical convolution complexity in males with attention-deficit/hyperactivity disorder using fractal information dimension. *Brain Dev.* **2007**, *29*, 649–655. [CrossRef] [PubMed]
26. Squarcina, L.; De Luca, A.; Bellani, M.; Brambilla, P.; Turkheimer, F.E.; Bertoldo, A. Fractal analysis of MRI data for the characterization of patients with schizophrenia and bipolar disorder. *Phys. Med. Biol.* **2015**, *60*, 1697–1716. [CrossRef] [PubMed]
27. Zhao, G.; Denisova, K.; Sehatpour, P.; Long, J.; Gui, W.; Qiao, J.; Javitt, D.C.; Wang, Z. Fractal dimension analysis of subcortical gray matter structures in schizophrenia. *PLoS ONE* **2016**, *11*, 1–23. [CrossRef]
28. Nickel, K.; Joos, A.; Tebartz van Elst, L.; Holovics, L.; Endres, D.; Zeeck, A.; Maier, S. Altered cortical folding and reduced sulcal depth in adults with anorexia nervosa. *Eur. Eat. Disord. Rev.* **2019**, *27*, 655–670. [CrossRef]
29. Favaro, A.; Clementi, M.; Manara, R.; Bosello, R.; Forzan, M.; Bruson, A.; Tenconi, E.; Degortes, D.; Titton, F.; Di Salle, F.; et al. Catechol-O-methyltransferase genotype modifies executive functioning and prefrontal functional connectivity in women with anorexia nervosa. *J. Psychiatry Neurosci.* **2013**, *38*, 241–248. [CrossRef]
30. American Psychiatric Association. *Diagnostic and Statistical Manual of Mental Disorders*; American Psychiatric Association: Virginia, VA, USA, 2013; ISBN 0-89042-555-8.
31. Favaro, A.; Santonastaso, P.; Manara, R.; Bosello, R.; Bommarito, G.; Tenconi, E.; Di Salle, F. Disruption of visuospatial and somatosensory functional connectivity in anorexia nervosa. *Biol. Psychiatry* **2012**, *72*, 864–870. [CrossRef]
32. Derogatis, L.R.; Lipman, R.S.; Rickels, K.; Uhlenhuth, E.H.; Covi, L. The Hopkins Symptom Checklist (HSCL): A Self Report Symptom Inventory. *Behav. Sci.* **1974**, *19*, 1–15. [CrossRef]
33. Garner, D.M.; Olmstead, M.P.; Polivy, J. Development and validation of a multidimensional eating disorder inventory for anorexia nervosa and bulimia. *Int. J. Eat. Disord.* **1983**, *2*, 15–34. [CrossRef]
34. Oldfield, R.C. The assessment and analysis of handedness: The Edinburgh inventory. *Neuropsychologia* **1971**, *9*, 97–113. [CrossRef]
35. Fischl, B. FreeSurfer. *Neuroimage* **2012**, *62*, 774–781. [CrossRef] [PubMed]
36. Destrieux, C.; Fischl, B.; Dale, A.; Halgren, E. Automatic parcellation of human cortical gyri and sulci using standard anatomical nomenclature. *Neuroimage* **2010**, *53*, 1–15. [CrossRef]
37. Madan, C.R.; Kensinger, E.A. Test–retest reliability of brain morphology estimates. *Brain Inform.* **2017**, *4*, 107–121. [CrossRef]

38. Madan, C.R. Age differences in head motion and estimates of cortical morphology. *PeerJ* **2018**, *6*, e5176. [CrossRef]
39. Benjamini, Y.; Hochberg, Y. Controlling the False Discovery Rate—A Practical and Powerful Approach to Multiple Testing. *J. R. Stat. Soc. Ser. B* **1995**, *57*, 289–300. [CrossRef]
40. Madan, C.R.; Kensinger, E.A. Predicting age from cortical structure across the lifespan. *Eur. J. Neurosci.* **2018**, *47*, 399–416. [CrossRef]
41. Favaro, A. Brain development and neurocircuit modeling are the interface between genetic/environmental risk factors and eating disorders. A commentary on keel & forney and friederich et al. *Int. J. Eat. Disord.* **2013**, *46*, 443–446.
42. Sandu, A.-L.; Izard, E.; Specht, K.; Beneventi, H.; Lundervold, A.; Ystad, M. Post-adolescent developmental changes in cortical complexity. *Behav. Brain Funct.* **2014**, *10*, 44. [CrossRef]

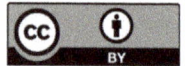

© 2020 by the authors. Licensee MDPI, Basel, Switzerland. This article is an open access article distributed under the terms and conditions of the Creative Commons Attribution (CC BY) license (http://creativecommons.org/licenses/by/4.0/).

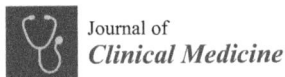

Article

Insular Cell Integrity Markers Linked to Weight Concern in Anorexia Nervosa—An MR-Spectroscopy Study

Simon Maier [1,2,*], Kathrin Nickel [2], Evgeniy Perlov [2,3], Alina Kukies [1], Almut Zeeck [1], Ludger Tebartz van Elst [2], Dominique Endres [2], Derek Spieler [1], Lukas Holovics [1], Armin Hartmann [1], Michael Dacko [4], Thomas Lange [4] and Andreas Joos [1,5]

[1] Department of Psychosomatic Medicine and Psychotherapy, Medical Center—University of Freiburg, Faculty of Medicine, University of Freiburg, 79104 Freiburg, Germany; alinakukies@hotmail.com (A.K.); almut.zeeck@uniklinik-freiburg.de (A.Z.); derek.spieler@uniklinik-freiburg.de (D.S.); lukas.holovics@uniklinik-freiburg.de (L.H.); armin.hartmann@uniklinik-freiburg.de (A.H.); andreas.joos@uniklinik-freiburg.de (A.J.)

[2] Department of Psychiatry and Psychotherapy, Medical Center—University of Freiburg, Faculty of Medicine, University of Freiburg, 79104 Freiburg, Germany; kathrin.nickel@uniklinik-freiburg.de (K.N.); evgeniy.perlov@lups.ch (E.P.); tebartzvanelst@uniklinik-freiburg.de (L.T.v.E.); dominique.endres@uniklinik-freiburg.de (D.E.)

[3] Luzerner Psychiatrie, Hospital St. Urban, 4915 St. Urban, Switzerland

[4] Department of Radiology, Medical Physics, Medical Center—University of Freiburg, Faculty of Medicine, University of Freiburg, 79106 Freiburg, Germany; michael.dacko@uniklinik-freiburg.de (M.D.); thomas.lange@uniklinik-freiburg.de (T.L.)

[5] Department of Psychosomatic Medicine and Psychotherapy, Ortenau Klinikum, Teaching Hospital of University of Freiburg, 77654 Offenburg, Germany

* Correspondence: simon.maier@uniklinik-freiburg.de

Received: 31 March 2020; Accepted: 28 April 2020; Published: 30 April 2020

Abstract: Objective: An insular involvement in the pathogenesis of anorexia nervosa (AN) has been suggested in many structural and functional neuroimaging studies. This magnetic resonance spectroscopy (MRS) study is the first to investigate metabolic signals in the anterior insular cortex in patients with AN and recovered individuals (REC). Method: The MR spectra of 32 adult women with AN, 21 REC subjects and 33 healthy controls (HC) were quantified for absolute N-acetylaspartate (NAA), glutamate + glutamine (Glx), total choline, myo-inositol, creatine concentrations (mM/L). After adjusting the metabolite concentrations for age and partial gray/white matter volume, group differences were tested using one-way multivariate analyses of variance (MANOVA). Post-hoc analyses of variance were applied to identify those metabolites that showed significant group effects. Correlations were tested for associations with psychometric measures (eating disorder examination), duration of illness, and body mass index. Results: The MANOVA exhibited a significant group effect. The NAA signal was reduced in the AN group compared to the HC group. The REC and the HC groups did not differ in metabolite concentrations. In the AN group, lower NAA and Glx signals were related to increased weight concern. Discussion: We interpret the decreased NAA availability in the anterior insula as a signal of impaired neuronal integrity or density. The association of weight concern, which is a core feature of AN, with decreased NAA and Glx indicates that disturbances of glutamatergic neurotransmission might be related to core psychopathology in AN. The absence of significant metabolic differences between the REC and HC subjects suggests that metabolic alterations in AN represent a state rather than a trait phenomenon.

Keywords: anorexia nervosa; magnetic resonance spectroscopy; MRS; insula; glutamate; N-acetylaspartate; NAA

1. Introduction

Patients with anorexia nervosa (AN) persistently restricted their food intake because of severe weight concerns and body image disturbance. AN mainly affects young women [1–3] and has the highest mortality rate of all mental disorders [4,5], while only about half of such patients fully recover [1,2].

Two decades ago, the first magnetic resonance spectroscopy (MRS) studies searched for metabolic anomalies associated with AN. MRS is a non-invasive and nonradioactive method for the in vivo detection of several neurometabolites. MRS sequences that measure the ^{1}H chemical shift allow the simultaneous absolute quantification of the concentrations of N-acetylaspartate (NAA) + N-acetyl-aspartyl-glutamate (NAAG), glutamate (Glu) + glutamine (Gln), glycerophosphorylcholine + phosphocholine (total choline, t-Cho), myo-inositol (mI), phosphocreatine (PCre), and creatine (Cre).

NAA is relatively abundant in healthy neuronal tissue and is therefore often used as a marker for neuronal integrity and density [6]. However, it has also been detected in oligodendrocytes and myelin [7,8], and it is synthesized in the mitochondria. Decreased concentrations of NAA indicate a loss of neuronal cells. Although NAA signal differences have been reported in various studies on AN, the results were inconsistent regarding a diminished or elevated NAA level [9–13] (see Table 1).

Glu is the primary excitatory neurotransmitter in the human brain (~85% of all synapses in the central nervous system are glutamatergic) [14] and has been implicated in different psychiatric disorders associated with AN, including anxiety disorders, depression, and obsessive-compulsive disorder [15–18]. Elevated Glu has toxic effects on neurons as well as oligodendrocytes, astrocytes, and endothelial and immune cells [19]. The distinction of Glu from its precursor and the metabolite Gln is difficult because of a considerable overlap of the spectral peaks. Therefore, the combined Glu and Gln resonances are often denoted collectively as Glx [20]. Previous MRS studies have reported lower Glx [10,12,21] and Glu [22] in the AN group compared to HC subjects or in response to AN-related symptoms; while this has mainly been in frontal cortices, it has also been in the basal ganglia and occipital lobe [22]. Notably, one study reported higher Glx signals in AN [9].

The major part of the t-Cho signal results from glycerophosphorylcholine and phosphocholine, but it also comes from other choline-containing compounds. Glycerophosphorylcholine and phosphocholine are integral components of the cell membrane and are more highly concentrated in glial cells than they are in neurons [23]. Changes in the t-Cho signal have been associated with changes in cell proliferation or cell degeneration [24]. MRS studies that detected t-Cho differences in AN or in relation to anorectic symptoms reported increased concentrations [9,11–13,25].

Creatine and phosphocreatine are measured as combined resonances (Cre) and are involved in the creatine kinase cycle. Despite their important role in energy metabolism, the level of the Cre signal remains relatively constant, even under conditions of increased energy demand [26]. Therefore, the Cre signal is widely used as an internal reference in MRS studies. While MRS studies reporting Cre signal differences in AN mostly showed increased Cre [9,12,25] in the anterior cingulate and frontal cortices, lower Cre was observed in the dorsolateral prefrontal cortex (dlPFC) [21].

The concentration of the sugar mI is thought to be increased in glial cells compared to neurons, and it serves as an intracellular second messenger. For this reason, mI is used as a glial marker [27]. In AN, mI was found to be decreased [10,21,22,28] whenever mI differences were detected.

Table 1. Overview of previous magnetic resonance spectroscopy (MRS) studies in anorexia nervosa.

Author	Patient Collective	Age	Sex	Patients/Controls	MR Method	Target Region	Results
Kato et al. (1997) [29]	AN (3 comorbid BN)	18–32	female	4 (2 longitudinal)/13	Localized ^{31}P (TE = 20 ms) 1.5T	Frontal lobe	PDE/P total + decreasing after gaining weight
Schlemmer et al. (1998) [3] *	AN	16 ± 1.9	female	10/17	^{1}H SVS STEAM (TE = 50 ms) 1.5T	(1) Thalamus (2) parieto-occipital WM	(1) Cho/Cr+, NAA/Cho−
Möckel et al. (1999) [30] *	AN	15.7 ± 1.7	female	22/17 (11 longitudinal)	^{1}H SVS STEAM (TE = 50 ms) 1.5T	(1) Thalamus (2) parieto-occipital WM	Both: Cho/Cr+ normalization with recovery
Hentschel et al. (1999) [11] *	AN	15.7 ± 1.7	female	15/17	^{1}H SVS STEAM (TE = 50 ms) 1.5T	(1) Thalamus (2) parieto-occipital WM	(1) Cho/Cr+ NAA/Cr+
Roser et al. (1999) [28]	AN and BN	10–28	19 female 1 male	20/15	^{1}H SVS STEAM (TE = 20 ms) 1.5T	(1) Frontal white matter (2) occipital gray matter, (3) cerebellum	(1) mI/Cr− lipid/Cr− (2) lipid/Cr− (3) all metabolites + except lipids
Rzanny et al. (2003) [31]	AN	12–20	female	10/10	Localized ^{31}P (TE = 16 ms) 1.5T	Frontal lobe	PDE/P total−
Ohrmann et al. (2004) [21]	AN	22.7 ± 3.8	female	10/12	^{1}H SVS STEAM (TE = 20 ms) 1.5T	(1) Rostral ACC (2) dlPFC	(1) Glx− (2) Cr−, mI−
Grzelak et al. (2005) [32]	AN	16–22	female	10/10	^{1}H SVS STEAM (TE = 20 ms) 1.5T	Parietal WM, parietal GM	WM: lipid−
Castro-Fornieles et al. (2007) [10]	AN	11–17	female	12/12	^{1}H SVS PRESS (TE = 35 ms) 1.5T	Frontal grey matter	NAA−, Glx−, mI− 7 months follow-up NAA+
Castro-Fornieles et al. (2010) [25]	AN vs. short-term recovered	13–18	female	32/20	^{1}H SVS PRESS (TE = 35 ms) 1.5T	prefrontal	Cho+, Cr+
Joos et al. (2011) [12]	10 BN 7AN	24.8 ± 4.9	female	17/14	^{1}H SVS PRESS (TE = 30 ms) 3T	ACC	No difference: NAA, Cho, Cr, mI, Glu, Glx
Blasel et al. (2012) [9]	AN	14.4 ± 1.9	female	21/29	^{1}H SVS PRESS (TE = 30 ms) ^{31}P (TE = 2.3 ms) 3T	centrum semiovale (including ACC)	GM: Glx+, NAA+, Cr+, Cho+, lipid catabolites−
Godlewska et al. (2017) [22]	AN	18–41	female	13/12	^{1}H SVS STEAM (TE = 11 ms) 7T	ACC, occipital cortex and putamen	Glu− in all areas mI− in ACC and occipital lobe

Abbreviations: ACC = anterior cingulate cortex; AN = anorexia nervosa; BN = bulimia nervosa; Cho = choline; re = creatine; dlPFC = dorsolateral prefrontal cortex; Glx = glutamate+glutamine; GM = grey matter; HC = healthy control; mI = myo-inositol; NAA = N-acetylaspartate; P total = total phosphate; PDE = phosphodiesters; SVS = single voxel spectroscopy; TE = echo time; WM = white matter; ^{1}H = proton spectroscopy; ^{31}P = phosphate spectroscopy. * overlapping samples.

Small sample sizes, low MR field strengths, and differences in voxel positioning are likely to be the main cause of the heterogeneous results of previous ^{1}H-MRS studies (Table 1). Given that higher field strengths are particularly recommended for the quantification of Glx, and considering that the Cre signal, which was often used as a reference in earlier studies [9,21,25], often reveals inconsistent results, older studies must be interpreted cautiously.

In conclusion, no metabolite was consistently altered across all studies, but increased t-Cho and Cre and decreased mI were the most consistent findings (Table 1). In general, the results of newer studies with higher field strengths and more advanced MRS protocols in combination with larger sample sizes are more reliable.

A longitudinal ^{1}H-MRS study reported a normalization of increased t-Cho/Cre ratios with recovery [29], while a small study of adolescent females with AN also indicated normalization, which was (in this case) decreased NAA in the frontal gray matter (GM) [10].

In terms of region of interest (ROI) localization, the anterior insular cortex appears to be of importance. The relevance of this region in AN has been emphasized in various brain structural [33–37] and functional [38–41] studies, and it even led to the postulation of the so-called *"insula hypothesis"* of AN [42,43]. This hypothesis states that early developmental damage in combination with socio-cultural and other stressors, such as dieting and hormonal changes, may lead to an impairment of insula function. The insula, as a central hub, conveys the information of numerous cortical and subcortical brain areas and therefore plays a central role in the interoceptional awareness and monitoring of the bodily state (somatic marker hypothesis) [44,45]. This includes, among other functions, the experience of physiological correlates of fear and anxiety [46] as well as taste [47,48], hunger [49], disgust [50], and visceral information [51]. Hence, altered insula functioning could explain the dysfunction of interoceptive awareness in AN in turn by not only biasing the experience of one's own bodily condition or the pleasantness/valence of consumed food but also the reward-related and motivational aspects of food intake [52]. Despite the high relevance of the insular lobe in AN pathomechanism, this area has never been targeted by previous MRS studies.

Rationale of our Study

This study examined female adults with AN, female adults who had recovered (REC) from AN, and healthy controls (HC) via MRS, which targeted the insular cortex. Considering the results of earlier studies, we expected to observe increased Cre and t-Cho signals in women with AN and decreased mI, while no clear hypothesis regarding NAA and Glx could be derived from previous studies. All hypothetical differences were expected to normalize in the REC subjects.

2. Methods and Materials

2.1. Participants

The MR spectra of 35 female patients with AN were acquired. Patients were recruited at the in- and outpatient units of the Department of Psychosomatic Medicine and Psychotherapy at the University of Freiburg as well as cooperating hospitals. Diagnoses were made by experienced and board-certified psychiatrists and psychologists and were confirmed by the structured clinical interviews SCID-I and SCID-II [53,54]. Diagnostic criteria according to the DSM-5 [55] were relevant for study inclusion. All AN patients met the weight criterion of a body mass index (BMI) < 18.5 kg/m^2. Three patients had to be excluded because of either data loss or corruption. Of the 32 remaining AN patients, 3 were of the binge eating/purging subtype, while all others were of the restrictive subtype.

Twenty-two REC were recruited for MRS acquisition and fulfilled the following recovery criteria [56]: No eating disorder symptomatology for at least 12 months with a conservative eating disorder examination total score (EDE) total score [57,58] within 1 standard deviation of normal. For study inclusion, a minimal BMI of >20 kg/m^2 was envisaged, which most REC participants met. However, the BMI of four REC subjects was slightly below 20 kg/m^2 (19.3–19.8 kg/m^2).

These participants were clinically completely recovered and had never exceeded a BMI >20 kg/m^2. In addition, 2 REC subjects had a BMI of 18.5–19.0 kg/m^2 with similar features, while 1 REC participant had to be excluded because of data loss or corruption, resulting in a final sample size of 21 individuals for the REC group. Finally, 1 REC participant was of the binge eating/purging subtype, while all others were of the restrictive subtype.

HC subjects were recruited via advertisements in local newspapers and announcements on the notice board of the participating hospital. The MR spectra of 40 age-matched female HC subjects were available. Mental disorders in HC subjects were ruled out by SCID-I and II interviews. After 7 HC participants were excluded because of either data loss or corruption, the final HC sample size was 33 individuals.

The general exclusion criteria included any history of head injury or surgery, neurological disorders, severe psychiatric comorbidities (psychosis, bipolar disorders, substance abuse), current regular psychotropic medication, and an inability to undergo MRI scans (e.g., metal implants, claustrophobia). In total, 7 AN, 17 HC, and 10 REC subjects took hormonal contraceptives. One woman with AN had only just started a minor dose of citalopram (10 mg/day; serum level of 31 ng/mL, which is below the therapeutic range) and was thus considered appropriate to be included.

The participants who took no hormonal contraceptives were studied in the luteal phase of the menstrual cycle. Regarding hormonal contraception, they had to be in the progesterone and estrogen phase (i.e., similar to the physiology of the luteal phase). Given that, the AN participants were mostly amenorrhoeic, the phase of their menstrual cycle could not be assessed.

2.2. Ethics Statement

All subjects gave written informed consent prior to participation, and the study was approved by the ethics committee of the University Medical Center Freiburg (Approval ID: EK-Freiburg 520/13 June 2013).

2.3. Psychometric Assessment

Apart from the SCID interviews [53,54] and the EDE interviews [57,58] mentioned above, the participants completed self-report questionnaires to assess their eating disorder pathology using the Eating Disorder Inventory–2 [59,60] and to assess any depression using the Beck Depression Inventory-II, BDI-II [61–63].

2.4. Procedure Before Scanning

Starting between 7:30 a.m. and 8:00 a.m., participants received a standardized breakfast, and their consumed calories were assessed. The participants read study-relevant information and completed an MR-safety questionnaire.

2.5. Data Acquisition and Processing

All measurements were performed at the University Medical Center of Freiburg using a 3T MAGNETOM Prisma scanner (Siemens Healthineers, Erlangen, Germany), which was equipped with a 20-channel head coil.

Before the MRS measurement was taken, a T1-weighted MPRAGE sequence (repetition time: 2000 ms, echo time: 4.11 ms, flip angle: 12°, field of view: 256 × 256 mm, 160 slices, voxel size: 1 × 1 × 1 mm) was performed and used for manual localization of spectroscopic voxels in the left insular cortex (size: 20 × 20 × 20 mm). A point resolved spectroscopy (PRESS) sequence with an echo time of 30 ms, a relaxation time of 3000 ms, 256 averages, and with water saturation was used. The water reference spectrum was obtained using 16 averages of the same PRESS sequence without water saturation. Shimming parameters were further manually adjusted to minimize the full-width at half maximum of the water peak. The established linear combination of model spectra (LCModel 6.3, Oakville, ON, Canada) software was used for spectra fitting and quantification [64]. The absolute metabolite concentrations of Cre, NAA, Cho, Glx, and mI were estimated [64–66]. All spectra were visually controlled to fulfill the internal criterion of quality (i.e., adequate visible peaks of main metabolites), and only spectra with Cramér-Rao lower bounds (CRLBs) for the main metabolites below 20% were included in further analyses. All voxels were segmented into GM, white matter (WM), and cerebrospinal fluid (CSF) using the statistical parametric mapping software SPM12 (Wellcome Trust Centre of Imaging Neuroscience, London, United Kingdom; for details, see [67]), according to the co-registered voxel position of the corresponding morphological T1-weighted image.

2.6. Statistical Analyses

The metabolite concentrations, as assessed in the LCModel, were transferred to a data table together with all clinical and psychometric data. All statistical analyses were performed using R statistical computing (version 3.4, R Foundation for Statistical Computing, Vienna, Austria [68]). All dependent variables of interest (metabolite concentrations) were first linearly adjusted for differences in age and partial GM+WM volume using the "predict" function of the R stats package. The resulting adjusted metabolite concentrations were then tested for normality of distribution using the Shapiro–Wilk test of normality. Subsequently, the Levene's test for homogeneity of variance across groups was computed for the adjusted metabolite concentrations.

Because the adjusted metabolite concentrations of NAA/NAAG, Cre/PCre and mI were not normally distributed, we tested group differences with a robust one-way MANOVA [69] using the rrcov package (version 1.4–3) in R [70]. In the robust MANOVA, a classical Wilk's Lambda statistic for testing the equality of the group means was modified into a robust one through substituting the classical estimates by the highly robust and efficiently reweighted minimum covariance determinant estimators for mean and variances. The procedure used 10,000 trials for the simulations to compute the multiplication factor for the approximate distribution of the robust Lambda statistic and the degrees of freedom.

To determine which metabolites significantly differed between groups, a post-hoc heteroscedastic one-way ANOVA for trimmed means was carried out with the WRS2 package [71,72]. A p-level of <0.05 was chosen as the criterion for significance. The explanatory power is reported using ξ as a robust measure of effect size [73]. A post-hoc Lincon test (with robustness equivalent to the Tukey-Kramer test) was carried out to assess the direction of the effects [71].

The robust MANOVA was repeated with adjusted metabolite concentrations after additionally correcting for the influence contraceptive use.

Finally, the adjusted metabolite concentrations were correlated with psychometric measures of AN (EDE scores, BMI, and duration of illness) using robust correlations (pbcor function of the WRS2 package [72]) independently for the AN group and across all groups (but not for duration of illness). The resulting p-values of the correlation analyses were corrected for multiple comparisons using the Benjamini and Hochberg False Discovery Rate [74].

3. Results

3.1. Demographic and Psychometric Data

The demographic and psychometric data of the participants are summarized in Table 2. For the final data analysis, 32 patients with AN, 21 REC participants, and 33 HCs were included in the study. The REC group was older than were both the AN and HC participants. As expected, there was a difference with respect to BMI between all three groups, with the lowest BMI in patients with AN (AN < REC < HC). The AN group showed more depressive symptoms in the BDI-II than did the REC and HC participants (HC > REC > AN). Diagnoses in the AN group included seven participants with depression, one with a specific phobia, one with obsessive-compulsive disorder, and two with generalized anxiety disorder. Two participants of the REC group had specific phobias. One participant of the AN, two of the HC, and none of the REC group were left-handed.

Table 2. Overview of demographic and psychometric data.

	Anorexia (n = 32)		Recovered (n = 21)		Healthy Controls (n = 33)		ANOVA	Post hoc t-Test Tukey-Kramer *
	Mean	SD	Mean	SD	Mean	SD	(d.f.; F; p)	
Age (Years)	23.7	4.2	27.6	5.2	23.2	3.4	2, 83; 5.8, 0.004 *	REC > AN, HC
Current BMI (kg/m^2)	16.2	1.3	20.6	1.3	22.1	2.4	2, 83; 91.0; <0.001 *	HC > REC > AN
Lowest-Lifetime BMI (kg/m^2)	14.8	1.4	15.1	2.2	-	-	2, 49; 0.5; 0.5	-
Calorie Intake at Breakfast (kcal)	135.9	161.9	297.7	128.1	399.3	86.4	2, 83; 23.7; <0.001 *	HC, RE > AN
EDE Total Score	3.2	1.2	0.6	0.4	0.4	0.3	2, 83; 119.9; <0.001 *	AN > REC, HC
EDE Restraint	3.4	1.4	0.5	0.7	0.4	0.5	2, 79; 90.2; <0.001 *	AN > REC, HC
EDE Eating Concern	2.6	1.5	0.1	0.2	0.0	0.1	2, 79; 76.3; <0.001 *	AN > REC, HC
EDE Weight Concern	3.1	1.4	0.7	0.5	0.4	0.3	2, 79; 76.4; <0.001 *	AN > REC, HC
EDE Shape Concern	3.5	1.4	0.8	0.7	0.6	0.5	2, 79; 88.1; <0.001 *	AN > REC, HC
EDI- Total Score	61.8	9.9	47.2	5.1	44.1	2.8	2, 83; 61.4; <0.001 *	AN > REC, HC
Duration of Illness (Years)	6.4	3.9	6.1	5.4	-	-	2, 46; 0.6; 0.5	-
SIAB III	7.4	4.8	4.5	5.5	2.7	3.2	2, 83; 9.1; <0.001 *	AN > REC, HC
BDI-II	21.7	9.7	6.5	6.1	1.6	2.3	2, 83; 75.6; <0.001 *	AN > REC, HC
MWTB	27.9	5.2	29.2	4.8	28.3	4.8	2, 83; 0.5; 0.6	-
Partial GM Volume **	0.59	0.1	0.63	0.1	0.59	0.1	2, 83; 2.3, 0.112	-
Partial WM Volume **	0.30	0.1	0.27	0.1	0.32	0.1	2, 83; 2.1, 0.134	-
Partial CSF Volume **	0.11	0.0	0.11	0.1	0.10	0.0	2, 83; 1.6, 0.202	-

Abbreviation: BMI = body mass index, d.f. = degrees of freedom, EDE = eating disorder examination, EDI = Eating Disorder Inventory-2, SIAB III = Structured Interview for Anorexic and Bulimic Syndromes, Subscale III, BDI-II = Beck Depression Inventory-II, MWT-B = Multiwortwahltest for IQ assessment, AN = anorexia nervosa; HC = healthy control; REC = recovered. * significant group effects, ** partial volume of the left insular MRS voxel.

3.2. MRS

After filtering all CRLBs above 20%, the Cho signal of one HC had to be removed from further analyses.

The robust one-way MANOVA model with the five metabolites as independent variables revealed a significant group effect ($\Lambda = 0.712$, χ^2 (8.41) = 17.1, $p = 0.036$). The robust one-way ANOVAs performed post-hoc were significant for the NAA peak (F (2,31.4) = 3.760; $p = 0.034$, $\xi = 0.35$), with the AN group showing lower NAA concentrations (Table 3, Figure 1). These differences remained significant after applying false discovery rate (FDR) correction for multiple comparisons. When comparing the AN group to the REC group the NAA peak differences reached the trend level, but this result failed to survive FDR correction. Both the REC and HC groups exhibited no significant differences in any metabolites. The robust one-way MANOVA model did still show a significant group effect after adjusting the data for the influence of contraceptive use ($\Lambda = 0.723$, χ^2 (8.41) = 16.3, $p = 0.047$).

Partial GM, WM, and CSF volumes of the left insular MRS voxel exhibited no significant group differences (Table 2).

Table 3. Robust one-way ANOVA results for the five metabolites compared across groups and *p*-value adjusted for multiple comparisons using false discovery rate (FDR) correction.

Metabolite	ANOVA	Post-Hoc Lincon
Cho	F (2.32) = 0.53; $p = 0.593$; $\xi = 0.17$	-
mI	F (2.31) = 1.06; $p = 0.360$; $\xi = 0.22$	-
NAA	F (2.31) = 3.76; $p = 0.034$ *; $\xi = 0.36$	AN < HC
Glx	F (2.28) = 0.39; $p = 0.678$; $\xi = 0.11$	-
Cre	F (2.33) = 0.04; $p = 0.963$; $\xi = 0.11$	-

Abbreviations: Cho = choline; mI = myo-inositol; NAA = N-acetylaspartate; lx = glutamate+glutamine; Cre = creatine. AN = anorexia nervosa; HC = healthy control; ξ = effect size. * significant group effects.

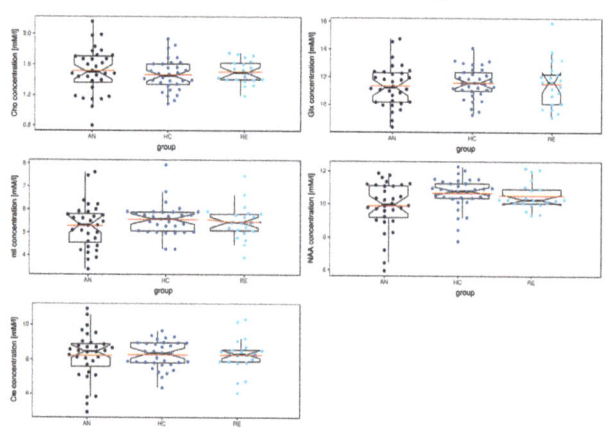

Figure 1. Boxplot of left insula metabolite concentrations across the anorexia nervosa (AN), healthy control (HC) and recovered group (RE). Red lines indicate mean metabolite concentrations. Abbreviations: Cho = choline; mI = myo-inositol; NAA = N-acetylaspartate; Glx = glutamate+glutamine; Cre = creatine.

In the AN group, correlation analyses with dimensional measures of AN severity showed a significant negative association of Glx concentrations with EDE shape concern as well as NAA and Glx concentrations with the EDE weight concern score (Table 4, Figure 2). There were no correlations with either the BMI (Cho: $p = 0.835$, Ins: $p = 0.361$, NAA: $p = 0.870$, Glx: $p = 0.557$, Cre: $p = 0.664$) or the duration of illness (Cho: $p = 0.397$, Ins: $p = 0.508$, NAA: $p = 0.275$, Glx: $p = 0.016$, Cre: $p = 0.223$). Only the correlation of NAA and Glx signals with the EDE weight concern score remained significant after FDR correction.

Table 4. Robust correlation results for the five metabolites with eating disorder symptom severity according to the eating disorder examination (EDE) scale in the AN group. p-values adjusted for multiple comparisons using FDR correction.

Metabolite	Total Score	Restrain	Eating Concern	Weight Concern	Shape Concern
Cho	$r = -0.09$ $p = 0.643$ $p_{FDR} = 0.804$	$r = -0.18$ $p = 0.315$ $p_{FDR} = 0.525$	$r = -0.09$ $p = 0.636$ $p_{FDR} = 0.655$	$r = -0.17$ $p = 0.365$ $p_{FDR} = 0.457$	$r = -0.12$ $p = 0.510$ $p_{FDR} = 0.616$
mI	$r = 0.03$ $p = 0.868$ $p_{FDR} = 0.868$	$r = 0.31$ $p = 0.080$ $p_{FDR} = 0.398$	$r = 0.08$ $p = 0.655$ $p_{FDR} = 0.655$	$r = -0.06$ $p = 0.733$ $p_{FDR} = 0.733$	$r = -0.09$ $p = 0.616$ $p_{FDR} = 0.616$
NAA	$r = -0.28$ $p = 0.120$ $p_{FDR} = 0.300$	$r = -0.06$ $p = 0.745$ $p_{FDR} = 0.849$	$r = -0.25$ $p = 0.174$ $p_{FDR} = 0.655$	$r = -0.46$ $p = 0.008*$ $p_{FDR} = 0.020$	$r = -0.25$ $p = 0.171$ $p_{FDR} = 0.322$
Glx	$r = -0.33$ $p = 0.061$ $p_{FDR} = 0.300$	$r = -0.04$ $p = 0.849$ $p_{FDR} = 0.849$	$r = -0.16$ $p = 0.377$ $p_{FDR} = 0.655$	$r = -0.48$ $p = 0.005*$ $p_{FDR} = 0.020$	$r = -0.40$ $p = 0.025*$ $p_{FDR} = 0.126$
Cre	$r = -0.15$ $p = 0.423$ $p_{FDR} = 0.705$	$r = -0.23$ $p = 0.215$ $p_{FDR} = 0.525$	$r = -0.13$ $p = 0.489$ $p_{FDR} = 0.655$	$r = -0.25$ $p = 0.169$ $p_{FDR} = 0.281$	$r = -0.23$ $p = 0.193$ $p_{FDR} = 0.322$

Abbreviations: Cho = choline; mI = myo-inositol; NAA = N-acetylaspartate; Glx = glutamate+glutamine; Cre = creatine. AN = anorexia nervosa; FDR = false discovery rate. * significant correlations.

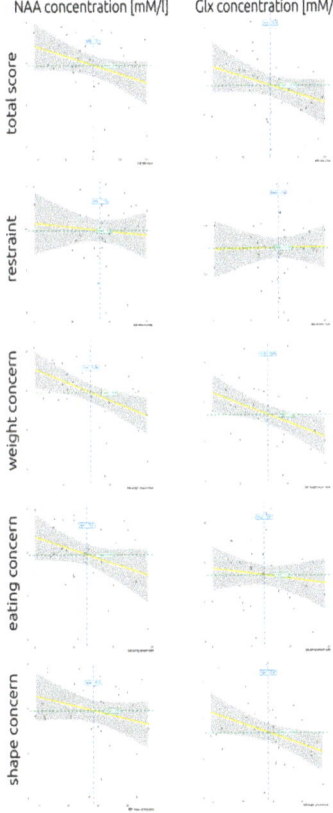

Figure 2. Scatterplot of eating disorder examination (EDE) total scores and subscores of the Anorexia group with left insular N-acetylaspartate (NAA) and glutamate + glutamine (Glx) concentrations, respectively. Blue lines indicate mean EDE scores. Green lines indicate mean metabolite concentrations. Regression lines are depicted in yellow with the 95% confidence interval as grey area. Significant correlations are NAA with weight concerns and Glx with weight and shape concerns.

Additional robust correlations between the five different metabolites showed a significant correlation across the concentration of all metabolites (Table S1).

4. Discussion

This MRS study is the largest to date to investigate insular metabolic alterations in women with acute AN and individuals who had recovered from AN. It was found that AN patients exhibited a significantly lower concentration of NAA in the anterior insular cortex in comparison to the REC and HC subjects, while the concentrations of all other investigated metabolites (t-Cho, mI, Glx, Cre) were unaltered. The REC and HC subjects showed no differences in the concentration of metabolites.

In the AN group, concerns about body weight (as measured with the EDE) were associated with lower NAA and Glx availability in the insular cortex. Prior to correction for multiple comparisons, shape concerns also showed a negative association with Glx concentration. It might be questioned whether this finding is due to a very low BMI or a long illness duration. Neither the BMI nor the duration of illness was associated with insular NAA concentrations.

4.1. Comparison to Earlier MRS Studies

A comparison to earlier MRS studies is complicated by the fact that this study is the first to target the anterior insular cortex in AN. Only two earlier studies reported lower NAA signals in WM and frontal GM [10,13], while one reported increased NAA in anorectic women in the anterior cingulate cortex and parieto-occipital WM [9]. Our findings complement previous studies that showed a reduction in the GM and WM volumes and the integrity during the acute stage of AN [35,75–77]. The detected decreased NAA signal as a marker of neuronal integrity and density [6] in AN might therefore support these earlier results. Structural changes during acute AN appear to be more pronounced in some cortical areas, including the insula [34,78]. Brooks et al. [34] found reduced GM in the right insular cortex in restrictive AN patients. Although the insular cortex has not been consistently affected across structural studies [35,79], in a study of our group with largely overlapping samples, reduced insular volumes and cortical thinning could be observed [78]. Regionally different concentrations of metabolites could thus, in principle, result from differently pronounced structural changes. To determine whether there are changes in metabolite concentration that go beyond known GM/WM volume changes in AN, one has to correct for partial GM/WM volume effects, which was done in the current study. Not all earlier MRS studies statistically controlled for partial GM and WM volume content of the MRS voxel. Metabolic differences that survive such a correction indicate a metabolic disturbance beyond the direct GM or WM volume effect and might therefore be associated with a loss of neuronal integrity, density, or other metabolic changes, some of which might not be known.

4.2. Possible Implications of the Findings: Beyond Density, Volume, and Integrity Effects

Our data indicated that lower NAA concentrations were associated with increased concerns about body weight (according to the EDE), which is a core feature of AN. The Glx signal showed a similar association with weight concerns and both NAA and Glx availability were important for glutamatergic neurotransmission [80,81]. Glx was also associated with shape concern, which did not survive the correction for multiple comparisons. Weight and shape concerns are central constructs of AN psychopathology and are part of a disturbed processing of body signals and integration of one's own body perception. Weight concern refers to the importance of body weight, dissatisfaction with one's own body weight, and the desire to lose weight as well as the preoccupation with shape and weight. Shape concerns imply feelings of fatness, fear of weight gain, and discomfort when looking at one's own body (for further details see: [57,58]). Therefore, the lower the Glx and NAA levels are, the more serious are these concerns.

Importantly, because there were no correlations of NAA and Glx with the BMI and we have corrected for the partial GM and WM volume, the correlation most likely does not simply reflect GM or body weight-related deficits. The associations of insular NAA and Glx availability with weight problems and, in the case of Glx, shape concerns, suggest that a lack of Glx or loss of neuronal density/integrity (which are predominantly glutamatergic in the neocortex) may be related to an exacerbation of AN symptoms, presumably because of a decreased glutamatergic effect.

Disturbed glutamatergic action in the insular cortex might therefore be related to AN's symptoms of "bodily awareness," such as perception of one's own body weight, state, and shape [43,82] and reflect dysregulation within the insular lobe (particularly in anterior parts), which serve to integrate multiple pieces of information. The insular cortex is highly connected and, according to Damasio's somatic marker hypothesis, the insula plays a central role in integrating various perceptions into a cognitive representational map. These perceptions include the information on the bodily state, the state of the autonomic nervous system, appetite, hunger, and disgust [43,44]. Although these are possible associations, no causal relationships can be deduced from these cross-sectional data (i.e., that cerebral dysfunction causes AN psychopathology). Conversely, aberrant perceptions and behavior in AN might lead to metabolic anomalies. A unifying explanation could be that both initially mild behavioral or perceptual abnormalities and initially minor cerebral aberrations reinforce each other in a kind of vicious circle until a full-blown psychopathology and pathophysiology manifests itself.

The absence of the NAA signal reductions in women who had recovered from AN compared to those with AN suggests that the apparent loss of neuronal density/integrity (apart from volume changes, e.g., due to dehydration effects) seem to be of particular importance in acute patients. This aligns with brain volumetric and other structural studies, which report a normalization of WM and GM changes after recovery [37,75,78,83]. Importantly, these patients also recovered with regard to psychopathology—as did our sample—which therefore does not allow any definite conclusions on causality between metabolic changes and psychopathology. At least in the AN group, a simple association with body weight seems unlikely.

However, we cannot completely rule out that the signal similarities of the REC and HC subjects can be attributed to a REC subgroup with a particularly good forecast; only long-term follow-up studies would be able to clarify this point [84].

A recent functional study on anxiety processing in AN showed marked dysfunction of key areas of the so-called "fear network," including the anterior insula cortex. [84]. Other studies have shown that functional abnormalities in the insula are not only in acute AN but also in REC subjects [38,39,41,85]. These observations suggest that NAA changes are likely to reflect anomalies of neurochemical processes beyond cell density or volume effects [37,75,78,83]. NAA is synthesized in neuronal mitochondria and finally absorbed and metabolized by glial cells. For example, in a longitudinal study on bipolar depression in which the NAA signal was regarded as a state marker for the disorder, the reduced NAA levels were interpreted as a dysregulation of the glial function [86].

4.3. Limitations

A longitudinal study design to test for the reversibility of the metabolic differences within the subjects would have been preferable and is envisaged for a subgroup of the AN patients of this study. Another problem was the presence of GM and WM volume effects after correcting for the volume of CSF in the LCModel. To the best of our knowledge there are no biological models available to adjust the concentrations of the different metabolites according to their abundance in GM or WM tissue, respectively. The overlap of the reported structural, functional, and metabolic alterations in the insular cortex in AN, which was investigated in the same subjects, should be confirmed in an independent sample.

5. Summary

In this study, we found decreased NAA signals in the anterior insular cortex of women with AN and lower NAA and Glx concentrations in patients with stronger AN symptoms. These changes cannot be explained by mere GM and WM volume changes, but they could be an expression of reduced neuronal and glial cell density, integrity, or function. These metabolic changes may reflect altered neurotransmission; thus, they may be related to anomalies of insula functioning that are known from functional MRI studies. This possible association should be further investigated in future combined MRS+fMRI studies. The REC and HC participants showed no differences in metabolite concentrations, which is encouraging for both patients and therapists. These data also improve our understanding of the pathophysiology of acute and recovered patients with AN, which can influence both our clinical thinking and psychoeducational interventions [87].

Supplementary Materials: The following are available online at http://www.mdpi.com/2077-0383/9/5/1292/s1, Table S1: Mutual correlation of MRS metabolites. The numbers indicate the correlation coefficient r.

Author Contributions: Conceptualization, S.M., E.P., A.Z., L.T.v.E., and A.J.; data curation, S.M., A.K., L.H., and M.D.; formal analysis, A.H.; funding acquisition, A.Z. and A.J.; investigation, S.M., K.N., and A.K.; methodology, S.M., E.P., D.E., L.H., A.H., M.D., and T.L.; project administration, S.M. and A.J.; resources, A.J.; software, M.D. and T.L.; visualization, S.M.; writing—original draft, S.M. and A.K.; writing—review and editing, K.N., A.Z., L.T.v.E., D.E., D.S., and A.J. All authors have read and agreed to the published version of the manuscript.

Funding: Financial support: Part of project DFG JO 744-2/1.

Acknowledgments: This study was carried out as part of the study DFG (German Research Foundation) of DFG-Grant JO 744-2/1. D.E. and D.S. were supported by the Berta-Ottenstein-Program for Advanced Clinician Scientists, Faculty of Medicine, University of Freiburg. "The article processing charge was funded by the Baden-Wuerttemberg Ministry of Science, Research and Art and the University of Freiburg in the funding program Open Access Publishing.

Conflicts of Interest: The authors declare no conflict of interest.

References

1. Roux, H.; Chapelon, E.; Godart, N. Epidemiology of anorexia nervosa: A review. *Encephale* **2013**, *39*, 85–93. [CrossRef] [PubMed]
2. Smink, F.R.E.; van Hoeken, D.; Hoek, H.W. Epidemiology of Eating Disorders: Incidence, Prevalence and Mortality Rates. *Curr. Psychiatry Rep.* **2012**, *14*, 406–414. [CrossRef] [PubMed]
3. Swanson, S.A.; Crow, S.J.; Le Grange, D.; Swendsen, J.; Merikangas, K.R. Prevalence and correlates of eating disorders in adolescents. Results from the national comorbidity survey replication adolescent supplement. *Arch. Gen. Psychiatry* **2011**, *68*, 714–723. [CrossRef] [PubMed]
4. Arcelus, J.; Mitchell, A.J.; Wales, J.; Nielsen, S. Mortality rates in patients with anorexia nervosa and other eating disorders. A meta-analysis of 36 studies. *Arch. Gen. Psychiatry* **2011**, *68*, 724–731. [CrossRef]
5. Sullivan, P.F. Mortality in anorexia nervosa. *Am. J. Psychiatry* **1995**, *152*, 1073–1074.
6. Birken, D.L.; Oldendorf, W.H. N-Acetyl-L-Aspartic acid: A literature review of a compound prominent in 1H-NMR spectroscopic studies of brain. *Neurosci. Biobehav. Rev.* **1989**, *13*, 23–31. [CrossRef]
7. Baslow, M.H. Evidence supporting a role for N-acetyl-l-aspartate as a molecular water pump in myelinated neurons in the central nervous system: An analytical review. *Neurochem. Int.* **2002**, *40*, 295–300. [CrossRef]
8. Bhakoo, K.K.; Pearce, D. In Vitro Expression of N-Acetyl Aspartate by Oligodendrocytes. *J. Neurochem.* **2000**, *74*, 254–262. [CrossRef]
9. Blasel, S.; Pilatus, U.; Magerkurth, J.; Stauffenberg, M. von; Vronski, D.; Mueller, M.; Woeckel, L.; Hattingen, E. Metabolic gray matter changes of adolescents with anorexia nervosa in combined MR proton and phosphorus spectroscopy. *Neuroradiology* **2012**, *54*, 753–764. [CrossRef]
10. Castro-Fornieles, J.; Bargalló, N.; Lázaro, L.; Andrés, S.; Falcon, C.; Plana, M.T.; Junqué, C. Adolescent anorexia nervosa: Cross-sectional and follow-up frontal gray matter disturbances detected with proton magnetic resonance spectroscopy. *J. Psychiatr. Res.* **2007**, *41*, 952–958. [CrossRef]
11. Hentschel, J.; Möckel, R.; Schlemmer, H.P.; Markus, A.; Göpel, C.; Gückel, F.; Köpke, J.; Georgi, M.; Schmidt, M.H. 1H-MR spectroscopy in anorexia nervosa: The characteristic differences between patients and healthy subjects. *ROFO Fortschr. Geb. Rontgenstr. Nuklearmed.* **1999**, *170*, 284–289. [CrossRef] [PubMed]
12. Joos, A.A.B.; Perlov, E.; Büchert, M.; Hartmann, A.; Saum, B.; Glauche, V.; Freyer, T.; Weber-Fahr, W.; Zeeck, A.; Tebartz van Elst, L. Magnetic resonance spectroscopy of the anterior cingulate cortex in eating disorders. *Psychiatry Res. Neuroimag.* **2011**, *191*, 196–200. [CrossRef] [PubMed]

13. Schlemmer, H.P.; Möckel, R.; Marcus, A.; Hentschel, F.; Göpel, C.; Becker, G.; Köpke, J.; Gückel, F.; Schmidt, M.H.; Georgi, M. Proton magnetic resonance spectroscopy in acute, juvenile anorexia nervosa. *Psychiatry Res.* **1998**, *82*, 171–179. [CrossRef]
14. Braitenberg, V.; Schüz, A. Cortical Architectonics. In *Cortex: Statistics and Geometry of Neuronal Connectivity*; Springer: Berlin/Heidelberg, Germany, 1998; pp. 135–137. ISBN 978-3-662-03735-5.
15. Hasler, G.; Veen, J.W.; van der Tumonis, T.; Meyers, N.; Shen, J.; Drevets, W.C. Reduced Prefrontal Glutamate/Glutamine and γ-Aminobutyric Acid Levels in Major Depression Determined Using Proton Magnetic Resonance Spectroscopy. *Arch. Gen. Psychiatry* **2007**, *64*, 193–200. [CrossRef] [PubMed]
16. Naaijen, J.; Lythgoe, D.J.; Amiri, H.; Buitelaar, J.K.; Glennon, J.C. Fronto-striatal glutamatergic compounds in compulsive and impulsive syndromes: A review of magnetic resonance spectroscopy studies. *Neurosci. Biobehav. Rev.* **2015**, *52*, 74–88. [CrossRef]
17. Pollack, M.H.; Jensen, J.E.; Simon, N.M.; Kaufman, R.E.; Renshaw, P.F. High-field MRS study of GABA, glutamate and glutamine in social anxiety disorder: Response to treatment with levetiracetam. *Prog. Neuropsychopharmacol. Biol. Psychiatry* **2008**, *32*, 739–743. [CrossRef]
18. Yüksel, C.; Öngür, D. Magnetic resonance spectroscopy studies of glutamate-related abnormalities in mood disorders. *Biol. Psychiatry* **2010**, *68*, 785–794. [CrossRef]
19. Macrez, R.; Stys, P.K.; Vivien, D.; Lipton, S.A.; Docagne, F. Mechanisms of glutamate toxicity in multiple sclerosis: Biomarker and therapeutic opportunities. *Lancet Neurol.* **2016**, *15*, 1089–1102. [CrossRef]
20. Bartha, R.; Williamson, P.C.; Drost, D.J.; Malla, A.; Carr, T.J.; Cortese, L.; Canaran, G.; Rylett, R.J.; Neufeld, R.W.J. Measurement of Glutamate and Glutamine in the Medial Prefrontal Cortex of Never-Treated Schizophrenic Patients and Healthy Controls by Proton Magnetic Resonance Spectroscopy. *Arch. Gen. Psychiatry* **1997**, *54*, 959–965. [CrossRef]
21. Ohrmann, P.; Kersting, A.; Suslow, T.; Lalee-Mentzel, J.; Donges, U.-S.; Fiebich, M.; Arolt, V.; Heindel, W.; Pfleiderer, B. Proton magnetic resonance spectroscopy in anorexia nervosa: Correlations with cognition. *Neuroreport* **2004**, *15*, 549–553. [CrossRef]
22. Godlewska, B.R.; Pike, A.; Sharpley, A.L.; Ayton, A.; Park, R.J.; Cowen, P.J.; Emir, U.E. Brain glutamate in anorexia nervosa: A magnetic resonance spectroscopy case control study at 7 Tesla. *Psychopharmacology* **2017**, *234*, 421–426. [CrossRef] [PubMed]
23. Plitman, E.; de la Fuente-Sandoval, C.; Reyes-Madrigal, F.; Chavez, S.; Gómez-Cruz, G.; León-Ortiz, P.; Graff-Guerrero, A. Elevated Myo-Inositol, Choline, and Glutamate Levels in the Associative Striatum of Antipsychotic-Naive Patients With First-Episode Psychosis: A Proton Magnetic Resonance Spectroscopy Study With Implications for Glial Dysfunction. *Schizophr. Bull.* **2015**, *42*, 415–424. [CrossRef] [PubMed]
24. Baek, H.-M.; Chen, J.-H.; Nalcioglu, O.; Su, M.-Y. Choline as a Biomarker for Cell Proliferation: Do the Results from Proton MR Spectroscopy Show Difference between HER2/neu Positive and Negative Breast Cancers? *Int. J. Cancer J. Int. Cancer* **2008**, *123*, 1219–1221. [CrossRef]
25. Castro-Fornieles, J.; Garcia, A.I.; Lazaro, L.; Andrés-Perpiñá, S.; Falcón, C.; Plana, M.T.; Bargallo, N. Prefrontal brain metabolites in short-term weight-recovered adolescent anorexia nervosa patients. *Prog. Neuropsychopharmacol. Biol. Psychiatry* **2010**, *34*, 1049–1053. [CrossRef] [PubMed]
26. Wyss, M.; Kaddurah-Daouk, R. Creatine and Creatinine Metabolism. *Physiol. Rev.* **2000**, *80*, 1107–1213. [CrossRef]
27. Soares, D.P.; Law, M. Magnetic resonance spectroscopy of the brain: Review of metabolites and clinical applications. *Clin. Radiol.* **2009**, *64*, 12–21. [CrossRef]
28. Roser, W.; Bubl, R.; Buergin, D.; Seelig, J.; Radue, E.W.; Rost, B. Metabolic changes in the brain of patients with anorexia and bulimia nervosa as detected by proton magnetic resonance spectroscopy. *Int. J. Eat. Disord.* **1999**, *26*, 119–136. [CrossRef]
29. Kato, T.; Shioiri, T.; Murashita, J.; Inubushi, T. Phosphorus-31 magnetic resonance spectroscopic observations in 4 cases with anorexia nervosa. *Prog. Neuropsychopharmacol. Biol. Psychiatry* **1997**, *21*, 719–724. [CrossRef]
30. Möckel, R.; Schlemmer, H.P.; Gückel, F.; Göpel, C.; Becker, G.; Köpke, J.; Hentschel, F.; Schmidt, M.; Georgi, M. 1H-MR spectroscopy in anorexia nervosa: Reversible cerebral metabolic changes. *ROFO Fortschr. Geb. Rontgenstr. Nuklearmed.* **1999**, *170*, 371–377. [CrossRef]

31. Rzanny, R.; Freesmeyer, D.; Reichenbach, J.R.; Mentzel, H.J.; Pfleiderer, S.O.R.; Klemm, S.; Gerhard, U.J.; Blanz, B.; Kaiser, W.A. 31P-MR spectroscopy of the brain in patients with anorexia nervosa: Characteristic differences in the spectra between patients and healthy control subjects. *ROFO Fortschr. Geb. Rontgenstr. Nuklearmed.* **2003**, *175*, 75–82. [CrossRef]
32. Grzelak, P.; Gajewicz, W.; Wyszogrodzka-Kucharska, A.; Rotkiewicz, A.; Stefańczyk, L.; Góraj, B.; Rabe-Jabłońska, J. Brain metabolism alterations in patients with anorexia nervosa observed in 1H-MRS. *Psychiatr. Pol.* **2005**, *39*, 761–771. [PubMed]
33. Bomba, M.; Riva, A.; Morzenti, S.; Grimaldi, M.; Neri, F.; Nacinovich, R. Global and regional brain volumes normalization in weight-recovered adolescents with anorexia nervosa: Preliminary findings of a longitudinal voxel-based morphometry study. *Neuropsychiatr. Dis. Treat.* **2015**, *11*, 637–645. [CrossRef] [PubMed]
34. Brooks, S.J.; Barker, G.J.; O'Daly, O.G.; Brammer, M.; Williams, S.C.; Benedict, C.; Schiöth, H.B.; Treasure, J.; Campbell, I.C. Restraint of appetite and reduced regional brain volumes in anorexia nervosa: A voxel-based morphometric study. *BMC Psychiatry* **2011**, *11*, 179. [CrossRef] [PubMed]
35. Frank, G.K.W.; Shott, M.E.; Hagman, J.O.; Yang, T.T. Localized Brain Volume and White Matter Integrity Alterations in Adolescent Anorexia Nervosa. *J. Am. Acad. Child Adolesc. Psychiatry* **2013**, *52*, 1066–1075. [CrossRef] [PubMed]
36. Friederich, H.-C.; Walther, S.; Bendszus, M.; Biller, A.; Thomann, P.; Zeigermann, S.; Katus, T.; Brunner, R.; Zastrow, A.; Herzog, W. Grey matter abnormalities within cortico-limbic-striatal circuits in acute and weight-restored anorexia nervosa patients. *NeuroImage* **2012**, *59*, 1106–1113. [CrossRef] [PubMed]
37. Wagner, A.; Greer, P.; Bailer, U.F.; Frank, G.K.; Henry, S.E.; Putnam, K.; Meltzer, C.C.; Ziolko, S.K.; Hoge, J.; McConaha, C.; et al. Normal Brain Tissue Volumes after Long-Term Recovery in Anorexia and Bulimia Nervosa. *Biol. Psychiatry* **2006**, *59*, 291–293. [CrossRef] [PubMed]
38. Kerr, K.L.; Moseman, S.E.; Avery, J.A.; Bodurka, J.; Zucker, N.L.; Simmons, W.K. Altered Insula Activity during Visceral Interoception in Weight-Restored Patients with Anorexia Nervosa. *Neuropsychopharmacology* **2016**, *41*, 521–528. [CrossRef]
39. Kim, K.R.; Ku, J.; Lee, J.-H.; Lee, H.; Jung, Y.-C. Functional and effective connectivity of anterior insula in anorexia nervosa and bulimia nervosa. *Neurosci. Lett.* **2012**, *521*, 152–157. [CrossRef]
40. Oberndorfer, T.; Simmons, A.; McCurdy, D.; Strigo, I.; Matthews, S.; Yang, T.; Irvine, Z.; Kaye, W. Greater anterior insula activation during anticipation of food images in women recovered from anorexia nervosa versus controls. *Psychiatry Res. Neuroimag.* **2013**, *214*, 132–141. [CrossRef]
41. Strigo, I.A.; Matthews, S.C.; Simmons, A.N.; Oberndorfer, T.; Klabunde, M.; Reinhardt, L.E.; Kaye, W.H. Altered insula activation during pain anticipation in individuals recovered from anorexia nervosa: Evidence of interoceptive dysregulation. *Int. J. Eat. Disord.* **2013**, *46*, 23–33. [CrossRef]
42. Nunn, K.; Frampton, I.; Gordon, I.; Lask, B. The fault is not in her parents but in her insula—A neurobiological hypothesis of anorexia nervosa. *Eur. Eat. Disord. Rev. J. Eat. Disord. Assoc.* **2008**, *16*, 355–360. [CrossRef] [PubMed]
43. Nunn, K.; Frampton, I.; Fuglset, T.S.; Törzsök-Sonnevend, M.; Lask, B. Anorexia nervosa and the insula. *Med. Hypotheses* **2011**, *76*, 353–357. [CrossRef]
44. Craig, A.D.B. How do you feel now? The anterior insula and human awareness. *Nat. Rev. Neurosci.* **2009**, *10*, 59–70. [CrossRef] [PubMed]
45. Craig, A.D. Interoception: The sense of the physiological condition of the body. *Curr. Opin. Neurobiol.* **2003**, *13*, 500–505. [CrossRef]
46. Paulus, M.P.; Stein, M.B. An insular view of anxiety. *Biol. Psychiatry* **2006**, *60*, 383–387. [CrossRef]
47. Mazzola, L.; Royet, J.-P.; Catenoix, H.; Montavont, A.; Isnard, J.; Mauguière, F. Gustatory and olfactory responses to stimulation of the human insula. *Ann. Neurol.* **2017**, *82*, 360–370. [CrossRef]
48. Small, D.M. Taste representation in the human insula. *Brain Struct. Funct.* **2010**, *214*, 551–561. [CrossRef]
49. Haase, L.; Cerf-Ducastel, B.; Murphy, C. Cortical activation in response to pure taste stimuli during the physiological states of hunger and satiety. *NeuroImage* **2009**, *44*, 1008–1021. [CrossRef]
50. Pujol, J.; Blanco-Hinojo, L.; Coronas, R.; Esteba-Castillo, S.; Rigla, M.; Martínez-Vilavella, G.; Deus, J.; Novell, R.; Caixàs, A. Mapping the sequence of brain events in response to disgusting food: Brain Response to Disgusting Food. *Hum. Brain Mapp.* **2018**, *39*, 369–380. [CrossRef]
51. Critchley, H.D.; Harrison, N.A. Visceral Influences on Brain and Behavior. *Neuron* **2013**, *77*, 624–638. [CrossRef]

52. Kaye, W.H.; Fudge, J.L.; Paulus, M. New insights into symptoms and neurocircuit function of anorexia nervosa. *Nat. Rev. Neurosci.* **2009**, *10*, 573–584. [CrossRef] [PubMed]
53. Fydrich, T.; Renneberg, B.; Schmitz, B.; Wittchen, H.U. *SKID-II. Strukturiertes Klinisches Interview für DSM-IV. Achse II: Persönlichkeitsstörungen, Interviewheft*; Hogrefe: Gottingen, Germany, 1997.
54. Wittchen, H.U.; Zaudig, M.; Fydrich, T. *SKID. Strukturiertes Klinisches Interview für DSM-IV. Achse I und II, Handanweisung*; Hogrefe: Gottingen, Germany, 1997.
55. American Psychiatric Association. *The Diagnostic and Statistical Manual of Mental Disorders: DSM 5*; American Psychiatric Publishing: Arlington, TX, USA, 2013.
56. Couturier, J.; Lock, J. What is remission in adolescent anorexia nervosa? A review of various conceptualizations and quantitative analysis. *Int. J. Eat. Disord.* **2006**, *39*, 175–183. [CrossRef] [PubMed]
57. Hilbert, A.; Tuschen-Caffier, B.; Karwautz, A.; Niederhofer, H.; Munsch, S. Eating Disorder Examination-Questionnaire. *Diagnostica* **2007**, *53*, 144–154. [CrossRef]
58. Hilbert, A.; Tuschen-Caffier, B.; Ohms, M. Eating Disorder Examination: Deutschsprachige Version des strukturierten Essstörungsinterviews. *Diagnostica* **2004**, *50*, 98–106. [CrossRef]
59. Garner, D.M. *Eating Disorder Inventory-2*; Psychological Assessment Resources: Odessa, TX, USA, 1991.
60. Meermann, R.; Napierski, C.; Schulenkorf, E. *Eating Disorder Inventory (German Version)*; Walter de Gruyter: Berlin, Germany, 1987.
61. Hautzinger, M.; Keller, F.; Kühner, C. *Beck Depressions-Inventar (BDI-II)*; Harcourt Test Services: Frankfurt, Germany, 2006.
62. Beck, A.T.; Steer, R.A. *Beck Depression Inventory*; The Psychological Corporation: San Antonio, TX, USA, 1987.
63. Herzberg, P.; Goldschmidt, S.; Heinrichs, N. Beck Depressions-Inventar (BDI-II). *Revis. Rep. Psychol.* **2008**, *33*, 301–302.
64. Provencher, S.W. Estimation of metabolite concentrations from localized in vivo proton NMR spectra. *Magn. Reason. Med.* **1993**, *30*, 672–679. [CrossRef]
65. Provencher, S.W. Automatic quantitation of localized in vivo 1H spectra with LCModel. *NMR Biomed.* **2001**, *14*, 260–264. [CrossRef]
66. Endres, D.; Perlov, E.; Maier, S.; Feige, B.; Nickel, K.; Goll, P.; Bubl, E.; Lange, T.; Glauche, V.; Graf, E.; et al. Normal Neurochemistry in the Prefrontal and Cerebellar Brain of Adults with Attention-Deficit Hyperactivity Disorder. *Front. Behav. Neurosci.* **2015**, *9*, 242. [CrossRef]
67. Friston, K.J. *Statistical Parametric Mapping: The Analysis of Functional Brain Images*; Elsevier: Amsterdam, The Netherlands, 2008.
68. R Core Team. *R: A Language and Environment for Statistical Computing*; R Foundation for Statistical Computing: Vienna, Austria, 2016.
69. Todorov, V.; Filzmoser, P. Robust statistic for the one-way MANOVA. *Comput. Stat. Data Anal.* **2010**, *54*, 37–48. [CrossRef]
70. Todorov, V.; Filzmoser, P. An Object-Oriented Framework for Robust Multivariate Analysis. *J. Stat. Softw.* **2009**. [CrossRef]
71. Wilcox, R.R. *Introduction to Robust Estimation and Hypothesis Testing*; Academic Press: Cambridge, MA, USA, 2011.
72. Schoenbrodt, F.; Wilcox, R. *WRS2: Wilcox Robust Estimation and Testing*; Version 0.9; R Core Team: Vienna, Austria, 2017.
73. Wilcox, R.R.; Tian, T.S. Measuring effect size: A robust heteroscedastic approach for two or more groups. *J. Appl. Stat.* **2011**, *38*, 1359–1368. [CrossRef]
74. Benjamini, Y.; Hochberg, Y. Controlling the False Discovery Rate: A Practical and Powerful Approach to Multiple Testing. *J. R. Stat. Soc. Ser. B Methodol.* **1995**, *57*, 289–300. [CrossRef]
75. Bang, L.; Rø, Ø.; Endestad, T. Normal gray matter volumes in women recovered from anorexia nervosa: A voxel-based morphometry study. *BMC Psychiatry* **2016**, *16*, 144. [CrossRef] [PubMed]
76. Fuglset, T.S.; Endestad, T.; Hilland, E.; Bang, L.; Tamnes, C.K.; Landrø, N.I.; Rø, Ø. Brain volumes and regional cortical thickness in young females with anorexia nervosa. *BMC Psychiatry* **2016**, *16*, 404. [CrossRef] [PubMed]
77. King, J.A.; Geisler, D.; Ritschel, F.; Boehm, I.; Seidel, M.; Roschinski, B.; Soltwedel, L.; Zwipp, J.; Pfuhl, G.; Marxen, M.; et al. Global cortical thinning in acute anorexia nervosa normalizes following long-term weight restoration. *Biol. Psychiatry* **2015**, *77*, 624–632. [CrossRef]

78. Nickel, K.; Joos, A.; Elst, L.T.; van Matthis, J.; Holovics, L.; Endres, D.; Zeeck, A.; Hartmann, A.; Tüscher, O.; Maier, S. Recovery of cortical volume and thickness after remission from acute anorexia nervosa. *Int. J. Eat. Disord.* **2018**, *51*, 1056–1069. [CrossRef]
79. Lavagnino, L.; Amianto, F.; Mwangi, B.; D'Agata, F.; Spalatro, A.; Zunta Soares, G.B.; Daga, G.A.; Mortara, P.; Fassino, S.; Soares, J.C. The relationship between cortical thickness and body mass index differs between women with anorexia nervosa and healthy controls. *Psychiatry Res. Neuroimag.* **2016**, *248*, 105–109. [CrossRef]
80. Yan, H.-D.; Ishihara, K.; Serikawa, T.; Sasa, M. Activation by N-Acetyl-l-Aspartate of Acutely Dissociated Hippocampal Neurons in Rats via Metabotropic Glutamate Receptors. *Epilepsia* **2003**, *44*, 1153–1159. [CrossRef]
81. Reiner, A.; Levitz, J. Glutamatergic Signaling in the Central Nervous System: Ionotropic and Metabotropic Receptors in Concert. *Neuron* **2018**, *98*, 1080–1098. [CrossRef]
82. Hogeveen, J.; Bird, G.; Chau, A.; Krueger, F.; Grafman, J. Acquired alexithymia following damage to the anterior insula. *Neuropsychologia* **2016**, *82*, 142–148. [CrossRef]
83. Lázaro, L.; Andrés, S.; Calvo, A.; Cullell, C.; Moreno, E.; Plana, M.T.; Falcón, C.; Bargalló, N.; Castro-Fornieles, J. Normal gray and white matter volume after weight restoration in adolescents with anorexia nervosa. *Int. J. Eat. Disord.* **2013**, *46*, 841–848. [CrossRef] [PubMed]
84. Maier, S.; Schneider, K.; Stark, C.; Zeeck, A.; Tebartz van Elst, L.; Holovics, L.; Hartmann, A.; Lahmann, C.; Domschke, K.; Nickel, K.; et al. Fear Network Unresponsiveness in Women with Anorexia Nervosa. *Psychother. Psychosom.* **2018**. [CrossRef] [PubMed]
85. Leppanen, J.; Cardi, V.; Paloyelis, Y.; Simmons, A.; Tchanturia, K.; Treasure, J. Blunted neural response to implicit negative facial affect in anorexia nervosa. *Biol. Psychol.* **2017**, *128*, 105–111. [CrossRef] [PubMed]
86. Croarkin, P.E.; Thomas, M.A.; Port, J.D.; Baruth, J.M.; Choi, D.-S.; Abulseoud, O.A.; Frye, M.A. N-acetylaspartate normalization in bipolar depression after lamotrigine treatment. *Bipolar Disord.* **2015**, *17*, 450–457. [CrossRef]
87. Bang, L.; Treasure, J.; Rø, Ø.; Joos, A. Advancing our understanding of the neurobiology of anorexia nervosa: Translation into treatment. *J. Eat. Disord.* **2017**, *5*, 38. [CrossRef]

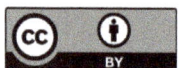

© 2020 by the authors. Licensee MDPI, Basel, Switzerland. This article is an open access article distributed under the terms and conditions of the Creative Commons Attribution (CC BY) license (http://creativecommons.org/licenses/by/4.0/).

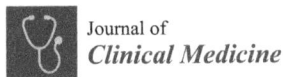

Article

A Randomized Trial of Deep Brain Stimulation to the Subcallosal Cingulate and Nucleus Accumbens in Patients with Treatment-Refractory, Chronic, and Severe Anorexia Nervosa: Initial Results at 6 Months of Follow Up

Gloria Villalba Martínez [1,2], Azucena Justicia [3,4,5], Purificación Salgado [4], José María Ginés [4], Rocío Guardiola [4], Carlos Cedrón [4], María Polo [4], Ignacio Delgado-Martínez [1], Santiago Medrano [6], Rosa María Manero [7], Gerardo Conesa [1,3,8], Gustavo Faus [9], Antoni Grau [9], Matilde Elices [3,5,*] and Víctor Pérez [2,3,4,5]

1. Department of Neurosurgery, Hospital del Mar, 08003 Barcelona, Spain; gloriavillabamartinez@gmail.com (G.V.M.); idelgadom@parcdesalutmar.cat (I.D.-M.); gconesa@parcdesalutmar.cat (G.C.)
2. Department of Psychiatry and Forensic Medicine, Universitat Autònoma de Barcelona, Cerdanyola del Vallès, 08193 Barcelona, Spain; vperezsola@parcdesalutmar.cat
3. Hospital del Mar Medical Research Institute (IMIM), 08003 Barcelona, Spain; ajusticia@imim.es
4. Institut de Neuropsiquiatria i Adiccions (INAD), Hospital del Mar, 08003 Barcelona, Spain; psalgado@parcdesalutmar.cat (P.S.); jgines@parcdesalutmar.cat (J.M.G.); rguardiola@parcdesalutmar.cat (R.G.); ccedron@parcdesalutmar.cat (C.C.); mpolo@parcdesalutmar.cat (M.P.)
5. Centro de Investigación Biomédica en Red de Salud Mental (CIBERSAM), 28029 Madrid, Spain
6. Department of Radiology, Hospital del Mar, 08003 Barcelona, Spain; santiago.medrano@upf.edu
7. Department of Neurology, Hospital del Mar, 08003 Barcelona, Spain; rmanero@parcdesalutmar.cat
8. Department of Surgery, Universitat Autònoma de Barcelona, Cerdanyola del Vallès, 08193 Barcelona, Spain
9. ITA, Mental Health Specialists, 08036 Barcelona, Spain; gfaus@ita.com (G.F.); agrau@ita.com (A.G.)
* Correspondence: melices@imim.es; Tel.: +34-933160

Received: 31 May 2020; Accepted: 16 June 2020; Published: 22 June 2020

Abstract: Background: The main objective of this study was to assess the safety and efficacy of deep brain stimulation (DBS) in patients with severe anorexia nervosa (AN). Methods: Eight participants received active DBS to the subcallosal cingulate (SCC) or nucleus accumbens (NAcc) depending on comorbidities (affective or anxiety disorders, respectively) and type of AN. The primary outcome measure was body mass index (BMI). Results: Overall, we found no significant difference ($p = 0.84$) between mean preoperative and postoperative (month 6) BMI. A BMI reference value (BMI-RV) was calculated. In patients that received preoperative inpatient care to raise the BMI, the BMI-RV was defined as the mean BMI value in the 12 months prior to surgery. In patients that did not require inpatient care, the BMI-RV was defined as the mean BMI in the 3-month period before surgery. This value was compared to the postoperative BMI (month 6), revealing a significant increase ($p = 0.02$). After 6 months of DBS, five participants showed an increase of ≥10% in the BMI-RV. Quality of life was improved ($p = 0.03$). Three cases presented cutaneous complications. Conclusion: DBS may be effective for some patients with severe AN. Cutaneous complications were observed. Longer term data are needed.

Keywords: anorexia nervosa; deep brain stimulation; psychosurgery; clinical trial; subcallosal cingulate; nucleus accumbens; body mass index

1. Introduction

Anorexia nervosa (AN) is a psychiatric disorder with an estimated prevalence of 0.7–3%. It primarily affects females and is usually diagnosed in adolescence and young adulthood [1,2]. AN is a life-threatening illness that can have a devastating impact on patients and their family [2,3]. The Diagnostic and Statistical Manual of Mental Disorders (DSM-5) criteria define two subtypes of AN: the restricting type and the binge-eating/purging type, with the latter type (purging) having a worse prognosis. Treatment of AN involves a combination of nutritional, pharmacological, psychological, and family interventions, all of which aim to restore normal weight, alter behavioural patterns, and address associated psychological issues. However, the optimal treatment for AN remains unclear and controversial [4,5].

Clear criteria to determine treatment refractoriness has not been fully established yet for this complex illness. Refractoriness in AN is currently defined as a failure to respond to repeated interventions over an extended time period (5–10 years), with recovery considered unlikely or, at best, limited in patients who have had AN for more than 10 years [3,6]. This condition is believed to be multifactorial, including neurobiological, environmental, and genetic factors, among others. Several studies seem to agree that AN is primarily caused by neurobiological alterations provoked by underlying dysfunction in the brain circuits. Although numerous models have been proposed to explain this dysfunction, most researchers agree that limbic system alterations are likely the main cause [7–13]. It has also been suggested that AN is, at least partially, maintained by dysfunctional activity in key neuroanatomic circuits [14–17], primarily those related to the modulation of reward and motivation, such as the mesolimbic cortex and the striatum [8,12].

Some authors have suggested that brain areas involved in the cognitive control of appetite (dorsolateral prefrontal and the parietal cortex) could also be involved in the pathophysiology of AN [10,13]. Morphological and functional studies in patients with AN have shown alterations in insular activity and in the prefrontal cortex, orbitofrontal, temporal, parietal, anterior cingulate, and ventral striatum (nucleus accumbens, NAcc) [18–20]. The available evidence suggests that the two most relevant targets for the surgical treatment of AN appear to be the NAcc [21] and the subcallosal cingulate (SCC), mainly due to the substantial involvement of these two structures in the reward circuits, but also because these two areas serve as communication links between the limbic and cortical systems [7,9].

Deep brain stimulation (DBS) is a surgical technique with a long history in the treatment of movement disorders such as Parkinson's disease, dystonia, and essential tremor, offering good outcomes with only minimal complications [10,22,23]. In recent decades, this technique has also been used to treat mental disorders such as obsessive-compulsive disorder (OCD), major depressive disorder (MDD), and schizophrenia [24,25]. However, OCD is the only mental disorder for which DBS is currently approved by both the United States Food and Drug Administration (FDA) and by the European Union (CE Marking certification) [24,26,27]. In other mental disorders, DBS has only been performed in the context of clinical trials or for compassionate use.

Although the precise mechanism of action of DBS remains unclear, several models and hypotheses have been proposed. Electrophysiological studies suggest that the effect of DBS depends on the type of stimulated brain tissue (e.g., grey or white matter) and on the type of fibers involved in the stimulation [13,28,29]. In addition, DBS is believed to alter neuronal discharge patterns in the target area (jamming effect). These different mechanisms may thus combine both inhibitory and excitatory processes, which could act simultaneously. Even though DBS is applied locally to a specific brain area, both focal and distal effects have been reported [29].

Experience with DBS in patients with AN is limited. To date, a total of 26 women with AN, with variable clinical characteristics (e.g., severity, chronicity) have participated in clinical studies. Moreover, those studies targeted different brain structures. McLaughlin et al. reported a case of a patient with comorbid AN and OCD (body mass index (BMI): 18.5) whose condition improved slightly after DBS to the ventral striatum [30]. Wang and colleagues described two cases of adolescent patients with AN who received bilateral DBS to the NAcc, with no complications; over the course of 12-month follow up, both patients in that study successfully reached a normal BMI and also showed improvements in psychopathological symptoms and quality of life. Wu et. al. [31] also reported results of a case series of four adolescents with AN in which DBS was applied to the NAcc. In all four cases, psychological symptoms improved and body weight increased by up to 65%, without complications over a follow-up period that ranged from 9 to 50 months. In that same year (2013), Lipsman et al. reported results from a phase 1 pilot trial in which DBS was applied to the subcallosal cingulate in 6 patients with AN [32]. At nine months of follow up, half of the patients showed a response to treatment (BMI above baseline values); in addition, four patients presented improved psychometric assessments. Israel et al. published a case report of a patient with MDD and comorbid AN, who received DBS to the SCC (unilateral, right side, intermittent). The results were good and the patient successfully maintained BMI = 19.6 for more than 30 months [33]. In 2017, the same research group reported the results of a 12-month clinical trial involving 16 patients with AN (including the six patients from the original study) who received DBS to the SCC. Mean BMI values and psychometric assessments improved in all 16 patients over time; moreover, a flurodeoxyglucose–positron-emission tomography (FDG-PET) scan showed metabolic changes in the brain after six months of DBS. However, several adverse events were reported, including one event of each of the following: air embolism, seizure, skin infection, worsening in mood, and intraoperative panic attack, and five of the patients also experienced pain [34]. Blomstedt and colleagues published a case report of a patient with MDD and comorbid AN in whom DBS was administered to the bed nucleus of the stria terminalis (BNST). Although the procedure did not significantly change the BMI, it did improve the patient's anxiety about food and eating [35]. Finally, the most recently published study was reported by Manuelli et al. (in 2019), who described the case of a patient with moderate AN who underwent DBS to the BNST. In that patient, BMI, core AN symptoms, and nutritional status all improved at six months of follow up [36].

Together, the limited evidence for DBS as a treatment for AN suggests that DBS appears to be a safe and effective treatment. However, due to the heterogeneity of this disorder, and the difficulty of recruiting patients to participate in clinical trials and studies, it is difficult to make definitive conclusions about the efficacy of DBS, the optimal target site, and the clinical and radiological variables that determine response. In this context, the main aim of the present clinical trial was to assess the efficacy and safety of DBS applied to two different targets (SCC and NAcc) to treat patients with chronic, severe, refractory AN. This study has been divided into three distinctive phases. Phase I involved the selection of participants and preoperative procedures. Phase II involved the surgical procedure itself, including a 6-month period of active stimulation. In phase III, patients considered responders to the DBS implant were randomized to one of two arms (ON/OFF or OFF/ON), while non-responders were not randomized, rather, they continued to be assessed monthly throughout the 12-month follow-up period. As phase III is currently ongoing, the current report presents data on phase I (preoperative) and phase II (6 months follow up).

2. Materials and Methods

2.1. Participants and Setting

A total of eight participants diagnosed with chronic, severe, refractory AN were included in this trial over a one-year period, which was conducted jointly by the Departments of Psychiatry and the Surgery Department of the Hospital del Mar in Barcelona, Spain, a tertiary care university hospital. Participants were recruited from collaborating sites around Spain, including the *Eating Disorders Institute, Mental Health Specialists* (in Spanish, *ITA Especialistas en Salud Mental*), a national network of hospitals and treatment centers across Spain providing specialized care for patients with eating disorders.

The inclusion criteria were as follows: age: 18–60 years, clinical diagnosis of any type of AN (DSM-5 criteria), duration of AN > 10 years, treatment-resistant AN, defined as follows: (a) lack of response to ≥3 voluntary intensive treatments (full or partial hospitalization) or (b) clinical worsening and unwillingness to receive any further treatment, including ≥2 hospital admissions for involuntary feeding, preoperative BMI between 13 and 15.99 (patients with BMI values outside this range could be included on case-by-case basis), and capacity to fully understand the study and to provide informed consent. Exclusion criteria: current or past psychotic episode, comorbid neurological illness, drug abuse in the last year, contraindications to undergo magnetic resonance imaging (MRI) or DBS, any medical condition involving a risk for the surgical procedure, and pregnancy.

Written informed consent was obtained from all participants before proceeding with any intervention. The study was performed according to the ethical standards stated in the Declaration of Helsinki and subsequent updates. The study was approved by the Ethics Committee of the Parc de Salut (Barcelona, Spain, approval number: 2016/6813/I). Trial registration: Clinicaltrials.gov: NCT03168893.

2.2. Design and Procedure

This is a randomized, double-blind, controlled crossover clinical trial consisting of two consecutive 6-month phases (total duration: 12 months). Target selection was based on the presence of comorbidities with other psychiatric conditions and the type of AN. Patients whose predominant comorbidity was an affective disorder received DBS to the SCC, while patients whose predominant comorbidity was an anxiety disorder received DBS to the NAcc. The predominant comorbidity was determined by a clinical psychiatrist based on the MINI International Neuropsychiatric Interview scores and a comprehensive clinical interview. Each case was then reviewed by the other members of the clinical research team (a psychologist and a psychiatrist) to ensure their assessments for each comorbidity were consistent. For patients that did not show any clear predominant comorbidity, the target was selected based on the type of AN: patients with binge-eating/purgative AN received DBS to the NAcc, and patients with restrictive AN received DBS to the SCC. If a patient presented criteria for both targets, the target that corresponded to the most severe comorbidity was selected.

Phase I of the study consisted of the patient recruitment and selection. Potential candidates were interviewed by a member of the research team (psychiatrist). After this initial screening, an independent, external psychiatrist confirmed that the patient met all inclusion criteria. Patients were required to present normal results on all of the following preoperative tests: chest x-ray, electrocardiogram, and anesthesia tolerance test. Minimal alterations in blood test results were allowed, provided that these were normalized prior to surgery. The optimal pre-operative BMI was set at ≥13; in cases with a BMI < 13, the participant was admitted to the inpatient ward to raise the BMI to meet the minimum threshold. A 1.5 T MRI with diffusion tensor imaging (DTI) was performed pre-operatively. Before study inclusion, the participants' BMI data in the previous year was registered (lowest, highest, and mean).

Phase II involved the surgical procedure and six-month follow-up. The DBS system was implanted using robotic stereotactic assistance (ROSA; Zimmer Biomet, Inc. Montpellier, France). The surgical procedure was performed under general anesthesia and divided into three steps: (1) fiducial markers were inserted followed by an intraoperative computerized tomography (CT) scan, (2) the ROSA robotic arm was prepared and electrodes (Infinity; Abbott Inc., Saint Paul, MN, USA) were placed on the selected target through two trephine holes, at the frontal level, bilaterally. The Infinity electrodes (Abbott Inc., Saint Paul, MN, USA) are directional electrodes with four contacts, 1.5 mm in diameter, with 1.5 mm spacing between contacts, with an inactive distal part, and (3) finally, a pulse generator was implanted subfascially at the right abdominal area and connected to the electrodes. A postoperative cranial CT scan was performed and fused with the preoperative MRI CT scan. Correct placement of the electrode contact points was verified. Next, monopolar stimulation was performed. The stimulation started at 3.5 milliamperes (MA) and was increased according to patient response. The frequency (130 Hz), pulse amplitude (90 micros), and contact were set to remain constant throughout the trial.

Stimulation began 24 hours after surgery and participants were discharged 72 hours after the intervention. At 10 days, an initial postoperative assessment was performed by the psychiatrist and neurosurgeon at the outpatient clinic, and subsequent evaluations were scheduled to be performed monthly. All participants were provided with contact details (telephone/email) for the surgeon and co-primary investigator to communicate any adverse events over the course of the trial.

A third and final phase (phase III) of this trial is still ongoing. Consequently, the present report focuses on describing phase I and on presenting the data from phase II (6-months follow up). A flowchart of the complete study design is shown in Figure 1.

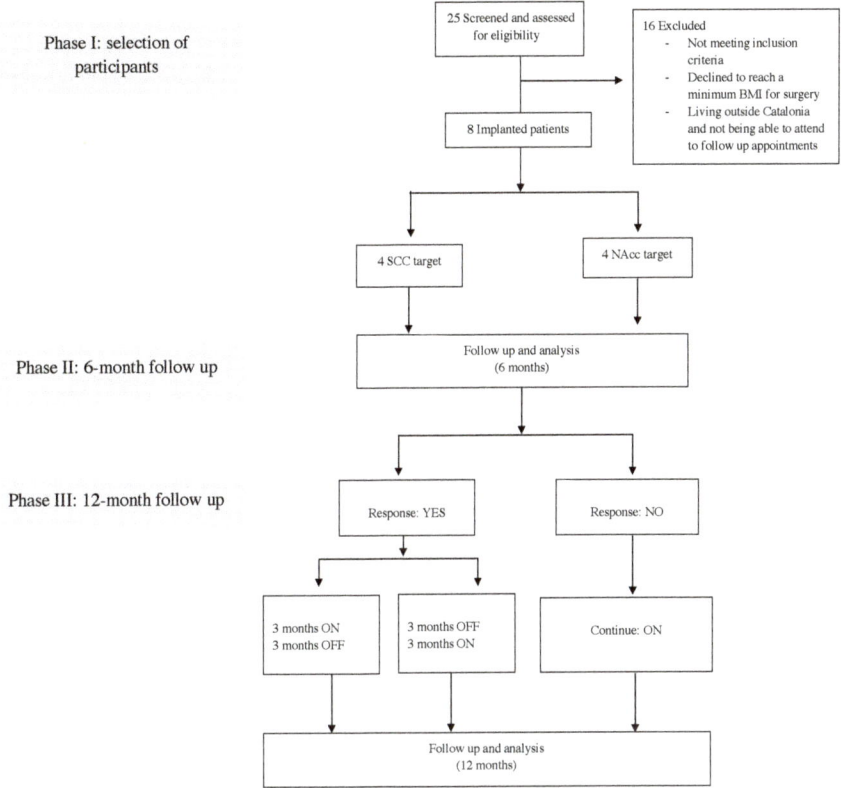

Figure 1. Participants' selection and pathway for the randomized crossover controlled clinical trial. Here, results are presented including the follow-up analysis at 6 months.

2.3. Measures

A wide range of variables were collected, including sociodemographic characteristics of the sample and a complete clinical history.

Primary outcome:

The primary outcome measure was BMI. Anthropometric measures (weight and BMI calculation) were collected at baseline, immediately before surgery, and monthly thereafter.

Secondary outcomes:

Secondary outcome measures include scores on a range of instruments described below.

Clinical outcome measures:

- The Mini-International Neuropsychiatric Interview (MINI) [37], a short diagnostic structured interview.

- The Hamilton Depression Rating Scale (HAMD$_{17}$) [38], designed to assess depressive symptoms. Each item on the questionnaire is scored on a 3- or 5-point scale, depending on the item. The original version contains 17 items (HAMD$_{17}$).
- Hamilton Anxiety Rating Scale (HAM-A) [39], a 14-item scale designed to rate the severity of anxiety symptoms. Each item contains a group of symptoms rated on a scale of 0–4, with 4 being the most severe.
- The Yale-Brown Obsessive Compulsive Scale (Y-BOCS) [40], a 10-item scale designed to measure the severity of illness in patients with obsessive-compulsive disorder, with a range of severity and types of obsessive-compulsive symptoms. Each item is rated from 0 (no symptoms) to 4 (extreme symptoms), with separate subtotals for severity of obsessions and compulsions.
- The Yale-Brown-Cornell Eating Disorders Scale (YBC-EDS) [41] is a semi-structured interview containing 8 items to assess the nature and severity of preoccupations and rituals related to the eating disorder.
- The Multidimensional Assessment of Interoceptive Awareness (MAIA) [42] is an 8-scale state-trait self-report questionnaire containing 32 items to measure multiple dimensions of interoception.
- Gardner Assessment of Body-Image [43] is a set of schematic contour scales to assess body disturbances.
- Barratt Impulsiveness Scale [44] is a 30-item self-report measure of impulsive personality traits.
- The Short Form Health Survey (SF-36) [45] is a 36-item instrument to assess quality of life.

Neuroimaging:

A brain MRI (1.5 T + DTI, 60 directions) was performed. Fractional anisotropy (FA), mean diffusivity (MD), axial diffusion (AD), radial diffusion (RD), and tractography were determined. The following target and stimulation parameters were registered: active contacts, voltage, frequency, pulse width, and amplitude.

2.4. Data Analyses

Considering the small sample size and that data showed a non-normal distribution, non-parametric tests were run.

2.4.1. Primary Outcome: change in BMI Value

To test the effects of DBS on the primary outcome measure (BMI), Friedman's non-parametric, repeated-measures analysis of variance (ANOVA) was used to compare BMI values at surgery to BMI values at each of the six-monthly postoperative determinations. As the main aim of the study was to evaluate treatment effects after 6 months of DBS, the Wilcoxon rank test was also used to compare two data points: pre-surgery BMI versus BMI at month 6.

Some participants required inpatient care before surgery to reach the minimum preoperative BMI value. Consequently, this preoperative BMI was not their "usual" BMI, but rather the result of inpatient treatment. To reflect this, we determined a BMI reference value (BMI-RV) for each patient, which was calculated differently depending on whether or not the patient required preoperative inpatient care. For patients who required preoperative inpatient care (patients 3, 4, 6 and 8), the BMI-RV was defined as the mean BMI achieved in the year prior to surgery (not including the BMI values obtained during inpatient care). For patients that did not require preoperative inpatient care (patients 1, 2, 5, 7), the BMI-RV was defined as the mean BMI achieved in the three-month period immediately prior to surgery. The same statistical analyses described above (Friedman's and Wilcoxon) were repeated, but this time based on the BMI-RV values. The BMI-RV value was used to determine treatment response, which was defined as an increase of ≥10% in the pre-treatment BMI-RV value.

For exploratory purposes, the sample was also divided into different subgroups (i.e., participants who received preoperative inpatient care versus those that did not and participants with SCC stimulation versus participants with NAcc stimulation) to test for possible changes in BMI values between those groups (Wilcoxon rank test).

2.4.2. Secondary Outcomes: Change in Anorexia Nervosa Behavior and Clinical Variables

Given the small sample size, the data on AN-related behaviors are given only as descriptive data. The Wilcoxon signed-rank test was used to compare scores obtained on the various instruments administered at baseline with the scores obtained at the end of month six of follow up. The results of this pre-post comparison were also used to determine whether participants who received DBS to the SCC or NAcc differed in terms of their relative improvement on depression and obsessive-compulsive scores (HAMD-17 and YBOCS, respectively).

3. Results

3.1. Participants Characteristics

The study sample included eight participants (7 female), with a mean age at surgery of 40.75 years (standard deviation (SD) = 15.49). Most patients ($n = 6$) had a primary diagnosis of AN-restrictive type. The mean time since disease onset was 25.25 years (SD = 11.25). Comorbidities with other psychiatric diagnoses were frequent, most commonly major depressive disorder (MDD, $n = 7$), followed by panic disorder (PD, $n = 3$), and obsessive-compulsive disorder (OCD, $n = 3$). Six of the eight patients (75%) were taking benzodiazepines, while three were under antidepressant treatment, and one was taking antipsychotic medication.

The minimum and maximum BMI values over the last five years were registered. We evaluated variability in the BMI values over the 15 months prior to DBS implantation. The patients presented three main BMI fluctuation patterns over this period, which we classified as pattern A, B, or C. Pattern A consisted of a stable BMI trajectory, observed in participants 1, 4, 5, 7, and 8. Pattern B was characterized by frequent hospital admissions and ascendant and descendent peaks in BMI (unstable BMI trajectory), which was observed in two patients (3 and 6). Finally, one patient (2) showed a stable but descendent weight trajectory, which was denominated pattern C. Preoperative inpatient care was required in four cases to achieve the minimum BMI (=13) level required for surgery. Of these four patients, only one (participant 4) did not achieve the minimum BMI; however, the patient's BMI (12.12) was considered acceptable and surgery was performed.

In participants 1, 2, 3, and 4, target selection was based on anatomical/stereotactic references; in participants 5, 6, 7, and 8, target selection was based on anatomical/stereotactic references as well as DTI data. Stimulation started at 3.5 MA for all patients and was maintained or increased accordingly to patient response, which was assessed monthly. The maximum stimulation was set at 8 MA.

Table 1 describes the demographic and clinical characteristics of the sample, with the active contacts and stimulation parameters. Figure 2 shows location of electrode active contacts.

Table 1. Participant's demographic and clinical characteristics, active contacts, and stimulating parameters.

Patient	Sex	Age	Type AN	AN Duration (Years)	Inpatient Care before Surgery	Minimum BMI	Maximum BMI	Reference BMI Value	Pharmacological Treatment	Main Comorbidity	Target	Active Contact (−), left	Active Contact (−), right	Maximum Intensity (MA)
1	Female	37	Restrictive	26	NO	14.64	16.22	16.22	Clonazepam	Affective Disorder	SCC	2	2	7
2	Male	45	Restrictive	32	NO	13.44	17.51	13.44	None	Anxiety Disorder	NAcc	1	1	8
3	Female	45	Restrictive	16	YES	10.06	11.72	10.94	Citalopram, Diazepam, Olanzapine, Lormetazepam	Affective Disorder	SCC	3	1	8
4	Female	39	Purgative	25	YES	11.47	12.55	11.83	Lorazepam Sertraline,	Anxiety Disorder	NAcc	2	1	8
5	Female	36	Restrictive	22	NO	13.07	15.18	13.07	Venlafaxine, Mirtazapine	Affective Disorder	SCC	2.3	2	7
6	Female	33	Restrictive	21	YES	9.64	12.73	11.57	Bromazepam	Affective Disorder	SCC	1.2	3.4	8
7	Female	57	Restrictive	41	NO	11.92	12.74	12.33	Venlafaxine, Mirtazapine, Bromazepam, Lormetazepam	Anxiety Disorder	NAcc	2	2.3	7.5
8	Female	34	Binge-Purge	19	YES	11.61	12.34	11.98	Lorazepam	Anxiety Disorder	NAcc	3.4	3.4	8

Note. AN = Anorexia Nervosa. MINI = International Psychiatric Interview for Mental Disorders. BMI = Body Mass Index. OCD = Obsessive Compulsive Disorder. MDD = Major Depressive Disorder. SCC = subcallosal cingulate. NAcc = Nucleus accumbens. MA = Milliampere. Minimum and maximum BMI refer to the last 5 years.

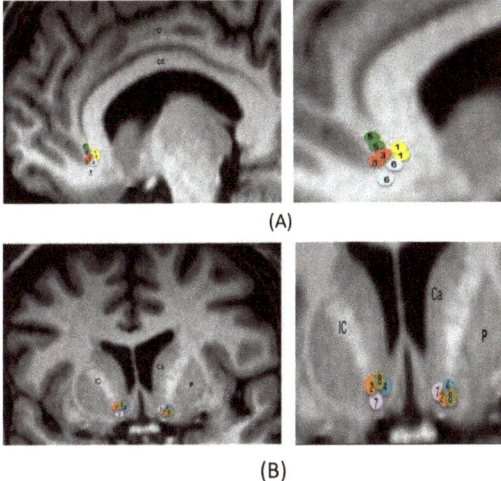

(A)

(B)

Figure 2. Location of electrode active contacts. (**A**) Location of electrode contacts on a sagittal view for patients with DBS on the subcallosal cingulate. Circles are schematic representations of electrode active contacts. Numbers within circles correspond to each patient. The figure at the right side is an enlargement. C = cingulate. CC = corpus callosum. (**B**) Location of electrode contacts on a coronal view for patients with DBS on the nucleus accumbens. Circles are schematic representations of electrode active contacts. Numbers within circles correspond to each patient. The figure at the right side is an enlargement. CA = caudate nucleus. CI = internal capsule. P = putamen. DBS = deep brain stimulation.

3.2. Primary Outcome: Change in Body Mass Index Values

To assess the effect of the DBS on BMI (the primary outcome measure), we compared the preoperative BMI for all patients (regardless of receiving inpatient care before surgery or not) to the BMI values measured at each postoperative time point (monthly). On this analysis, the Friedman repeated-measures ANOVA revealed no significant increase in BMI after surgery ($X^2 = 2.71$, $p = 0.84$). A Wilcoxon signed-rank test was performed to compare only two data points: preoperative BMI with BMI at month 6 of follow up, also revealing no significant changes ($Z = -0.28$, $p = 0.78$). Figure 3 shows the mean BMI scores for each patient over the six-month study period.

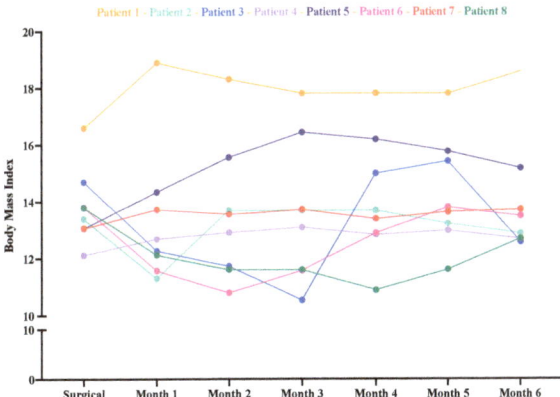

Figure 3. Individual changes in body mass index (BMI) during the six month follow-up period. BMI at surgery (criterion 1) was used as the reference value for this comparison.

These analyses were repeated using a BMI reference value (BMI-RV; see the Data Analyses Section for a description) for each patient as the pre-operative BMI measure. The Friedman repeated measures ANOVA showed no significant increase in BMI ($X^2 = 7.96$, $p = 0.24$). However, when we compared only two data points (BMI-RV with the BMI obtained at the six month follow up), the increase was significant (BMI-RV: M = 12.67, SD = 1.64 versus BMI value at month 6: M = 13.98, SD = 2.05, $Z = -2.38$, $p = 0.02$).

The data were analyzed again but using a different approach (as explained above), in which treatment response was defined as a ≥10% increase in BMI-RV. Patient 1 showed a sustained gain in BMI (10%) at all monthly time points throughout the six month follow up. By contrast, patients 2 and 8 did not achieve a 10% gain in BMI at any time point. Finally, the other three patients showed a variable pattern during the follow-up period. However, at month 6, five of the eight participants presented an increase of at least 10% in BMI. Table 2 shows the reference BMI values for each patient and their response.

Table 2. Participant response defined as a 10% increase in BMI during the six-month follow-up period.

Patient	Reference BMI Value	Response Value (10% Increase)	Months 1	2	3	4	5	6	Response to DBS (YES/NO)
1	16.22	17.842	G	G	G	G	G	G	YES
2	13.44	14.784	R	R	R	R	R	R	NO
3	10.94	12.034	R	R	G	G	R	G	YES
4	11.83	13.013	R	R	R	R	R	R	NO
5	13.07	14.377	R	G	G	R	G	G	YES
6	11.57	12.727	R	R	R	R	R	R	NO
7	12.33	13.563	R	R	G	G	R	G	YES
8	11.98	13.178	R	R	R	R	R	R	NO

Note. A green box indicates that the patient achieved a 10% increase in BMI at a given month while a red box means that the patient did not reach the 10% BMI gain threshold for that month. DBS = deep brain stimulation. BMI = body mass index.

Lastly, were performed other analyses (Wilcoxon rank test) to explore differences between the subgroups. No significant pre/post (6 months) differences in BMI were found for participants who received preoperative inpatient care ($Z = -1.09$, $p = 0.27$) versus those who did not ($Z = -1.46$, $p = 0.14$). Similarly, neither subgroup (SCC nor NAcc) showed a significant increase in BMI: SCC stimulation ($Z = 0.00$, $p = 1.00$) versus NAcc stimulation ($Z = 0.00$, $p = 1.0$).

3.3. Secondary Outcomes: Change in Anorexia Nervosa Behaviors and Clinical Variables

Patient 1 showed a reduction in daily physical activity (walking), which decreased from 6 hours per day to one hour/day at the one-month follow up. This reduction was maintained over the 6-month study period. Patient 2 also reduced the amount of daily physical activity from 6 hours to 3. Two patients (4 and 8) presented purging behavior prior to DBS. During the five years prior to DBS, patient 4 had maintained an exclusively liquid diet. After one month of DBS, the patient included two solid meals a day. Diuretic/laxative intake (patient 4) was significantly reduced from 40 tablets of furosemide a day to 5 tablets a day, and from 70 powder laxative sachets at baseline to complete abstinence. For patient 8, the purging frequency remained unchanged at month 6.

No significant improvement was observed (Wilcoxon signed-rank test) for most clinical variables. However, a significant change was found in SF-36 scores at month 6, indicating an improvement in the patients' quality of life ($Z = 2.10$, $p = 0.03$). Patients stimulated at the SCC (patients: 2, 4, 7, 8) whose predominant comorbidities were affective disorders presented larger improvements in depression scores (HAMD-17) than patients with SCC stimulation (SCC target: $M_{pre} = 13.50$, SD = 3.31 versus $M_{6months} = 4.75$, SD = 3.30, $Z = -1.82$, $p = 0.06$; NAcc target: $M_{pre} = 17.25$, SD = 7.13; $M_{6months} = 16.25$, SD = 11.32, $Z = 0.00$, $p = 1.00$); however, these differences were not statistically significant. In terms of YBOCs scores, no significant differences were found for patients with SCC stimulation or those who received NAcc stimulation (SCC target: $M_{pre} = 18.50$, SD = 6.60; $M_{6months} = 16.50$, SD = 11.61,

$Z = -0.55$, $p = 0.58$; NAcc target: $M_{pre} = 14.50$, $SD = 9.14$ versus $M_{6months} = 9.00$, $SD = 12.27$, $Z = 0.53$, $p = 0.59$). Table 3 shows the results of the secondary outcomes from baseline to the 6 months follow-up assessment. Figure 4A, B shows changes in depression (HAMD-17) and obsessive-compulsive (YBOCS) scores for each patient.

Table 3. Wilcoxon signed-rank test for secondary outcomes measured preoperatively (baseline) and at month 6 of follow up.

	Mean	Standard Deviation	Z	p
HAMD-17				
Pre-surgery	15.38	5.52	−1.47	0.14
Month 6	10.50	9.87		
YBOCS				
Pre-surgery	16.50	7.69	−0.85	0.39
Month 6	12.75	11.76		
HAM-A				
Pre-surgery	13.63	6.30	−1.26	0.21
Month 6	10.94	11.84		
YBC-EDS				
Pre-surgery	111.38	48.28	−1.54	0.12
Month 6	87.62	64.26		
MAIA				
Pre-surgery	15.53	7.11	0.42	0.67
Month 6	15.15	7.61		
Gardner—Distortion				
Pre-surgery	2.50	3.65	−0.70	0.48
Month 6	2.75	4.09		
Gardner—Dissatisfaction				
Pre-surgery	2.75	3.19	−0.32	0.74
Month 6	3.00	4.17		
SF36				
Pre-surgery	32.18	16.98	2.10	0.03
Month 6	60.56	22.40		
BIS-11				
Pre-surgery	43.88	19.66	−0.42	0.67
Month 6	42.25	10.06		

Note. HAMD-17 = Hamilton Depression Rating Scale. YBOCS = Yale-Brown Obsessive-Compulsive Scale. HAMA = Hamilton Anxiety Rating Scale. YBC-EDS = Yale-Brown-Cornell Eating Disorders Scale. MAIA = Multidimensional Assessment of Interoceptive Awareness. Gardner Assessment of Body-Image. SF36 = Short Form Health Survey. BIS-11 = Barrat Impulsivity Scale 11.

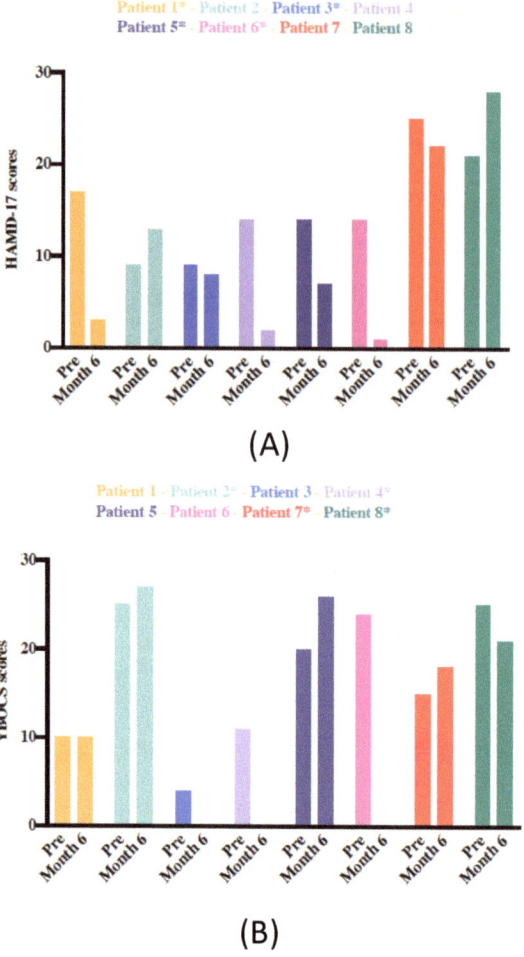

Figure 4. Changes in depression (HAMD-17) and obsessive-compulsive (YBOCS) scores for each patient. (**A**) Changes in depression scores based on the Hamilton Rating Scale for Depression (HAMD-17) from baseline to month 6 post-DBS. Patients identified with an asterisk (*) are those whose main comorbidity was an affective disorder, with SCC stimulation. (**B**) Changes in obsessive-compulsive symptoms based on the Yale-Brown Obsessive-Compulsive Scale (YBOCS) from baseline to month 6 post-DBS. Patients identified with an asterisk (*) are those whose main comorbidity was an anxiety disorder, with NAcc stimulation. HAMD-17 = Hamilton Depression Rating Scale. YBOCS = Yale-Brown Obsessive-Compulsive Scale.

3.4. Adverse Events

Cutaneous complications occurred in 3 patients (2, 5, and 6). Approximately 72 h after the procedure, patient 2 developed a greyish coloration in the area of the right electrode, potentially indicative of reduced blood flow; three days later (day 6), a necrotic eschar was observed, requiring skin flap surgery. Ten days after surgery, patient 5 developed skin dehiscence at the site of the incision for the surgical fiducial marker. The dehiscence did not respond to conservative treatment, and therefore the affected area was surgically cleaned to prevent infection. Patient 6 developed a chronic infection at the site of the skin incisions for surgical fiducial markers. The infection did not respond to

4. Discussion

Overall, the initial results of this study of six months of DBS to the NAcc and SCC in patients with severe and chronic AN show that DBS did not produce a statistically significant increase in BMI. Five out of eight patients achieved an increase of ≥10% in BMI (at month 6), and three out of eight presented changes in AN behaviors, including reduced physical activity and use of laxatives and diuretics. At month 6, DBS was associated with improvements in a patient-reported measure of quality of life (SF-36). Almost 40% of the patients treated developed skin complications that required treatment, including surgery.

As indicate above (in the Methods Section), we used two different criteria to assess the primary outcome (change in BMI). First, we compared preoperative BMI to postoperative BMI values obtained at the monthly assessments, finding no significant increase in body mass in the overall sample. This lack of a significant difference in BMI could be attributed to the particular characteristics of our patient sample versus other studies that did find significant differences in BMI after DBS [29,30,32,34]. First, unlike many of those studies, we included treatment-resistant, chronic patients. Second, we required a minimal preoperative BMI (13), which meant that half of the patients ($n = 4$) required inpatient intensive treatment to gain weight before they could undergo DBS implantation. Although we managed to recruit the sample over a one-year period, many patients with a severe AN profile declined to participate in the study due to this criterion (i.e., they were unwilling to gain weight). For some patients with AN, the idea of participating in a clinical trial whose main aim is to restore weight can seem to contradict their personal objectives. Third, we used different stimulation targets (SCC or NAcc) depending on the comorbid psychopathology (affective predominance or anxious predominance, respectively). Previous studies [29,31–34] have also evaluated DBS for AN, using the same targets (SCC and NAcc). However, to our knowledge, none of those studies considered comorbidities or the type of AN when selecting the DBS target. This is relevant given that data obtained from studies using functional MRI reveal differences between AN subtype (restrictive versus bingeing/purging) in terms of brain activation [12,14]. Moreover, in contrast to our study, most patients included in previous studies were characterized by less severe AN with a shorter time from diagnosis and/or were willing to achieve a BMI > 15 before undergoing surgery [30,31,36].

Interestingly, when we calculated a preoperative reference BMI value (BMI-RV) for each patient, we found a significant increase in BMI at month 6 (versus the preoperative BMI-RV), although the mean BMI at this follow-up assessment was still quite low (M = 13.98). Although the use of this novel value (BMI-RV) could be questioned, we believe that it better captures the patients' true BMI before surgery, as it reflects the mean BMI over a longer time frame beyond just the immediate preoperative period.

When we performed another analysis in which treatment response was defined as an increase in BMI ≥ 10% (considered sufficient in this group of chronic, severe patients), five of the eight participants met this objective at month 6 and were thus considered responders (Table 2). Using the 10% gain in BMI as the cut-off to define treatment response, we observed different patterns. Of the four patients who met this criterion and were thus considered responders (patients 1, 3, 5, and 7), three received DBS stimulation to the SCC. In addition, most of these patients (1,5, and 7) presented a pattern A BMI trajectory before surgery, while only one patient (3) was characterized in the "unstable BMI trajectory" group (pattern B). Patient 2 showed a clear pattern of no-response that was consistent with the preoperative BMI pattern (sustained disease severity with clinical worsening). Together, these findings seem to suggest a link between the BMI pattern (i.e., illness trajectory) and the impact of DBS; however, more data are needed to corroborate this potential association. AN-specific behaviors in our sample were inverse, as some patients (1, 2, 4) presented a decrease in physical activity and diuretic/laxative use.

Of the various secondary clinical outcomes evaluated in this study, most did not show statistically significant improvements, which could be due to the short follow-up [34]. However, two findings were particularly noteworthy. First, we observed a significant increase in SF-36 scores, which indicates that the patients perceived a subjective improvement in quality of life after the intervention (month 6). Second, as we expected, patients whose predominant comorbidities were affective disorders and received stimulation to the SCC presented larger improvements in depression scores, while those with NAcc stimulation presented a greater improvement in the YBOCS (although none reached statistical significance). However, a positive impact on these measures related to features of AN (YBC-EDS; MAIA and Gardner) was not evidenced, in contrast to the findings of Lipsman et al. [34], who reported significant reductions on several subscales of the YBC-EDS. Nevertheless, the results of our study and those of Lipsman and colleagues [34] are not directly comparable, as that study had a much longer (12 months) follow-up period.

These results must be interpreted in the context of the study limitations. First, the small sample size and preliminary findings. Nevertheless, our data were obtained from a real-world sample of patients with chronic AN, a population in urgent need of novel treatment options such as DBS. Second, a recommended cut-off point for inclusion in this trial was BMI ≥ 13. To reach this cut-off point, some participants required inpatient intensive care, and therefore, the BMI reached at pre-surgery reflected this time under treatment. This cut-off point was established because excessively thin patients are more likely to develop pressure ulcers caused by the pulse generator implanted under the skin (due to the decreased skin thickness and greater fragility of the subcutaneous tissue). Although a higher BMI cut-off point would reduce this risk even further, doing so would likely require the exclusion of very severe patients (which is why we offered inpatient treatment to raise the BMI in selected patients). Indeed, even though we provided preoperative inpatient care, one patient still underwent surgery despite not reaching the minimum BMI. The decision to allow this patient to participate was made after careful consideration. The research team concluded that the patient's safety could be ensured and therefore we decided to proceed. The patient did not experience any adverse events and, despite a lack of response in terms of BMI, her use of diuretics/laxatives decreased significantly, which we consider a good outcome. A third limitation is that we only included one male. Consequently, it was not possible to assess differences between men and women in treatment response. Fourth, the relatively short follow-up (6 months) is a limitation; however, the longer-term stability of our findings will be reported when data from the phase III part of this trial (12 months of follow up) become available. In addition, we observed cutaneous complications, which might be related to lower BMI and to other differences in the patients' characteristics. In some patients, resolution of the cutaneous complications required surgery, as less invasive treatments were unsuccessful. However, and in contrast with other studies, no devices needed to be explanted.

5. Conclusions

After 6 months of DBS, some patients in this study with severe, chronic AN showed some benefits: increase in BMI, reduction in AN behavior, and improvement in quality of life (regardless of whether or not BMI improved). The percentage of patients developing cutaneous complications was high, but effectively resolved. Due to the short follow-up (6 months), we cannot reach any conclusions regarding the superiority of the target site (NAcc versus SCC) in terms of treatment outcomes. However, in the future, we will report longer term outcomes (12 months), which will provide a clearer picture of the long-term stability of BMI. Studies that include larger samples are needed to clarify whether DBS in patients with AN is associated with an improvement in comorbid symptoms (i.e., depression, anxiety). Finally, more research is needed to better characterize the relationship between BMI fluctuations, comorbid symptoms, and DBS targets.

Author Contributions: Conceptualization, G.V.M. and V.P.; Formal analysis, M.E.; Funding acquisition, V.P.; Investigation, G.V.M., P.S., J.M.G., R.G., C.C., M.P., I.D.-M., S.M., R.M.M., G.C., G.F., and A.G.; Methodology,

G.V.M. and V.P.; Supervision, V.P.; Writing—original draft, G.V.M. and A.J.; Writing—review and editing, M.E. All authors have read and agreed to the published version of the manuscript.

Funding: This research was funded by the Instituto de Salud Carlos III, by a grant for research projects (PI16/00382) and co-financed with European Union ERDF funds.

Acknowledgments: M.E. has a Juan de la Cierva research contract awarded by the ISCIII (FJCI-2017-31738). V.P. and M.E. want to thank unrestricted research funding from "Secretaria d'Universitats i Recerca del Departament d'Economia i Coneixement (2017 SGR 134 to "Mental Health Research Group"), Generalitat de Catalunya (Government of Catalonia). We thank Bradley Londres for professional English language editing.

Conflicts of Interest: Perez has been a consultant to or has received honoraria or grants from AstraZeneca, Bristol-Myers-Squibb, Janssen Cilag, Lundbeck, Otsuka, Servier, Medtronicand Exeltis.

References

1. Hoek, H.W. Incidence, prevalence and mortality of anorexia nervosa and other eating disorders. *Curr. Opin. Psychiatry* **2006**, *19*, 389–394. [CrossRef] [PubMed]
2. Machado, P.P.; Machado, B.C.; Gonçalves, S.; Hoek, H.W. The prevalence of eating disorders not otherwise specified. *Int. J. Eat. Disord.* **2007**, *40*, 7–212. [CrossRef] [PubMed]
3. Bulik, C.M.; Reba, L.; Siega-Riz, A.M.; Reichborn-Kjennerud, T. Anorexia nervosa: Definition, epidemiology, and cycle of risk. *Int. J. Eat. Disord.* **2005**, *37*, S2–S9. [CrossRef] [PubMed]
4. Lock, J.; Kraemer, H.C.; Jo, B.; Couturier, J. When meta-analyses get it wrong: Response to 'treatment outcomes for anorexia nervosa: A systematic review and meta-analysis of randomized controlled trials'. *Psychol. Med.* **2019**, *49*, 697–698. [CrossRef] [PubMed]
5. Hay, P.J.; Touyz, S.; Sud, R. Treatment for severe and enduring anorexia nervosa: A review. *Aust. N. Z. J. Psychiatry* **2012**, *46*, 44–1136. [CrossRef]
6. Steinhausen, H.C. The outcome of anorexia nervosa in the 20th century. *Am. J. Psychiatry* **2002**, *159*, 93–1284. [CrossRef]
7. Avena, N.M.; Bocarsly, M.E. Dysregulation of brain reward systems in eating disorders: Neurochemical information from animal models of binge eating, bulimia nervosa, and anorexia nervosa. *Neuropharmacology* **2012**, *63*, 87–96. [CrossRef]
8. Fladung, A.K.; Grön, G.; Grammer, K.; Herrnberger, B.; Schilly, E.; Grasteit, S.; Wolf, R.C.; Walter, H.; von Wietersheim, J. A neural signature of anorexia nervosa in the ventral striatal reward system. *Am. J. Psychiatry* **2010**, *167*, 12–206. [CrossRef]
9. Friederich, H.C.; Wu, M.; Simon, J.J.; Herzog, W. Neurocircuit function in eating disorders. *Int. J. Eat. Disord.* **2013**, *46*, 32–425. [CrossRef]
10. Jauregui-Lobera, I.; Martinez-Quinones, J.V. Neuromodulation in eating disorders and obesity: A promising way of treatment? *Neuropsychiatr. Dis. Treat.* **2018**, *14*, 2817–2835. [CrossRef]
11. Keating, C.; Tilbrook, A.J.; Rossell, S.L.; Enticott, P.G.; Fitzgerald, P.B. Reward processing in anorexia nervosa. *Neuropsychologia* **2012**, *50*, 75–567. [CrossRef] [PubMed]
12. Lipsman, N.; Woodside, D.B.; Lozano, A.M. Neurocircuitry of limbic dysfunction in anorexia nervosa. *Cortex* **2015**, *62*, 18–109. [CrossRef] [PubMed]
13. Whiting, A.C.; Oh, M.Y.; Whiting, D.M. Deep brain stimulation for appetite disorders: A review. *Neurosurg. Focus* **2018**, *45*, E9. [CrossRef] [PubMed]
14. Kaye, W.H.; Wagner, A.; Fudge, J.L.; Paulus, M. Neurocircuity of eating disorders. *Curr. Top. Behav. Neurosci.* **2011**, *6*, 37–57.
15. Van Kuyck, K.; Gérard, N.; Van Laere, K.; Casteels, C.; Pieters, G.; Gabriëls, L.; Nuttin, B. Towards a neurocircuitry in anorexia nervosa: Evidence from functional neuroimaging studies. *J. Psychiatr. Res.* **2009**, *43*, 45–1133. [CrossRef]
16. Sodersten, P.; Bergh, C.; Ammar, A. Anorexia nervosa: Towards a neurobiologically based therapy. *Eur. J. Pharmacol.* **2003**, *480*, 67–74. [CrossRef]
17. Lozano, A.M.; Lipsman, N.; Bergman, H.; Brown, P.; Chabardes, S.; Chang, J.W.; Matthews, K.; McIntyre, C.C.; Schlaepfer, T.E.; Schulder, M.; et al. Deep brain stimulation: Current challenges and future directions. *Nat. Rev. Neurol.* **2019**, *15*, 148–160. [CrossRef]

18. Bar, K.J.; de la Cruz, F.; Berger, S.; Schultz, C.C.; Wagner, G. Structural and functional differences in the cingulate cortex relate to disease severity in anorexia nervosa. *J. Psychiatry Neurosci.* **2015**, *40*, 79–269. [CrossRef]
19. Gaudio, S.; Wiemerslage, L.; Brooks, S.J.; Helgi, B. A systematic review of resting-state functional-MRI studies in anorexia nervosa: Evidence for functional connectivity impairment in cognitive control and visuospatial and body-signal integration. *Neurosci. Biobehav. Rev.* **2016**, *71*, 578–589. [CrossRef]
20. Nico, D.; Claser, C.; Borja-Cabrera, G.P.; Travassos, L.R.; Palatnik, M.; da Silva Soares, I.; Rodrigues, M.M. Palatnik-de-Sousa, C.B. Adaptive immunity against Leishmania nucleoside hydrolase maps its c-terminal domain as the target of the CD4+ T cell-driven protective response. *PLoS Negl. Trop. Dis.* **2010**, *4*, e866. [CrossRef]
21. Blanchet, C.; Guillaume, S.; Bat-Pitault, F.; Carles, M.E.; Clarke, J.; Dodin, V.; Duriez, P.; Gerardin, P.; Hanachi-Guidoum, M.; Iceta, S.; et al. Medication in AN: A Multidisciplinary Overview of Meta-Analyses and Systematic Reviews. *J. Clin. Med.* **2019**, *8*. [CrossRef] [PubMed]
22. Pugh, J.; Maslen, H.; Savulescu, J. Deep Brain Stimulation, Authenticity and Value-CORRIGENDUM. *Camb. Q. Healthc. Ethics* **2018**, *27*, 179. [CrossRef] [PubMed]
23. Zrinzo, L.; Foltynie, T.; Limousin, P.; Hariz, M.I. Reducing hemorrhagic complications in functional neurosurgery: A large case series and systematic literature review. *J. Neurosurg.* **2012**, *116*, 84–94. [CrossRef]
24. Clair, A.H.; Haynes, W.; Mallet, L. Recent advances in deep brain stimulation in psychiatric disorders. *F1000Res* **2018**, *7*. [CrossRef]
25. Graat, I.; Figee, M.; Denys, D. The application of deep brain stimulation in the treatment of psychiatric disorders. *Int. Rev. Psychiatry* **2017**, *29*, 178–190. [CrossRef] [PubMed]
26. Arya, S.; Filkowski, M.M.; Nanda, P.; Sheth, S.A. Deep brain stimulation for obsessive-compulsive disorder. *Bull. Menn. Clin.* **2019**, *83*, 84–96. [CrossRef] [PubMed]
27. Naesstrom, M.; Blomstedt, P.; Bodlund, O. A systematic review of psychiatric indications for deep brain stimulation, with focus on major depressive and obsessive-compulsive disorder. *Nord. J. Psychiatry* **2016**, *70*, 91–483. [CrossRef]
28. Pugh, J.; Maslen, H.; Savulescu, J. Deep Brain Stimulation, Authenticity and Value. *Camb. Q. Healthc. Ethics* **2017**, *26*, 640–657. [CrossRef]
29. Wang, D.; Liu, X.; Zhou, B.; Kuang, W.; Guo, T. Advanced research on deep brain stimulation in treating mental disorders. *Exp. Ther. Med.* **2018**, *15*, 3–12. [CrossRef]
30. McLaughlin, N.C.; Didie, E.R.; Machado, A.G.; Haber, S.N.; Eskandar, E.N.; Greenberg, B.D. Improvements in anorexia symptoms after deep brain stimulation for intractable obsessive-compulsive disorder. *Biol. Psychiatry* **2013**, *73*, e29–31. [CrossRef]
31. Wu, H.; Van Dyck-Lippens, P.J.; Santegoeds, R.; van Kuyck, K.; Gabriëls, L.; Lin, G.; Pan, G.; Li, Y.; Li, D.; Zhan, S.; et al. Deep-brain stimulation for anorexia nervosa. *World Neurosurg.* **2013**, *80*, S29.e1-10. [CrossRef] [PubMed]
32. Lipsman, N.; Woodside, D.B.; Giacobbe, P.; Hamani, C.; Carter, J.C.; Norwood, S.J.; Sutandar, K.; Staab, R.; Elias, G.; Lyman, C.H.; et al. Subcallosal cingulate deep brain stimulation for treatment-refractory anorexia nervosa: A phase 1 pilot trial. *Lancet* **2013**, *381*, 1361–1370. [CrossRef]
33. Israel, M.; Steiger, H.; Kolivakis, T.; McGregor, L.; Sadikot, A.F. Deep brain stimulation in the subgenual cingulate cortex for an intractable eating disorder. *Biol. Psychiatry* **2010**, *67*, e4–53. [CrossRef] [PubMed]
34. Lipsman, N.; Lam, E.; Volpini, M.; Sutandar, K.; Twose, R.; Giacobbe, P.; Sodums, D.J.; Smith, G.S.; Woodside, D.B.; Lozano, A.M. Deep brain stimulation of the subcallosal cingulate for treatment-refractory anorexia nervosa: 1 year follow-up of an open-label trial. *Lancet. Psychiatry* **2017**, *4*, 285–294. [CrossRef]
35. Blomstedt, P.; Naesstrom, M.; Bodlund, O. Deep brain stimulation in the bed nucleus of the stria terminalis and medial forebrain bundle in a patient with major depressive disorder and anorexia nervosa. *Clin. Case Rep.* **2017**, *5*, 679–684. [CrossRef]
36. Manuelli, M.; Franzini, A.; Galentino, R.; Bidone, R.; Dell'Osso, B.; Porta, M.; Servello, D.; Cena, H. Changes in eating behavior after deep brain stimulation for anorexia nervosa. A case study. *Eat. Weight. Disord.* **2019**. [CrossRef]
37. Sheehan, D.V.; Lecrubier, Y.; Sheehan, K.H.; Amorim, P.; Janavs, J.; Weiller, E.; Hergueta, T.; Baker, R.; Dunbar, G.C. The Mini-International Neuropsychiatric Interview (M.I.N.I.): The development and validation of a structured diagnostic psychiatric interview for DSM-IV and ICD-10. *J. Clin. Psychiatry* **1998**, *59*, 22–33.

38. Hamilton, M. A rating scale for depression. *J. Neurol. Neurosurg. Psychiatry* **1960**, *23*, 56–62. [CrossRef]
39. Hamilton, M. The assessment of anxiety states by rating. *Br. J. Med Psychol.* **1959**, *32*, 5–50. [CrossRef]
40. Goodman, W.K.; Price, L.H.; Rasmussen, S.A.; Mazure, C.; Fleischmann, R.L.; Hill, C.L.; Heninger, G.R.; Charney, D.S. The Yale-Brown Obsessive Compulsive Scale. I. Development, use, and reliability. *Arch. Gen. Psychiatry* **1989**, *46*, 11–1006.
41. Mazure, C.M.; Halmi, K.A.; Sunday, S.R.; Romano, S.J.; Einhorn, A.M. The Yale-Brown-Cornell Eating Disorder Scale: Development, use, reliability and validity. *J. Psychiatr. Res.* **1994**, *28*, 45–425. [CrossRef]
42. Mehling, W.E.; Price, C.; Daubenmier, J.J.; Acree, M.; Bartmess, E.; Stewart, A. The Multidimensional Assessment of Interoceptive Awareness (MAIA). *PLoS ONE* **2012**, *7*, e48230. [CrossRef] [PubMed]
43. Gardner, R.M.; Stark, K.I.M.; Jackson, N.A.; Friedman, B.N. Development and validation of two new scales for assessment of body-image. *Percept. Mot. Ski.* **1999**, *89*, 93–981. [CrossRef] [PubMed]
44. Barratt, E.S. Violence and mental disorder: Developments in risk assessment. In *Impulsiveness and Aggression*; Monoham, J., Steadman, H.J., Eds.; University of Chicago Press: Chicago, IL, USA, 1994; pp. 61–79.
45. Ware, J.E.; Kosinski, M.; Gandek, B. *SF-36 Health Survey. Manual and Interpretation Guide*; The Health Institute, New England Medical Center: Boston, MA, USA, 1993.

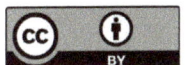

© 2020 by the authors. Licensee MDPI, Basel, Switzerland. This article is an open access article distributed under the terms and conditions of the Creative Commons Attribution (CC BY) license (http://creativecommons.org/licenses/by/4.0/).

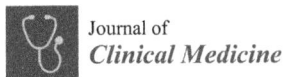

Review

Brain Stimulation in Eating Disorders: State of the Art and Future Perspectives

Philibert Duriez [1,2,†], Rami Bou Khalil [3,4,†], Yara Chamoun [3], Redwan Maatoug [5], Robertas Strumila [6], Maude Seneque [4,7], Philip Gorwood [1,2], Philippe Courtet [4,7] and Sébastien Guillaume [4,7,*]

1. GHU Paris Psychiatry and Neuroscience, Clinique des Maladies Mentales et de l'Encéphale (CMME), Sainte-Anne Hospital, 75014 Paris, France; phduriez@gmail.com (P.D.); P.GORWOOD@ghu-paris.fr (P.G.)
2. Institute of Psychiatry and Neurosciences of Paris (IPNP), UMR_S1266, INSERM, Université de Paris, 102-108 rue de la Santé, 75014 Paris, France
3. Department of Psychiatry, Hotel Dieu de France- Saint Joseph University, 166830 Beirut, Lebanon; ramiboukhalil@hotmail.com (R.B.K.); yara.chamoun@hotmail.com (Y.C.)
4. Neuropsychiatry: Epidemiological and Clinical Research, Université Montpellier, INSERM, CHU de Montpellier, 34295 Montpellier, France; maude.seneque@gmail.com (M.S.); p-courtet@chu-montpellier.fr (P.C.)
5. Sorbonne Université, AP-HP, Service de Psychiatrie Adulte de la Pitié-Salpêtrière, Institut du Cerveau, ICM, 75013 Paris, France; redwanmaatoug@gmail.com
6. Faculty of Medicine, Institute of Clinical Medicine, Psychiatric Clinic, Vilnius University, 03101 Vilnius, Lithuania; robertas.strumila@gmail.com
7. Department of Emergency Psychiatry and Post-Acute Care, CHRU Montpellier, 34295 Montpellier, France
* Correspondence: s-guillaume@chu-montpellier.fr; Tel.: +33-467-338-581
† These authors contributed equally to this work.

Received: 25 May 2020; Accepted: 20 July 2020; Published: 23 July 2020

Abstract: The management of eating disorders (EDs) is still difficult and few treatments are effective. Recently, several studies have described the important contribution of non-invasive brain stimulation (repetitive transcranial magnetic stimulation, transcranial direct current stimulation, and electroconvulsive therapy) and invasive brain stimulation (deep brain stimulation and vagal nerve stimulation) for ED management. This review summarizes the available evidence supporting the use of brain stimulation in ED. All published studies on brain stimulation in ED as well as ongoing trials registered at clinicaltrials.gov were examined. Articles on neuromodulation research and perspective articles were also included. This analysis indicates that brain stimulation in EDs is still in its infancy. Literature data consist mainly of case reports, cases series, open studies, and only a few randomized controlled trials. Consequently, the evidence supporting the use of brain stimulation in EDs remains weak. Finally, this review discusses future directions in this research domain (e.g., sites of modulation, how to enhance neuromodulation efficacy, personalized protocols).

Keywords: rTMS; deep brain stimulation; treatment; anorexia; bulimia; binge eating disorders

---

1. Introduction

Eating disorders (EDs) are serious psychiatric disorders characterized by abnormal eating or weight-control behaviors [1]. These disorders are most often chronic and relapsing, and this has a heavy impact on the patients' physical and mental health and life expectancy. Anorexia nervosa (AN) is a multifactorial ED characterized by significantly low body weight for the individual's height, age, and developmental stage, intense fear of gaining weight despite obvious thinness, and extreme behaviors designed to lose weight, such as food restriction with or without induced vomiting, or use of laxatives. The consequence is massive weight loss and/or pathological thinness. Binge eating disorder (BED) and bulimia nervosa (BN) are EDs characterized by recurrent episodes of binge eating and loss of personal control during binging. Individuals with BN counteract binge eating with compensatory behaviors to prevent weight gain, whereas individuals with BED do not exhibit recurrent compensatory behaviors. BED and BN are characterized by compulsive overeating, and shared neural alterations and neurobiological mechanisms underlie these EDs. EDs impair the quality of life of both patients and their families [2]. Among individuals with EDs, mortality and morbidity are increased and health service use is particularly high, resulting in elevated healthcare costs [3].

To date, ED management is still difficult, and few treatments have demonstrated their efficacy. In accordance with most guidelines, management programs are generally multidisciplinary. In AN, the available treatment recommendations aim at restoring normal weight, adapting and relaxing eating behaviors, improving social and interpersonal relationships, and improving the patient's self-image. Psychotherapy is the main therapeutic approach. However, data to guide the psychotherapy choice are limited and controversial [4]. Medication trials have been disappointing [5]. Overall, about one-third of patients will not recover, and the standardized mortality rate is 5.9 [6]. In patients with BN or BED, the best validated and most frequently used treatment is ED-specific cognitive behavioral therapy [7]. Nevertheless, a meta-analysis found that core BN symptoms are still present in more than 60% of patients, even after receiving the best available treatments [8]. Other psychotherapies have been proposed. Moreover, serotonergic antidepressants, the most frequently used pharmacological option, improve the medium-term symptomatology to some degree, but do not allow full remission. In this context, the development of alternative therapeutic strategies is crucial.

Brain stimulation is a therapeutic modality in which the activity of a specific neural circuit is modified by applying an electric current with predefined frequency, amplitude, and pulse width to restore the functional state without any tissue damage [9]. Brain stimulation is obtained by invasive and non-invasive interventions that stimulate or block the action potentials in the nervous system [9,10]. The ultimate aim of brain stimulation is to reverse maladaptive neurocircuitry changes in neural tissue and improve inter-neuronal connectivity [9–11]. These changes implicate synaptic potentiation or depression via regulation of neurotransmitters and ion channels and modification of the expression of intracellular second messengers [12,13]. In direct electrical stimulation, electrodes are used to apply a potential gradient across a neuron that induces intracellular ionic current flow, localized depolarization and hyperpolarization of the cell membrane, resulting in neural stimulation or inhibition [9]. The mechanism for magnetic stimulation is similar, except that the potential gradients are induced in the tissue by a rapidly changing strong magnetic field that is implemented transcutaneously [9]. Non-invasive brain stimulation (NIBS) techniques include electroconvulsive therapy (ECT), repetitive transcranial magnetic stimulation (rTMS), and transcranial direct current stimulation (tDCS). In ECT, seizures are induced by a direct current passing through the brain under general anesthesia [14]. In rTMS, excitability is induced by delivering magnetic stimulation pulses with a wire coil placed externally on the scalp above specific cortical regions [15]. In tDCS, direct current is delivered through electrodes implanted on the scalp, without seizure induction, with the aim of exciting (anodal stimulation) or inhibiting (cathodal stimulation) the activity in specific brain regions [16,17]. Invasive neuromodulation includes deep brain stimulation (DBS) and vagal nerve stimulation (VNS). In DBS, a pulse generator usually implanted in the subclavicular region delivers electrical current to the brain parenchyma through implanted electrodes. On the other hand, in VNS the left cervical vagal nerve is stimulated through a device implanted in the left chest wall [18].

The number of studies on brain stimulation in EDs and/or in dimensions associated with EDs is progressively increasing. In this review, we present the available data, issues, and future directions concerning the use of brain stimulation in EDs.

2. Methods

This is a non-systematic review of the literature on brain stimulation techniques used in patients with EDs. Nevertheless, a systematic research of the available literature was performed in the PubMed database by combining the search terms "eating disorders", "anorexia nervosa", "bulimia nervosa", "binge eating disorders" with the terms "neuromodulation", "rTMS", "tDCS", "DBS", "ECT", "VNS". All papers in English or French published up to June 2020 were retrieved. All original articles on brain stimulation in patients with EDs were included. Studies in high risk populations without EDs (e.g., patients with obesity or healthy subjects with high levels of food craving) were not included. This search was then supplemented by internet searches and manual search of the reference lists of potentially relevant articles and reviews, and by examining pertinent trials registered at clinicaltrial.gov. Among the 121 manuscripts identified, after duplicate removal, 72 were screened. All manuscripts are not cited because when a recent systematic review was available, it was included and prioritized in the synthesis of results. Additional studies on neuromodulation mechanisms, ED treatment, potential ED biomarkers, and mechanistic models of circuitries involved in EDs were also added. The search was performed independently by three researchers (P.D., R.B.K., Y.C.). Disagreements were resolved by consensus among all authors.

3. Results

3.1. rTMS in Eating Disorders

3.1.1. Anorexia Nervosa

As shown in Table 1, In 2008, the first published case on rTMS concerned a patient with AN and comorbid depression. The study reported weight gain and amelioration of the depressive symptoms after 41 sessions of rTMS over the left dorsolateral prefrontal cortex (DLPFC) [19]. This was followed by other case reports and case series on left DLPFC rTMS in patients with AN, often with comorbid depression [20–22]. The first case series on five patients with AN and without a clinically manifest comorbidity reported AN symptom improvement at 6 months but no longer at 12 months after 20 sessions of rTMS delivered over the left DLPFC [23]. A pilot study in which one session of high-frequency rTMS (10 Hz) was delivered to the left DLPFC in 10 patients showed that the procedure was well tolerated, leading to a reduction in the sensation of feeling full, fat, and anxious as well as in the urge to exercise after exposure to visual and real food stimuli [24]. These studies were followed by double-blind, controlled clinical trials [25–27]. In one of these trials, one rTMS session was delivered to the left DLPFC in 49 patients with AN, but the effect on AN core symptoms was not significant [25] compared with the sham session group. However, in the group analysis, AN core symptoms improved in the rTMS arm compared with baseline (before rTMS), and the results persisted at 24 h of follow-up [25]. Several studies suggest that a higher number of rTMS sessions give better clinical results [26,27]. An ancillary analysis of the sample of a randomized controlled feasibility trial on rTMS [26], using a food choice task, found a decrease in self-controlled food choices, suggesting than rTMS may promote more flexibility in relation to food choices [28]. Finally, the feasibility and safety of rTMS of DLPFC in patients with AN have been confirmed by these randomized controlled trials [25–27].

Table 1. Repetitive transcranial magnetic stimulation (rTMS) in eating disorders.

Reference	Type of Study	Participants	Modulation Target	Treatment Characteristics	Main Results
			Anorexia Nervosa		
Kamolz et al., 2008 [19]	Case report	24-year-old female with AN	Left DLPFC Manual targeting	41 sessions 100 × 2 s trains/10 s inter-train interval at 10 Hz = 2000 pulses per session, 110 % MT	Full remission
Van den Eynde et al., 2013 [24]	Case series (pilot study)	10 patients with AN	Left DLPFC Manual targeting	1 session, 20 × 5 s trains/55 s inter-train interval, 10 Hz, intensity of 110% MT, 1000 pulses over 20 min	Reduced levels of feeling full, feeling fat, and feeling anxious
McClelland et al., 2013 [20]	Case report	23-year-old and 52-year-old women with AN [1]	Left DLPFC Neuronavigation	20 and 19 sessions 20 × 5 s trains/55 s inter-train interval, 10 Hz, intensity of 110% MT, 1000 pulses over 20 min within each session	Significant improvement
McClelland et al., 2016 [23]	Case series	5 women with AN [1]	Left DLPFC Neuronavigation	~20 sessions, 20 × 5 s trains/55 s inter-train interval, 10 Hz, intensity of 110% MT, 1000 pulses over 20 min within each session	Significant improvement of ED and affective symptoms after 6 months, but positive results waned at 12 months follow-up
McClelland et al., 2016 [25]	RCT	49 patients with AN [1]	Left DLPFC Neuronavigation	1 session 5 s trains/55 s inter-train interval, 10 Hz, intensity of 110% MT, 1000 pulses over 20 min	No significant effect on core symptoms of ED compared to sham rTMS, but improvement in individuals who received real rTMS when compared before and after the session and the results persisted at 24 h of follow-up
Choudhary et al., 2017 [21]	Case report	23-year-old female with AN	Left DLPFC Manual targeting	21 sessions High-frequency rTMS (10 Hz) at 110% of resting MT, 1000 pulses	Significant improvement
Jaššová et al., 2018 [22]	Case report	25-year-old female with AN	Left DLPFC Targeting method not available	10 sessions, 10 Hz, 15 trains/day, 100 pulses/train, intertrain interval 107 s	No improvement of ED, anxiety, or depression
Woodside et al., 2017 [29]	Case series	Fourteen subjects with eating disorders (6 AN, 5 BN, and 3 ednos) and comorbid PTSD	DMPFC Neuronavigation	20–30 sessions 120% resting MT, at 10 Hz, 5 s on, 10 s off, 3000 pulses/hemisphere, with left then right lateralized coil orientation	Improvement in emotional regulation and PTSD symptoms
Dalton et al., 2018 [26]	RCT	30 patients (16 real, 14 sham) with AN [2]	Left DLPF CNeuronavigation	20 sessions, 20 × 5 s trains/55 s inter-train interval, 10 Hz, intensity of 110% MT, 1000 pulses over 20 min within each session	Between-group effect sizes of change scores (baseline to follow-up) were small for BMI (d = 0.2, 95% CI −0.49 to 0.90) and eating disorder symptoms (d = 0.1, 95% CI −0.60 to 0.79), medium for quality of life and moderate to large (d = 0.61 to 1.0) for mood outcomes, all favoring rTMS over sham

Table 1. Cont.

Reference	Type of Study	Participants	Modulation Target	Treatment Characteristics	Main Results
Knyahnytska et al., 2019 [30]	Case series (pilot study)	8 women with AN	Insula Manual targeting	42 sessions, H-coil dTMS 18 Hz, 2 s on, 20 s off, number of pulses 36, number of trains 80, over 20 min	Reduction in AN-related obsessions and compulsions, as well as depression and anxiety scores
Dalton et al., 2020 [28]	RCT	34 anorexic female patients (17 real, 17 sham) vs. 30 healthy controls [2]	Left DLPFC Neuronavigation	20 sessions 20×5 s trains/55 s inter-train interval, 10 Hz, intensity of 110% MT, 1000 pulses over 20 min within each session	No significant effect of rTMS nor time on food choices related to fat content. Among AN participants who received real rTMS, there was a decrease in self-controlled food choices at post-treatment
Bulimic Disorders (Bulimia and/or Binge Eating Disorders)					
Hausmann et al., 2004 [31]	Case report	One woman with BN and depression	Left DLPFC Neuronavigation	10 sessions, 20×5 s trains/55 s inter-train interval, 10 Hz, intensity of 110% MT	Significant improvement in BN symptoms
Walpoth et al., 2008 [32]	RCT	14 females with BN	Left DLPFC Manual targeting	15 sessions, 10×10 s trains/60 s inter-train interval at 20 Hz, = 2000 pulses; 120% MT	No difference between real and sham group
Van den Eynde et al., 2010 [33]	RCT	38 females with BN [3]	Left DLPFC Manual targeting	1 session, 20×5 s trains/55 s inter-train interval, 10 Hz, intensity of 110% MT, 1000 pulses over 20 min	Real rTMS associated with a decrease in self-reported urge to eat and binge eating
Van den Eynde et al., 2011 [34]	RCT	33 females with BN [3]	Left DLPFC Manual targeting	1 session, 20×5 s trains/55 s inter-train interval, 10 Hz, intensity of 110% MT, 1000 pulses over 20 min	No differences between the real and sham groups on stroop task
Van den Eynde et al., 2011 [35]	RCT	38 females with BN [3]	Left DLPFC Manual targeting	1 session, 20×5 s trains/55 s inter-train interval, 10 Hz, intensity of 110% MT, 1000 pulses over 20 min	TMS did not alter blood pressure or heart rate
Claudino et al., 2011 [36]	RCT	22 patients (11 real, 11 sham) with BN [3]	Left DLPFC Manual targeting	1 session, 20×5 s trains/55 s inter-train interval, 10 Hz, intensity of 110% MT, 1000 pulses over 20 min	Decreased salivary cortisol concentrations compared with sham rTMS
Van den Eynde et al., 2012 [37]	Case series	7 left-handed females with BN	Left DLPFCM anual targeting	1 session, 20×5 s trains/55 s inter-train interval, 10 Hz, intensity of 110% MT, 1000 pulses over 20 min	Different effects in left- and right-handed people
Downar et al., 2012 [38]	Case report	One woman with severe refractory BN and depression	DMPFC Neuronavigation	2×20 sessions 60 trains of 10 Hz stimulation at 120% of resting motor threshold in 5 s trains with a 10-s inter-train interval	Significant improvement in BN symptoms
Baczynski et al., 2014 [39]	Case report	One woman with BED and comorbid depression	Left DLPFC Manual targeting	20 sessions 20×4 s trains/26 s inter-train interval, 10 Hz, intensity of 110% MT	Improvement in binge eating scale

161

Table 1. Cont.

Reference	Type of Study	Participants	Modulation Target	Treatment Characteristics	Main Results
Dunlop, 2015 [40]	Case series	28 subjects with anorexia nervosa, binge-purge subtype or bulimia nervosa	DMPFC Neuronavigation	20–30 sessions 120% resting MT, at 10 Hz, 5 s on, 10 s off, 3000 pulses/hemisphere, with left then right lateralized coil orientation	Enhanced frontostriatal connectivity was associated with responders to DMPFC-rTMS for binge/purge behavior
Sutoh et al., 2016 [41]	Case series (pilot study)	8 women with BN	Left DLPFC Manual targeting	1 session, 15 × 5 s trains/55 s inter-train interval, 10 Hz, intensity of 110% MT, 1000 pulses over 20 min within each session	Significant reduction of food craving and decrease in cerebral oxygenation of the left DLPFC
Gay et al., 2016 [42]	RCT	47 women (23 real, 24 sham) with BN [4]	Left DLPFC Manual targeting	10 sessions, 20 × 5 s trains/55 s inter-train interval, 10 Hz intensity of 110% MT, 1000 pulses over 20 min within each session	No significant improvement of bingeing or purging
Guillaume et al., 2018 [43]	RCT	39 patients (22 real, 17 sham) with BN [4]	Left DLPFC Manual targeting	10 sessions, 20 × 5 s trains/55 s inter-train interval, 10 Hz, intensity of 110% MT	Improvement of inhibitory control and decision-making

Note: All studies are cited in bibliography, because when a recent systematic review was available, it was included and prioritized in the synthesis of results. [1,2,3,4]: Partial or total overlap on sample.

Besides DLPFC, one study on rTMS of the inferior parietal cortex was stopped for safety reasons (NCT01717079). The study promoter informed us that the study was halted following two suicide attempts after the first inclusions. Another pilot case series ($n = 8$ patients with long-lasting AN) used deep rTMS to target the insula and found that this approach was safe and well-tolerated. At the end of the 42 sessions, AN-related obsessions and compulsions were reduced, as were the depression and anxiety scores [30].

3.1.2. Bulimia Nervosa and Binge-Eating Disorder

In a recent review of the literature, Dalton et al. identified eight studies on rTMS for BN. The areas stimulated were mainly the left DLPFC, and the dorsomedial prefrontal cortex (DMPFC). The results showed a decrease in food craving, and in some studies a reduction in food binging or purging behavior (for review see Dalton et al. [44]). DLPFC stimulation may also improve the inhibitory control and decision making in patients with BN [43]. A study on the correlation between salivary cortisol and rTMS on the left DLPFC in BN showed that salivary cortisol concentrations were significantly lower in the rTMS arm compared with the sham rTMS arm. This suggests that stimulation of this area modifies the hypothalamic–pituitary–adrenal axis activity in people with BN [36]. Moreover, frontal lobe oxygenation is decreased after one rTMS session [41]. On the other hand, one randomized controlled trial showed no improvement of binge/purge behavior after 10 sessions of high-frequency rTMS on the left DLPFC [42]. A groundbreaking research study demonstrated that self-reported food craving during exposure to experimental foods remained stable before and after stimulation of the left DLPFC compared with the sham group in which craving increased [45].

Another interesting finding is the relationship between frontostriatal connectivity and response to 20 sessions of rTMS in patients with refractory binge/purge behavior. In this case series, enhanced frontostriatal connectivity was associated with binge/purge behavior improvement after DMPFC-rTMS. Conversely, in non-responders, who showed high connectivity on the resting-state fMRI, rTMS caused paradoxical suppression of frontostriatal connectivity [40]. Finally, in an open-label case series that included patients with various EDs (mainly binge form) and comorbid post-traumatic stress disorder, post-traumatic stress symptoms were improved after 20 to 30 sessions of high-frequency rTMS on the DMPFC [29].

Hence, rTMS is an important tool to explore the neurobiology of craving and binge eating (BE). An ongoing study is investigating rTMS tolerability and safety and its effects on food craving and BE behavior, and also on ED-related psychopathology (including depression, anxiety, and stress symptoms), anthropometric measures, cognition, brain structure and function, hormones, and inflammatory biomarkers [46].

3.1.3. rTMS and Site of Modulation

As shown in Table 1, most of the published studies targeted the left DLPFC with excitatory modulation. Nevertheless, other neuroanatomical targets should be investigated. The first is the DMPFC, which plays an important role in self-control, including self-inhibition of movements, self-cessation of loss-chasing in pathological gamblers, self-suppression of emotional responses, and impulse control. It has been hypothesized that DMPFC stimulation may alter the DMPFC top-down executive control of the striatal regions associated with the urge to binge, thereby improving binge symptoms. The available open label studies using 10 Hz stimulation [40] emphasize the interest of this target particularly in BN and BED, although more work is needed to allow definitive conclusions.

The insula has also been considered in one pilot study. The insula is involved in the process of imagination of food images and food intake, in the perception of taste during food intake and of satiety, and in the feeling of disgust after eating. The insular lobe plays a role in the disturbed body image perception in patients with AN and is implicated in the brain response to stress through its close connection with the hypothalamus–pituitary–adrenal axis [12]. This brain area is reduced in patients with AN [47]. Moreover, Kaye et al. demonstrated a functional disconnection between the insula and ventral caudal putamen in patients with AN in a hungry state [48]. All these findings suggest that insula is a potential target in AN.

The corticostriatal circuits through the orbitofrontal cortex (OFC) might also represent a valuable target. They play key roles in complex human behaviors, such as evaluation, affect regulation, and reward-based decision making, and have been implicated in all ED types [49]. A functional hyperconnectivity between NAcc and the orbitofrontal cortex has been shown in AN [50]. Few studies have targeted this area with NIBS, and to our knowledge, it has not been done in patients with ED. Nevertheless, the good response to inhibitory (1 Hz) rTMS in patients with obsessive-compulsive disorder (OCD) who share some features with ED (e.g., functional hyperconnectivity between NAcc and OFC) [51] supports testing this target in ED.

Finally, other targets have also been explored in patients with addictions with promising results, particularly high-frequency stimulation of the superior frontal gyrus [52] and inhibition of the medial prefrontal cortex in patients with cocaine use disorder [53]. All these areas might constitute interesting targets in bulimic disorders, but it is challenging to decide which region to stimulate to obtain the best results.

3.2. tDCS and Eating Disorders

As shown in Table 2, in AN, tDCS approaches on the right and left DLPFC have been tested [54]. In an open-label single-arm study, seven patients with AN underwent left DLPFC anodal tDCS for 25 min daily for 10 days. In three patients, the levels of eating and depressive symptoms improved immediately after the sessions, and the response was maintained at 1 month in one patient [55]. Of note, only patients concomitantly treated with selective serotonin reuptake inhibitors (SSRI) improved. In another open-label study, nine patients with AN received 20 sessions of tDCS (the anode over the left DLPFC and the cathode over the right DLPFC). The treatment was effective on several AN dimensions and the comorbid depression at 1 month of follow-up [56]. Finally, a pilot study is currently testing the efficacy and safety of high-definition tDCS over the left inferior parietal lobe [57].

Table 2. Transcranial direct current stimulation (tDCS) and eating disorders.

Reference	Type of Study	Participants	Modulation Target	Treatment Characteristics	Main Results
Khedr et al., 2014 [55]	Open-label, single arm study (pilot study)	7 patients with AN	Left DLPFC	10 sessions Anodal tDCS for 25 min at 2 mA (15 s ramp in and 15 s ramp out)	Immediate improvement in 3 patients after the sessions on eating and depressive symptoms, with one patient maintaining the response at 1 month
Burgess et al., 2016 [58]	RCT (proof-of-concept study)	30 participants with BED	Right DLPFC	1 session, 2 mA, 20 min	Decreased craving for sweets, savory proteins, and an all-foods category, with strongest reductions in men
Kekic et al., 2017 [59]	RCT	39 patients (2 male) with BN	Right and left DLPFC (3 montages: AR/CL; AL/CR; sham)	1 session 20 min, 2 mA, 10 s ramp on/off	Reduction in ED cognitions with AR/CL tDCS Suppression of urge to binge-eat and increased self-regulatory control with both active montages Improvement of mood with AR/CL
Sreeraj et al., 2018 [60]	Case report	37 year old female with schizophrenia and binge-eating	Right DLPFC	10 sessions, 2 mA, 30 min	Improvement in subjective reporting on cognitive restraint and control over eating as well as feeling of satiation and ability to eat after exposure to cues 3 kg weight loss by the end of the treatment, 7 kg at 10-month follow-up
Strumila et al., 2019 [56]	Open-label study	10 females with AN	Anode over left DLPFC and cathode over right DLPFC	20 sessions of anodal 2 mA stimulation during a period of two weeks	Improvement of anorexic and depressive symptoms

In BN and BED, suppression of the urge to binge eat and increased self-regulatory control were reported by the only double-blind sham-controlled proof-of-principle trial on the effects of bilateral tDCS over the DLPFC in 39 adults with BN [59]. Two electrode montages were tested: anode on the right and cathode on the left (AR/CL) and the reverse (AL/CR). One session of AR/CL led to bulimic cognition reduction and mood improvement, compared with the AL/CR and sham conditions [59]. A case report [60] and the study by Burgess et al. (n = 30 participants with BED) showed that compared with the sham arm, tDCS on the right DLPFC decreased cravings for sweets, savory proteins, and an all-food category with stronger reductions in men. A possible explanation of this finding is that stimulation of the right DLPFC enhances cognitive control and/or decreases the need for reward [58].

3.3. ECT in Eating Disorders

3.3.1. Anorexia Nervosa

As shown in Table 3, only case reports and case series have evaluated ECT in AN (n = 50 patients in total) [61]. In most cases, ECT was proposed to treat a comorbid major depressive disorder (MDD), especially treatment-refractory MDD or associated with suicide attempts or obsessive-compulsive disorder (OCD). Indeed, due to the high suicide rate in patients with EDs, intensive treatments, like ECT, are often proposed. The recent and largest case series on patients with AN treated by ECT concerned 30 adolescents with comorbid depression [62]. All were severely depressed and suicidal upon admission and resistant to antidepressants. Improvement in depressive and ED symptoms was observed after ECT with minimal adverse effects. Several years after discharge, 46.6% of patients had no evidence of depression, suicidality, and ED symptomatology, and 23% had only ED symptomatology. Due to the simultaneous improvement of AN symptoms, body weight, and depression, a specific effect on ED cannot be easily identified. Finally, two recent case reports show contradictory results of ECT in patients with AN without psychiatric comorbidity [63,64]. Specifically, Naguy et al. demonstrated a strong improvement of eating behaviors in a 16-year-old girl after only six ECT sessions. However, the absence of comorbid depression or OCD was not clearly stated, and high-dose antidepressant treatment was introduced during the ECT course. Duriez et al. reported that 10 sessions of ECT had a negative outcome and rapid relapse after discharge in patients with careful evaluation of depression, anxiety, and ED dimensions before and after ECT.

Table 3. Electroconvulsive therapy (ECT) and eating disorders.

Reference	Type of Study	Participants	Modulation Target	Treatment Characteristics	Main Results
		Anorexia Nervosa			
Davis et al., 1961 [65]	Case report	12-year-old girl with AN-R	-	12 sessions (bilateral)	Weight gain and discharge
Bernstein et al., 1964 [66]	Case report	20-year-old female with AN-R and personality disorder	-	21 sessions followed by maintenance ECT	Weight gain and mood improvement
Bernstein et al., 1972 [67]	Case report	94-year-old female with AN-R and psychotic disorder	-	5 sessions	Short term weight gain
Ferguson et al., 1993 [68]	Case series	3 patients with AN and MDD	-	11, 8 and 16 sessions (bilateral)	Transient improvement on weight and symptomatology for 2/3 patients
Bek et al., 1996 [69]	Case series	8 females with AN, one had psychosis and five had personality disorders	-	11 sessions	Modest weight gain
Hill et al., 2001 [70]	Case report	77-year-old female with AN-R and MDD	-	9 sessions	Modest weight gain and mood improvement
Poutanen et al., 2009 [71]	Case report	21-year-old female with AN-B/P and MDD	-	45 sessions in three courses (bilateral)	Modest thymic and eating amelioration. Cognitive impairment.

Table 3. Cont.

Reference	Type of Study	Participants	Modulation Target	Treatment Characteristics	Main Results
Andrews et al., 2014 [72]	Case report	17-year-old with AN-B/P, MDD, and NSSI	-	10 unilateral and 21 bilateral sessions/13 weeks	Mood improvement
Andersen et al., 2017 [73]	Case report	14-year-old girl with AN-R, MDD, and GAD	-	22 sessions (bilateral)	Weight gain
Saglam et al., 2018 [74]	Case report	24-year-old male with AN-B/P, OCD, and MDD	-	12 sessions (bitemporal)	Weight restoration and OCD improvement, stopped diuretic and laxative abuse.
Pacillio et al., 2019 [61]	Case report	30-year-old female patient with AN and MDD	-	11 sessions (unilateral)	Modest increase of eating disorder, mood improvement
Naguy et al., 2019 [63]	Case report	16-year-old female with AN and personality disorder	-	6 sessions (bitemporal)	Weight gain and improvement in eating behavior
Duriez et al., 2020 [75]	Case report	19-year-old female with AN	-	10 sessions	No improvement of AN symptoms
Shilton et al., 2020 [62]	Case series	30 female adolescents with AN and MDD	-	-	Mood improvement, treatment well tolerated, no specific improvement for eating disorder symptoms
Bulimic Disorders (Bulimia and/or Binge Eating Disorders)					
Rapinesi et al., 2013 [76]	Case report	41-year-old male with BED and bipolar disorder. Personal history of AN	-	8 sessions (bitemporal)	Important weight loss and decrease of psychotic symptoms

AN: anorexia nervosa; AN-R: anorexia nervosa restricting subtype; AN-B/P: anorexia nervosa binge/purge subtype; BED: binge eating disorder; OCD: obsessive-compulsive disorder; MDD: major depressive disorder; NSSI: non-suicidal self-injury.

To our knowledge, no controlled trial is currently testing ECT efficacy in AN. Furthermore, as only case series have been published, no standardized evaluation has been provided, thus preventing the precise comparison of patients with different AN profiles. Moreover, we hypothesize a strong publication bias towards ECT in severe and enduring AN without comorbid psychiatric disorders.

Nevertheless, the available results suggest that ECT is safe in this population and might improve AN symptomatology in addition to its positive effects on comorbid mood disorders. ECT appears to be well tolerated in this population, and it is even used in late-onset AN in older adults [67,70].

3.3.2. Bulimia Nervosa and Binge Eating Disorder

MDD is more frequent in patients with BN than in AN [77]. According to a recent systematic review [61], only one case report described ECT use in BED and none in BN. In this patient with a psychiatric comorbidity, ECT was safe and effective on bulimic symptoms.

3.4. VNS in Eating Disorders

To date, no study assessed VNS effects in patients with EDs [78]. However, a growing body of evidence suggests the relevance of VNS in patients with ED. Some studies in animal models showed an association between VNS and reduction in food intake and/or weight loss, suggesting that vagal stimulation might mediate satiety signals (for review see McClelland 2013 [79]). Several fMRI studies have also shown that VNS modulates the activity in brain regions related to the processing of afferent vagal signals and interoception, such as the thalamus, precentral gyrus, and insular cortex [80–82]. A recent study demonstrated that transcutaneous VNS improves interoceptive accuracy [83]. This is a very valuable point given the central role of interoception in ED [84–86].

3.5. Deep Brain Stimulation in Eating Disorders

3.5.1. Deep Brain Stimulation in Anorexia Nervosa

In a recent review, Sobstyl et al. described all trials on DBS in patients with AN [87]. Ten years ago, the first description of DBS in a patient with severe and treatment-resistant MDD and comorbid AN opened the way to a new therapeutic modality [88]. To date, 58 case reports on DBS in AN have been published (Table 4). The first studies concerned well known targets in MDD or OCD, mostly in the limbic system linked to the anxiety and emotion pathways. Barbier et al. [89] described AN remission and complete weight recovery in a patients with comorbid OCD/AN after treatment first by bilateral stimulation of the anterior limb of the internal capsule and then of the bed nucleus of the stria terminalis. In 2012, McLaughlin et al. reported the improvement of severe OCD in a patient with comorbid AN treated by DBS of the ventral capsule and ventral striatum [90]. Moreover, they observed a small weight gain, but less distress about caloric intake. Blomstedt et al. [91] showed that bilateral stimulation of the medial forebrain bundle (MFB) and then of the bed nucleus of the stria terminalis (BNST) improved MDD and AN. However, it should be noted that this 60-year-old woman lost weight during the procedure. The first case series came from an open-label trial involving 16 patients with AN, among whom 14 had comorbid depression or other major psychiatric comorbidities [92]. The primary outcomes were acceptability and safety of DBS applied to the subgenual cingulate cortex (SCC), a validated target for the treatment of resistant depression [93]. After 1 year, patients exhibited weight gain and improvement in depressive and anxious symptoms. In 2013, AN remission was observed in four patients after implanting electrodes bilaterally in the nucleus accumbens (NAcc) [94]. Wang et al. [95] used the same method in two patients with AN and a comorbid psychiatric disorder (OCD, generalized anxiety disorder, or MDD). These two trials also demonstrated glucose metabolism changes after DBS in the NAcc and SCC by positron emission tomography [96,97]. Recently, the Shanghai group published the largest series on DBS in AN involving 28 patients with refractory AN who were followed for at least 2 years after electrode implantation in the NAcc [98]. All patients had a major psychiatric comorbidity at inclusion ($n = 9$ OCD, $n = 7$ severe anxiety, and $n = 12$ MDD). Post-hoc analysis suggests that NAcc DBS is less effective for weight restoration in the binge/purge AN subtype than in the restrictive subtype [98]. Another recent preliminary study proposes for the first time two targets in the same trial chosen according to the main psychiatric comorbidities associated with AN: SCC for affective disorder ($n = 4$) and NAcc for anxiety disorder ($n = 4$) (Martinez et al., 2020). Four patients considered as responders after 6 months will be randomized in two arms (ON/OFF or OFF/ON) for a double-blind controlled cross over trial.

Regarding tolerance and safety, DBS is a reversible procedure, and the device can be removed if requested by the patient [93,96]. The clinical situation of malnutrition is a key issue for surgical procedures, like DBS [92]. The existing studies did not report any permanent neurological deficit after the procedure. In one patient, the device was removed due to infection (new implantation 6 months later). Moreover, Lipsman et al. observed excessive pain at the incision site in five patients, treatment withdrawal by two patients (device off or removal) without any precise reason, and seizures in two patients. Liu et al. reported device removal in one patient (3%) at 18 months due to rejection. It has been suggested that the surgical risk is higher in patients with severe AN and BMI lower than 14 kg/m^2 due to malnutrition. These first findings are encouraging, but more investigations and controlled trials are needed. Nevertheless, the high mortality and morbidity in severe and enduring AN and the increasing knowledge of AN functional neuroanatomy give strong ethical support for this procedure.

Table 4. Deep brain stimulation (DBS) in eating disorders.

Reference	Type of Study	Participants	Modulation Target	Treatment Characteristics *	Main Results
Anorexia Nervosa					
Israël et al., 2010 [88]	Case report	56-year-old female with AN and severe depression	SCC (bilateral)	Intermittent stimulation 2 min on/1 min off 5 mA/91 µs/130 Hz	Maintenance of normal BMI (average 19.1 kg/m^2) at 3 years, normal scores in restraint and weight and shape concerns
Barbier et al., 2011 [89]	Case report	39-year-old female with AN and severe OCD	ALIC and BNST (bilateral)	Unknown	Full recovery of AN and strong improvement of OCD
McLaughlin et al., 2012 [90]	Case report	52-year-old female with refractory OCD and AN	Ventral capsule and ventral striatum (bilateral)	Left unilateral, monopolar 7.5 V/120 µs/120 Hz	Significant weight improvement, reduction in AN-related obsession and patient can go out to eat
Wu et al., 2013 and Sun et al., 2012 [94,99]	Case series	4 females with AN (3 OCD, 1 GAD) [1]	NAcc (bilateral)	Unknown	Full remission of AN, restoration of menstrual cycle and return to school for 3 patients
Wang et al., 2013 [95]	Case series	2 females with AN, depression, and OCD	NAcc (bilateral)	2.5–3.8 V/120–210 µs/135–185 Hz	Significant weight gain and affective improvement
Lipsman et al., 2013 [96]	Open label clinical trial	6 females with AN, 5 with psychiatric comorbidities (MDD, OCD, SUD, PTSD) [2]	SCC (bilateral)	5–7 V/90 µs/130 Hz	Weight gain in 3 patients, changes in brain metabolism
Hayes et al., 2015 [100]	Ancillary Study	8 females with AN, 7 with psychiatric comorbidities (MDD, OCD, GAD, PTSD, BPD) [2]	SCC (bilateral)	Unknown	Weight loss in 3 patients, weight gain in 5 patients
Lipsman et al., 2017 [93]	Open label clinical trial	16 females with AN, 14 with psychiatric comorbidities (MDD, OCD, SUD, PTSD, GAD, BPD) [2]	SCC (bilateral)	5–6.5 V/90 µs/130 Hz	Significant weight gain for 8 patients Adverse effects: 1 surgical-site infection, 2 devices explanted at patient request, 1 seizure
Blomstedt et al., 2017 [91]	Case report	60-year-old female with AN and depression	MFB (bilateral) and subsequent BNST (bilateral)	Bipolar MFB stimulation 3 V/60 µs/130 Hz two years later: monopolar BNST stimulation 4.3 V/120 µs/130 Hz	Improvement of affective symptoms Weight stabilization Target change due to blurred vision
Manuelli et al., 2019 [101]	Case report	37-year-old female with AN-BP	BNST (bilateral)	4 V/60 µs/130 Hz	Full weight restoration after 4 months
Wei Liu et al., 2020 [98]	Open label clinical trial	29 females with AN, 28 with psychiatric comorbidities (12 MDD, 9 OCD, 7 GAD)	NAcc (bilateral)	2.5–4 V/120–150 µs/160–180 Hz	12 patients obtained full weight restoration and 5 significant weight increase after 2 years of follow up Less effective with AN-BP than AN-R
Martinez et al., 2020 [102]	Open label clinical trial [3]	7 female and 1 male with AN, 4 with affective disorder and 4 with anxiety disorder as main psychiatric comorbidities	SCC (bilateral) or NAcc (bilateral)	7–8 mA/90 µs/130 Hz	No weight gain. Subjective improvement of quality of life

Table 4. *Cont.*

Reference	Type of Study	Participants	Modulation Target	Treatment Characteristics *	Main Results
Bulimic Disorders (Bulimia and/or Binge Eating Disorders)					
Whiting et al., 2013 [103]	Case series	3 patients with BED	LHA (bilateral)	Monopolar unknown V/90 µs/185 Hz	1/3 significantly improvement in binge eating Significant weight loss in 2/3
Tronnier et al., 2018 [104]	Case report	47-year-old female with BED and severe depression	NAcc (bilateral)	Bipolar 3 V/90 µs/130 Hz	Weight loss (2.8 kg/month), affective improvement and decrease of binge eating behaviors

AN: anorexia nervosa; AN-R: anorexia nervosa restricting subtype; AN-BP: anorexia nervosa binge/purge subtype; BED: binge eating disorder; OCD: obsessive-compulsive disorder; MDD: major depressive disorder; GAD: generalized anxiety disorder; SUD: substance use disorder; PTSD: post traumatic stress disorder; BMI: body mass index; BNST: bed nucleus of the stria terminalis; SCC: subgenual cingulate cortex; NAcc: nucleus accumbens; MFB: medial forebrain bundle; ALIC: anterior limb of internal capsule; LHA: lateral hypothalamus; PET: positron emission tomography. * We retained the main stimulation parameter after adjustments: amplitude/pulse width/frequency. 1,2: Partial overlap on sample; 3: in a second phase, patients will be included in a randomized trial with two arms (ON/OFF or OFF/ON).

3.5.2. Deep Brain Stimulation in Bulimia Nervosa and Binge Eating Disorder

As shown in Table 4, several patients have been treated by DBS of the hypothalamus or NAcc for severe obesity [105]. In some cases, binge eating behaviors were mentioned, but without a clear ED diagnosis. A pilot study with a 2-year follow-up assessed DBS of the lateral hypothalamic area in three patients with refractory obesity [103]. Only one patient reported binge eating reduction. Tronier et al. observed a reduction of binge eating behaviors after bilateral DBS of NAcc in one patient with treatment-resistant depression and severe obesity previously treated by gastric bypass [104].

3.5.3. Neuroanatomical Targets in DBS

SCC was the first DBS target tested in AN by Andres Lozano's group after their extensive experience with DBS in depression. This region is an affective regulatory center [106]. Substantial evidence indicates the main role of dysregulated emotional processing in AN pathogenesis [107]. SCC stimulation in AN also benefits from the experience in refractory MDD, and is an extensively interconnected component of the limbic system.

Other limbic regions have also been targeted. The BNST is a center of integration for limbic information and valence monitoring [108]. The MFB is a key structure of the reward-seeking circuitry and is highly connected to the limbic system [109]. Preclinical data supports the interest of NAcc modulation in EDs and the stimulation of the ventral striatum. NAcc stimulation increased food intake and weight gain in a rodent model of food restriction and hyperactivity [110,111]. Abnormalities in goal-directed behavior and the establishment of a compulsive/restrictive behavior might be the consequences of dysregulation of neurocircuits that control positive/negative valence as well as reward and decision-making behaviors [112]. A recent study highlighted the role of the mesolimbic reward circuitry in a rodent model of AN [113].

It is important to stress that when choosing targets for brain stimulation, the dysfunctional networks in EDs must be taken into account, as illustrated by recent studies on DBS. Lipsman et al. and Zhang et al. observed broad changes in glucose metabolism in many brain regions after DBS of the SCC and NAcc, respectively. Specifically, SCC stimulation increases activity in the insula and glucose metabolism in parietal and temporal regions, and decreases cingulate activity [93]. NAcc stimulation decreases activity in the frontal lobe, lentiform nucleus (putamen), and hippocampus [97]. More studies are needed to investigate the influence of ventral striatum (NAcc) stimulation and dorsal striatum (caudate nucleus and putamen) on habit formation. The DBS mechanism of action on neuronal pathways is only partially understood, but the target choice is the focus of the current research because a highly focal intervention can have a very broad effect.

4. Discussion

4.1. Current Evidence and Issues

Altogether, the evidence for the use of brain stimulation in EDs is promising, but more studies are needed before it will be considered an effective intervention. Indeed, the literature consists mainly of case reports, cases series, and open studies, and only a few randomized controlled trials. Most studies had small samples and focused mainly on the immediate effects on craving or neurocognition, without follow-up data. Moreover, methodologies were very heterogeneous among studies. For instance, some studies on rTMS effects on craving did not use cues to induce craving, while others used them only during stimulation or for pre-stimulation craving induction, but not for post-stimulation craving assessment. Some studies assessed craving using a visual analogic scale, whereas other used questionnaires. Moreover, only a few studies assessed the (immediate and long-term) clinical effects of brain stimulation. Yet, a crucial question is whether brain stimulation can induce lasting changes in a well-established behavior. Studies using ECT are limited to case reports. Nevertheless, there have been more studies on ECT in AN in the past two years than in the previous thirty years. This is probably due to a global increase of interest in ECT after years of stigma and the recent demonstration of neurogenesis induction by ECT [114]. Although the level of evidence is low, ECT may be useful and safe for the management of severe and treatment-resistant MDD in patients with AN. Its wider accessibility compared to other brain stimulation techniques should facilitate the organization of a prospective trial, particularly in patients with severe comorbid MDD, given the lower efficacy of SSRI in AN [5]. The cognitive and memory effects of ECT are a challenging aspect. They are the strongest limiting factors of ECT use in MDD and should be thoroughly evaluated in the specific metabolic context of AN. DBS is the most recent and promising brain stimulation technique for severe and enduring AN (due to the ethical issues linked to an invasive procedure). Although the lack of consensus on the best neuroanatomical target strongly limits the level of evidence, there are already prospective studies and a few randomized trials currently recruiting. Park et al. proposed a double-blind cross-over study that includes a sham-stimulation phase [92]. Perez et al. are currently recruiting for a cross-over trial in Spain (NCT03168893) [102].

The main issue of the reviewed studies is that many of them were underpowered. Therefore, their findings must interpreted with caution due to the high risk of type II error and inflated effect sizes. Future studies should include larger samples, and the number of patients needed for a robust statistical analysis should be calculated in advance. In rTMS, most studies used manual methods rather than MRI-based methods to locate the target, particularly those on rTMS of the DLPFC. As the location of the intended target region varied across individuals, this might have affected the results and resulted in low effect-size. Moreover, the standard figure-8-shaped rTMS coil, used in most studies, allows a relatively limited and shallow stimulation area that does not induce direct stimulation of deep cortical areas [115]. Stimulation of deeper areas using an H coil might be more effective, leading to enduring benefits. With the exception of Dalton et al. [28,44], the randomized controlled studies only proposed a limited number of pulses and 1 to 10 sessions (i.e., about 10,000 pulses maximum). It is likely that more sessions are needed to modify neural programs and their associated behaviors. Future studies should determine the optimal dose of neuromodulation and duration (for example by comparing different rTMS durations or by investigating in ancillary studies non-responders to a specific program).

Psychiatric comorbidities are the norm in people with eating disorders (>70%) [1]. Binge disorders are often comorbid with a substance use disorders [1]. Binge eating is also frequently compared to addictions, based on the evidence that they share common characteristics, such as escalating frequency of the behavior, ambivalence towards treatments, and frequent relapses [116,117]. In addition, brain stimulation is a successful strategy in MDD. ECT is recommended in most guideline and rTMS in some of them [118]. Given the high rate of these comorbid disorders in patients with EDs, some of the published studies were built on this background. Protocols targeting DMPFC in BN were adapted from substance use disorders studies, ECT studies on severe MDD have been one of the main drivers to begin ECT in patients with MDD and AN. In DBS, AN comorbid with MDD and OCD was one of the reasons to target the SCC. In their study targeting two areas in the same trial for the first time, the targets were chosen based on two of the major psychiatric comorbidities associated with AN: SCC for affective disorder ($n = 4$) and NAcc for anxiety disorder ($n = 4$) [102]. Indeed, most studies reported positive effects on depressive symptoms with rTMS [26], tDCS [56], ECT [62], and DBS [93]. Future studies in EDs might benefit from this knowledge in brain target selection (Figure 1), in studies design (add-on with another modalities of treatment, inclusion and exclusion criteria, etc.), or in the stimulation parameters: number of sessions, type of coil or electrode, stimulation duration, etc. Nevertheless, regarding the mood component, there is a crucial methodological problem: because of the simultaneous improvement of ED weight and mood features, a specific effect on ED cannot be identified. Systematic measurement of depressive symptoms associated with subgroup analyses of patients without depression will make it possible to address this problem.

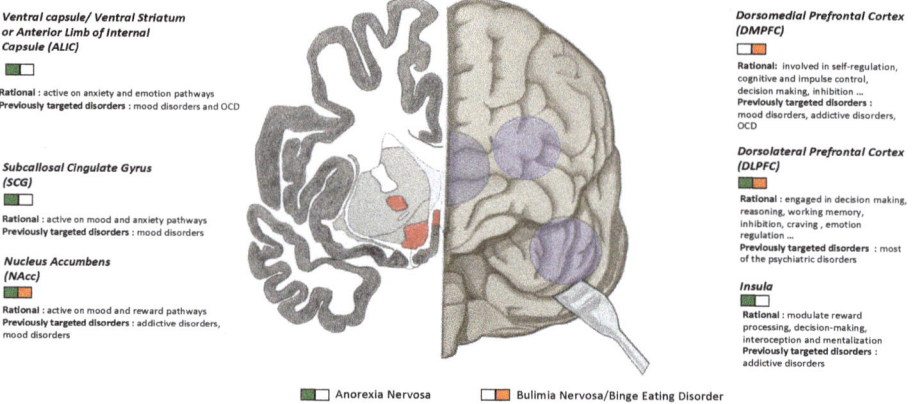

Figure 1. Overview of main neuromodulation targets in eating disorders. Schematic coronal section of right brain and front view of left brain. DBS: deep brain stimulation; rTMS: repetitive transcranial magnetic stimulation; tDCS: transcranial direct current stimulation; OCD: obsessive-compulsive disorder.

Another factor that should be considered is the variability in brain activity related to the metabolic state. The nutritional state in patients with ED might affect brain functions more than in any other psychiatric disorder. Starvation and nutritional status affect behavior, cognition, and disease symptoms. The nutritional status also influences the treatment response, especially to antidepressants that are less effective in acutely ill and underweight patients [5]. To the best of our knowledge, no study has determined whether the nutritional status affects the resting brain state and the neuromodulatory response. Nevertheless, it is possible that the nutritional status influences the response/non-response to a treatment and acts as a confounding factor on brain stimulation efficiency. Better metabolic monitoring could be useful to limit some central deficit that might affect the stimulation response, as reported for folate deficiency in people with comorbid depression [119] and for kynurenic pathway defects [120]. This should be investigated in view of personalized treatment programs.

Finally, in most of the studies reviewed here, samples only included adults and mainly patients with severe, chronic ED. However, due to the good safety and acceptability profile of NIBS, it would be interesting to assess their effects in patients with less severe ED forms, as is usually done in studies on SSRI efficiency in bulimia [121].

4.2. Perspectives

4.2.1. Improving Brain Stimulation Efficiency

A promising strategy consists in stimulating a specific disorder-related circuitry involved in ED using NIBS and in functionally engaging the targeted circuit through cognitive tasks or therapies. This is particularly relevant for neurocognition.

Behavioral abnormalities driven by cognitive processes are a prominent ED feature. For instance, studies in adults with AN suggest poor set-shifting [122], weak central coherence [123], and impaired decision making [124]. Similarly, in BN and BED, decision making and cognitive inhibition seem to be impaired [94,124]. Cognitive remediation programs that target specifically some of these functions have been developed, and some have proved their effectiveness, notably in AN [125]. NIBS also may modulate some of these cognitive functions [126]. It would be interesting to determine whether concomitant brain stimulation might enhance cognitive remediation training. This is especially true for tDCS, which is easier to administer and does not interfere with the psychotherapy sessions. Some proof of concept studies are currently testing them in EDs [127]. Moreover, studies on other disorders showed that when a patient experiences salient cues before modulation with TMS, the benefits increase significantly compared with patients who receive no provocation task [128]. An optimized provocation task before or during brain stimulation is one of the future challenges. In this context, the widespread availability of virtual reality gaming environments that could be customized and adapted to EDs (for example with cues related to food or body shape) might be an opportunity.

In DBS, the stimulation parameters also may be critical. This includes frequency, voltage, pulse width, and also number of contacts and number of directions depending on the electrode model. The choice of parameters remains challenging [129] because symptom improvement cannot be immediately monitored, in contrast to movement disorders. None of the reviewed studies on DBS evaluated the stimulation parameters, although this is a crucial issue. Awake surgery, proposed by Lipsman to increase the procedure safety, could be used also to optimize the target location by testing during implantation [93]. Alternatively, deep electroencephalography during a neurocognitive task immediately before electrode positioning may help to precisely choose the target. In addition, in the currently used open-loop DBS, the medical team can modify the stimulation parameters at different times based on clinical changes. In closed-loop DBS, the stimulation parameters are programmed automatically based on the measured biomarker. Closed-loop devices could adapt the stimulation as a function of the eating behaviors during food consumption or food deprivation. External interventions can modulate some therapeutic strategies to model behaviors like exposition work during specific cognitive behavioral therapy. Finally, the current brain stimulation strategies have little access to important therapeutic targets, deep within the brain. Recent NIBS studies [130,131] in rodent models suggest that deep-brain areas could be targeted in a non-invasive manner, potentially enlarging the number of patients who might benefit from deep-brain stimulation due to the reduction of risk and the perspective of mapping deep-brain targets. Currently, this promising technique has only shown its effectiveness on rodent brains. Its relevance and spatial resolution in human brains, which are much larger, are unknown. Resolution might be increased also using optogenetic techniques, but these methods raise ethical questions linked to their translation from animals to humans [132,133].

4.2.2. Toward More Personalized Protocols

As EDs and each subtype are highly heterogeneous and have many overlapping features, finding a single "optimal" protocol is highly unlikely. Moreover, it has been suggested that there are distinct neural endophenotypes, not readily apparent when using standard diagnostic criteria, but with differential neural and clinical responses to interventions.

Targeting specific subgroups is a valuable option. For instance, many findings support a specific disease trajectory, and preliminary evidence suggests that interventions should be matched to the disease stage [134]. Interventions tailored according to ED stage or to the developmental trajectory were tested in a recent pilot study [30]. Some clinical features could also be considered because they are associated with a specific disease form or poorer prognosis, such as ED subtype (restrictive versus binge), age, gender, associated personality traits, psychiatric comorbidities, or history of childhood abuse. Latent class and profile analyses have been performed and could be a starting point for patient stratification.

Another possible solution is to move from a categorical to a dimensional approach and to target relevant dimensions associated with the disorders rather than with the specific diagnosis. This might be particularly relevant within the research domain criteria (RDoC) research framework. This project seeks to characterize the fundamental domains of cognitive, perceptual, and social processing with the aim of identifying novel targets for mental health disorder treatment. It integrates many levels of information (from genomics and circuits to behavior and self-reports) to assess basic dimensions of functioning that span the full range of human behavior from normal to abnormal. These basic dimensions, independent of DSM diagnoses, are then used to describe the pathological behaviors of psychiatric disorders. Many dimensions associated with EDs can be studied within the RDoC matrix, such as delay discounting, sensitivity to reward/punishment, compulsive behavior, and cognitive functions [135,136]. Brain stimulation is a tremendously interesting approach to modulate the cerebral circuits involved in these dimensions and to assess the impact of this modulation in an integrative way from the molecular level to behavior.

The effects of a given protocol can vary widely across individuals. Some patients will drastically improve, whereas others will not improve, or will even worsen. ED heterogeneity and the potential confounding factors might play a major role, and therefore it is crucial to identify predictors and correlates of the response to a treatment. The perfect illustration of this is the study by Dunlop et al. [40] where enhanced frontostriatal connectivity was associated with response to DMPFC rTMS for binge/purge behavior. rTMS caused paradoxical suppression of frontostriatal connectivity in non-responders who had a high connectivity on resting-state fMRI. Thus, resting-state fMRI could be a key tool to optimize the stimulation parameters. Moreover, in a study on cocaine users treated by continuous theta-burst stimulation of the medial prefrontal cortex, the effects on the neural circuitry of cravings were not uniform and may depend on the individual baseline frontal-striatal reactivity to cues [137]. Hayes et al. also demonstrate that presurgical fornix and anterior limb of internal capsule (ALIC) connectivity are correlated with DBS response [100]. If these results are replicated, this feature might be useful in selecting potential responders. These examples indicate that future studies should include as secondary objectives the profiles of responders/non-responders. It also illustrates the relevance of fMRI neuromodulation studies for patient selection and for investigating the neuromodulatory mechanism. Martinez et al. adapted the DBS target depending on the main comorbidity in patients with severe and resistant AN: SCC for affective disorder or NAcc for anxiety disorder [102]. Finally, all DBS studies defined a minimal illness duration (from 7 to 10 years) as eligibility criterion. Better evidence for choosing the criteria of ED severity, based on neurocognitive tasks, neuroimaging, neuronal metabolism, genetic, or other metabolic patterns, is needed to allow evaluating DBS in patients with shorter illness duration [138]. More precise neurocognitive analyses correlated with neurophysiological measures are also needed.

5. Conclusions

Brain stimulation techniques in EDs are still in their infancy. Different potential targets have been considered (Figure 1), but the literature includes mainly open studies with only a few randomized controlled trials, and many issues remain to be addressed. At this time, the evidence for using brain stimulation as a routine treatment in ED management is weak. However, several ongoing studies should bring new information on optimal stimulation protocols and targets. This is a major source of hope for EDs where the development of alternative treatments is crucial.

Author Contributions: Conceptualization, P.D., R.B.K., S.G.; methodology P.D., R.B.K., P.G., P.C., S.G.; validation P.G., P.C., S.G.; investigation, P.D., R.B.K., Y.C., R.S., M.S., R.M., S.G.; resources, R.S., M.S., R.M.; writing—original draft preparation P.D., R.B.K., S.G.; writing—review and editing, all co-authors; supervision P.C., S.G.; project administration, M.S.; All authors have read and agreed to the published version of the manuscript.

Funding: This research received no external funding.

Conflicts of Interest: The authors declare no conflict of interest.

References

1. Treasure, J.; Duarte, T.A.; Schmidt, U. Eating disorders. *Lancet* **2020**, *395*, 899–911. [CrossRef]
2. Zabala, M.J.; Macdonald, P.; Treasure, J. Appraisal of caregiving burden, expressed emotion and psychological distress in families of people with eating disorders: A systematic review. *Eur. Eat. Disord. Rev. Prof. J. Eat. Disord. Assoc.* **2009**, *17*, 338–349. [CrossRef] [PubMed]
3. Striegel-Moore, R.H.; DeBar, L.; Wilson, G.T.; Dickerson, J.; Rosselli, F.; Perrin, N.; Lynch, F.; Kraemer, H.C. Health services use in eating disorders. *Psychol. Med.* **2008**, *38*, 1465–1474. [CrossRef] [PubMed]
4. Mitchell, J.E.; Peterson, C.B. Anorexia Nervosa. *N. Engl. J. Med.* **2020**, *382*, 1343–1351. [CrossRef] [PubMed]

5. Blanchet, C.; Guillaume, S.; Bat-Pitault, F.; Carles, M.E.; Clarke, J.; Dodin, V.; Duriez, P.; Gerardin, P.; Hanachi-Guidoum, M.; Iceta, S.; et al. Medication in AN: A Multidisciplinary Overview of Meta-Analyses and Systematic Reviews. *J. Clin. Med.* **2019**, *8*, 278. [CrossRef]
6. Treasure, J.; Claudino, A.M.; Zucker, N. Eating disorders. *Lancet* **2015**, *375*, 375–583. [CrossRef]
7. Eating Disorders: Recognition and Treatment (NICE Guideline 69). Available online: https://www.nice.org.uk/guidance/ng69 (accessed on 8 June 2020).
8. Slade, E.; Keeney, E.; Mavranezouli, I.; Dias, S.; Fou, L.; Stockton, S.; Saxon, L.; Waller, G.; Turner, H.; Serpell, L.; et al. Treatments for bulimia nervosa: A network meta-analysis. *Psychol. Med.* **2018**, *48*, 2629–2636. [CrossRef]
9. Luan, S.; Williams, I.; Nikolic, K.; Constandinou, T.G. Neuromodulation: Present and emerging methods. *Front. Neuroeng.* **2014**, *7*, 27. [CrossRef]
10. De Pitta, M.; Brunel, N.; Volterra, A. Astrocytes: Orchestrating synaptic plasticity? *Neuroscience* **2016**, *323*, 43–61. [CrossRef]
11. Gomez-Fernandez, L. Cortical plasticity and restoration of neurologic functions: An update on this topic. *Rev. Neurol.* **2000**, *31*, 749–756.
12. Pascual-Leone, A.; Tormos-Munoz, J.M. Transcranial magnetic stimulation: The foundation and potential of modulating specific neuronal networks. *Rev. Neurol.* **2008**, *46* (Suppl. 1), S3–S10. [PubMed]
13. Lopez-Rojas, J.; Almaguer-Melian, W.; Bergado-Rosado, J.A. Synaptic tagging and memory trace. *Rev. Neurol.* **2007**, *45*, 607–614. [PubMed]
14. Read, J.; Bentall, R. The effectiveness of electroconvulsive therapy: A literature review. *Epidemiol. Psichiatr. Soc.* **2010**, *19*, 333–347. [CrossRef] [PubMed]
15. Klomjai, W.; Katz, R.; Lackmy-Vallee, A. Basic principles of transcranial magnetic stimulation (TMS) and repetitive TMS (rTMS). *Ann. Phys. Rehabil. Med.* **2015**, *58*, 208–213. [CrossRef]
16. Impey, D.; de la Salle, S.; Knott, V. Assessment of anodal and cathodal transcranial direct current stimulation (tDCS) on MMN-indexed auditory sensory processing. *Brain Cogn.* **2016**, *105*, 46–54. [CrossRef]
17. Uher, R.; Murphy, T.; Brammer, M.J.; Dalgleish, T.; Phillips, M.L.; Ng, V.W.; Andrew, C.M.; Williams, S.C.; Campbell, I.C.; Treasure, J. Medial prefrontal cortex activity associated with symptom provocation in eating disorders. *Am. J. Psychiatry* **2004**, *161*, 1238–1246. [CrossRef]
18. Marangell, L.B.; Martinez, M.; Jurdi, R.A.; Zboyan, H. Neurostimulation therapies in depression: A review of new modalities. *Acta Psychiatr. Scand.* **2007**, *116*, 174–181. [CrossRef]
19. Kamolz, S.; Richter, M.M.; Schmidtke, A.; Fallgatter, A.J. Transcranial magnetic stimulation for comorbid depression in anorexia. *Nervenarzt* **2008**, *79*, 1071–1073. [CrossRef]
20. McClelland, J.; Bozhilova, N.; Nestler, S.; Campbell, I.C.; Jacob, S.; Johnson-Sabine, E.; Schmidt, U. Improvements in symptoms following neuronavigated repetitive transcranial magnetic stimulation (rTMS) in severe and enduring anorexia nervosa: Findings from two case studies. *Eur. Eat. Disord. Rev.* **2013**, *21*, 500–506. [CrossRef]
21. Choudhary, P.; Roy, P.; Kumar Kar, S. Improvement of weight and attitude towards eating behaviour with high frequency rTMS augmentation in anorexia nervosa. *Asian J. Psychiatr* **2017**, *28*, 160. [CrossRef]
22. Jassova, K.; Albrecht, J.; Papezova, H.; Anders, M. Repetitive Transcranial Magnetic Stimulation (rTMS) Treatment of Depression and Anxiety in a Patient with Anorexia Nervosa. *Med. Sci. Monit.* **2018**, *24*, 5279–5281. [CrossRef] [PubMed]
23. McClelland, J.; Kekic, M.; Campbell, I.C.; Schmidt, U. Repetitive Transcranial Magnetic Stimulation (rTMS) Treatment in Enduring Anorexia Nervosa: A Case Series. *Eur. Eat. Disord. Rev.* **2016**, *24*, 157–163. [CrossRef] [PubMed]
24. Van den Eynde, F.; Guillaume, S.; Broadbent, H.; Campbell, I.C.; Schmidt, U. Repetitive transcranial magnetic stimulation in anorexia nervosa: A pilot study. *Eur Psychiatry* **2013**, *28*, 98–101. [CrossRef] [PubMed]
25. McClelland, J.; Kekic, M.; Bozhilova, N.; Nestler, S.; Dew, T.; Van den Eynde, F.; David, A.S.; Rubia, K.; Campbell, I.C.; Schmidt, U. A Randomised Controlled Trial of Neuronavigated Repetitive Transcranial Magnetic Stimulation (rTMS) in Anorexia Nervosa. *PLoS ONE* **2016**, *11*, e0148606. [CrossRef] [PubMed]
26. Dalton, B.; Bartholdy, S.; McClelland, J.; Kekic, M.; Rennalls, S.J.; Werthmann, J.; Carter, B.; O'Daly, O.G.; Campbell, I.C.; David, A.S.; et al. Randomised controlled feasibility trial of real versus sham repetitive transcranial magnetic stimulation treatment in adults with severe and enduring anorexia nervosa: The TIARA study. *BMJ Open* **2018**, *8*, e021531. [CrossRef]

27. Bartholdy, S.; McClelland, J.; Kekic, M.; O'Daly, O.G.; Campbell, I.C.; Werthmann, J.; Rennalls, S.J.; Rubia, K.; David, A.S.; Glennon, D.; et al. Clinical outcomes and neural correlates of 20 sessions of repetitive transcranial magnetic stimulation in severe and enduring anorexia nervosa (the TIARA study): Study protocol for a randomised controlled feasibility trial. *Trials* **2015**, *16*, 548. [CrossRef]
28. Dalton, B.; Foerde, K.; Bartholdy, S.; McClelland, J.; Kekic, M.; Grycuk, L.; Campbell, I.C.; Schmidt, U.; Steinglass, J.E. The effect of repetitive transcranial magnetic stimulation on food choice-related self-control in patients with severe, enduring anorexia nervosa. *Int. J. Eat. Disord.* **2020**, 1–11. [CrossRef]
29. Woodside, D.B.; Colton, P.; Lam, E.; Dunlop, K.; Rzeszutek, J.; Downar, J. Dorsomedial prefrontal cortex repetitive transcranial magnetic stimulation treatment of posttraumatic stress disorder in eating disorders: An open-label case series. *Int. J. Eat. Disord.* **2017**, *50*, 1231–1234. [CrossRef]
30. Knyahnytska, Y.O.; Blumberger, D.M.; Daskalakis, Z.J.; Zomorrodi, R.; Kaplan, A.S. Insula H-coil deep transcranial magnetic stimulation in severe and enduring anorexia nervosa (SE-AN): A pilot study. *Neuropsychiatr. Dis. Treat.* **2019**, *15*, 2247–2256. [CrossRef]
31. Hausmann, A.; Mangweth, B.; Walpoth, M.; Hoertnagel, C.; Kramer-Reinstadler, K.; Rupp, C.I.; Hinterhuber, H. Repetitive transcranial magnetic stimulation (rTMS) in the double-blind treatment of a depressed patient suffering from bulimia nervosa: A case report. *Int. J. Neuropsychopharmacol.* **2004**, *7*, 371–373. [CrossRef]
32. Walpoth, M.; Hoertnagl, C.; Mangweth-Matzek, B.; Kemmler, G.; Hinterholzl, J.; Conca, A.; Hausmann, A. Repetitive transcranial magnetic stimulation in bulimia nervosa: Preliminary results of a single-centre, randomised, double-blind, sham-controlled trial in female outpatients. *Psychother. Psychosom.* **2008**, *77*, 57–60. [CrossRef] [PubMed]
33. Van den Eynde, F.; Claudino, A.M.; Mogg, A.; Horrell, L.; Stahl, D.; Ribeiro, W.; Uher, R.; Campbell, I.; Schmidt, U. Repetitive transcranial magnetic stimulation reduces cue-induced food craving in bulimic disorders. *Biol. Psychiatry* **2010**, *67*, 793–795. [CrossRef]
34. Van den Eynde, F.; Samarawickrema, N.; Kenyon, M.; DeJong, H.; Lavender, A.; Startup, H.; Schmidt, U. A study of neurocognition in bulimia nervosa and eating disorder not otherwise specified-bulimia type. *J. Clin. Exp. Neuropsychol.* **2012**, *34*, 67–77. [CrossRef] [PubMed]
35. Van den Eynde, F.; Claudino, A.M.; Campbell, I.; Horrell, L.; Andiappan, M.; Stahl, D.; Schmidt, U. Cardiac safety of repetitive transcranial magnetic stimulation in bulimic eating disorders. *Brain Stimul.* **2011**, *4*, 112–114. [CrossRef] [PubMed]
36. Claudino, A.M.; Van den Eynde, F.; Stahl, D.; Dew, T.; Andiappan, M.; Kalthoff, J.; Schmidt, U.; Campbell, I.C. Repetitive transcranial magnetic stimulation reduces cortisol concentrations in bulimic disorders. *Psychol. Med.* **2011**, *41*, 1329–1336. [CrossRef] [PubMed]
37. Van den Eynde, F.; Broadbent, H.; Guillaume, S.; Claudino, A.; Campbell, I.C.; Schmidt, U. Handedness, repetitive transcranial magnetic stimulation and bulimic disorders. *Eur. Psychiatry* **2012**, *27*, 290–293. [CrossRef]
38. Downar, J.; Sankar, A.; Giacobbe, P.; Woodside, B.; Colton, P. Unanticipated Rapid Remission of Refractory Bulimia Nervosa, during High-Dose Repetitive Transcranial Magnetic Stimulation of the Dorsomedial Prefrontal Cortex: A Case Report. *Front. Psychiatry* **2012**, *3*, 30. [CrossRef]
39. Baczynski, T.P.; de Aquino Chaim, C.H.; Nazar, B.P.; Carta, M.G.; Arias-Carrion, O.; Silva, A.C.; Machado, S.; Nardi, A.E. High-frequency rTMS to treat refractory binge eating disorder and comorbid depression: A case report. *CNS Neurol. Disord. Drug Targets* **2014**, *13*, 771–775. [CrossRef]
40. Dunlop, K.; Woodside, B.; Lam, E.; Olmsted, M.; Colton, P.; Giacobbe, P.; Downar, J. Increases in frontostriatal connectivity are associated with response to dorsomedial repetitive transcranial magnetic stimulation in refractory binge/purge behaviors. *Neuroimage Clin.* **2015**, *8*, 611–618. [CrossRef]
41. Sutoh, C.; Koga, Y.; Kimura, H.; Kanahara, N.; Numata, N.; Hirano, Y.; Matsuzawa, D.; Iyo, M.; Nakazato, M.; Shimizu, E. Repetitive Transcranial Magnetic Stimulation Changes Cerebral Oxygenation on the Left Dorsolateral Prefrontal Cortex in Bulimia Nervosa: A Near-Infrared Spectroscopy Pilot Study. *Eur. Eat. Disord. Rev.* **2016**, *24*, 83–88. [CrossRef]
42. Gay, A.; Jaussent, I.; Sigaud, T.; Billard, S.; Attal, J.; Seneque, M.; Galusca, B.; Van Den Eynde, F.; Massoubre, C.; Courtet, P.; et al. A Lack of Clinical Effect of High-frequency rTMS to Dorsolateral Prefrontal Cortex on Bulimic Symptoms: A Randomised, Double-blind Trial. *Eur. Eat. Disord. Rev.* **2016**, *24*, 474–481. [CrossRef] [PubMed]

43. Guillaume, S.; Gay, A.; Jaussent, I.; Sigaud, T.; Billard, S.; Attal, J.; Seneque, M.; Galusca, B.; Thiebaut, S.; Massoubre, C.; et al. Improving decision-making and cognitive impulse control in bulimia nervosa by rTMS: An ancillary randomized controlled study. *Int. J. Eat. Disord.* **2018**, *51*, 1103–1106. [CrossRef] [PubMed]
44. Dalton, B.; Bartholdy, S.; Campbell, I.C.; Schmidt, U. Neurostimulation in Clinical and Sub-clinical Eating Disorders: A Systematic Update of the Literature. *Curr. Neuropharmacol.* **2018**, *16*, 1174–1192. [CrossRef] [PubMed]
45. Uher, R.; Yoganathan, D.; Mogg, A.; Eranti, S.V.; Treasure, J.; Campbell, I.C.; McLoughlin, D.M.; Schmidt, U. Effect of left prefrontal repetitive transcranial magnetic stimulation on food craving. *Biol. Psychiatry* **2005**, *58*, 840–842. [CrossRef]
46. Maranhao, M.F.; Estella, N.M.; Cury, M.E.; Amigo, V.L.; Picasso, C.M.; Berberian, A.; Campbell, I.; Schmidt, U.; Claudino, A.M. The effects of repetitive transcranial magnetic stimulation in obese females with binge eating disorder: A protocol for a double-blinded, randomized, sham-controlled trial. *BMC Psychiatry* **2015**, *15*, 194. [CrossRef]
47. Titova, O.E.; Hjorth, O.C.; Schioth, H.B.; Brooks, S.J. Anorexia nervosa is linked to reduced brain structure in reward and somatosensory regions: A meta-analysis of VBM studies. *BMC Psychiatry* **2013**, *13*, 110. [CrossRef]
48. Kaye, W.H.; Wierenga, C.E.; Bischoff-Grethe, A.; Berner, L.A.; Ely, A.V.; Bailer, U.F.; Paulus, M.P.; Fudge, J.L. Neural Insensitivity to the Effects of Hunger in Women Remitted From Anorexia Nervosa. *Am. J. Psychiatry* **2020**. [CrossRef]
49. Steward, T.; Menchon, J.M.; Jimenez-Murcia, S.; Soriano-Mas, C.; Fernandez-Aranda, F. Neural Network Alterations Across Eating Disorders: A Narrative Review of fMRI Studies. *Curr. Neuropharmacol.* **2018**, *16*, 1150–1163. [CrossRef]
50. Cha, J.; Ide, J.S.; Bowman, F.D.; Simpson, H.B.; Posner, J.; Steinglass, J.E. Abnormal reward circuitry in anorexia nervosa: A longitudinal, multimodal MRI study. *Hum. Brain Mapp.* **2016**, *37*, 3835–3846. [CrossRef]
51. Ruffini, C.; Locatelli, M.; Lucca, A.; Benedetti, F.; Insacco, C.; Smeraldi, E. Augmentation effect of repetitive transcranial magnetic stimulation over the orbitofrontal cortex in drug-resistant obsessive-compulsive disorder patients: A controlled investigation. *Prim. Care Companion J. Clin. Psychiatry* **2009**, *11*, 226–230. [CrossRef]
52. Rose, J.E.; McClernon, F.J.; Froeliger, B.; Behm, F.M.; Preud'homme, X.; Krystal, A.D. Repetitive transcranial magnetic stimulation of the superior frontal gyrus modulates craving for cigarettes. *Biol. Psychiatry* **2011**, *70*, 794–799. [CrossRef] [PubMed]
53. Hanlon, C.A.; Dowdle, L.T.; Austelle, C.W.; DeVries, W.; Mithoefer, O.; Badran, B.W.; George, M.S. What goes up, can come down: Novel brain stimulation paradigms may attenuate craving and craving-related neural circuitry in substance dependent individuals. *Brain Res.* **2015**, *1628*, 199–209. [CrossRef] [PubMed]
54. Hecht, D. Transcranial direct current stimulation in the treatment of anorexia. *Med. Hypotheses* **2010**, *74*, 1044–1047. [CrossRef]
55. Khedr, E.M.; Elfetoh, N.A.; Ali, A.M.; Noamany, M. Anodal transcranial direct current stimulation over the dorsolateral prefrontal cortex improves anorexia nervosa: A pilot study. *Restor. Neurol. Neurosci.* **2014**, *32*, 789–797. [CrossRef] [PubMed]
56. Strumila, R.; Thiebaut, S.; Jaussent, I.; Seneque, M.; Attal, J.; Courtet, P.; Guillaume, S. Safety and efficacy of transcranial direct current stimulation (tDCS) in the treatment of Anorexia Nervosa. The open-label STAR study. *Brain Stimul.* **2019**, *12*, 1325–1327. [CrossRef]
57. Phillipou, A.; Kirkovski, M.; Castle, D.J.; Gurvich, C.; Abel, L.A.; Miles, S.; Rossell, S.L. High-definition transcranial direct current stimulation in anorexia nervosa: A pilot study. *Int. J. Eat. Disord.* **2019**, *52*, 1274–1280. [CrossRef]
58. Burgess, E.E.; Sylvester, M.D.; Morse, K.E.; Amthor, F.R.; Mrug, S.; Lokken, K.L.; Osborn, M.K.; Soleymani, T.; Boggiano, M.M. Effects of transcranial direct current stimulation (tDCS) on binge eating disorder. *Int. J. Eat. Disord.* **2016**, *49*, 930–936. [CrossRef]
59. Kekic, M.; McClelland, J.; Bartholdy, S.; Boysen, E.; Musiat, P.; Dalton, B.; Tiza, M.; David, A.S.; Campbell, I.C.; Schmidt, U. Single-Session Transcranial Direct Current Stimulation Temporarily Improves Symptoms, Mood, and Self-Regulatory Control in Bulimia Nervosa: A Randomised Controlled Trial. *PLoS ONE* **2017**, *12*, e0167606. [CrossRef]

60. Sreeraj, V.S.; Masali, M.; Shivakumar, V.; Bose, A.; Venkatasubramanian, G. Clinical Utility of Add-On Transcranial Direct Current Stimulation for Binge Eating Disorder with Obesity in Schizophrenia. *Indian J. Psychol. Med.* **2018**, *40*, 487–490. [CrossRef]
61. Pacilio, R.M.; Livingston, R.K.; Gordon, M.R. The Use of Electroconvulsive Therapy in Eating Disorders: A Systematic Literature Review and Case Report. *J. ECT* **2019**, *35*, 272–278. [CrossRef]
62. Shilton, T.; Enoch-Levy, A.; Giron, Y.; Yaroslavsky, A.; Amiaz, R.; Gothelf, D.; Weizman, A.; Stein, D. A retrospective case series of electroconvulsive therapy in the management of comorbid depression and anorexia nervosa. *Int. J. Eat. Disord.* **2020**, *53*, 210–218. [CrossRef] [PubMed]
63. Naguy, A.; Al-Tajali, A.; Alamiri, B. An Adolescent Case of Treatment-Refractory Anorexia Nervosa Favorably Responded to Electroconvulsive Therapy. *J. ECT* **2019**, *35*, 217–218. [CrossRef] [PubMed]
64. Duriez, P.; Ramoz, N.; Gorwood, P.; Viltart, O.; Tolle, V. A Metabolic Perspective on Reward Abnormalities in Anorexia Nervosa. *Trends Endocrinol. Metab.* **2019**, *30*, 915–928. [CrossRef] [PubMed]
65. Davis, H.K. Anorexia nervosa: Treatment with hypnosis and ECT. *Dis. Nerv. Syst.* **1961**, *22*, 627–631. [PubMed]
66. Bernstein, I.C. Anorexia Nervosa Treated Successfully with Electroshock Therapy and Subsequently Followed by Pregnancy. *Am. J. Psychiatry* **1964**, *120*, 1023–1024. [CrossRef]
67. Bernstein, I.C. Anorexia nervosa, 94-year-old woman treated with electroshock. *Minn. Med.* **1972**, *55*, 552–553.
68. Ferguson, J.M. The use of electroconvulsive therapy in patients with intractable anorexia nervosa. *Int. J. Eat. Disord.* **1993**, *13*, 195–201. [CrossRef]
69. Bek, R.; Hotujak, L. Clinical characteristics of female patients suffering from anorexia nervosa. *Soc. Psihijat.* **1996**, *24*, 159–161.
70. Hill, R.; Haslett, C.; Kumar, S. Anorexia nervosa in an elderly woman. *Aust. N. Z. J. Psychiatry* **2001**, *35*, 246–248. [CrossRef]
71. Poutanen, O.; Huuhka, K.; Perko, K. Severe anorexia nervosa, co-occurring major depressive disorder and electroconvulsive therapy as maintenance treatment: A case report. *Cases J.* **2009**, *2*, 9362. [CrossRef]
72. Andrews, J.T.; Seide, M.; Guarda, A.S.; Redgrave, G.W.; Coffey, D.B. Electroconvulsive therapy in an adolescent with severe major depression and anorexia nervosa. *J. Child. Adolesc. Psychopharmacol.* **2014**, *24*, 94–98. [CrossRef] [PubMed]
73. Andersen, L.; LaRosa, C.; Gih, D.E. Reexamining the Role of Electroconvulsive Therapy in Anorexia Nervosa in Adolescents. *J. ECT* **2017**, *33*, 294–296. [CrossRef] [PubMed]
74. Saglam, T.; Aksoy Poyraz, C.; Poyraz, B.C.; Tosun, M. Successful use of electroconvulsive therapy in a patient with anorexia nervosa and severe acute-onset obsessive-compulsive disorder. *Int. J. Eat. Disord.* **2018**, *51*, 1026–1028. [CrossRef] [PubMed]
75. Duriez, P.; Maatoug, R.; Verbe, J. Failure of Electroconvulsive Therapy to Improve Anorexia Nervosa in the Absence of Other Psychiatric Comorbidities: A Case Report. *J. ECT* **2020**. [CrossRef] [PubMed]
76. Rapinesi, C.; Del Casale, A.; Serata, D.; Caccia, F.; Di Pietro, S.; Scatena, P.; Carbonetti, P.; Fensore, C.; Angeletti, G.; Tatarelli, R.; et al. Electroconvulsive therapy in a man with comorbid severe obesity, binge eating disorder, and bipolar disorder. *J. ECT* **2013**, *29*, 142–144. [CrossRef] [PubMed]
77. Jaite, C.; Hoffmann, F.; Glaeske, G.; Bachmann, C.J. Prevalence, comorbidities and outpatient treatment of anorexia and bulimia nervosa in German children and adolescents. *Eat. Weight Disord.* **2013**, *18*, 157–165. [CrossRef]
78. Val-Laillet, D.; Aarts, E.; Weber, B.; Ferrari, M.; Quaresima, V.; Stoeckel, L.E.; Alonso-Alonso, M.; Audette, M.; Malbert, C.H.; Stice, E. Neuroimaging and neuromodulation approaches to study eating behavior and prevent and treat eating disorders and obesity. *Neuroimage Clin.* **2015**, *8*, 1–31. [CrossRef]
79. McClelland, J.; Bozhilova, N.; Campbell, I.; Schmidt, U. A systematic review of the effects of neuromodulation on eating and body weight: Evidence from human and animal studies. *Eur. Eat. Disord. Rev.* **2013**, *21*, 436–455. [CrossRef]
80. Badran, B.W.; Dowdle, L.T.; Mithoefer, O.J.; LaBate, N.T.; Coatsworth, J.; Brown, J.C.; DeVries, W.H.; Austelle, C.W.; McTeague, L.M.; George, M.S. Neurophysiologic effects of transcutaneous auricular vagus nerve stimulation (taVNS) via electrical stimulation of the tragus: A concurrent taVNS/fMRI study and review. *Brain Stimul.* **2018**, *11*, 492–500. [CrossRef]

81. Dietrich, S.; Smith, J.; Scherzinger, C.; Hofmann-Preiss, K.; Freitag, T.; Eisenkolb, A.; Ringler, R. A novel transcutaneous vagus nerve stimulation leads to brainstem and cerebral activations measured by functional MRI. *Biomed. Tech.* **2008**, *53*, 104–111. [CrossRef]
82. Yakunina, N.; Kim, S.S.; Nam, E.C. Optimization of Transcutaneous Vagus Nerve Stimulation Using Functional MRI. *Neuromodulation* **2017**, *20*, 290–300. [CrossRef] [PubMed]
83. Villani, V.; Tsakiris, M.; Azevedo, R.T. Transcutaneous vagus nerve stimulation improves interoceptive accuracy. *Neuropsychologia* **2019**, *134*, 107201. [CrossRef] [PubMed]
84. Kaye, W.H.; Wagner, A.; Fudge, J.L.; Paulus, M. Neurocircuity of eating disorders. *Curr. Top. Behav. Neurosci.* **2011**, *6*, 37–57. [CrossRef] [PubMed]
85. Khalsa, S.S.; Adolphs, R.; Cameron, O.G.; Critchley, H.D.; Davenport, P.W.; Feinstein, J.S.; Feusner, J.D.; Garfinkel, S.N.; Lane, R.D.; Mehling, W.E.; et al. Interoception and Mental Health: A Roadmap. *Biol Psychiatry Cogn. Neurosci. Neuroimaging* **2018**, *3*, 501–513. [CrossRef] [PubMed]
86. Berner, L.A.; Simmons, A.N.; Wierenga, C.E.; Bischoff-Grethe, A.; Paulus, M.P.; Bailer, U.F.; Kaye, W.H. Altered anticipation and processing of aversive interoceptive experience among women remitted from bulimia nervosa. *Neuropsychopharmacology* **2019**, *44*, 1265–1273. [CrossRef]
87. Sobstyl, M.; Stapinska-Syniec, A.; Sokol-Szawlowska, M.; Kupryjaniuk, A. Deep brain stimulation for the treatment of severe intractable anorexia nervosa. *Br. J. Neurosurg.* **2019**, *33*, 601–607. [CrossRef] [PubMed]
88. Israel, M.; Steiger, H.; Kolivakis, T.; McGregor, L.; Sadikot, A.F. Deep brain stimulation in the subgenual cingulate cortex for an intractable eating disorder. *Biol. Psychiatry* **2010**, *67*, e53–e54. [CrossRef]
89. Barbier, J.; Gabriels, L.; van Laere, K.; Nuttin, B. Successful anterior capsulotomy in comorbid anorexia nervosa and obsessive-compulsive disorder: Case report. *Neurosurgery* **2011**, *69*, E745–E751, discussion E751. [CrossRef]
90. McLaughlin, N.C.; Didie, E.R.; Machado, A.G.; Haber, S.N.; Eskandar, E.N.; Greenberg, B.D. Improvements in anorexia symptoms after deep brain stimulation for intractable obsessive-compulsive disorder. *Biol. Psychiatry* **2013**, *73*, e29–e31. [CrossRef]
91. Blomstedt, P.; Naesstrom, M.; Bodlund, O. Deep brain stimulation in the bed nucleus of the stria terminalis and medial forebrain bundle in a patient with major depressive disorder and anorexia nervosa. *Clin. Case Rep.* **2017**, *5*, 679–684. [CrossRef]
92. Park, R.J.; Singh, I.; Pike, A.C.; Tan, J.O. Deep Brain Stimulation in Anorexia Nervosa: Hope for the Hopeless or Exploitation of the Vulnerable? The Oxford Neuroethics Gold Standard Framework. *Front. Psychiatry* **2017**, *8*, 44. [CrossRef] [PubMed]
93. Lipsman, N.; Lam, E.; Volpini, M.; Sutandar, K.; Twose, R.; Giacobbe, P.; Sodums, D.J.; Smith, G.S.; Woodside, D.B.; Lozano, A.M. Deep brain stimulation of the subcallosal cingulate for treatment-refractory anorexia nervosa: 1 year follow-up of an open-label trial. *Lancet Psychiatry* **2017**, *4*, 285–294. [CrossRef]
94. Wu, H.; Van Dyck-Lippens, P.J.; Santegoeds, R.; van Kuyck, K.; Gabriels, L.; Lin, G.; Pan, G.; Li, Y.; Li, D.; Zhan, S.; et al. Deep-brain stimulation for anorexia nervosa. *World Neurosurg.* **2013**, *80*, S29.e1–S29.e10. [CrossRef] [PubMed]
95. Wang, J.; Chang, C.; Geng, N.; Wang, X.; Gao, G. Treatment of intractable anorexia nervosa with inactivation of the nucleus accumbens using stereotactic surgery. *Stereotact. Funct. Neurosurg.* **2013**, *91*, 364–372. [CrossRef]
96. Lipsman, N.; Woodside, D.B.; Giacobbe, P.; Lozano, A.M. Neurosurgical treatment of anorexia nervosa: Review of the literature from leucotomy to deep brain stimulation. *Eur. Eat. Disord. Rev.* **2013**, *21*, 428–435. [CrossRef]
97. Zhang, H.W.; Li, D.Y.; Zhao, J.; Guan, Y.H.; Sun, B.M.; Zuo, C.T. Metabolic imaging of deep brain stimulation in anorexia nervosa: A 18F-FDG PET/CT study. *Clin. Nucl. Med.* **2013**, *38*, 943–948. [CrossRef]
98. Liu, W.; Zhan, S.; Li, D.; Lin, Z.; Zhang, C.; Wang, T.; Pan, S.; Zhang, J.; Cao, C.; Jin, H.; et al. Deep brain stimulation of the nucleus accumbens for treatment-refractory anorexia nervosa: A long-term follow-up study. *Brain Stimul.* **2020**, *13*, 643–649. [CrossRef]
99. Sun, B.; Liu, W. Stereotactic surgery for eating disorders. *Surg. Neurol. Int.* **2013**, *4*, S164–S169. [CrossRef]
100. Hayes, D.J.; Lipsman, N.; Chen, D.Q.; Woodside, D.B.; Davis, K.D.; Lozano, A.M.; Hodaie, M. Subcallosal Cingulate Connectivity in Anorexia Nervosa Patients Differs From Healthy Controls: A Multi-tensor Tractography Study. *Brain Stimul.* **2015**, *8*, 758–768. [CrossRef]

101. Manuelli, M.; Franzini, A.; Galentino, R.; Bidone, R.; Dell'Osso, B.; Porta, M.; Servello, D.; Cena, H. Changes in eating behavior after deep brain stimulation for anorexia nervosa. A case study. *Eat. Weight Disord.* **2019**. [CrossRef]
102. Villalba Martinez, G.; Justicia, A.; Salgado, P.; Gines, J.M.; Guardiola, R.; Cedron, C.; Polo, M.; Delgado-Martinez, I.; Medrano, S.; Manero, R.M.; et al. A Randomized Trial of Deep Brain Stimulation to the Subcallosal Cingulate and Nucleus Accumbens in Patients with Treatment-Refractory, Chronic, and Severe Anorexia Nervosa: Initial Results at 6 Months of Follow Up. *J. Clin. Med.* **2020**, *9*, 1946. [CrossRef] [PubMed]
103. Whiting, D.M.; Tomycz, N.D.; Bailes, J.; de Jonge, L.; Lecoultre, V.; Wilent, B.; Alcindor, D.; Prostko, E.R.; Cheng, B.C.; Angle, C.; et al. Lateral hypothalamic area deep brain stimulation for refractory obesity: A pilot study with preliminary data on safety, body weight, and energy metabolism. *J. Neurosurg.* **2013**, *119*, 56–63. [CrossRef] [PubMed]
104. Tronnier, V.M.; Rasche, D.; Thorns, V.; Alvarez-Fischer, D.; Munte, T.F.; Zurowski, B. Massive weight loss following deep brain stimulation of the nucleus accumbens in a depressed woman. *Neurocase* **2018**, *24*, 49–53. [CrossRef] [PubMed]
105. Formolo, D.A.; Gaspar, J.M.; Melo, H.M.; Eichwald, T.; Zepeda, R.J.; Latini, A.; Okun, M.S.; Walz, R. Deep Brain Stimulation for Obesity: A Review and Future Directions. *Front. Neurosci.* **2019**, *13*, 323. [CrossRef] [PubMed]
106. Mayberg, H.S.; Liotti, M.; Brannan, S.K.; McGinnis, S.; Mahurin, R.K.; Jerabek, P.A.; Silva, J.A.; Tekell, J.L.; Martin, C.C.; Lancaster, J.L.; et al. Reciprocal limbic-cortical function and negative mood: Converging PET findings in depression and normal sadness. *Am. J. Psychiatry* **1999**, *156*, 675–682. [CrossRef]
107. Lipsman, N.; Woodside, D.B.; Lozano, A.M. Neurocircuitry of limbic dysfunction in anorexia nervosa. *Cortex* **2015**, *62*, 109–118. [CrossRef]
108. Lebow, M.A.; Chen, A. Overshadowed by the amygdala: The bed nucleus of the stria terminalis emerges as key to psychiatric disorders. *Mol. Psychiatry* **2016**, *21*, 450–463. [CrossRef]
109. Coenen, V.A.; Panksepp, J.; Hurwitz, T.A.; Urbach, H.; Madler, B. Human medial forebrain bundle (MFB) and anterior thalamic radiation (ATR): Imaging of two major subcortical pathways and the dynamic balance of opposite affects in understanding depression. *J. Neuropsychiatry Clin. Neurosci.* **2012**, *24*, 223–236. [CrossRef]
110. van der Plasse, G.; Schrama, R.; van Seters, S.P.; Vanderschuren, L.J.; Westenberg, H.G. Deep brain stimulation reveals a dissociation of consummatory and motivated behaviour in the medial and lateral nucleus accumbens shell of the rat. *PLoS ONE* **2012**, *7*, e33455. [CrossRef]
111. Guercio, L.A.; Schmidt, H.D.; Pierce, R.C. Deep brain stimulation of the nucleus accumbens shell attenuates cue-induced reinstatement of both cocaine and sucrose seeking in rats. *Behav. Brain Res.* **2015**, *281*, 125–130. [CrossRef]
112. Steding, J.; Boehm, I.; King, J.A.; Geisler, D.; Ritschel, F.; Seidel, M.; Doose, A.; Jaite, C.; Roessner, V.; Smolka, M.N.; et al. Goal-directed vs. habitual instrumental behavior during reward processing in anorexia nervosa: An fMRI study. *Sci. Rep.* **2019**, *9*, 13529. [CrossRef] [PubMed]
113. Foldi, C.J.; Milton, L.K.; Oldfield, B.J. The Role of Mesolimbic Reward Neurocircuitry in Prevention and Rescue of the Activity-Based Anorexia (ABA) Phenotype in Rats. *Neuropsychopharmacology* **2017**, *42*, 2292–2300. [CrossRef]
114. Joshi, S.H.; Espinoza, R.T.; Pirnia, T.; Shi, J.; Wang, Y.; Ayers, B.; Leaver, A.; Woods, R.P.; Narr, K.L. Structural Plasticity of the Hippocampus and Amygdala Induced by Electroconvulsive Therapy in Major Depression. *Biol. Psychiatry* **2016**, *79*, 282–292. [CrossRef] [PubMed]
115. Zangen, A.; Roth, Y.; Voller, B.; Hallett, M. Transcranial magnetic stimulation of deep brain regions: Evidence for efficacy of the H-coil. *Clin. Neurophysiol.* **2005**, *116*, 775–779. [CrossRef] [PubMed]
116. Gearhardt, A.N.; White, M.A.; Potenza, M.N. Binge eating disorder and food addiction. *Curr. Drug Abuse Rev.* **2011**, *4*, 201–207. [CrossRef] [PubMed]
117. Volkow, N.D.; Wang, G.J.; Fowler, J.S.; Tomasi, D.; Baler, R. Food and drug reward: Overlapping circuits in human obesity and addiction. *Curr. Top. Behav. Neurosci.* **2012**, *11*, 1–24. [CrossRef] [PubMed]
118. Bayes, A.J.; Parker, G.B. Comparison of guidelines for the treatment of unipolar depression: A focus on pharmacotherapy and neurostimulation. *Acta Psychiatr. Scand.* **2018**, *137*, 459–471. [CrossRef]
119. Pan, L.A.; Martin, P.; Zimmer, T.; Segreti, A.M.; Kassiff, S.; McKain, B.W.; Baca, C.A.; Rengasamy, M.; Hyland, K.; Walano, N.; et al. Neurometabolic Disorders: Potentially Treatable Abnormalities in Patients With Treatment-Refractory Depression and Suicidal Behavior. *Am. J. Psychiatry* **2017**, *174*, 42–50. [CrossRef]

120. Schwieler, L.; Samuelsson, M.; Frye, M.A.; Bhat, M.; Schuppe-Koistinen, I.; Jungholm, O.; Johansson, A.G.; Landen, M.; Sellgren, C.M.; Erhardt, S. Electroconvulsive therapy suppresses the neurotoxic branch of the kynurenine pathway in treatment-resistant depressed patients. *J. Neuroinflamm.* **2016**, *13*, 51. [CrossRef]
121. Romano, S.J.; Halmi, K.A.; Sarkar, N.P.; Koke, S.C.; Lee, J.S. A placebo-controlled study of fluoxetine in continued treatment of bulimia nervosa after successful acute fluoxetine treatment. *Am. J. Psychiatry* **2002**, *159*, 96–102. [CrossRef]
122. Roberts, M.E.; Tchanturia, K.; Stahl, D.; Southgate, L.; Treasure, J. A systematic review and meta-analysis of set-shifting ability in eating disorders. *Psychol. Med.* **2007**, *37*, 1075–1084. [CrossRef] [PubMed]
123. Lang, K.; Lopez, C.; Stahl, D.; Tchanturia, K.; Treasure, J. Central coherence in eating disorders: An updated systematic review and meta-analysis. *World J. Biol. Psychiatry* **2014**, *15*, 586–598. [CrossRef] [PubMed]
124. Guillaume, S.; Gorwood, P.; Jollant, F.; Van den Eynde, F.; Courtet, P.; Richard-Devantoy, S. Impaired decision-making in symptomatic anorexia and bulimia nervosa patients: A meta-analysis. *Psychol. Med.* **2015**, *45*, 3377–3391. [CrossRef] [PubMed]
125. Leppanen, J.; Adamson, J.; Tchanturia, K. Impact of Cognitive Remediation Therapy on Neurocognitive Processing in Anorexia Nervosa. *Front. Psychiatry* **2018**, *9*, 96. [CrossRef] [PubMed]
126. Brevet-Aeby, C.; Brunelin, J.; Iceta, S.; Padovan, C.; Poulet, E. Prefrontal cortex and impulsivity: Interest of noninvasive brain stimulation. *Neurosci. Biobehav. Rev.* **2016**, *71*, 112–134. [CrossRef]
127. Gordon, G.; Brockmeyer, T.; Schmidt, U.; Campbell, I.C. Combining cognitive bias modification training (CBM) and transcranial direct current stimulation (tDCS) to treat binge eating disorder: Study protocol of a randomised controlled feasibility trial. *BMJ Open* **2019**, *9*, e030023. [CrossRef]
128. Dinur-Klein, L.; Dannon, P.; Hadar, A.; Rosenberg, O.; Roth, Y.; Kotler, M.; Zangen, A. Smoking cessation induced by deep repetitive transcranial magnetic stimulation of the prefrontal and insular cortices: A prospective, randomized controlled trial. *Biol. Psychiatry* **2014**, *76*, 742–749. [CrossRef]
129. Karas, P.J.; Lee, S.; Jimenez-Shahed, J.; Goodman, W.K.; Viswanathan, A.; Sheth, S.A. Deep Brain Stimulation for Obsessive Compulsive Disorder: Evolution of Surgical Stimulation Target Parallels Changing Model of Dysfunctional Brain Circuits. *Front. Neurosci.* **2018**, *12*, 998. [CrossRef]
130. Grossman, N.; Bono, D.; Dedic, N.; Kodandaramaiah, S.B.; Rudenko, A.; Suk, H.J.; Cassara, A.M.; Neufeld, E.; Kuster, N.; Tsai, L.H.; et al. Noninvasive Deep Brain Stimulation via Temporally Interfering Electric Fields. *Cell* **2017**, *169*, 1029–1041. [CrossRef]
131. Lozano, A.M. Waving Hello to Noninvasive Deep-Brain Stimulation. *N. Engl. J. Med.* **2017**, *377*, 1096–1098. [CrossRef]
132. Delbeke, J.; Hoffman, L.; Mols, K.; Braeken, D.; Prodanov, D. And Then There Was Light: Perspectives of Optogenetics for Deep Brain Stimulation and Neuromodulation. *Front. Neurosci.* **2017**, *11*, 663. [CrossRef]
133. Gradinaru, V.; Mogri, M.; Thompson, K.R.; Henderson, J.M.; Deisseroth, K. Optical deconstruction of parkinsonian neural circuitry. *Science* **2009**, *324*, 354–359. [CrossRef] [PubMed]
134. Treasure, J.; Stein, D.; Maguire, S. Has the time come for a staging model to map the course of eating disorders from high risk to severe enduring illness? An examination of the evidence. *Early Interv. Psychiatry* **2015**, *9*, 173–184. [CrossRef] [PubMed]
135. Dunlop, K.A.; Woodside, B.; Downar, J. Targeting Neural Endophenotypes of Eating Disorders with Non-invasive Brain Stimulation. *Front. Neurosci.* **2016**, *10*, 30. [CrossRef] [PubMed]
136. Wildes, J.E.; Marcus, M.D. Application of the Research Domain Criteria (RDoC) framework to eating disorders: Emerging concepts and research. *Curr. Psychiatry Rep.* **2015**, *17*, 30. [CrossRef] [PubMed]
137. Kearney-Ramos, T.E.; Dowdle, L.T.; Mithoefer, O.J.; Devries, W.; George, M.S.; Hanlon, C.A. State-Dependent Effects of Ventromedial Prefrontal Cortex Continuous Thetaburst Stimulation on Cocaine Cue Reactivity in Chronic Cocaine Users. *Front. Psychiatry* **2019**, *10*, 317. [CrossRef]
138. Wonderlich, S.A.; Bulik, C.M.; Schmidt, U.; Steiger, H.; Hoek, H.W. Severe and enduring anorexia nervosa: Update and observations about the current clinical reality. *Int. J. Eat. Disord.* **2020**. [CrossRef]

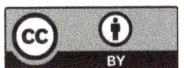

© 2020 by the authors. Licensee MDPI, Basel, Switzerland. This article is an open access article distributed under the terms and conditions of the Creative Commons Attribution (CC BY) license (http://creativecommons.org/licenses/by/4.0/).

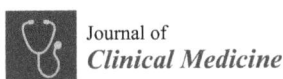

Article

Clinical and Neurophysiological Correlates of Emotion and Food Craving Regulation in Patients with Anorexia Nervosa

Nuria Mallorquí-Bagué [1,2,3,*,†], María Lozano-Madrid [1,2,†], Giulia Testa [1,2], Cristina Vintró-Alcaraz [1,2], Isabel Sánchez [1], Nadine Riesco [1], José César Perales [4], Juan Francisco Navas [5,6], Ignacio Martínez-Zalacaín [1,7], Alberto Megías [4], Roser Granero [2,8], Misericordia Veciana De Las Heras [9], Rayane Chami [10], Susana Jiménez-Murcia [1,2,7], José Antonio Fernández-Formoso [2], Janet Treasure [10] and Fernando Fernández-Aranda [1,2,7,*]

1. Department of Psychiatry, University Hospital of Bellvitge-IDIBELL, 08907 Barcelona, Spain; maria.lozano@bellvitgehospital.cat (M.L.-M.); gtesta@idibell.cat (G.T.); cvintro@bellvitgehospital.cat (C.V.-A.); isasanchez@bellvitgehospital.cat (I.S.); nriesco@bellvitgehospital.cat (N.R.); imartinezz@outlook.es (I.M.-Z.); sjimenez@bellvitgehospital.cat (S.J.-M.)
2. CIBER Fisiopatologia Obesidad y Nutrición (CIBERobn), Instituto de Salud Carlos III, 28029 Madrid, Spain; Roser.Granero@uab.cat (R.G.); tono.fernandez@ciberisciii.es (J.A.F.-F.)
3. Addictive Behavior Unit, Department of Psychiatry, Hospital de la Santa Creu i Sant Pau, 08001 Barcelona, Spain
4. Department of Experimental Psychology, Mind, Brain, and Behavior Research Centre, University of Granada, 18071 Granada, Spain; jcesar@ugr.es (J.C.P.); megiasrobles@gmail.com (A.M.)
5. Department of Basic Psychology, Autonomous University of Madrid, 28049 Madrid, Spain; juan.fco.navas@gmail.com
6. Universitat Oberta de Catalunya, 08018 Barcelona, Spain
7. Clinical Sciences Department, School of Medicine, University of Barcelona, 08907 Barcelona, Spain
8. Department of Psychobiology and Methodology, Autonomous University of Barcelona, 08035 Barcelona, Spain
9. Neurophysiology Unit, Neurology Department, Hospital Universitari de Bellvitge, 08907 Barcelona, Spain; mveciana@bellvitgehospital.cat
10. Section of Eating Disorders, Institute of Psychiatry, Psychology & Neuroscience (IoPPN), King's College London, London SE5 8AF, UK; rayane.chami@kcl.ac.uk (R.C.); janet.treasure@kcl.ac.uk (J.T.)
* Correspondence: nmallorqui@santpau.cat (N.M.-B.); ffernandez@bellvitgehospital.cat (F.F.-A.)
† Shared First authorship: Nuria Mallorquí-Bagué and María Lozano-Madrid.

Received: 6 February 2020; Accepted: 27 March 2020; Published: 31 March 2020

Abstract: Background: Difficulties in emotion regulation and craving regulation have been linked to eating symptomatology in patients with anorexia nervosa (AN), contributing to the maintenance of their eating disorder. Methods: To investigate clinical and electrophysiological correlates of these processes, 20 patients with AN and 20 healthy controls (HC) completed a computerized task during EEG recording, where they were instructed to down-regulate negative emotions or food craving. Participants also completed self-report measures of emotional regulation and food addiction. The P300 and Late Positive Potential (LPP) ERPs were analysed. Results: LPP amplitudes were significantly smaller during down-regulation of food craving among both groups. Independent of task condition, individuals with AN showed smaller P300 amplitudes compared to HC. Among HC, the self-reported use of re-appraisal strategies positively correlated with LPP amplitudes during emotional regulation task, while suppressive strategies negatively correlated with LPP amplitudes. The AN group, in comparison to the HC group, exhibited greater food addiction, greater use of maladaptive strategies, and emotional dysregulation. Conclusions: Despite the enhanced self-reported psychopathology among AN, both groups indicated neurophysiological evidence of food craving regulation as evidenced by blunted LPP amplitudes in the relevant task condition. Further research is required to delineate the mechanisms associated with reduced overall P300 amplitudes among individuals with AN.

Keywords: food craving; food addiction; emotion regulation; eating disorders; anorexia nervosa; event related potentials; EEG; neurophysiology; psychopathology

1. Introduction

Anorexia nervosa (AN) is recognized as a severe mental disorder characterized by restrained eating, dysfunctional thoughts, preoccupation concerning food and body image disturbance [1,2]. In addition to maladaptive cognitions and behaviours, difficulties in emotion regulation and food craving regulation have been linked to disordered eating symptomatology (i.e., binging, purging, or restriction), which are considered to be contributing factors to the maintenance of eating disorders [3–5].

Emotion regulation is understood as the process by which individuals are able to modulate the way they experience and express their emotions [6]. Two strategies have been of special interest when studying emotion regulation: suppression and reappraisal. Suppression consists of inhibiting the behavioural expression of an emotional response to a stressor, while reappraisal implicates reinterpreting the meaning of an emotional event [7]. Although the former is considered to be a maladaptive response, the latter is considered to be an adaptive strategy used to reduce the impact of negative emotional states evoked during stressful situations. In this sense, reappraisal appears to be particularly effective because it implies less physiological and cognitive costs, as well as less negative impact on memory compared to suppression [8].

It is hardly surprising that dysfunctional emotion regulation is considered to be a key mechanism underpinning numerous psychopathologies [9–12], among which we can find the whole spectrum of eating disorders [13–15]. Several studies suggest that, due to emotion regulation being adopted as a means of regulating negative emotions, difficulties in this area could be involved in the development and maintenance of problematic eating disorder-related behaviours [16,17]. Accordingly, emotion dysregulation has been exhibited as a trait among patients with AN, and also as a key element of their therapy [18,19].

Interestingly, food craving (i.e., intense desire for specific food), which is considered a hallmark of food addiction, has been recently proposed as an affective state involving behavioural and physiological changes [20]. Food craving is not necessary followed by increasing eating [21] and can be regulated like other affective states as suggested in recent studies in the non-clinical population [22–24]. In the eating disorder population, food craving and the related food addiction have been frequently reported [25], with a few studies suggesting the presence of these features even in patients with AN, especially those with binging/purging symptoms [26,27]. However, to our best knowledge, there is a lack of studies investigating food craving regulation in eating disorders, including AN.

Event-related potentials (ERPs) are electrical changes in electroencephalographic (EEG) recordings that are time-locked to sensory or cognitive events. Given the excellent time resolution, the event-related potential (ERP) technique has been adopted to investigate the time course of emotion regulation and craving regulation [28]. During late processing, the P300 component has been relevant to attention research as it increases with stimulus salience. Following it, the late positive potential (LPP) is thought to reflect motivated attention [7,29].

Previous ERP studies in the non-clinical population showed that the amplitude of the P300 and LPP components can be modulated by different emotion regulation strategies [30–38]. Due to the clinical relevance of emotions in daily life, numerous EEG studies have focused on down-regulation of P300 and LPP amplitudes in response to negative and positive emotions [30–38]. Although most studies point to a reduction of LPP amplitudes when participants try to down-regulate their negative emotions [30–33,39,40], other research studies have found no significant modulation of this component [35,38], or even a modulation in the opposite direction [41]. Focusing on the eating disorders field, several ERP studies have shown emotion regulation difficulties among individuals with comorbidities, such as anxiety disorders and alexithymia [42,43]. Nevertheless, no studies to date have examined ERP modulations by emotion regulation in specific eating disorder populations such as AN.

On the other hand, several ERP studies have strived to demonstrate the efficacy of different emotion regulation techniques in modulating food craving in healthy individuals. For instance, using reappraisal in order to change the emotional meaning of food increased LPP amplitude when participants tried to focus on the long-term consequences of eating high-caloric food [44]. Reappraisal was also employed in another study in which participants were instructed to increase or decrease the appetitive value of food. Results showed that P300 and LPP amplitudes to food cues were larger when participants tried to increase the appetitive value of food in comparison to the condition of decreasing or just watching the images [45]. Moreover, research instructing restrained eaters to either reappraise cravings, suppress cravings, or watch food during a food task found that engaging in cognitive reappraisal or suppression significantly reduced ERP amplitudes compared to the food watch condition [46]. Although research has demonstrated the efficacy of emotion regulation techniques in normal-weight healthy individuals, up to date there is a lack of ERP research assessing regulation of food craving in AN patients [47]. Elucidating neurophysiological mechanisms of food craving regulation could pave the way for new treatment approaches for anorexia nervosa, in which emotion regulation techniques might be employed to alter the motivational value of certain foods.

The primary aims of the study were to explore clinical and electrophysiological features of emotion regulation and food craving regulation among patients with AN. As for the clinical profile, we hypothesized that individuals with AN would present higher self-reported emotion dysregulation and food addiction compared to a group of healthy control (HC). Regarding electrophysiological data, we hypothesize that there will be a significant reduction in LPP amplitudes during conditions requiring participants to down-regulate negative emotions or food craving, as opposed to neutral conditions. Based on previous clinical research reporting emotion and food craving regulation difficulties in AN, we also aim to explore between-group differences in ERP during down-regulation of emotion or food craving. Finally, we explored to which extent self-reported emotion regulation strategies (adaptive or maladaptive) correlates with ERP (i.e., P300, LPP) during down-regulation of food craving or negative emotions. Maladaptive strategies are expected to be predominant in AN and possibly correlate with brain response during down-regulation of emotions/food craving.

2. Materials and Methods

2.1. Participants

The present study involved two different groups: a clinical group of patients with anorexia nervosa (AN) and a healthy control group (HC). The AN clinical group was comprised of 20 female treatment-seeking patients diagnosed with AN (60% AN restrictive subtype, 40% AN binge/purging subtype) according to DSM-5 criteria (Body Mass Index (BMI) < 18.5) [48]. Recruitment was conducted at the Eating Disorders Unit within the Department of Psychiatry at Bellvitge University Hospital, a public health hospital certified as a tertiary care centre with a highly specialised unit for the treatment of eating disorders in Barcelona (Spain). The HC group consisted of 21 female participants who had no history of an eating disorder. Participant groups were matched by age and education level. All participants were recruited between June 2016 and July 2018.

Data from one healthy control participant had to be excluded due to poor EEG data quality. The final sample size consisted of 40 participants, of whom 20 were patients with AN (mean age = 22.7 years, SD = 6.51, age range 18 to 43, mean BMI = 16.6 kg/m^2, SD = 1.1), and 20 were HC (mean age = 21.0 years, SD = 5.12, age range 18 to 39; mean BMI = 20.7 kg/m^2, SD = 1.78). Among AN group, 9 patients (45%) reported psychotropic treatment (antidepressants: n = 4, 20%; anxiolytics: n = 1 5%; both: n =

4, 20%). Exclusion criterion for all participants were: (a) being male, (b) younger than 18 years, (c) current or life-time history of chronic illness or neurological condition (abnormal EEG activity), which could influence electrophysiology and/or the neuropsychological assessment, (c) lifetime diagnosis of a severe mental health condition (bipolar disorder, lifetime diagnosis of psychotic disorder), (d) current substance dependence or any other mental disorder that could interfere cortical activity or the assessment. Additionally, in the HC group, an exclusion criteria was a lifetime diagnosis of any eating disorder, assessed by means of the Mini International Neuropsychiatric Interview (MINI) [49], being overweight/obese (Body Mass Index (BMI) $\geq$ 25), or underweight (BMI < 18.5).

Written informed consent was obtained before participation in the study, which was approved by the Ethics Committee of University Hospital of Bellvitge in accordance with the Helsinki Declaration of 1975 as revised in 1983. Participants received no compensation for taking part in the study.

2.2. Procedure

Patients who sought treatment for AN as their primary health concern were assessed by an experienced clinical psychologist as part of the Eating Disorders Unit protocol, which is based on DSM-5 criteria and includes height and weight measurements. All patients consecutively diagnosed with AN were screened for the inclusion criteria of the study and gave informed consent for voluntarily accepting to be part of the study. HC participants were recruited within a university campus and, if they were interested in taking part in the study, an eligibility screening was conducted prior to the initial face-to-face assessment session.

The variables explored in the present study were assessed in two separate sessions of approximately 90 minutes each. Firstly, participants were evaluated with the MINI to exclude those patients with any severe psychiatric condition. Afterwards, they completed a battery of self-reported questionnaires (DERS, ERQ, SCL-90-R, YFAS-2). Next, participants performed the experimental tasks (food craving and emotion regulation) during EEG acquisition. Participants were instructed to have a 'normal' meal 90 minutes before the session and then to refrain from eating or drinking coffee. Additional information was collected on the day of the experimental session, in order to control for a set of variables (i.e., food consumed on the day of the session, menstrual cycle, and alcohol or drugs consumption in the last 24h). In a second session, participants completed a different set of experimental neurophysiological tests (data will be reported in separate manuscript).

2.3. Clinical Assessment

The *Mini-International Neuropsychiatric Interview* (MINI) [49] is a short structured diagnostic interview for the major psychiatric disorders in DSM-III-R [50], DSM-IV [51] and DSM-5 [16] and ICD-10 [52]. Validation and reliability studies have been done comparing the MINI to the Structured Clinical Interview (SCID-P) [53] based on DSM-III-R [50] and the Composite International Diagnostic Interview (CIDI) [54], which is a structured interview developed by the World Health Organization. These studies showed that the MINI has similar reliability and validity properties to both instruments. With an administration time of approximately 15 minutes, it was designed to meet the needs for a short, yet accurate, structured psychiatric interview for multicentre clinical trials and epidemiology studies and to be used as a first step in outcome tracking in non-research clinical settings. The standard MINI assesses the 17 most common disorders in mental health. The disorders were selected based on current prevalence rates of 0.5% or higher in the general population in epidemiology studies. In the interest of brevity, it uses branching tree logic.

Difficulties in Emotion Regulation Scale (DERS; Spanish validation) [15,55,56] is a 36-item self-report scale that assesses relevant difficulties in emotion regulation on six subscales: non-acceptance of emotional responses, difficulties engaging in goal directed behaviour, impulse control difficulties, lack of emotional awareness, limited access to emotion regulation strategies and lack of emotional clarity. The measure yields a total score as well as scores on the six subscales. Higher scores indicate greater problems with emotion regulation. Cronbach's α for the total score in the present study was 0.91.

Emotion Regulation Questionnaire, Spanish version (ERQ) [57] is a 10-item questionnaire to assess the respondents' tendency to implement two emotion regulation strategies: reappraisal and emotional suppression. For the present study it shows a Cronbach's α of 0.76 for the suppression scale, and 0.85 for the reappraisal scale.

Symptom Checklist-90 Revised (SCL-90; Spanish validation) [58,59] is a 90-item questionnaire which evaluates psychopathological symptoms. It also includes a global severity index (GSI), designed to measure overall psychological distress. Internal consistency for GSI scale in the present study sample was 0.98.

The Yale Food Addiction Scale Version 2.0 (YFAS-2) [25] is a 25 item self-report questionnaire to measure addictive food behaviours. It consists of seven scales which refer to the criteria for substance dependence: (1) tolerance, (2) withdrawal, (3) substance taken in larger amount/period of time than intended, (4) persistent desire/unsuccessful efforts to cut down, (5) great deal of time spent to obtain substance, (6) important activities given up to obtain substance, (7) use continued despite psychological/physical problems. The Cronbach's α value for the present study was 0.97.

2.4. Electrophysiological Assessment

Participants completed an emotion regulation task and a food craving regulation task during continuous EEG recording.

Emotion regulation task: The task stimuli consisted of 180 images, of which 120 were negative images distributed in two blocks of 60 images each and 60 were neutral images grouped in a third block. Stimuli were presented for 3000 ms, with an inter-trial interval ranging from 3500 ms to 4500 ms. Negative images and neutral images were matched on contrast, brightness, resolution and complexity. Images were taken from the International Affective Picture System (IAPS) [60] and each image was presented only once during the task. Stimulus presentation was carried out by Presentation®software (Version 16.0) [61]. Participants were seated approximately 60 cm in front of a computer screen and the images were shown serially and occupied 35.1° of visual angle horizontally and 28.1° vertically.

For negative images, participants were instructed to either view each picture and allow themselves to feel any emotional response it might elicit (from now on referred to as Observe Negative) or to view each picture and try to reduce the emotional response that it might elicit (from now on referred to as Regulate Negative). For neutral images, participants were instructed to view each picture and allow themselves to feel any emotional response it might elicit (from now on referred to as Observe Neutral) while viewing the images and feeling the elicited emotion.

Food craving regulation task: Task stimuli consisted of 180 images, of which 120 were highly palatable food images distributed in two blocks of 60 images each and 60 were neutral images (i.e., office items) grouped in a third block. Stimuli were presented for 3000 ms, with an inter-trial interval ranging from 3500 ms to 4500 ms. Food images and neutral images were matched on contrast, brightness, resolution and complexity. Images were taken from Food Pics [62] and each image was presented only once during the task. Stimulus presentation was carried out by Presentation®software (Version 16.0) [61]. Participants were seated approximately 60 cm in front of a computer screen. The images were shown serially and occupied 18.9° of visual angle horizontally and 17.1° vertically.

For food images, participants were instructed to either view each picture and allow themselves to feel any emotional response it might elicit (from now on referred to as Observe Negative) or to view each picture and try to reduce the emotional response that it might elicit (from now on referred to as Regulate Negative). For neutral images, participants were instructed to view each picture and allow themselves to feel any emotional response it might elicit (from now on referred to as Observe Neutral).

2.5. Electrophysiological Recording and Analysis

The electroencephalogram (EEG) was recorded continuously throughout the experimental task using PyCorder (BrainVision). 60 active Ag/AgCI electrodes were inserted into an EEG recording cap (EASYCAP GmbH), distributed after the 10–20 system; additional three electrodes were adopted for recording vertical and horizontal electrooculogram (EOG) and Cz was used as online reference. Impedances were kept below 20 KOhm using the SuperVisc high-viscosity electrolyte gel for active electrodes. Signals from all channels were digitized with a sampling rate of 500 Hz and 24 bit/channel resolution and online filtered between 0.1 and 100 Hz.

Offline EEG analyses were performed with Brain Vision Analyzer (Version 2.2.0) [63] consisting of the following steps: high pass filtering 0.1 Hz, low pass filtering at 30 Hz (Butterworth zero phase filter; 24 dB/octave slope) and notch filter at 50 Hz; raw data inspection for manual detection of artefact and screening for bad channels, semi-automatic eye-blink correction using independent component analysis (ICA); artefact rejection of trials with an amplitude exciding ±80 µV; and baseline correction adopting the pre-stimulus interval between −200 and 2000 ms. EEG data were segmented into 2200 ms epochs from 200 ms before to 2000 ms after stimulus onset. Data were baseline corrected against the mean voltage during the −200 pre stimulus period. Artefact free epochs were separately averaged for each subject in each experimental condition for each paradigm.

ERP analyses were based on visual inspection of the grand average waveforms and the existing literature [45,46]. ERP components were analysed in a central-parietal cluster (CP1, CP5, P3, P7, CP2, CP6, P4, P8). P300 mean amplitude (µV) was computed in the time-window between 280 and 400 ms; LPP mean amplitude (µV) was measured within two time-windows: at 500-1000 ms (LPP1) and 1000-1500 ms (LPP2) [64–66].

2.6. Statistical Analysis

Statistical analysis was carried out with Stata Statistical Software: Release 15 for Windows [67]. The variables of the study (ERQ, YFAS, DERS and SCL-90-R) were compared between groups using t-tests for quantitative measures and chi square (χ^2) tests for categorical measures. Comparisons were considered significant with $p < 0.05$ after Bonferroni-Finner correction to avoid Type-I errors (Finner, 1993). The effect size for the mean differences/proportions was measured through Cohen's-*d* coefficient (low/small effect size was considered for $|d| > 0.2$, moderate for $|d| > 0.5$ and large/high for $|d| > 0.8$; Kelly and Preacher, 2012). In this study, different dimensional and categorical measures for the YFAS 2.0 were analysed: firstly, the YFAS 2.0 dimensional symptom count, which measures the 11 DSM-5 SRAD criteria (raw scores are in the range of 0–11); and secondly, the categorical classification based on the dimensional symptom count, a threshold for food addiction (presents for individuals with at least two symptoms plus self-reported clinically significant impairment or distress, and absent for participants who did not meet these criteria). The capacity of the dimensional YFAS 2.0 symptom count to discriminate between the groups was tested through two sample T-test, and the capacity of the YFAS 2.0 categorical classifications to discriminate between the diagnostic sub-types was tested through chi-square tests (χ^2).

The mean amplitudes (µV) of the emotion regulation and food craving regulation tasks were analysed for each ERP component (P300, LPP1, LPP2) with independent 3 × 2 mixed design analyses of variance (ANOVA), with condition as the within-subject variable (Regulate Negative/Food, Observe Negative/Food, Observe Neutral) and group as the between subject variable (HC versus AN). Pairwise comparisons were used to follow up main effects (for non-significant interaction condition-by-group) and single effects (for significant interaction condition-by-group).

Pearson's correlations were calculated for each group to estimate correlations between ERPs in the "regulation" condition of the emotion/food craving regulation tasks and ERQ subscales (ERQ-suppression; ERQ-reappraisal). Due to the strong association between this model and the sample size, practical relevance was based on the own coefficient measure (effect size was considered low/poor for $|R| > 0.10$, moderate for $|R| > 0.24$ and large/high for $|R| > 0.37$) [66].

3. Results

3.1. Comparison of Clinical Profiles

There were no significant between-group differences in age ($p = 0.364$, $|d| = 0.29$). As expected, the HC group had significantly greater BMIs ($p < 0.001$, $|d| = 2.79$), lower mean scores on psychopathological self-report measures (i.e., the SCL-90-R GSI, DERS and YFAS), and higher mean scores on ERQ-Reappraisal. The prevalence of participants with food addiction positive screening score was also higher in the AN group (70% vs. 0%, $p < 0.001$, $|d| = 2.16$) (See Table 1). When comparing food addiction between AN sub-types, significant higher scores were displayed by the AN-BP subtype on the YFAS total score ($p = 0.031$, $|d| = 1.00$) and in all the YFAS criteria with exception of "withdrawal symptoms" (See Table 2).

Table 1. Comparison of the clinical profile between groups.

	HC (n = 20)		AN (n = 20)		T-stat	p	|d|
	Mean	(SD)	Mean	(SD)			
Age (years-old)	21.00	(5.12)	22.70	(6.51)	0.92	0.364	0.29
BMI (current, kg/m²)	20.72	(1.78)	16.63	(1.06)	8.82	<0.001 *	2.79 †
SCL-90-R: GSI score	0.65	(0.45)	1.59	(0.70)	5.10	<0.001 *	1.61 †
DERS: Total score	73.30	(16.12)	114.25	(23.36)	6.45	<0.001 *	2.04 †
ERQ: Reappraisal	33.50	(5.94)	24.25	(6.69)	4.62	<0.001 *	1.46 †
ERQ: Suppression	13.45	(5.71)	15.75	(4.64)	1.40	0.170	0.51 †
YFAS2 total score	0.75	(1.12)	4.35	(3.73)	4.13	<0.001 *	1.31 †
	n	(%)	n	(%)	χ^2	p	|d|
FA positive screening (YFAS-2)	0	(0.0%)	14	(70.0%)	21.54	<0.001 *	2.16 †

Note. SD: standard deviation. HC: healthy control. AN: anorexia. FA: food addiction. * Bold: significant parameter (.05 level). † Bold: effect size into the mild/moderate ($|d| > 0.80$) to large/good range ($|d| > 0.80$).

Table 2. Comparison of the FA measures between AN sub-types.

	AN-R (n = 12)		AN-BP (n = 8)		χ^2	p	|d|
	n	(%)	n	(%)			
Substance taken in larger amount	4	33.3%	4	50.0%	0.56	0.456	0.34
Persistent desire	3	25.0%	4	50.0%	1.32	0.251	0.53 †
Much time-activity to obtain, use, recover	5	41.7%	6	75.0%	2.15	0.142	0.72 †
Social or occupational affectation	7	58.3%	7	87.5%	1.94	0.163	0.69 †
Use continues despite consequences	4	33.3%	5	62.5%	1.65	0.199	0.61 †
Tolerance	0	0.0%	5	62.5%	10.00	0.002 *	1.83 †
Withdrawal symptoms	5	41.7%	5	62.5%	0.83	0.361	0.43
Continued use despite social problems	1	8.3%	4	50.0%	4.44	0.035 *	1.03 †
Failure to fulfil major rule obligations	1	8.3%	4	50.0%	4.44	0.035 *	1.03 †
Use in physically hazardous situations	3	25.0%	4	50.0%	1.32	0.251	0.53 †
Craving, or a strong desire or urge to use	2	16.7%	4	50.0%	2.54	0.111	0.76 †
Clinically significant impairment-distress	8	66.7%	7	87.5%	1.11	0.292	0.51 †
FA positive screening score	8	66.7%	6	75.0%	0.16	0.690	0.18
	Mean	(SD)	Mean	(SD)	T-stat	P	|d|
FA dimensional (YFAS2 total)	2.92	2.39	6.50	4.47	2.34	0.031 *	1.00 †

Note. AN-R: anorexia restrictive subtype. AN-BP: anorexia bulimic-purgative subtype. FA: food addiction. SD: standard deviation. * Bold: significant parameter (.05 level). † Bold: effect size into the mild/moderate ($|d| > 0.80$) to large/good range ($|d| > 0.80$).

3.2. ERP Results: Emotion Regulation Task

P300. The mixed design ANOVA yielded a significant main effect of condition (Regulate Negative, Observe Negative, Observe Neutral; F:27.7, df = 2/38, $p < 0.001$; $\eta^2 = 0.421$) and a significant main effect of group (HC versus AN; F = 10.9, df = 1/38, $p = 0.002$; $\eta^2 = 0.223$). No significant group x condition interaction was detected (F = 1.51, df = 2/37, $p = 0.229$; $\eta^2 = 0.038$). Post-hoc t-tests revealed that the main effect of condition was due to higher P300 mean amplitude in Observe Negative and in Regulate Negative conditions compared to the neutral one (Observe Negative vs. Observe Neutral $p < 0.001$; Regulate vs. Observe Neutral $p < 0.001$). With regards to the main effect of group, the AN group showed significantly smaller mean P300 amplitudes compared to HC group ($p = 0.002$).

LPP1. The mixed design ANOVA showed a significant main effect of condition (F = 51.7, df = 2/38, $p < 0.001$; $\eta^2 = 0.577$), but no significant main effect for group (F = 3.04, df = 1/38 $p = 0.089$; $\eta^2 = 0.074$) or group x condition interaction (F = 1.01, df = 2/37, $p = 0.369$; $\eta^2 = 0.026$). Post hoc t-tests for the main effect of condition showed higher LPP1 amplitudes in the Observe Negative and Regulate Negative conditions, compared to Neutral condition (Observe Negative vs. Observe Neutral $p < 0.001$; Regulate vs. Observe Neutral $p < 0.001$).

LPP2. The mixed design ANOVA showed a significant main effect of condition (F = 13.1, df = 2/38, $p < 0.001$; $\eta^2 = 0.256$), but no main significant effect of group (F = 0.22, df = 1/38, $p = 0.643$; $\eta^2 = 0.006$) or group x condition interaction (F = 0.05, df = 2/37, $p = 0.954$; $\eta^2 = 0.001$). Post-hoc t-tests revealed that the effect of condition was due to higher mean LPP2 amplitudes in both the Observe Negative and Regulate Negative conditions, compared to the neutral one (Observe Negative vs. Observe Neutral $p = 0.002$; Regulate Negative vs. Observe Neutral $p < 0.001$).

Means and standard deviations of the ERP amplitudes (µV) for each component (P300, LPP1, LPP2) are reported in Table 3 (see also Figure 1).

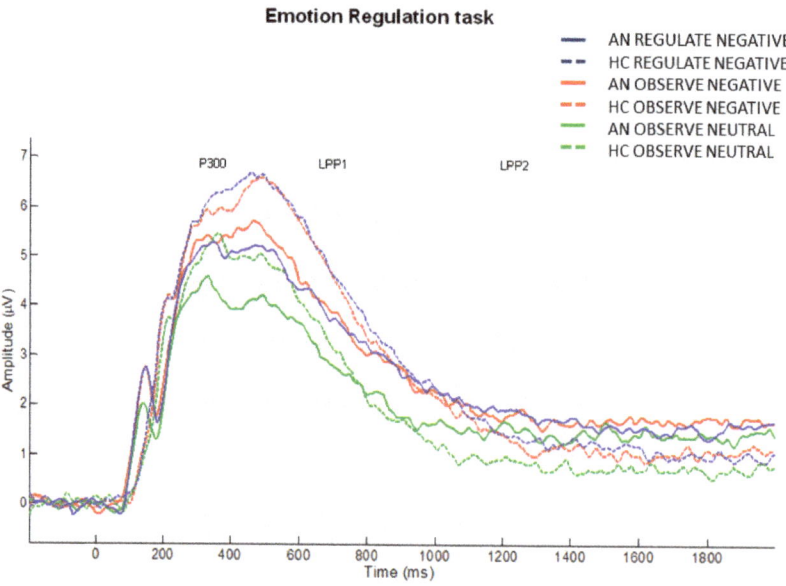

Figure 1. Grand average waveforms of the ER task, for each experimental condition (Regulate Negative, Observe Negative, Observe Neutral) and group (HC, AN), in the centro-parietal cluster of electrodes.

Table 3. Mean (SD) amplitudes (µV) of P300, LPP1 and LPP2 during the emotion regulation task.

	HC (n = 20)		AN (n = 20)	
	Mean	(SD)	Mean	(SD)
P300:				
observe negative	6.53	(2.72)	4.85	(1.97)
regulate negative	6.96	(2.93)	4.44	(1.84)
observe neutral	5.17	(1.86)	3.10	(1.44)
LPP1:				
observe negative	4.71	(2.59)	3.69	(1.63)
regulate negative	4.81	(2.27)	3.65	(1.49)
observe neutral	2.34	(1.53)	1.83	(1.20)
LPP2:				
observe negative	1.77	(2.16)	2.03	(1.48)
regulate negative	2.04	(2.04)	2.16	(1.11)
observe neutral	0.86	(1.47)	1.08	(1.10)

Note. HC: healthy control. AN: anorexia. SD: standard deviation.

3.3. ERP Results: Food Craving Regulation Task

P300. The mixed design ANOVA showed a significant main effect of condition (Regulate Food, Observe Food, Observe Neutral; $F = 47.2$, $df = 2/38$, $p < 0.001$; $\eta^2 = 0.560$) and a significant main effect of group (HC versus AN; $F = 6.72$, $df = 1/38$, $p = 0.014$; $\eta^2 = 0.154$), but no significant group x condition interaction ($F = 1.40$, $df = 2/37$, $p = 0.252$; $\eta^2 = 0.037$). Post-hoc t-tests for the main effect of condition showed higher amplitude in Observe Food and Regulate Food compared to the Observe Neutral condition (Observe Food vs. Observe Neutral $p < 0.001$; Regulate Food vs. Observe Neutral $p < 0.001$). Moreover, the AN group showed significantly smaller mean P300 amplitudes compared to the HC group ($p = 0.014$).

LPP1. The mixed design ANOVA showed a significant main effect of condition ($F = 38.5$, $df = 2/38$, $p < 0.001$; $\eta^2 = 0.504$), but no significant main effect of group ($F = 0.73$, $df = 1/38$, $p = 0.397$, $\eta^2 = 0.019$) or a significant group x condition interaction ($F = 0.25$, $df = 2/37$, $p = 0.778$; $\eta^2 = 0.007$). Post-hoc t-tests for condition revealed higher LPP1 in both Observe Food and Regulate Food compared to the Observe Neutral condition (Observe Food vs. Observe Neutral $p < 0.001$; Regulate Food vs. Observe Neutral $p < 0.001$), and higher LPP1 in Observe Food compared to Regulate Food ($p = 0.040$).

LPP2. The mixed design ANOVA showed a significant main effect of condition ($F = 23.3$, $df = 2/38$, $p < 0.001$; $\eta^2 = 0.380$), but no significant main effect of group ($F = 0.13$, $df = 1/38$, $p = 0.911$, $\eta^2 = 0.001$) or group x condition interaction ($F = 0.10$, $df = 2/37$, $p = 0.906$, $\eta^2 = 0.003$). Post-hoc t-tests for condition revealed higher LPP1 in both Observe and Regulate compared to the Observe Neutral condition (Observe Food vs. Observe Neutral $p < 0.001$; Regulate Food vs. Regulate Neutral $p < 0.001$), and higher LPP1 in Observe Food compared to Regulate Food ($p = 0.008$).

Mean and standard deviations of the ERP amplitudes (µV) for each component (P300, LPP1, LPP2) are reported in Table 4 (see also Figure 2).

Table 4. Mean (SD) amplitudes (μV) of P300, LPP1 and LPP2 during the food craving regulation task.

	HC (n = 20)		AN (n = 20)	
	Mean	(SD)	Mean	(SD)
P300:				
observe food	5.23	(2.39)	3.82	(1.47)
regulate food	5.60	(2.64)	3.67	(1.52)
observe neutral	3.68	(2.46)	2.32	(1.13)
LPP1:				
observe food	3.20	(1.91)	2.73	(1.38)
regulate food	2.86	(2.14)	2.38	(1.38)
observe neutral	1.49	(1.59)	1.25	(0.97)
LPP2:				
observe food	1.71	(1.45)	1.75	(1.19)
regulate food	1.26	(1.62)	1.21	(1.07)
observe neutral	0.42	(1.24)	0.54	(0.83)

Note. HC: healthy control. AN: anorexia. SD: standard deviation.

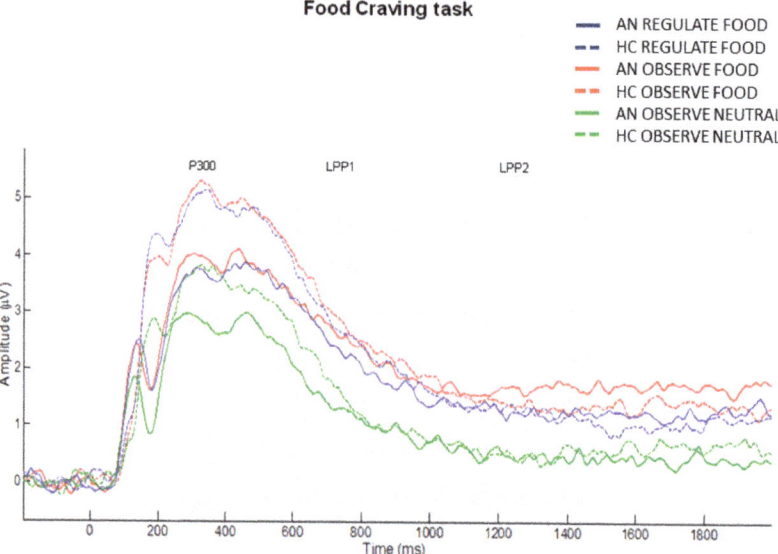

Figure 2. Grand average waveforms of the FRC task, for each experimental condition (Regulate Food, Observe Food, Observe Neutral) and group (HC, AN), in the centro-parietal cluster of electrodes.

3.4. Correlations between ERPs and Self-reported Emotional Regulation Strategies

Emotion Regulation Task and ERQ. In the HC group, reappraisal, as measured using the ERQ, was positively correlated with mean LPP1 amplitudes, while suppression was negatively correlated with mean LPP2 amplitudes. No significant correlations were found in the AN group.

Food Craving Regulation Task and ERQ. ERQ-reappraisal was positively correlated with mean LPP2 in the HC group, but not in the AN group. ERQ-suppression was negatively correlated with mean LPP1 and LPP2 amplitudes among patients with AN, but not in the HC group.

Table 5 shows the correlation matrix measuring the correlation between self-report measures of emotion regulation strategies (ERQ-suppression; ERQ-reappraisal) and ERPs amplitudes during emotion regulation (Regulate Negative) and food craving regulation (Regulate Food).

Table 5. Pearson's correlation between the amplitudes (µV) of the P300, LPP1, LPP2 during the "regulate" condition of the emotion regulation and the food craving regulation tasks.

	Emotion Regulation Task				Food Craving Regulation Task			
	HC (n = 20)		AN (n = 20)		HC (n = 20)		AN (n = 20)	
	ERQ reappr.	ERQ suppr.	ERQ reappr.	ERQ suppr.	ERQ reappr.	ERQ suppr.	ERQ reappr.	ERQ suppr.
P300	0.003	−0.195	0.119	−0.051	0.201	−0.187	0.101	0.018
LPP1	0.247 [†]	−0.205	0.130	−0.103	0.144	−0.207	0.204	−0.258 [†]
LPP2	0.196	−0.281 [†]	0.173	−0.058	0.396 [†]	−0.129	0.215	−0.370 [†]

Note. HC: healthy control. AN: anorexia. [†] Bold: effect size into the mild/moderate ($|R| > 0.24$) to large/good range ($|R| > 0.37$). Sample size: Healthy control = 20; Anorexia = 20.

4. Discussion

In the present study, clinical and electrophysiological features of emotion regulation and food craving regulation among patients with AN were investigated by means of self-report and ERP measures.

Results from self-report measures of emotion regulation, confirmed greater difficulties in emotion regulation in patients with AN compared to the HC group (as suggested by DERS scores). This is in line with previous studies comparing AN with HC using the same questionnaire [5,68–70]. In addition, in the ERQ subscales, differences between groups were found, suggesting that patients with AN most frequently implemented maladaptive strategies (i.e., suppression) than adaptive strategies (i.e., reappraisal). This latter results corroborated previous findings suggesting dysfunctional emotion regulation strategies (e.g. suppression, avoidance) in populations with eating disorder [71–73], as is the case with other psychiatric disorders [74]. Moreover, problematic eating behaviours, such as binging, purging, and restriction, can be seen as maladaptive strategies to avoid or suppress negative emotions [68,75,76]. With regards to food addiction, a higher score was detected in the AN, as opposed to the HC group. Additional comparisons within the AN sub-types suggested higher scores in multiple dimensions of food addiction in AN-BP compared to AN-R. The present findings portray evidence of the relevance of food addiction to AN, specifically in patients with binging/purging symptoms. It is important to note that food addiction scores have been more typically described in patients with binge-subtype eating disorder [77–80], with some inconclusive or less evident results in AN. In a previous study exploring food addiction in eating disorders, patients with AN binge/purging subtype showed the highest prevalence of food addiction although half of the AN patients with restrictive type also positively scored for food addiction [27].

Results from electrophysiological measures collected in the emotional regulation task indicated enhanced mean P300 and LPP amplitudes in presence of pictures depicting negative emotions compared to neutral pictures in both AN and HC groups. This suggested enhanced processing of emotional stimuli, potentially due to their evolutionary salience, in accordance with previous ERP literature on 'healthy' populations [7,81–85]. Based on our results, we can suggest that, similarly to HC, patients with AN display a facilitated processing of stimuli with negative emotional valence. Although a previous ERP study reported altered processing of emotional stimuli in patients with AN [86], these controversial findings could be explained by the use of different types of stimuli and task (i.e., recognition of emotional faces).

Despite of the reported ERP indices of emotional processing, the instruction to down-regulate negative emotions did not elicit significant differences in mean P300 and LPP amplitudes when compared to passive viewing of negatively valenced emotional stimuli in any group. Since a reduction in LPP amplitude has been previously shown during emotion down-regulation in healthy population [30–33,39,40], the lack of this effect can be explained by a failure in emotion down-regulation that occurred in both AN patients and controls. This can be due to the fact that participants were not instructed to adopt a specific regulation strategy (e.g. reappraisal; suppression), which makes it more difficult to successfully achieve emotion regulation. However, adopting visual analogue scales to measure self-reported down-regulation is necessary to avoid premature conclusions.

During the food craving regulation task, pictures of food elicited greater mean P300 and LPP amplitudes compared to neutral non-food pictures in both AN and HC groups. This can be interpreted as motivated attention, meaning a higher amount of attentional resources allocated to process food stimuli [87]. However, we did not find higher motivated attention toward food in patients with AN when compared to HC, suggesting similar allocation of attentional resources toward food-stimuli, at latest stages of attentional processing. This is in accordance with a previous study in which patients with AN did not display enhanced P300/LPP toward high-caloric food, but only for low-caloric food pictures when compared with HC [88]. Since we were interested in investigating regulation of food craving, which is generally experienced in response to "forbidden foods" (i.e., high caloric), low-caloric food was not included in our study.

Interestingly, smaller LPP amplitudes were detected during down-regulation of craving compared to passing viewing food pictures, possibly suggesting successful down-regulation of food craving in both groups. This result is in line with a previous study in non-clinical 'restrained' eaters, showing that P300 and LPP amplitudes were reduced during down-regulation of food craving compared to the passive viewing of food-related pictures [46]. As the first ERP study which explores food craving regulation in patients with AN, we could observe that, despite AN reported greater "food addiction" symptomatology, these subjects were able to regulate food craving, as depicted at a neurophysiological level. Nevertheless, differential ERP response during food craving regulation may be expected between AN-BP and AN-R. Thus, further research in larger sample sized including different AN sub-types is needed to deeply understand the neurophysiological mechanisms underpinning this craving modulation in AN.

Finally, differences in ERP between patients and controls were depicted by smaller P300 amplitudes in the AN group. This overall reduction in mean P300 amplitudes was consistent in both tasks and regardless of experimental condition. Reduced neurophysiological response in AN could reflect neurocognitive alterations, possibly as a secondary effect of malnutrition which consequently affect cognitive functioning [89]. Accordingly, cognitive difficulties have been suggested in patients with AN, especially in memory, attention and executive functions (i.e. decision-making, set-shifting [90–92]. Similarly to our findings, previous ERP studies adopting different tasks showed reduced P300 in AN compared to controls, regardless of the emotional relevance of the stimuli [93,94].

Exploratory correlations in each group were performed in order to explore how emotion regulation strategies modulate both emotion and food craving regulation at a neurophysiological level. As for the emotion regulation task, our findings suggest that, only among HC, the tendency to suppress emotions correlated with larger LPP amplitudes, while the tendency to reappraise emotions correlated with lower LPP amplitudes. This may suggest that the tendency to adopt different emotion regulation strategies (i.e. reappraisal or suppression) is related with different modulation of the LPP amplitude while regulating emotions, at least in healthy individuals. Since the modulation of LPP amplitude has been linked to reappraisal of negative emotions in HC [30–33,39,40], the present results may further suggest a link between neurophysiological markers of emotion regulation and the tendency to adopt reappraisal as cognitive strategy to down-regulate negative emotions in the non-clinical population. By contrast, LPP response did not significantly correlate with emotion regulation strategies among patients with AN.

Similarly to the emotion regulation task, the LPP amplitude during down-regulation of food craving was positively related to ERQ-reappraisal in HC. By contrast, LPP amplitudes negatively correlated with ERQ-suppression in patients with AN. These latter results could suggest that neurophysiological response during down-regulation of food craving is related to different emotion regulation strategies in patients as compared to controls, which is in line with the differences observed in ERQ scores among groups. Interestingly, significant correlations with suppression in AN were specifically present in the food craving regulation task, and this can be linked to the fact that patients tend to adopt dysfunctional eating behaviours (e.g. bingeing/purging, restriction) as maladaptive strategies to regulate negative emotions, as showed by higher scores in ERQ-suppression.

It is important to consider some limitations when interpreting the results of the present study. Firstly, our sample size is rather low, which might have decreased the likelihood of detecting a significant difference if it existed [95]. Further studies with larger samples would be required to confirm our findings. Moreover, the small size of the sample did not allow us to distinguish and compare restrictive and purging AN sub-types. Given that different AN sub-types may exhibit different neurobiological correlates [96], future studies with larger samples should explore neural correlates of emotion regulation and food craving in different AN sub-types. In addition, our sample only consisted of female participants, which limits the generalizability of the results to a wider population. Additionally, we did not expose individuals to real food stimuli, which would have mimicked real-life situations and perhaps elicited stronger emotional and physiological reactions than food pictures [97]. Given the nature of the paradigms, another limitation of the study is the lack of eye-tracking and the lack of arousal tracing. Additional studies should further control eye-movements and attention focus during the image presentation. Furthermore, a proportion of patients with AN were under psychopharmacological medication (i.e., antidepressants, neuroleptic drugs, and benzodiazepines) and our sample did not allow us to control for medication. Finally, the present study design is cross-sectional in nature and claims regarding causality cannot be made. Future longitudinal studies are required to examine the extent to which the repetitive use of emotion regulation and food craving regulation techniques might modify the long-term neurophysiological responses in AN patients.

5. Conclusions

To conclude, previous ERP findings did not appear to mirror clarifying findings regarding eating disorders' aetiology and functioning. Therefore, to this date, they might not be used as accurate parameters or biomarkers that could be directly employed in the diagnosis or treatment of eating disorders [98]. To our knowledge, this is the first study which has examined the electrophysiological features of emotion and food craving regulation among patients with AN. Interestingly, ERP results suggest a successful down-regulation of food craving in AN, despite the fact that AN reported greater food addiction symptomatology. Nevertheless, further research including different AN sub-types is needed to deeply understand the neurophysiological mechanisms underpinning this craving modulation in AN.

Furthermore, although ERP did not depict differential response between AN and HC while down-regulating emotions or food craving, reduced P300 mean amplitudes were detected in AN when compared to HC. This result might reflect a general alteration in the neurophysiological responses of AN patients, which is possibly related to their prolonged state of malnutrition [99]. In this regard, this study provides an objective parameter of those impairments which long-lasting malnutrition might be occasioning in the neural systems of AN patients. Previous research has also found neurophysiological dysfunctions in AN, which do not always seem to be normalised after weight gain [98]. In that respect, it would be of great interest that future studies explore not only if neurophysiological alterations remain or, on the contrary, are ameliorated after patients' recovery, but also investigate the factors which might contribute to normalise neural responses in AN (e.g., weight gain, pharmacological treatments, specific psychological interventions, etc.).

On the other hand, clinical measures showed that patients with AN were characterized by food addiction symptoms and difficulties in emotion regulation with the tendency to use maladaptive techniques (i.e., suppression) to manage negative emotions. Moreover, this is the first study which relates the use of suppression strategies to smaller ERP amplitudes during food craving regulation in AN patients. This possibly reflects their tendency to adopt dysfunctional eating behaviours as maladaptive strategies to regulate negative emotions. Future interventions should focus on implementing more effective emotion regulation techniques such as reappraisal, which act through a reinterpretation of emotional situation in order to reduce its emotional impact. Reappraisal has shown a better capacity to decrease negative emotional experience, consequently reducing distress [100].

Further research with larger samples and considering AN sub-types is needed to deeply understand the neurophysiological mechanisms underpinning emotion and food craving modulation in AN.

Author Contributions: N.M.-B., J.C.P., S.J.-M. and F.F.-A. conceived and designed the study; N.M.-B., M.L.-M. and G.T. curated the data; G.T. and R.G. analysed the data; F.F.-A. acquired the fundings; N.M.-B., M.L.M., C.V.-A., I.S., N.R. and J.F.N. collected the data; J.C.P., S.J.-M., J.T. and F.F.-A. supervised this study; N.M.-B., M.L.M., G.T. and R.G. wrote the original draft; N.M.-B., M.L.M., G.T., J.C.P., J.F.N., I.M.-Z., A.M., M.V.D.L.H., R.C., S.J.-M., J.A.F.-F., J.T. and F.F.-A. reviewed and edited the manuscript. All authors have read and agreed to the published version of the manuscript.

Funding: This manuscript and research were supported by grants from the Instituto de Salud Carlos III (ISCIII) [FIS PI14/00290, PI17/01167 and cofounded by FEDER funds/European Regional Development Fund (ERDF), a way to build Europe]. CIBER Fisiopatología de la Obesidad y Nutrición (CIBERobn) is an initiative of ISCIII. M.L-M and C.V-A are supported by a predoctoral grants of the Ministerio de Educación, Cultura y Deporte (FPU15/02911 and FPU16/01453). Study resulting from the SLT006/17/00246 grant, funded by the Department of Health of the Generalitat de Catalunya by the call "Acció instrumental de programes de recerca orientats en l'àmbit de la recerca i la innovació en salut". We thank CERCA Programme / Generalitat de Catalunya for Institutional support.

Conflicts of Interest: The authors declare no conflict of interest. The funders had no role in the design of the study; in the collection, analyses, or interpretation of data; in the writing of the manuscript, or in the decision to publish the results.

References

1. Schaumberg, K.; Welch, E.; Breithaupt, L.; Hübel, C.; Baker, J.H.; Munn-Chernoff, M.A.; Yilmaz, Z.; Ehrlich, S.; Mustelin, L.; Ghaderi, A.; et al. The Science Behind the Academy for Eating Disorders' Nine Truths About Eating Disorders. *Eur. Eat. Disord. Rev.* **2017**, *25*, 432–450. [CrossRef]
2. Glashouwer, K.A.; van der Veer, R.M.L.; Adipatria, F.; de Jong, P.J.; Vocks, S. The role of body image disturbance in the onset, maintenance, and relapse of anorexia nervosa: A systematic review. *Clin. Psychol. Rev.* **2019**, *74*. [CrossRef]
3. Giel, K.E.; Teufel, M.; Friederich, H.-C.; Hautzinger, M.; Enck, P.; Zipfel, S. Processing of pictorial food stimuli in patients with eating disorders-A systematic review. *Int. J. Eat. Disord.* **2010**, *44*, 105–117. [CrossRef]
4. Aviram-Friedman, R.; Astbury, N.; Ochner, C.N.; Contento, I.; Geliebter, A. Neurobiological evidence for attention bias to food, emotional dysregulation, disinhibition and deficient somatosensory awareness in obesity with binge eating disorder. *Physiol. Behav.* **2018**, *184*, 122–128. [CrossRef]
5. Harrison, A.; Sullivan, S.; Tchanturia, K.; Treasure, J. Emotional functioning in eating disorders: Attentional bias, emotion recognition and emotion regulation. *Psychol. Med.* **2010**, *40*, 1887–1897. [CrossRef]
6. Gross, J.J. The emerging field of emotion regulation: An integrative review. *Rev. Gen. Psychol.* **1998**, *2*, 271–299. [CrossRef]
7. Hajcak, G.; MacNamara, A.; Olvet, D.M. Event-Related Potentials, Emotion, and Emotion Regulation: An Integrative Review. *Dev. Neuropsychol.* **2010**, *35*, 129–155. [CrossRef]
8. Richards, J.M.; Gross, J.J. Emotion regulation and memory: The cognitive costs of keeping one's cool. *J. Pers. Soc. Psychol.* **2000**, *79*, 410–424. [CrossRef]
9. Daros, A.R.; Rodrigo, A.H.; Norouzian, N.; Darboh, B.S.; McRae, K.; Ruocco, A.C. Cognitive Reappraisal of Negative Emotional Images in Borderline Personality Disorder: Content Analysis, Perceived Effectiveness, and Diagnostic Specificity. *J. Pers. Disord.* **2018**, 1–17. [CrossRef]
10. Tenenbaum, R.B.; Musser, E.D.; Morris, S.; Ward, A.R.; Raiker, J.S.; Coles, E.K.; Pelham, W.E. Response Inhibition, Response Execution, and Emotion Regulation among Children with Attention-Deficit/Hyperactivity Disorder. *J. Abnorm. Child Psychol.* **2018**. [CrossRef]
11. Joormann, J.; Quinn, M.E. Cognitive processes and emotion regulation in depression. *Depress. Anxiety* **2014**, *31*, 308–315. [CrossRef] [PubMed]
12. Malik, S.; Wells, A.; Wittkowski, A. Emotion regulation as a mediator in the relationship between attachment and depressive symptomatology: A systematic review. *J. Affect. Disord.* **2015**, *172*, 428–444. [CrossRef] [PubMed]

13. Mallorquí-Bagué, N.; Vintró-Alcaraz, C.; Sánchez, I.; Riesco, N.; Agüera, Z.; Granero, R.; Jiménez-Murcia, S.; Menchón, J.M.; Treasure, J.; Fernández-Aranda, F.; et al. Emotion Regulation as a Transdiagnostic Feature Among Eating Disorders: Cross-sectional and Longitudinal Approach. *Eur. Eat. Disord. Rev.* **2018**, *26*, 53–61. [CrossRef] [PubMed]
14. Monell, E.; Clinton, D.; Birgegård, A. Emotion dysregulation and eating disorders-Associations with diagnostic presentation and key symptoms. *Int. J. Eat. Disord.* **2018**. [CrossRef]
15. Wolz, I.; Agüera, Z.; Granero, R.; Jiménez-Murcia, S.; Gratz, K.L.; Menchón, J.M.; Fernández-Aranda, F. Emotion regulation in disordered eating: Psychometric properties of the Difficulties in Emotion Regulation Scale among Spanish adults and its interrelations with personality and clinical severity. *Front. Psychol.* **2015**, *6*, 907. [CrossRef]
16. Engel, S.G.; Wonderlich, S.A.; Crosby, R.D.; Mitchell, J.E.; Crow, S.; Peterson, C.B.; Le Grange, D.; Simonich, H.K.; Cao, L.; Lavender, J.M.; et al. The role of affect in the maintenance of anorexia nervosa: Evidence from a naturalistic assessment of momentary behaviors and emotion. *J. Abnorm. Psychol.* **2013**, *122*, 709–719. [CrossRef]
17. Haynos, A.F.; Roberto, C.A.; Martinez, M.A.; Attia, E.; Fruzzetti, A.E. Emotion regulation difficulties in anorexia nervosa before and after inpatient weight restoration. *Int. J. Eat. Disord.* **2014**, *47*, 888–891. [CrossRef]
18. Adamson, J.; Leppanen, J.; Murin, M.; Tchanturia, K. Effectiveness of emotional skills training for patients with anorexia nervosa with autistic symptoms in group and individual format. *Eur. Eat. Disord. Rev.* **2018**, *26*, 367–375. [CrossRef]
19. Oldershaw, A.; Lavender, T.; Schmidt, U. Are socio-emotional and neurocognitive functioning predictors of therapeutic outcomes for adults with anorexia nervosa? *Eur. Eat. Disord. Rev.* **2018**, *26*, 346–359. [CrossRef]
20. Giuliani, N.R.; Berkman, E.T. Craving Is an Affective State and Its Regulation Can Be Understood in Terms of the Extended Process Model of Emotion Regulation. *Psychol. Inq.* **2015**, *26*, 48–53. [CrossRef]
21. Hill, A.J. Symposium on "molecular mechanisms and psychology of food intake"—The psychology of food craving. *Proc. Nutr. Soc.* **2007**, *66*, 277–285. [CrossRef]
22. Giuliani, N.R.; Calcott, R.D.; Berkman, E.T. Piece of cake. Cognitive reappraisal of food craving. *Appetite* **2013**, *64*, 56–61. [CrossRef]
23. Giuliani, N.R.; Mann, T.; Tomiyama, A.J.; Berkman, E.T. Neural Systems Underlying the Reappraisal of Personally Craved Foods. *J. Cogn. Neurosci.* **2014**, *26*, 1390–1402. [CrossRef]
24. Siep, N.; Roefs, A.; Roebroeck, A.; Havermans, R.; Bonte, M.; Jansen, A. Fighting food temptations: The modulating effects of short-term cognitive reappraisal, suppression and up-regulation on mesocorticolimbic activity related to appetitive motivation. *Neuroimage* **2012**, *60*, 213–220. [CrossRef]
25. Granero, R.; Jiménez-Murcia, S.; Gerhardt, A.N.; Agüera, Z.; Aymamí, N.; Gómez-Peña, M.; Lozano-Madrid, M.; Mallorquí-Bagué, N.; Mestre-Bach, G.; Neto-Antao, M.I.; et al. Validation of the Spanish version of the Yale Food Addiction Scale 2.0 (YFAS 2.0) and clinical correlates in a sample of eating disorder, gambling disorder, and healthy control participants. *Front. Psychiatry* **2018**, *9*, 1–11. [CrossRef]
26. Gendall, K.A.; Sullivan, P.F.; Joyce, P.R.; Bulik, C.M. Food cravings in women with a history of anorexia nervosa. *Int. J. Eat. Disord.* **1997**, *22*, 403–409. [CrossRef]
27. Granero, R.; Hilker, I.; Agüera, Z.; Jiménez-Murcia, S.; Sauchelli, S.; Islam, M.A.; Fagundo, A.B.; Sánchez, I.; Riesco, N.; Dieguez, C.; et al. Food Addiction in a Spanish Sample of Eating Disorders: DSM-5 Diagnostic Subtype Differentiation and Validation Data. *Eur. Eat. Disord. Rev.* **2014**, *22*, 389–396. [CrossRef]
28. Blackwood, D.H.; Muir, W.J. Cognitive brain potentials and their application. *Br. J. Psychiatry. Suppl.* **1990**, 96–101. [CrossRef]
29. Wolz, I.; Sauvaget, A.; Granero, R.; Mestre-Bach, G.; Baño, M.; Martín-Romera, V.; Veciana de las Heras, M.; Jiménez-Murcia, S.; Jansen, A.; Roefs, A.; et al. Subjective craving and event-related brain response to olfactory and visual chocolate cues in binge-eating and healthy individuals. *Sci. Rep.* **2017**, *7*, 41736. [CrossRef]
30. Moser, J.S.; Hajcak, G.; Bukay, E.; Simons, R.F. Intentional modulation of emotional responding to unpleasant pictures: An ERP study. *Psychophysiology* **2006**, *43*, 292–296. [CrossRef]
31. Hajcak, G.; Nieuwenhuis, S. Reappraisal modulates the electrocortical response to unpleasant pictures. *Cogn. Affect. Behav. Neurosci.* **2006**, *6*, 291–297. [CrossRef]

32. Blechert, J.; Sheppes, G.; Di Tella, C.; Williams, H.; Gross, J.J. See What You Think. *Psychol. Sci.* **2012**, *23*, 346–353. [CrossRef]
33. Moser, J.S.; Krompinger, J.W.; Dietz, J.; Simons, R.F. Electrophysiological correlates of decreasing and increasing emotional responses to unpleasant pictures. *Psychophysiology* **2009**, *46*, 17–27. [CrossRef]
34. Baur, R.; Conzelmann, A.; Wieser, M.J.; Pauli, P. Spontaneous emotion regulation: Differential effects on evoked brain potentials and facial muscle activity. *Int. J. Psychophysiol.* **2015**, *96*, 38–48. [CrossRef]
35. Gardener, E.K.T.; Carr, A.R.; Macgregor, A.; Felmingham, K.L. Sex differences and emotion regulation: An event-related potential study. *PLoS ONE* **2013**, *8*, e73475. [CrossRef]
36. Yang, Q.; Gu, R.; Tang, P.; Luo, Y.-J. How does cognitive reappraisal affect the response to gains and losses? *Psychophysiology* **2013**, *50*, 1094–1103. [CrossRef]
37. Shafir, R.; Zucker, L.; Sheppes, G. Turning off hot feelings: Down-regulation of sexual desire using distraction and situation-focused reappraisal. *Biol. Psychol.* **2018**, *137*, 116–124. [CrossRef]
38. Langeslag, S.J.E.; van Strien, J.W. Cognitive reappraisal of snake and spider pictures: An event-related potentials study. *Int. J. Psychophysiol.* **2018**, *130*, 1–8. [CrossRef]
39. Yang, B.; Cao, J.; Zhou, T.; Dong, L.; Zou, L.; Xiang, J. Exploration of Neural Activity under Cognitive Reappraisal Using Simultaneous EEG-fMRI Data and Kernel Canonical Correlation Analysis. *Comput. Math. Methods Med.* **2018**, *2018*, 1–11. [CrossRef]
40. Reva, N.V.; Pavlov, S.V.; Korenek, V.V.; Loktev, K.V.; Tumialis, A.V.; Brak, I.V.; Aftanas, L.I. The regulation of negative and positive emotions during picture viewing: An ERP study. *Ross. Fiziol. zhurnal Im. I.M. Sechenova* **2015**, *101*, 114–122.
41. Langeslag, S.J.E.; Surti, K. The effect of arousal on regulation of negative emotions using cognitive reappraisal: An ERP study. *Int. J. Psychophysiol.* **2017**, *118*, 18–26. [CrossRef]
42. Han, H.Y.; Gan, T.; Li, P.; Li, Z.J.; Guo, M.; Yao, S.M. Attentional bias modulation by reappraisal in patients with generalized anxiety disorder: An event-related potential study. *Brazilian J. Med. Biol. Res. = Rev. Bras. Pesqui. medicas e Biol.* **2014**, *47*, 576–583. [CrossRef]
43. Pollatos, O.; Gramann, K. Attenuated modulation of brain activity accompanies emotion regulation deficits in alexithymia. *Psychophysiology* **2012**, *49*, 651–658. [CrossRef]
44. Meule, A.; Kübler, A.; Blechert, J. Time course of electrocortical food-cue responses during cognitive regulation of craving. *Front. Psychol.* **2013**, *4*. [CrossRef]
45. Sarlo, M.; Übel, S.; Leutgeb, V.; Schienle, A. Cognitive reappraisal fails when attempting to reduce the appetitive value of food: An ERP study. *Biol. Psychol.* **2013**, *94*, 507–512. [CrossRef]
46. Svaldi, J.; Tuschen-Caffier, B.; Biehl, S.C.; Gschwendtner, K.; Wolz, I.; Naumann, E. Effects of two cognitive regulation strategies on the processing of food cues in high restrained eaters. An event-related potential study. *Appetite* **2015**, *92*, 269–277. [CrossRef]
47. Wolz, I.; Fagundo, A.B.; Treasure, J.; Fernández-Aranda, F. The processing of food stimuli in abnormal eating: A systematic review of electrophysiology. *Eur. Eat. Disord. Rev.* **2015**, *23*, 251–261. [CrossRef]
48. APA. *Diagnostic and Statistical Manual of Mental Disorders*, 5th ed.; American Journal of Psychiatry: Washington, DC, USA, 2013; ISBN 9780890425541.
49. Sheehan, D.V.; Lecrubier, Y.; Sheehan, K.H.; Amorim, P.; Janavs, J.; Weiller, E.; Hergueta, T.; Baker, R.; Dunbar, G.C. The Mini-International Neuropsychiatric Interview (M.I.N.I.): The development and validation of a structured diagnostic psychiatric interview for DSM-IV and ICD-10. *J. Clin. Psychiatry* **1998**, *59* (Suppl. 2), 22–33; quiz 34-57.
50. APA. *DSM-III-R: Diagnostic and Statistical Manual of Mental Disorders (Rev.)*; APA: Washington, DC, USA, 1987.
51. APA. *American Psychiatric Association, Diagnostic and Statistical Manual of Mental Disorders*, 4th ed.; American Psychiatric Association: Washington, DC, USA, 1994.
52. World Health Organization. *International Statistical Classification of disease and related health problems, Tenth Revision (ICD-10)*; World Health Organization: Geneva, Switzerland, 1992.
53. Spitzer, R.L.; Williams, J.B.W.; Gibbon, M.; First, M.B. The Structured Clinical Interview for DSM-III-R (SCID). *Arch. Gen. Psychiatry* **1992**, *49*, 624. [CrossRef]
54. World Health Organization. *Composite international diagnostic interview (CIDI)*; World Health Organization: Geneva, Switzerland, 1993.

55. Gratz, K.L.; Roemer, L. Multidimensional Assessment of Emotion Regulation and Dysregulation: Development, Factor Structure, and Initial Validation of the Difficulties in Emotion Regulation Scale. *J. Psychopathol. Behav. Assess.* **2004**, *26*, 41–54. [CrossRef]
56. Hervás, G.; Jódar, R. Adaptación al castellano de la Escala de Dificultades en la Regulación Emocional The spanish version of the Difficulties in Emotion Regulation Scale. *Clínica y Salud* **2008**, *19*, 139–156.
57. Cabello, R.; Salguero, J.M.; Fernández-Berrocal, P.; Gross, J.J. A Spanish Adaptation of the Emotion Regulation Questionnaire. *Eur. J. Psychol. Assess.* **2013**, *29*, 234–240. [CrossRef]
58. Derogatis, L. *SCL-90-R. Cuestionario de 90 síntomas. [SCL-90-R. 90-Symptoms Questionnaire]*; TEA Ediciones: Madrid, Spain, 1994.
59. González de Rivera, J.L.; de las Cuevas, C.; Rodríguez Abuín, M.; y Rodríguez Pulido, F. *SCL-90-R. Cuestionario de 90 síntomas. Manual*; TEA Ediciones: Madrid, Spain, 2002.
60. Lang, P.J. *International Affective Picture System (IAPS): Affective Ratings of Pictures and Instruction Manual*; University of Florida: Gainesville, FL, USA, 2005.
61. *Presentation®Software (Version 16.0)*, Neurobehavioral Systems, Inc.: Berkeley, CA, USA.
62. Blechert, J.; Meule, A.; Busch, N.A.; Ohla, K. Food-pics: An image database for experimental research on eating and appetite. *Front. Psychol.* **2014**, *5*, 617. [CrossRef]
63. *Brain Vision Analyzer (Version 2.2.0) [Computer Software]*, Brain Products GmbH: Gilching, Germany, 2019.
64. Finner, H. On a Monotonicity Problem in Step-Down Multiple Test Procedures. *J. Am. Stat. Assoc.* **1993**, *88*, 920–923. [CrossRef]
65. Kelley, K.; Preacher, K.J. On effect size. *Psychol. Methods* **2012**, *17*, 137–152. [CrossRef]
66. Rosnow, R.L.; Rosenthal, R. Computing contrasts, effect sizes, and counternulls on other people's published data: General procedures for research consumers. *Psychol. Methods* **1996**, *1*, 331–340. [CrossRef]
67. StataCorp. *Stata Statistical Software: Release 15*; StataCorp LLC: College Station, TX, USA, 2017.
68. Harrison, A.; Sullivan, S.; Tchanturia, K.; Treasure, J. Emotion recognition and regulation in anorexia nervosa. *Clin. Psychol. Psychother.* **2009**, *16*, 348–356. [CrossRef]
69. Rowsell, M.; Macdonald, D.E.; Carter, J.C. Emotion regulation difficulties in anorexia nervosa: Associations with improvements in eating psychopathology. *J. Eat. Disord.* **2016**, *7*. [CrossRef]
70. Oldershaw, A.; Lavender, T.; Sallis, H.; Stahl, D.; Schmidt, U. Emotion generation and regulation in anorexia nervosa: A systematic review and meta-analysis of self-report data. *Clin. Psychol. Rev.* **2015**, *39*, 83–95. [CrossRef]
71. Svaldi, J.; Griepenstroh, J.; Tuschen-Caffier, B.; Ehring, T. Emotion regulation deficits in eating disorders: A marker of eating pathology or general psychopathology? *Psychiatry Res.* **2012**, *197*, 103–111. [CrossRef]
72. Aldao, A.; Nolen-Hoeksema, S.; Schweizer, S. Emotion-regulation strategies across psychopathology: A meta-analytic review. *Clin. Psychol. Rev.* **2010**, *30*, 217–237. [CrossRef] [PubMed]
73. Meule, A.; Richard, A.; Schnepper, R.; Reichenberger, J.; Georgii, C.; Naab, S.; Voderholzer, U.; Blechert, J. Emotion regulation and emotional eating in anorexia nervosa and bulimia nervosa. *Eat. Disord.* **2019**, 1–17. [CrossRef] [PubMed]
74. Sloan, E.; Hall, K.; Moulding, R.; Bryce, S.; Mildred, H.; Staiger, P.K. Emotion regulation as a transdiagnostic treatment construct across anxiety, depression, substance, eating and borderline personality disorders: A systematic review. *Clin. Psychol. Rev.* **2017**, *57*, 141–163. [CrossRef]
75. Brockmeyer, T.; Skunde, M.; Wu, M.; Bresslein, E.; Rudofsky, G.; Herzog, W.; Friederich, H.-C. Difficulties in emotion regulation across the spectrum of eating disorders. *Compr. Psychiatry* **2014**, *55*, 565–571. [CrossRef]
76. Lavender, J.M.; Wonderlich, S.A.; Peterson, C.B.; Crosby, R.D.; Engel, S.G.; Mitchell, J.E.; Crow, S.J.; Smith, T.L.; Klein, M.H.; Goldschmidt, A.B.; et al. Dimensions of Emotion Dysregulation in Bulimia Nervosa. *Eur. Eat. Disord. Rev.* **2014**, *22*, 212–216. [CrossRef]
77. Cassin, S.E.; von Ranson, K.M. Is binge eating experienced as an addiction? *Appetite* **2007**, *49*, 687–690. [CrossRef]
78. Gearhardt, A.N.; White, M.A.; Masheb, R.M.; Morgan, P.T.; Crosby, R.D.; Grilo, C.M. An examination of the food addiction construct in obese patients with binge eating disorder. *Int. J. Eat. Disord.* **2012**, *45*, 657–663. [CrossRef]
79. Meule, A.; von Rezori, V.; Blechert, J. Food Addiction and Bulimia Nervosa. *Eur. Eat. Disord. Rev.* **2014**, *22*, 331–337. [CrossRef]

80. Gearhardt, A.N.; White, M.A.; Masheb, R.M.; Grilo, C.M. An examination of food addiction in a racially diverse sample of obese patients with binge eating disorder in primary care settings. *Compr. Psychiatry* **2013**, *54*, 500–505. [CrossRef]
81. Lang, P.J.; Bradley, M.M.; Cuthbert, B.N. Motivated attention: Affect, activation, and action. In *Attention and Orienting: Sensory and Motivational Processes*; Psychology Press: East Sussex, UK, 1997; pp. 97–135. ISBN 9781135808273.
82. Schupp, H.T.; Markus, J.; Weike, A.I.; Hamm, A.O. Emotional Facilitation of Sensory Processing in the Visual Cortex. *Psychol. Sci.* **2003**, *14*, 7–13. [CrossRef]
83. Schupp, H.T.; Flaisch, T.; Stockburger, J.; Junghöfer, M. Emotion and attention: Event-related brain potential studies. *Prog. Brain Res.* **2006**, *156*, 31–51.
84. Cuthbert, B.N.; Schupp, H.T.; Bradley, M.M.; Birbaumer, N.; Lang, P.J. Brain potentials in affective picture processing: Covariation with autonomic arousal and affective report. *Biol. Psychol.* **2000**, *52*, 95–111. [CrossRef]
85. Amrhein, C.; Mühlberger, A.; Pauli, P.; Wiedemann, G. Modulation of event-related brain potentials during affective picture processing: A complement to startle reflex and skin conductance response? *Int. J. Psychophysiol.* **2004**, *54*, 231–240. [CrossRef]
86. Pollatos, O.; Herbert, B.M.; Schandry, R.; Gramann, K. Impaired Central Processing of Emotional Faces in Anorexia Nervosa. *Psychosom. Med.* **2008**, *70*, 701–708. [CrossRef]
87. Bradley, M.M.; Sabatinelli, D.; Lang, P.J.; Fitzsimmons, J.R.; King, W.; Desai, P. Activation of the visual cortex in motivated attention. *Behav. Neurosci.* **2003**, *117*, 369–380. [CrossRef]
88. Novosel, A.; Lackner, N.; Unterrainer, H.F.; Dunitz-Scheer, M.; Scheer, P.J.Z.; Wallner-Liebmann, S.J.; Neuper, C. Motivational processing of food cues in anorexia nervosa: A pilot study. *Eat. Weight Disord.* **2014**, *19*, 169–175. [CrossRef]
89. Micali, N.; Kothari, R.; Nam, K.W.; Gioroukou, E.; Walshe, M.; Allin, M.; Rifkin, L.; Murray, R.M.; Nosarti, C. Eating Disorder Psychopathology, Brain Structure, Neuropsychological Correlates and Risk Mechanisms in Very Preterm Young Adults. *Eur. Eat. Disord. Rev.* **2015**, *23*, 147–155. [CrossRef]
90. Fagundo, A.B.; de la Torre, R.; Jiménez-Murcia, S.; Agüera, Z.; Granero, R.; Tárrega, S.; Botella, C.; Baños, R.; Fernández-Real, J.M.; Rodríguez, R.; et al. Executive Functions Profile in Extreme Eating/Weight Conditions: From Anorexia Nervosa to Obesity. *PLoS ONE* **2012**, *7*, e43382. [CrossRef]
91. Tchanturia, K.; Liao, P.-C.; Forcano, L.; Fernández-Aranda, F.; Uher, R.; Treasure, J.; Schmidt, U.; Penelo, E.; Granero, R.; Jiménez-Murcia, S.; et al. Poor Decision Making in Male Patients with Anorexia Nervosa. *Eur. Eat. Disord. Rev.* **2012**, *20*, 169–173. [CrossRef]
92. Tchanturia, K.; Campbell, I.C.; Morris, R.; Treasure, J. Neuropsychological studies in anorexia nervosa. *Int. J. Eat. Disord.* **2005**, *37*, S72–S76. [CrossRef]
93. Nikendei, C.; Friederich, H.C.; Weisbrod, M.; Walther, S.; Sharma, A.; Herzog, W.; Zipfel, S.; Bender, S. Event-related potentials during recognition of semantic and pictorial food stimuli in patients with anorexia nervosa and healthy controls with varying internal states of hunger. *Psychosom. Med.* **2012**, *74*, 136–145. [CrossRef] [PubMed]
94. Hatch, A.; Madden, S.; Kohn, M.R.; Clarke, S.; Touyz, S.; Gordon, E.; Williams, L.M. Emotion brain alterations in anorexia nervosa: A candidate biological marker and implications for treatment. *J. Psychiatry Neurosci.* **2010**, *35*, 267–274. [CrossRef] [PubMed]
95. Ellis, P.D. *The Essential Guide to Effect Sizes: Statistical Power, Meta-analysis, and the Interpretation of Research Results*; Cambridge University Press: Cambridge, MA, USA, 2010; ISBN 0521142466.
96. Van Autreve, S.; De Baene, W.; Baeken, C.; van Heeringen, C.; Vervaet, M. Do Restrictive and Bingeing/Purging Subtypes of Anorexia Nervosa Differ on Central Coherence and Set Shifting? *Eur. Eat. Disord. Rev.* **2013**, *21*, 308–314. [CrossRef] [PubMed]
97. Gorini, A.; Griez, E.; Petrova, A.; Riva, G. Assessment of the emotional responses produced by exposure to real food, virtual food and photographs of food in patients affected by eating disorders. *Ann. Gen. Psychiatry* **2010**, *9*, 30. [CrossRef] [PubMed]
98. Jáuregui-Lobera, I. Electroencephalography in eating disorders. *Neuropsychiatr. Dis. Treat.* **2012**, *8*, 1–11. [CrossRef]

99. Tóth, E.; Kondákor, I.; Túry, F.; Gáti, Á.; Weisz, J.; Molnár, M. Nonlinear and linear EEG complexity changes caused by gustatory stimuli in anorexia nervosa. *Int. J. Psychophysiol.* **2004**, *51*, 253–260. [CrossRef]
100. Wang, Y.; Yang, L.; Wang, Y. Suppression (but Not Reappraisal) Impairs Subsequent Error Detection: An ERP Study of Emotion Regulation's Resource-Depleting Effect. *PLoS ONE* **2014**, *9*, e96339. [CrossRef]

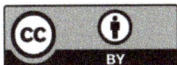

© 2020 by the authors. Licensee MDPI, Basel, Switzerland. This article is an open access article distributed under the terms and conditions of the Creative Commons Attribution (CC BY) license (http://creativecommons.org/licenses/by/4.0/).

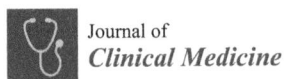

Article

Impulsivity, Emotional Dysregulation and Executive Function Deficits Could Be Associated with Alcohol and Drug Abuse in Eating Disorders

María Lozano-Madrid [1,2,3], Danielle Clark Bryan [4], Roser Granero [3,5], Isabel Sánchez [1,2,3], Nadine Riesco [1,2,3], Núria Mallorquí-Bagué [3,6], Susana Jiménez-Murcia [1,2,3,7], Janet Treasure [4] and Fernando Fernández-Aranda [1,2,3,7,*]

1. Department of Psychiatry, Bellvitge University Hospital-IDIBELL, 08907 L'Hospitalet de Llobregat, Barcelona, Spain; maria.lozano@bellvitgehospital.cat (M.L.-M.); isasanchez@bellvitgehospital.cat (I.S.); nriesco@bellvitgehospital.cat (N.R.); sjimenez@bellvitgehospital.cat (S.J.-M.)
2. Psychiatry and Mental Health Group, Neuroscience Program, Institut d'Investigació Biomèdica de Bellvitge—IDIBELL, 08907 L'Hospitalet de Llobregat, Barcelona, Spain
3. Ciber Fisiopatología Obesidad y Nutrición (CIBERobn), Instituto Salud Carlos III, 28029 Madrid, Spain; Roser.Granero@uab.cat (R.G.); nmallorqui@live.com (N.M.-B.)
4. Department of Psychological Medicine, Section of Eating Disorders, Institute of Psychiatry, Psychology and Neuroscience, King's College London, SE5 8AF London, UK; danielle.clarkbryan@kcl.ac.uk (D.C.B.); janet.treasure@kcl.ac.uk (J.T.)
5. Departament de Psicobiologia i Metodologia. Universitat Autònoma de Barcelona, 08035 Barcelona, Spain
6. Department of Psychiatry, Addictive Behavior Unit, Hospital de la Santa Creu i Sant Pau, Biomedical Research Institute Sant Pau, 08001 Barcelona, Spain
7. Department of Clinical Sciences, School of Medicine and Health Sciences, University of Barcelona, 08907 L'Hospitalet de Llobregat, Barcelona, Spain
* Correspondence: ffernandez@bellvitgehospital.cat; Tel.: +34-93-2607227; Fax: +34-93-2607193

Received: 28 May 2020; Accepted: 18 June 2020; Published: 21 June 2020

Abstract: Background: Empirical data suggests a high comorbid occurrence of eating disorders (EDs) and substance use disorders (SUDs), as well as neurological and psychological shared characteristics. However, no prior study has identified the neuropsychological features of this subgroup. This study examines the prevalence of alcohol and/or drug abuse (A/DA) symptoms in ED patients. It also compares the clinical features and neuropsychological performance of ED patients with and without A/DA symptoms. Methods: 145 participants (74.5% females) with various forms of diagnosed EDs underwent a comprehensive clinical (TCI-R, SCL-90-R and EDI-2) and neuropsychological assessment (Stroop, WCST and IGT). Results: Approximately 19% of ED patients (across ED subtypes) had A/DA symptoms. Those with A/DA symptoms showed more impulsive behaviours and higher levels of interoceptive awareness (EDI-2), somatisation (SCL-90-R) and novelty seeking (TCI-R). This group also had a lower score in the Stroop-words measure, made more perseverative errors in the WCST and showed a weaker learning trajectory in the IGT. Conclusions: ED patients with A/DA symptoms display a specific phenotype characterised by greater impulsive personality, emotional dysregulation and problems with executive control. Patients with these temperamental traits may be at high risk of developing a SUD.

Keywords: eating disorder; alcohol and/or drug abuse; substance use disorder; executive functions; impulsivity; emotional dysregulation

1. Introduction

Eating disorders (EDs) are mental illnesses characterized by abnormal eating behaviours, which normally lead to significant impairments in physical health and psychosocial functioning [1]. EDs often co-occur with other untreated mental conditions such as substance use disorders (SUDs) [2], summarised as the inability to control the usage or craving of substances despite problems related to their use [1]. A recent meta-analysis of 43 studies estimated that the lifetime prevalence of any SUD among adults with EDs is 25.4%, with tobacco, caffeine and alcohol most commonly abused [2]. The prevalence of substance abuse varies according to demographic factors (e.g., age, sex, ethnicity) and ED diagnostic subtype [2–4]. According to the above-mentioned meta-analysis [2], the lifetime prevalence of SUDs seems to be higher in female-sample studies (26%) compared to mixed studies (15%), in adult populations (26%) compared to young adults (19%) and in primarily Caucasian samples (24%) compared to Asian samples (7%). Similarly, several studies have reported a stronger association between substance abuse and bulimia nervosa (BN) compared to anorexia nervosa (AN) [3,4]. Overall, it seems that those ED patients with purging behaviours are at higher risk of developing a comorbid SUD [2,5].

This comorbidity might be due to shared biological and psychological endophenotypes [6]. Genetic studies reveal that EDs and SUDs share overlapping genetic risk factors, especially those ED subtypes characterized by binge-purge behaviours [7,8]. Personality traits such as impulsivity are also shared [9–11], as are the elevated rates of psychopathology (especially social anxiety, antisocial behaviour, and cluster B and C personality disorders) and emotional dysregulation [12–14]. Neuropsychological impairments are another common feature [15–27], especially in executive functions (i.e., high-level cognitive processes implicated in the formation of successful goal-directed behaviours [28]). Difficulties in decision-making, cognitive flexibility and inhibitory control have been reported in all ED subtypes [15–20], as well as in SUD patients [21–27]. However, no studies have explored neuropsychological performance in ED patients with substance abuse comorbidity.

Empirical data on the comorbidity of EDs and SUDs, as well as their biological and psychological shared characteristics are available. However, there are no prior studies which have assessed the neuropsychological profile in ED patients with substance abuse symptomatology. Identifying these neuropsychological features might help to develop specific treatments that target these deficits with the purpose of preventing the later evolution into a SUD. As such, the first aim of this study was to examine the prevalence of alcohol and/or drug abuse (A/DA) symptoms in a heterogeneous series of ED patients. Our hypothesis was that A/DA symptoms would be most common in those with binge-purge behaviours. A second aim was to compare clinical (i.e., eating symptomatology, general psychopathology and personality traits) and neuropsychological features (i.e., decision-making, cognitive flexibility and inhibitory control) of patients with or without A/DA symptoms. Our hypothesis was that ED patients with A/DA symptoms will display higher impulsivity and emotional dysregulation, along with poorer executive functions.

2. Materials and Methods

2.1. Participants

The total sample comprised of 145 participants (74.5% females) aged between 18 and 60 years old. All participants were diagnosed with an ED by experienced clinicians according to the DSM-5 diagnostic criteria [1]. The final sample included: AN-restrictive subtype [AN-R] ($n = 57$), AN-binge/purge subtype [AN-BP] ($n = 26$), BN ($n = 28$), binge eating disorder [BED] ($n = 22$) and other specified feeding or eating disorder [OSFED] ($n = 12$).

Participants were recruited at the *Eating Disorders Unit* within the Department of Psychiatry at Bellvitge University Hospital (Barcelona, Spain), where they were receiving outpatient treatment. All participants were informed about the research procedures and gave their informed consent in writing. Procedures were approved by the Ethical Committee of the above-mentioned institution in accordance with the Helsinki Declaration of 1975 as revised in 1983 (reference: PR146/14). Exclusion criteria were the following: (1) history of chronic medical illness or neurological condition that might affect cognitive function; (2) head trauma with loss of consciousness for more than 2 min, learning disability or intellectual disability; (3) use of psycho-active medications or drugs; (4) age under 18 or over 60 (to discard neuropsychological deficits associated with the age).

2.2. Procedure and Assessment

As part of the protocol, all patients who arrived at the *Eating Disorders Unit* seeking treatment for an ED were assessed by experienced clinicians using a semi-structured clinical interview based on the DSM-5 diagnostic criteria [1]. All patients consecutively diagnosed with an ED were screened for the inclusion criteria of the study. Those who met the criteria and voluntarily accepted to be part of the study underwent a comprehensive neuropsychological and clinical assessment within the first week of their outpatient treatment. Weight and Body Mass Index (BMI) were measured for all subjects on the day of assessment. Additional sociodemographic information was also taken. The neuropsychological tests were selected to cover various aspects of executive functions including decision-making, response inhibition, strategic planning and cognitive flexibility and were administered by a trained psychologist in a single session and in a randomised order. Finally, information regarding the presence or absence of impulsive behaviours (including alcohol abuse, drugs abuse, binge episodes, theft, kleptomania and compulsive buying) was taken from the semi-structured clinical interview. The presence of A/DA symptoms was defined as the confirmation of current or lifetime behaviours of alcohol abuse, illicit drug abuse or both, causing significant distress or impairments in daily functioning.

2.2.1. Psychopathological/Personality Measures

Semi-structured clinical interview: This interview is based on the ED module of the Structured Clinical Interview for DSM-5 (SCID-5 [29]) and is used to ascertain the presence of a current ED according to the DSM-5 criteria. It provides specific information regarding the symptomatology and course of the ED. It also includes other questions in relation to the impulsive behaviours frequently found in ED patients, such us alcohol abuse, drug abuse, theft, compulsive buying, etc.

The *Temperament and Character Inventory-Revised* (TCI-R [30]; Spanish validation [31]) is a reliable and valid 240-item questionnaire that measures seven personality dimensions: four temperament dimensions (novelty seeking, harm avoidance, reward dependence and persistence) and three about character (self-directedness, cooperativeness and self-transcendence). The scales in the revised version showed a mean internal consistency of 0.87 (α coefficient).

The *Symptom Checklist-90 Revised* (SCL-90-R [32]; Spanish validation [33]) is a 90-item questionnaire which evaluates psychopathological symptoms; these are grouped as follows: somatization, obsessive-compulsive, interpersonal sensitive, depression, anxiety, hostility, phobic anxiety, paranoia and psychotic. It also includes a global severity index (GSI), designed to measure overall psychological distress. This instrument has demonstrated satisfactory psychometric properties in the Spanish version, obtaining a mean internal consistency of 0.75 (α coefficient).

The *Eating Disorders Inventory-2* (EDI-2 [34]; Spanish validation [35]) is a 91-item self-report questionnaire that assesses the following ED factors: drive for thinness, bulimia, body dissatisfaction, ineffectiveness, perfectionism, interpersonal distrust, interoceptive awareness, maturity fears, asceticism, impulse regulation and social insecurity. This instrument was validated in a Spanish population with a mean internal consistency of 0.63 (α coefficient).

2.2.2. Neuropsychological Measures

The Stroop Colour and Word Test (SCWT [36]; Spanish version [37]) is an extensively used neuropsychological test to assess inhibitory control (including response inhibition and interference control). It consists of three different lists: a word list containing the names of colours printed in black ink, a colour list that comprises letter Xs printed in colour and a colour-word list comprised of names of colours in a colour ink that does not match the written name. Three final scores are obtained based on the number of items that the participant is able to read on each of the three lists in a time window of 45 s. An interference score is computed from all three lists. A higher score is interpreted as better inhibitory control.

The Wisconsin Card Sorting Test (WCST [38]) is a computerized set-shifting task for assessing cognitive flexibility. It includes 128 cards that vary according to three attributes: number (N), colour (C) and shape (S). The participant has to pile the cards beneath four reference cards that also vary along these same dimensions, and in order to succeed, they have to settle upon a predetermined sorting rule. The only feedback given to the participant is the word "right" or "wrong" after each sorting. Initially, C is the correct sorting category, and positive feedback is given only if the card is placed in the pile with the same colour. After 10 consecutive correct sorts, the rule changes. Thus, the positive feedback is only given when the sorting matches the new category. By trial and error, the participant must learn to change the sorting categories according to the given feedback. There are up to six attempts to derive a rule, providing rule shifts in the following category sequence: C-S-N-C-S-N. Participants are not informed of the correct sorting principle and that the sorting principle shifts during the test. The test is completed when all 128 cards are sorted or after the six full categories are completed. The number of completed categories, the percentage of perseverative errors (i.e., failures to change sorting strategy after negative feedback) and the percentage of non-perseverative errors are recorded.

The Iowa Gambling Task (IGT [39]) is a computerized task to evaluate decision-making, which has also been proposed as a measure of choice impulsivity [40]. It involves a total of 100 turns distributed across four decks of cards (A, B, C and D), and each time the participant selects a deck, a specified amount of play money is awarded. The interspersed rewards among these decks are probabilistic punishments (monetary losses with different amounts). Participants are instructed that the final aim of the task is to win as much money as possible and to avoid losing as much money as possible. Moreover, they may choose cards from any deck, and switch decks at any time. This test is scored by subtracting the number of cards selected from decks A and B from the number of cards selected from decks C and D. Decks A and B are not advantageous as the final loss is higher than the final gain; however, decks C and D are advantageous since the punishments are smaller. Higher scores indicate better performance on the task.

2.3. Statistical Analyses

Statistical analysis was carried out with Stata16 for Windows [41]. The comparisons between the groups with and without A/DA symptoms were based on T-TEST procedures for quantitative variables and chi-square tests (χ^2) for categorical variables. The effect size of the mean differences in the clinical variables was estimated with Cohen's-d coefficient, considering null effect for $|d| < 0.20$, low-poor for $|d| > 0.20$, moderate-medium for $|d| > 0.5$ and large-high for $|d| > 0.8$ [42]. The significance tests were complemented with other standardised measures of the effect size: partial eta-squared coefficients (η^2), which measures the proportion of the total variance in a criterion associated with the membership of the different groups, defined by the independent variable once the potential effects of other predictors and interactions are partialled out (in one way ANOVA, eta-squared and partial eta-squared come out the same, but in multivariate ANOVA, their values differ). The comparisons between the proportions were based on the Cohen's-h coefficient, a standardised measure of the distance between the proportions obtained in two groups; it is estimated as the difference of the arcsine transformation for the two probabilities [43]. In addition, and due the multiple statistical comparisons performed on the clinical and neuropsychological variables, Finner-correction was used to control the increase in the Type-I error [44]. Finner-method uses a stepwise multiple comparisons procedure, which solves the monotonicity of the critical values by means of an inequality for the distribution function of the statistic range, using the principle of family-wise Type I correction. The post-hoc power calculation was also conducted for each observed effect based on the sample size and the parameter estimates, defining an alpha value $\alpha = 0.05$.

A 2 × 5 mixed analysis of variance was obtained to analyse the learning curve in the IGT test. For this analysis, the group was defined as the between-subjects factor (2 levels: with versus without

A/DA) and the IGT-block as the within-subjects factor (5 levels: blocks 1 to 5). Tests of within-subjects included polynomial contrasts for assessing the presence of trends in the mean estimates (linear, quadratic, cubic and order-4). Effect size of the parameter estimates were assessed with eta-squared values (η^2).

3. Results

3.1. Characteristics of the Sample

Most participants were women (108, 74.5%), born in Spain (130, 89.7%) and single (105, 72.4%). Mean chronological age was 30.3 years (SD = 10.3), age of ED onset was 22.7 years (SD = 9.1) and duration of the ED symptoms 7.7 years (SD = 7.4). The prevalence of impulsive behaviours was 43.1% for binges episodes, 18.6% for theft, 3.4% for kleptomania and 11.0% for compulsive buying. No participants reported instances of problematic gambling behaviours.

Table 1 shows the comparison between the groups with and without A/DA symptoms. Statistical differences were found for the presence of impulsive behaviours (higher prevalence among patients with A/DA).

Table 1. Descriptive of the sample.

		Without A/DA		With A/DA		p
		n = 118		n = 27		
		n	%	n	%	
Sex	Women	88	74.6%	20	74.1%	0.957
	Men	30	25.4%	7	25.9%	
ED subtype	Anorexia restrictive	49	41.5%	8	29.6%	0.751
	Anorexia binge/purge	20	16.9%	6	22.2%	
	Bulimia	21	17.8%	7	25.9%	
	Binge eating disorder	18	15.3%	4	14.8%	
	Other specified feeding eating dis.	10	8.5%	2	7.4%	
Education	Primary	30	25.4%	10	37.0%	0.438
	Secondary	52	44.1%	11	40.7%	
	University	36	30.5%	6	22.2%	
		Mean	SD	Mean	SD	p
	Age (years-old)	30.30	10.13	30.56	11.22	0.907
	Onset of the ED (years-old)	22.94	8.99	21.59	9.83	0.491
	Duration of the ED (years)	7.36	7.58	8.96	6.72	0.312
	BMI (kg/m^2)	21.70	8.47	22.50	8.87	0.663
	Other impulsive behaviours	n	%	n	%	p
	Binges episodes	46	39.3%	16	59.3%	0.049 *
	Theft	18	15.3%	9	33.3%	0.029 *
	Kleptomania	2	1.7%	3	11.1%	0.045 *
	Compulsive buying	10	8.5%	6	22.2%	0.040 *

A/DA: alcohol and/or drugs abuse symptoms. ED: eating disorder. BMI: body mass index. SD: standard deviation.
*: significant comparison (0.05 level).

3.2. Prevalence of A/DA in ED Patients

The number of patients with A/DA symptoms was 27 (prevalence = 18.6%). Table 2 compares prevalence estimates between ED subtypes and gender. No differences by gender (women (18.5%) and men (18.9%) ($\chi^2 = 0.01$, $df = 1$, $p = 0.957$)) or subtype (14.0% for AN-R, 23.1% for AN-BP, 25.0% for BN, 18.2% for BED and 16.7% for OSFED ($\chi^2 = 1.92$, $df = 4$, $p = 0.751$)) were found. The highest effect size for the comparison between AN-R and BN was a Cohen's-h into the low range $|h| = 0.28$.

Table 2. Prevalence estimate of A/DA depending on ED subtype and gender.

Total		AN-R		AN-BP		BN		BED		OSFED		Women		Men	
$n = 145$		$n = 57$		$n = 26$		$n = 28$		$n = 22$		$n = 12$		$n = 108$		$n = 37$	
n	%	n	%	n	%	n	%	n	%	n	%	n	%	n	%
27	18.6%	8	14.0%	6	23.1%	7	25.0%	4	18.2%	2	16.7%	20	18.5%	7	18.9%
χ^2	1.92	(df = 4)										0.01	(df = 1)		
p	0.751											0.957			

AN-R: anorexia restrictive. AN-BP: anorexia binge/purge. BN: bulimia. BED: binge eating disorder. OSFED: other specified feeding eating disorder. df: degrees of freedom.

3.3. Comparison of the Clinical and Neuropsychological Profile of Patients with and without A/DA

Table 3 compares the clinical measures of patients with and without A/DA symptoms. Those with A/DA had higher levels of interoceptive awareness (EDI-2), somatisation (SCL-90-R) and novelty seeking (TCI-R). Internal consistency in the sample of the study was between good to excellent for all the psychometrical scales (Cronbach's alpha values).

Table 3. Comparison of the clinical profile between groups with and without A/DA.

		Without A/DA		With A/DA					
	α	$n = 118$		$n = 27$		p	|d|	η^2	Power
		Mean	SD	Mean	SD				
EDI Drive for thinness	0.846	11.24	6.65	12.10	6.50	0.544	0.13	0.003	0.093
EDI Body dissatisfaction	0.922	13.35	8.86	15.66	7.70	0.213	0.28	0.011	0.237
EDI Interoceptive awareness	0.868	8.98	7.13	12.10	5.95	0.036 *	0.52 †	0.030	0.556
EDI Bulimia	0.791	4.92	5.20	6.51	4.83	0.148	0.32	0.015	0.303
EDI Interpersonal distrust	0.824	5.59	4.84	5.92	4.47	0.752	0.07	0.001	0.061
EDI Ineffectiveness	0.905	8.61	6.89	10.78	6.91	0.142	0.32	0.015	0.312
EDI Maturity fears	0.841	7.54	5.08	7.58	5.89	0.975	0.01	0.001	0.050
EDI Perfectionism	0.842	5.31	4.40	5.16	4.54	0.878	0.03	0.001	0.053
EDI Impulse regulation	0.850	5.43	5.85	5.60	4.43	0.886	0.03	0.001	0.052
EDI Ascetic	0.703	5.99	4.37	6.92	3.76	0.307	0.23	0.007	0.175
EDI Social insecurity	0.825	6.37	5.17	7.28	5.72	0.417	0.17	0.005	0.127
EDI Total score	0.974	83.33	48.73	95.62	42.19	0.228	0.27	0.010	0.225
SCL-90R Somatization	0.857	1.45	0.90	1.82	0.77	0.049 *	0.44	0.026	0.497
SCL-90-R Obsessive-compulsive	0.909	1.57	0.98	1.78	0.89	0.308	0.22	0.007	0.174
SCL-90-R Interpersonal sensitive	0.912	1.76	1.04	1.94	0.91	0.416	0.18	0.005	0.128
SCL-90-R Depression	0.946	2.00	1.05	2.21	0.82	0.329	0.22	0.007	0.164
SCL-90-R Anxiety	0.911	1.38	0.95	1.66	0.74	0.145	0.34	0.015	0.307
SCL-90-R Hostility	0.774	1.17	0.88	1.25	0.97	0.672	0.09	0.001	0.071
SCL-90-R Phobic anxiety	0.854	0.78	0.87	0.86	0.73	0.667	0.10	0.001	0.072
SCL-90-R Paranoia	0.875	1.27	0.89	1.32	0.81	0.821	0.05	0.001	0.056
SCL-90-R Psychotic	0.893	1.17	0.77	1.28	0.67	0.529	0.14	0.003	0.096
SCL-90-R GSI	0.980	1.50	0.82	1.69	0.68	0.257	0.26	0.009	0.204
SCL-90-R PST	0.980	56.61	19.91	63.15	17.64	0.119	0.35	0.017	0.345
SCL-90-R PSDI	0.980	2.20	0.66	2.32	0.42	0.383	0.21	0.005	0.140
TCI-R Novelty seeking	0.797	94.68	13.80	103.37	13.83	0.004 *	0.63 †	0.057	0.834
TCI-R Harm avoidance	0.925	112.31	20.84	116.07	21.50	0.402	0.18	0.005	0.133
TCI-R Reward dependence	0.700	101.21	15.47	102.56	17.33	0.691	0.08	0.001	0.068
TCI-R Persistence	0.860	114.12	20.30	107.33	24.13	0.133	0.30	0.016	0.323
TCI-R Self-directedness	0.908	125.72	21.84	119.33	24.19	0.181	0.28	0.012	0.266
TCI-R Cooperativeness	0.831	136.66	17.28	135.89	15.97	0.832	0.05	0.001	0.055
TCI-R Self-transcendence	0.893	63.16	15.28	63.37	18.91	0.951	0.01	0.001	0.050

SD: standard deviation. Cronbach's alpha in the sample. *: significant comparison (0.05 level). †: effect size into the moderate (|d| > 0.50) to high range (|d| > 0.80). p-values with Finner-correction.

Table 4 shows the comparison of the neuropsychological profile. Higher scores in perseverative errors (WCST) and in the first block of the IGT and lower scores in the Stroop-words measure were found.

Table 4. Comparison of the neuropsychological profile between groups with and without A/DA.

	Without A/DA n = 118		With A/DA n = 27		p	|d|	η^2	Power
	Mean	SD	Mean	SD				
Stroop Words	104.43	19.39	95.61	24.53	0.045 *	0.40	0.028	0.521
Stroop Colour	75.84	16.06	80.24	19.74	0.221	0.24	0.010	0.231
Stroop Words-colour	48.27	11.75	46.50	9.33	0.467	0.17	0.004	0.112
Stroop Interference	5.09	8.99	4.42	7.92	0.725	0.08	0.001	0.064
WCST Total trials	94.42	20.72	100.55	20.70	0.168	0.30	0.013	0.280
WCST Correct	67.83	10.87	68.06	14.02	0.924	0.02	0.001	0.051
WCST Perseverative errors	12.40	10.33	18.54	19.41	0.023 *	0.39	0.036	0.629
WCST Non-perseverative errors	14.20	15.25	14.22	11.91	0.993	0.01	0.001	0.050
WCST Conceptual	60.64	16.54	59.18	19.97	0.692	0.08	0.001	0.068
WCST Categories completed	5.10	1.80	4.88	1.98	0.577	0.12	0.002	0.086
WCST Trials completed 1st categ.	20.36	24.17	26.73	31.78	0.248	0.23	0.009	0.210
IGT Block 1	−2.59	4.21	−0.62	2.84	0.023 *	0.55 †	0.036	0.629
IGT Block 2	−1.11	4.91	0.32	4.41	0.165	0.31	0.013	0.284
IGT Block 3	0.29	5.80	−1.39	3.55	0.152	0.35	0.014	0.298
IGT Block 4	0.38	6.69	0.68	6.67	0.834	0.04	0.001	0.055
IGT Block 5	0.51	7.78	0.06	5.42	0.777	0.07	0.001	0.059
IGT Total	−2.52	20.79	−0.95	11.51	0.704	0.09	0.001	0.067

SD: standard deviation. *: significant comparison (0.05 level). †: effect size into the moderate (|d| > 0.50) to high range (|d| > 0.80). p-values with Finner-correction.

The results of the mixed ANOVA obtained to analyse the learning curve in the IGT showed a quasi-significant interaction parameter IGT-by-Group ($F_{(3.42;488.5)}$ = 2.02, p = 0.091, η^2 = 0.014; Greenhouse–Geisser adjusted) as well as a main effect of the IGT-block ($F_{(3.42;488.5)}$ = 2.65, p = 0.041, η^2 = 0.018). Figure 1 shows the adjusted mean net scores in the blocks, showing a learning trajectory only for patients without A/DA symptoms: Among this group, polynomial contrasts for the IGT-block showed a significant linear trend ($F_{(1;117)}$ = 18.3, p < 0.001, η^2 = 0.135) and a significant quadratic trend ($F_{(1;117)}$ = 6.97, p = 0.009, η^2 = 0.056), while non-significant results were found for the cubic ($F_{(1;117)}$ = 0.01, p = 0.931 η^2 = 0.001) and order 4 ($F_{(1;117)}$ = 0.59, p = 0.442, η^2 = 0.005) trends. In patients without A/DA symptoms, post-hoc pairwise comparisons defining the difference-type contrasts (based on comparing each block with the previous) showed statistical differences between blocks 2 versus block 1 (p = 0.008) and block 3 versus block 2 (p = 0.011), while no statistical differences were found between blocks 4 versus block 3 (p = 0.886) and block 5 versus block 4 (p = 0.832). However, patients with A/DA symptoms did not have significant results (linear: $F_{(1;26)}$ = 0.27, p = 0.607, η^2 = 0.010; quadratic: $F_{(1;26)}$ = 0.06, p = 0.815, η^2 = 0.002; cubic: $F_{(1;26)}$ = 0.01, p = 0.988, η^2 = 0.001; order 4: $F_{(1;26)}$ = 2.30, p = 0.141, η^2 = 0.081). No statistical differences were found in the post-hoc pairwise comparisons comparing the IGT blocks among patients who reported the presence of A/DA.

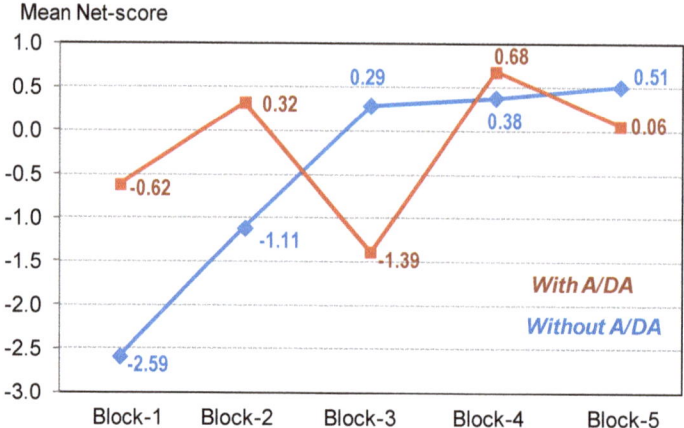

Figure 1. Learning curve in the IGT measure. Note. A/DA: alcohol and/or drug abuse. Sample size: $n = 145$.

4. Discussion

The first aim of this study was to assess the prevalence of A/DA symptoms in a sample of patients across the range of ED diagnoses. The lifetime A/DA prevalence was similar to that found previously in ED patients [2], although slightly lower. This small difference could be explained by the fact that we only assessed symptoms of alcohol and illicit drugs abuse, whereas previous studies considered other substances such as tobacco and caffeine [2]. Although this study had insufficient power to detect differences between subtypes, the trends were in the same direction as previous studies, with BN patients showing the highest prevalence [2–5] and those with AN-BP higher than those with AN-R [45], confirming our first hypothesis based on previous studies. We failed to find the gender difference in prevalence observed in a previous systematic review [2]; however, this might be a question of low power and methodology. While our study compares female and male patients within the same sample, Bahji et al. [2] compared the prevalence observed in female sample studies to mixed studies.

When comparing the clinical profile, the A/DA group scored higher on interoceptive awareness subscale (EDI-2), which indicates a poorer ability to recognise and differentiate between hunger and satiety and emotional states [34]. In ED patients, emotional dysregulation is associated with difficulties in controlling impulsive behaviours (e.g., compulsive binging, purging and overeating) in both negative and positive states [46,47], and this may lead to abuse of alcohol and drugs [13,14]. Indeed, the weaker interoceptive awareness previously found in individuals with BN [48] may explain their higher vulnerability to develop comorbid A/DA symptoms [3,4].

Moreover, the A/DA group had higher levels of somatisation (SCL-90-R), the experience of psychological distress in the presence of unexplained physical symptoms [49]. It is suggested that patients experiencing high levels of somatising symptoms use substances to numb uncomfortable experiences [49]. Furthermore, somatising symptoms are closely associated with symptoms of substance intoxication or withdrawal, but whether they are a cause or effect of substance abuse remains unclear [50]. In any case, our results seem to reflect this association between somatising and substance abuse symptoms, yet longitudinal studies would be needed to clarify the direction of these interactions.

The group with A/DA symptoms had higher scores for the novelty seeking trait (TCI-R), mainly related to impulsivity [30]. Our findings align with other neurobehavioural research, which suggests that novelty seeking is associated with vulnerability to substance abuse [10,11] and with the finding of a higher prevalence of binge episodes, theft, kleptomania and compulsive buying in this subgroup. Strong associations among all the impulsive behaviours mentioned above are documented in the literature. For instance, ED patients who engage in binge-purge behaviours frequently display high prevalence of SUD [2–5,45] and compulsive buying [51,52]. Similarly, several studies have reported high rates of SUDs in individuals with kleptomania and compulsive buying [53,54].

The neuropsychological assessment results revealed that ED patients with A/DA symptoms display significantly lower scores in the Stroop-words measure, demonstrating a poorer reading ability in terms of speed and accuracy [36]. Contrary to expectations, no differences between groups were found in the Stroop-interference measure, meaning no differences in inhibitory control [36]. Impairments in inhibitory control are found to be a core deficit among binge/purge-type EDs [15,16] and SUDs [21,23], especially when examining stimuli related to each disorder (e.g., food, body shape, use of substances, etc.) [15,55,56]. Since inhibitory deficits seem to represent a risk factor for the development of both disorders separately, we expected to find greater inhibitory control impairments when both disorders co-occur. The fact that we failed to find this result might be explained because of the limited statistical power of this study. Further studies with larger samples are needed to clarify this issue.

In addition, patients with A/DA symptoms made more perseverative errors (WCST). Previous research demonstrated that individuals with EDs perform worse on set-shifting tasks than healthy individuals, which translates to poorer cognitive flexibility and higher rigidity [17,18]. Reduced cognitive flexibility has also been observed in individuals with SUDs, which may negatively impact on their problem-solving strategies [24,25]. In summary, poor cognitive flexibility is shown to be a common feature in EDs and SUDs, and our results point out that it might be highlighted when both disorders are present at the same time. However, due to the relatively small sample size of one of the groups and the low statistical power, our results should be interpreted with caution until more evidence is available.

Lastly, even though no differences between groups were found on the IGT total score, both groups displayed an impaired decision-making performance in comparison to healthy population [18,57,58]. However, when comparing the learning curve of both groups, patients with A/DA symptoms showed a weaker learning trajectory and greater difficulties to learn the reward/punishment contingencies of their choices [59]. Our results point out that decision-making problems seem to be present in ED patients [18–20], particularly in those with comorbid substance abuse symptomatology. Once again, future studies are needed to confirm this finding.

The results of this study should be interpreted in the context of some limitations. First, although our sample size is relatively large, the subgroups vary in size, and one of them is relatively small, leading to a low statistical power. Studies with small samples are severely underpowered, which might represent a concern if the "null hypothesis" cannot be rejected. For this reason, the significance tests were complemented with other standardized measure of the effect size. In any case, the results of this study should be interpreted with caution and considering this limitation. Furthermore, because the design is cross-sectional, claims regarding causality cannot be made. Future longitudinal studies should examine the extent to which psychopathology and cognitive function improve after treatment. Another limitation was the lack of a formal diagnosis of SUD in our sample. Finally, our sample was largely made up of young adults, and it would be of clinical interest to explore whether similar impairments in neuropsychological functioning are present in older samples.

5. Conclusions

To conclude, although previous studies have explored comorbidity between EDs and SUDs, this is the first study to explore gender differences. Moreover, it is the first to assess the neuropsychological profile in ED patients with A/DA symptoms. We found that this subgroup displays a specific phenotype characterised by greater impulsivity (i.e., high novelty seeking and difficulties to control impulsive behaviours), noticeable emotional dysregulation (i.e., decreased interoceptive awareness) and more impaired executive control (i.e., low cognitive flexibility and poor decision-making). Of future benefit would be the consolidation of our findings in larger samples and clarifying if these deficits are involved in the development and maintenance of substance abuse comorbidity. As such, this subgroup of ED patients might benefit from augmented treatment that targets these problems, such as inhibitory control training [60], emotion regulation training [61] or cognitive remediation therapy [62]. This may reduce the present substance abuse symptomatology and prevent later evolution into a SUD, as previous studies have reported that ED patients who do not receive any adjunctive treatment for substance abuse are at high risk for switching from one problematic behaviour to the other, especially during the recovery process [2].

Author Contributions: Conceptualization, M.L.-M., F.F.-A., S.J.-M. and J.T.; methodology, M.L.-M. and F.F.-A.; formal analysis, R.G.; data curation, M.L.-M. and N.M.-B.; investigation, I.S. and N.R.; writing—original draft preparation, M.L.-M. and D.C.B.; writing—review and editing, M.L.-M., D.C.B., F.F.-A. and J.T.; funding acquisition, F.F.-A., M.L.-M. and J.T. All authors have read and agreed to the published version of the manuscript.

Funding: We thank CERCA Program/Generalitat de Catalunya for institutional support. This manuscript and research were supported by grants from the Instituto de Salud Carlos III (ISCIII) [FIS PI17/01167] and cofounded by FEDER funds/European Regional Development Fund (ERDF), a way to build Europe. CIBER Fisiopatología de la Obesidad y Nutrición (CIBERobn) is an initiative of ISCIII. M.L.-M. is supported by a predoctoral grant of the Ministerio de Educación, Cultura y Deporte (FPU15/02911). J.T. acknowledges financial support from the National Institute for Health Research (NIHR), Specialist Biomedical Research Centre for Mental Health award to the South London and Maudsley NHS Foundation Trust and the Institute of Psychiatry, King's College London.

Conflicts of Interest: The authors declare no conflicts of interest. The funders had no role in the design of the study; in the collection, analyses or interpretation of data; in the writing of the manuscript or in the decision to publish the results.

References

1. American Psychiatric Association. *Diagnostic and Statistical Manual of Mental Disorders*, 5th ed.; American Psychiatric Association: Washington, DC, USA, 2013.
2. Bahji, A.; Mazhar, M.N.; Hudson, C.C.; Nadkarni, P.; MacNeil, B.A.; Hawken, E. Prevalence of substance use disorder comorbidity among individuals with eating disorders: A systematic review and meta-analysis. *Psychiatry Res.* **2019**, *273*, 58–66. [CrossRef] [PubMed]
3. Hudson, J.I.; Hiripi, E.; Pope, H.G.; Kessler, R.C. The Prevalence and Correlates of Eating Disorders in the National Comorbidity Survey Replication. *Biol. Psychiatry* **2007**, *61*, 348–358. [CrossRef] [PubMed]
4. Fouladi, F.; Mitchell, J.E.; Crosby, R.D.; Engel, S.G.; Crow, S.; Hill, L.; Le Grange, D.; Powers, P.; Steffen, K.J. Prevalence of Alcohol and Other Substance Use in Patients with Eating Disorders. *Eur. Eat. Disord. Rev.* **2015**, *23*, 531–536. [CrossRef] [PubMed]
5. Dennis, A.B.; Pryor, T. The Complex Relationship between Eating Disorders and Substance Use Disorders. In *Clinical Handbook of Complex and Atypical Eating Disorders*; Anderson, L.K., Murray, S.B., Kaye, W.H., Eds.; Oxford University Press: New York, NY, USA, 2017; pp. 60–78.
6. Harrop, E.N.; Marlatt, G.A. The comorbidity of substance use disorders and eating disorders in women: Prevalence, etiology, and treatment. *Addict. Behav.* **2010**, *35*, 392–398. [CrossRef] [PubMed]
7. Munn-Chernoff, M.A.; Baker, J.H. A Primer on the Genetics of Comorbid Eating Disorders and Substance Use Disorders. *Eur. Eat. Disord. Rev.* **2016**, *24*, 91–100. [CrossRef] [PubMed]
8. Munn-Chernoff, M.A.; Johnson, E.C.; Chou, Y.L.; Coleman, J.R.I.; Thornton, L.M.; Walters, R.K.; Yilmaz, Z.; Baker, J.H.; Hübel, C.; Gordon, S.; et al. Shared genetic risk between eating disorder- and substance-use-related phenotypes: Evidence from genome-wide association studies. *Addict. Biol.* **2020**. [CrossRef]
9. Krug, I.; Pinheiro, A.P.; Bulik, C.; Jiménez-Murcia, S.; Granero, R.; Penelo, E.; Masuet, C.; Agüera, Z.; Fernández-Aranda, F. Lifetime substance abuse, family history of alcohol abuse/dependence and novelty seeking in eating disorders: Comparison study of eating disorder subgroups. *Psychiatry Clin. Neurosci.* **2009**, *63*, 82–87. [CrossRef]
10. Fernández-Mondragón, S.; Adan, A. Personality in male patients with substance use disorder and/or severe mental illness. *Psychiatry Res.* **2015**, *228*, 488–494. [CrossRef]
11. Wingo, T.; Nesil, T.; Choi, J.S.; Li, M.D. Novelty Seeking and Drug Addiction in Humans and Animals: From Behavior to Molecules. *J. Neuroimmune Pharmcol.* **2016**, *11*, 456–470. [CrossRef]
12. Lilenfeld, L.R.; Kaye, W.H.; Greeno, C.G.; Merikangas, K.R.; Plotnicov, K.; Pollice, C.; Rao, R.; Strober, M.; Bulik, C.M.; Nagy, L. Psychiatric disorders in women with bulimia nervosa and their first-degree relatives: Effects of comorbid substance dependence. *Int. J. Eat. Disord.* **1997**, *22*, 253–264. [CrossRef]

13. Sloan, E.; Hall, K.; Moulding, R.; Bryce, S.; Mildred, H.; Staiger, P.K. Emotion regulation as a transdiagnostic treatment construct across anxiety, depression, substance, eating and borderline personality disorders: A systematic review. *Clin. Psychol. Rev.* **2017**, *57*, 141–163. [CrossRef]
14. Aldao, A.; Nolen-Hoeksema, S. Specificity of cognitive emotion regulation strategies: A transdiagnostic examination. *Behav. Res. Ther.* **2010**, *48*, 974–983. [CrossRef]
15. Wu, M.; Hartmann, M.; Skunde, M.; Herzog, W.; Friederich, H.-C. Inhibitory Control in Bulimic-Type Eating Disorders: A Systematic Review and Meta-Analysis. *PLoS ONE* **2013**, *8*, e83412. [CrossRef]
16. Lavagnino, L.; Arnone, D.; Cao, B.; Soares, J.C.; Selvaraj, S. Inhibitory control in obesity and binge eating disorder: A systematic review and meta-analysis of neurocognitive and neuroimaging studies. *Neurosci. Biobehav. Rev.* **2016**, *68*, 714–726. [CrossRef]
17. Roberts, M.E.; Tchanturia, K.; Treasure, J.L. Overlapping neurocognitive inefficiencies in anorexia nervosa: A preliminary investigation of women with both poor set-shifting and weak central coherence. *Eat. Weight Disord. Stud. Anorex. Bulim. Obes.* **2016**, *21*, 725–729. [CrossRef]
18. Aloi, M.; Rania, M.; Caroleo, M.; Bruni, A.; Palmieri, A.; Cauteruccio, M.A.; De Fazio, P.; Segura-García, C. Decision making, central coherence and set-shifting: A comparison between Binge Eating Disorder, Anorexia Nervosa and Healthy Controls. *BMC Psychiatry* **2015**, *15*, 1–10. [CrossRef]
19. Fagundo, A.B.; de la Torre, R.; Jiménez-Murcia, S.; Agüera, Z.; Granero, R.; Tárrega, S.; Botella, C.; Baños, R.; Fernández-Real, J.M.; Rodríguez, R.; et al. Executive Functions Profile in Extreme Eating/Weight Conditions: From Anorexia Nervosa to Obesity. *PLoS ONE* **2012**, *7*, e43382. [CrossRef]
20. Guillaume, S.; Gorwood, P.; Jollant, F.; Van den Eynde, F.; Courtet, P.; Richard-Devantoy, S. Impaired decision-making in symptomatic anorexia and bulimia nervosa patients: A meta-analysis. *Psychol. Med.* **2015**, *45*, 3377–3391. [CrossRef]
21. Luijten, M.; Machielsen, M.W.J.; Veltman, D.J.; Hester, R.; de Haan, L.; Franken, I.H.A. Systematic review of ERP and fMRI studies investigating inhibitory control and error processing in people with substance dependence and behavioural addictions. *J. Psychiatry Neurosci.* **2014**, *39*, 149–169. [CrossRef]
22. Allen, D.N.; Woods, S.P. *Neuropsychological Aspects of Substance Use Disorders: Evidence-Based Perspectives*; Oxford University Press: New York, NY, USA, 2014; ISBN 9780199930838.
23. Ersche, K.D.; Turton, A.J.; Chamberlain, S.R.; Müller, U.; Bullmore, E.T.; Robbins, T.W. Cognitive dysfunction and anxious-impulsive personality traits are endophenotypes for drug dependence. *Am. J. Psychiatry* **2012**, *169*, 926–936. [CrossRef]
24. Fernández-Serrano, M.J.; Pérez-García, M.; Verdejo-García, A. What are the specific vs. generalized effects of drugs of abuse on neuropsychological performance? *Neurosci. Biobehav. Rev.* **2011**, *35*, 377–406. [CrossRef]
25. Henry, B.L.; Minassian, A.; Perry, W. Effect of methamphetamine dependence on everyday functional ability. *Addict. Behav.* **2010**, *35*, 593–598. [CrossRef]
26. Ersche, K.D.; Sahakian, B.J. The neuropsychology of amphetamine and opiate dependence: Implications for treatment. *Neuropsychol. Rev.* **2007**, *17*, 317–336. [CrossRef] [PubMed]
27. Fernández-Serrano, M.J.; Perales, J.C.; Moreno-López, L.; Pérez-García, M.; Verdejo-García, A. Neuropsychological profiling of impulsivity and compulsivity in cocaine dependent individuals. *Psychopharmacology* **2012**, *219*, 673–683. [CrossRef]
28. Lezak, M.D.; Howieson, D.B.; Bigler, E.D.; Tranel, D. *Neuropsychological Assessment*, 5th ed.; Oxford University Press: New York, NY, USA, 2012; ISBN 9780195395525.
29. First, M.; Williams, J.; Karg, R.; Spitzer, R. *Structured Clinical Interview for DSM-5 Disorders, Clinician Version (SCID-5-CV)*; American Psychiatric Association: Arlington, VA, USA, 2016.
30. Cloninger, C.R.; Przybeck, T.R.; Svrakic, D.M.; Wetzel, R.D. *The Temperament and Character Inventory (TCI): A Guide to Its Development and Use*; Center for Psychobiology of Personality, Washington University: St. Louis, MO, USA, 1994; ISBN 0-9642917-03.
31. Gutiérrez-Zotes, J.A.; Bayón, C.; Montserrat, C.; Valero, J.; Labad, A.; Cloninger, C.; Fernández-Aranda, F. Temperament and Character Inventory-Revised (TCI-R). Standardization and normative data in a general population sample. *Actas Esp Psiquiatr* **2004**, *32*, 8–15.
32. Derogatis, L.R. *Symptom Checklist-90-R (SCL-90-R): Administration, scoring, and procedures manual*, 3rd ed.; NCS Pearson: Minneapolis, MN, USA, 1994; ISBN 2090-6684 (Print) 2090-6692.
33. González de Rivera, J.L.; de las Cuevas, C.; Rodríguez-Abuín, M.; y Rodríguez-Pulido, F. *SCL-90-R. Cuestionario de 90 Síntomas. Manual*; TEA Ediciones: Madrid, Spain, 2002.

34. Garner, D.M. *Eating Disorder Inventory-2*; Psychological Assessment Resources: Odessa, Ukraine, 1991.
35. Garner, D.M. *Inventario de Trastornos de la Conducta Alimentaria (EDI-2)-Manual*; TEA: Madrid, Spain, 1998.
36. Golden, C.J. Stroop colour and word test. *Age* **1978**, *15*, 90.
37. Golden, C.J. *Stroop: Test de Colores y Palabras: Manual*; TEA Ediciones: Madrid, Spain, 2001.
38. Heaton, R.K. *PAR Staff Wisconsin Card Sorting TestTM: Computer Version 4, Research Edition*; Psychological Assessment Resources: Lutz, FL, USA, 2003.
39. Bechara, A.; Damasio, A.R.; Damasio, H.; Anderson, S.W. Insensitivity to future consequences following damage to human prefrontal cortex. *Cognition* **1994**, *50*, 7–15. [CrossRef]
40. Eisinger, A.; Magi, A.; Gyurkovics, M.; Szabo, E.; Demetrovics, Z.; Kokonyei, G. Iowa Gambling Task: Illustration of a behavioral measurement. *Neuropsychopharmacol. Hung.* **2016**, *18*, 45–55.
41. *StataCorp Stata Statistical Software: Release 16*; StataCorp LLC.: College Station, TX, USA, 2019.
42. Kelley, K.; Preacher, K.J. On effect size. *Psychol. Methods* **2012**, *17*, 137–152. [CrossRef]
43. Cohen, J. *Statistical Power Analysis for Behavioural Sciences*; Lawrence Earlbaum Associates: Hillsdale, NJ, USA, 1998; ISBN 0805802835.
44. Finner, H. On a Monotonicity Problem in Step-Down Multiple Test Procedures. *J. Am. Stat. Assoc.* **1993**, *88*, 920. [CrossRef]
45. Root, T.L.; Pinheiro, A.P.; Thornton, L.; Strober, M.; Fernandez-Aranda, F.; Brandt, H.; Crawford, S.; Fichter, M.M.; Halmi, K.A.; Johnson, C.; et al. Substance use disorders in women with anorexia nervosa. *Int. J. Eat. Disord.* **2010**, *43*, 14–21. [CrossRef] [PubMed]
46. Bongers, P.; Jansen, A.; Houben, K.; Roefs, A. Happy eating: The single target implicit association test predicts overeating after positive emotions. *Eat. Behav.* **2013**, *14*, 348–355. [CrossRef] [PubMed]
47. Leehr, E.J.; Krohmer, K.; Schag, K.; Dresler, T.; Zipfel, S.; Giel, K.E. Emotion regulation model in binge eating disorder and obesity-a systematic review. *Neurosci. Biobehav. Rev.* **2015**, *49*, 125–134. [CrossRef] [PubMed]
48. Fassino, S.; Pierò, A.; Gramaglia, C.; Abbate-Daga, G. Clinical, psychopathological and personality correlates of interoceptive awareness in anorexia nervosa, bulimia nervosa and obesity. *Psychopathology* **2004**, *37*, 168–174. [CrossRef]
49. Hasin, D.; Katz, H. Somatoform and substance use disorders. *Psychosom. Med.* **2007**, *69*, 870–875. [CrossRef]
50. Kanner, R. Substance Abuse, Somatization, and Personality Disorders. In *Emergency Neurology*; Roos, K.L., Ed.; Elseiver: Boston, MA, USA, 2012; pp. 375–384. ISBN 9780387885858.
51. Fernández-Aranda, F.; Jiménez-Murcia, S.; Álvarez-Moya, E.M.; Granero, R.; Vallejo, J.; Bulik, C.M. Impulse control disorders in eating disorders: Clinical and therapeutic implications. *Compr. Psychiatry* **2006**, *47*, 482–488. [CrossRef]
52. Jiménez-Murcia, S.; Granero, R.; Moragas, L.; Steiger, H.; Israel, M.; Aymamí, N.; Gómez-Peña, M.; Sauchelli, S.; Agüera, Z.; Sánchez, I.; et al. Differences and similarities between bulimia nervosa, compulsive buying and gambling disorder. *Eur. Eat. Disord. Rev.* **2015**, *23*, 126–132. [CrossRef]
53. Grant, J.E. Impulse control disorders, a clinician's guide to understanding and treating behavi oral addictions. *Psicoter. Cogn. E Comport.* **2011**, *17*, 130–131. [CrossRef]
54. Schreiber, L.; Odlaug, B.L.; Grant, J.E. Impulse control disorders: Updated review of clinical characteristics and pharmacological management. *Front. Psychiatry* **2011**, *2*. [CrossRef]
55. Schag, K.; Schönleber, J.; Teufel, M.; Zipfel, S.; Giel, K.E. Food-related impulsivity in obesity and Binge Eating Disorder-a systematic review. *Obes. Rev.* **2013**, *14*, 477–495. [CrossRef]
56. Wrege, J.; Schmidt, A.; Walter, A.; Smieskova, R.; Bendfeldt, K.; Radue, E.-W.; Lang, U.; Borgwardt, S. Effects of Cannabis on Impulsivity: A Systematic Review of Neuroimaging Findings. *Curr. Pharm. Des.* **2014**, *20*, 2126–2137. [CrossRef] [PubMed]
57. Verdejo-Garcia, A.; Benbrook, A.; Funderburk, F.; David, P.; Cadet, J.L.; Bolla, K.I. The differential relationship between cocaine use and marijuana use on decision-making performance over repeat testing with the Iowa Gambling Task. *Drug Alcohol Depend.* **2007**, *90*, 2–11. [CrossRef] [PubMed]
58. Bechara, A.; Tranel, D.; Damasio, H. Characterization of the decision-making deficit of patients with ventromedial prefrontal cortex lesions. *Brain* **2000**, *123*, 2189–2202. [CrossRef] [PubMed]
59. Bechara, A.; Damasio, H.; Damasio, A.R.; Lee, G.P. Different contributions of the human amygdala and ventromedial prefrontal cortex to decision-making. *J. Neurosci.* **1999**, *19*, 5473–5481. [CrossRef] [PubMed]

60. Turton, R.; Nazar, B.P.; Burgess, E.E.; Lawrence, N.S.; Cardi, V.; Treasure, J.; Hirsch, C.R. To Go or Not to Go: A Proof of Concept Study Testing Food-Specific Inhibition Training for Women with Eating and Weight Disorders. *Eur. Eat. Disord. Rev.* **2018**, *26*, 11–21. [CrossRef] [PubMed]
61. Claudat, K.; Brown, T.A.; Anderson, L.; Bongiorno, G.; Berner, L.A.; Reilly, E.; Luo, T.; Orloff, N.; Kaye, W.H. Correlates of co-occurring eating disorders and substance use disorders: A case for dialectical behavior therapy. *Eat. Disord.* **2020**, *28*, 142–156. [CrossRef]
62. Hagan, K.E.; Christensen, K.A.; Forbush, K.T. A preliminary systematic review and meta-analysis of randomized-controlled trials of cognitive remediation therapy for anorexia nervosa. *Eat. Behav.* **2020**, *37*. [CrossRef]

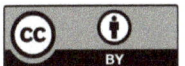

© 2020 by the authors. Licensee MDPI, Basel, Switzerland. This article is an open access article distributed under the terms and conditions of the Creative Commons Attribution (CC BY) license (http://creativecommons.org/licenses/by/4.0/).

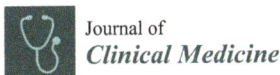

Article

Emotion Recognition Abilities in Adults with Anorexia Nervosa are Associated with Autistic Traits

Jess Kerr-Gaffney [1], Luke Mason [2], Emily Jones [2], Hannah Hayward [3], Jumana Ahmad [4], Amy Harrison [5,6], Eva Loth [3], Declan Murphy [3] and Kate Tchanturia [1,6,7,*]

1. Department of Psychological Medicine, Institute of Psychiatry, Psychology and Neuroscience, King's College London, London SE5 8AB, UK; jess.kerr-gaffney@kcl.ac.uk
2. Centre for Brain & Cognitive Development, Birkbeck, University of London, London WC1E 7JL, UK
3. Department of Forensic & Neurodevelopmental Sciences, Institute of Psychiatry, Psychology and Neuroscience, King's College London, London SE5 8AB, UK
4. School of Human Sciences, University of Greenwich, London SE10 9LS, UK
5. Department of Psychology and Human Development, University College London, London WC1H 0AA, UK
6. South London and Maudsley NHS Trust, National Eating Disorders Service, Psychological Medicine Clinical Academic Group, London SE5 8AZ, UK
7. Department of Psychology, Ilia State University, Tbilisi 0162, Georgia
* Correspondence: kate.tchanturia@kcl.ac.uk

Received: 20 February 2020; Accepted: 3 April 2020; Published: 8 April 2020

Abstract: Difficulties in socio-emotional functioning are proposed to contribute to the development and maintenance of anorexia nervosa (AN). This study aimed to examine emotion recognition abilities in individuals in the acute and recovered stages of AN compared to healthy controls (HCs). A second aim was to examine whether attention to faces and comorbid psychopathology predicted emotion recognition abilities. The films expressions task was administered to 148 participants (46 AN, 51 recovered AN, 51 HC) to assess emotion recognition, during which attention to faces was recorded using eye-tracking. Comorbid psychopathology was assessed using self-report questionnaires and the Autism Diagnostic Observation Schedule–2nd edition (ADOS-2). No significant differences in emotion recognition abilities or attention to faces were found between groups. However, individuals with a lifetime history of AN who scored above the clinical cut-off on the ADOS-2 displayed poorer emotion recognition performance than those scoring below cut-off and HCs. ADOS-2 scores significantly predicted emotion recognition abilities while controlling for group membership and intelligence. Difficulties in emotion recognition appear to be associated with high autism spectrum disorder (ASD) traits, rather than a feature of AN. Whether individuals with AN and high ASD traits may require different treatment strategies or adaptations is a question for future research.

Keywords: anorexia nervosa; ASD; comorbidity; emotion recognition; attention

---

1. Introduction

Anorexia nervosa (AN) is a severe psychiatric disorder characterised by an intense fear of weight gain, persistent behaviour to restrict energy intake, and a disturbance in the way one's body weight or shape are experienced [1]. Difficulties in social functioning have been identified as key factors in the development and maintenance of AN [2]. For example, before illness onset, individuals with AN report more social difficulties, fewer childhood friends, and engage in more solitary activities than healthy controls (HCs) [3–6]. During the illness, a variety of difficulties are seen, including high social anxiety, poorer social skills and social problem-solving abilities, loss of interest in social activities, and reduced social networks [7–14]. Given that interpersonal difficulties are associated with poorer outcomes in those with AN [15–17], it is important to understand potential underlying socio-cognitive mechanisms.

One area that has received considerable attention is emotion recognition. Given that up to two-thirds of human communication occurs through non-verbal means, recognising emotions from faces is considered key to successful social interaction [18]. Findings from studies in individuals with AN are mixed, with some reporting those with AN are significantly less accurate at inferring emotions from faces than HCs [19–22], and others reporting no differences [23–26]. A meta-analysis of 10 studies found that individuals with AN were significantly poorer at recognising basic and complex emotions relative to HCs, with small-to-medium and large effect sizes, respectively [27]. Given the effects of starvation on higher level cognitive processes, it is important to establish whether these effects may be a result of the ill state in AN. However, very few studies have examined emotion recognition performance in those recovered from AN, and results are equally mixed. While some report performance similar to that of HCs [28], others have reported poorer emotion recognition abilities, similar to those who are acutely unwell [20,29]. It is therefore not known whether potential differences in emotion recognition abilities are a result of the ill state in AN. However, one study found that emotion recognition difficulties were also present in unaffected twins of those with AN, suggesting that difficulties in this domain might represent an endophenotype for the disorder [30].

Clinical presentation of AN is associated with high levels of depression [31], anxiety [32], alexithymia [7], and autism spectrum disorder (ASD) traits [33], factors which by themselves may alter social-cognitive abilities. It is therefore possible that comorbid psychopathology might moderate emotion recognition abilities in those with AN. Although few studies have directly investigated this issue, a few have examined the impact of alexithymia. Alexithymia is a sub-clinical trait also present within the general population, describing an inability to recognise or describe one's own emotions. When matched for levels of alexithymia, individuals with AN or bulimia nervosa (BN) have been found to show similar emotion recognition abilities to HCs [34,35], suggesting that emotion recognition difficulties may be attributable to alexithymia rather than the eating disorder (ED) per se. However, the use of mixed ED groups and small sample sizes limit interpretation of the results for AN specifically. Given the profound effects of ASD on social cognitive abilities, it is perhaps surprising that very few studies have examined the impact of ASD traits on emotion recognition in individuals with AN. Dinkler and colleagues [28] reported that individuals recovered from AN with comorbid ASD were more accurate at recognising low intensity emotional expressions than those without ASD, who did not differ from HCs. However, due to the very small sample size in the AN+ASD group ($n = 6$), analyses were treated as exploratory only. Nonetheless, these findings support the proposition that AN with or without comorbid ASD may be two qualitatively different forms of the illness [36].

Another variable that has received little attention in emotion recognition research in AN is social attention. Attending to nonverbal social cues provided by others, such as eye gaze, gestures, and facial expressions, is a necessary precursor to higher-order social cognitive abilities such as emotion recognition [37]. In typical human development, social information in the environment is highly salient, and stimuli such as faces and eyes hold particular importance [38]. This attentional bias towards social information is demonstrated from infancy, and reductions in this capacity are among one of the first signs of socio-communicative disorders such as ASD [39]. There is also emerging evidence to suggest that individuals with AN show reduced attention to faces [40] and eyes [41]. Reduced attention to facial features has been found to predict the degree of emotion recognition impairment and lower social competence in individuals with ASD [37,42,43], however only a few studies have measured attention during emotion recognition in individuals with AN. Phillipou and colleagues [44] demonstrated that while individuals with AN and HCs did not differ in their ability to recognise basic emotions, AN displayed more fixations of shorter duration to faces, indicating a "hyperscanning" strategy. Unfortunately, this study did not examine whether eye movements were associated with emotion recognition performance. In a mixed ED sample (AN or BN), Fujiwara and colleagues [35] found that difficulties in emotion recognition were predicted by less visual attention to faces in those with an ED, but not in HCs. This raises the possibility that difficulties in emotion recognition sometimes associated with EDs are a result of differences in spontaneous social attention, rather than misinterpretation of emotional displays. Finally, Dinkler et al. [28] found no differences in eye movements between those recovered from AN and HCs, and accuracy was not associated with attention to facial features. Together, these findings suggest there may be differences in the relationship between emotion recognition and attention in the acute stage of AN compared to the recovered stage or those who have never had an ED. However, studies including an acute AN group (rather than AN and BN together) are required to test this hypothesis.

The current study aimed to examine emotion recognition performance in adults in the acute and recovered stages of AN compared to HCs. It has been suggested that difficulties in this area in those with AN may be more subtle and less detectable using basic emotions [27], therefore a paradigm allowing for assessment of both basic and complex emotion recognition was selected. In order to understand why individuals with AN might display emotion recognition deficits, a secondary aim was to examine whether visual attention to faces predicted emotion recognition performance. Relatedly, a third aim was to examine whether levels of comorbid psychopathology were associated with emotion recognition performance. As well as including measures of alexithymia and ASD traits, we included depression, anxiety, and social anxiety due to their high co-occurrence with AN [8,32,45] and potential effects on social cognition [46–51]. We hypothesised that individuals with AN would be less accurate at recognising complex emotions compared to HCs, and that those recovered from AN would show intermediate levels of performance. No significant differences in basic emotion recognition were predicted. Finally, we predicted that more attention to faces, as well as lower alexithymia and ASD traits would be associated with better emotion recognition performance.

2. Methods

Ethical approval was obtained from the National Health Service (NHS) Research Ethics Committee (Camberwell St Giles, 17/LO/1960).

2.1. Participants

All participants were required to be between 18 and 55 years old and fluent in English. Exclusion criteria were a history of brain trauma or learning disability. HC participants were recruited through a King's College London email circular and posters around campuses. Before taking part, HC participants were screened using the Structured Clinical Interview for DSM-5 Disorders, research version (SCID-5-RV) [52], to ensure they did not meet criteria for any psychiatric disorders. HCs were required to have a body mass index (BMI) between 19 and 27.

In addition to the university advertisements, participants with a lifetime history of AN were recruited through online advertisements (B-eat, call for participants, MQ Mental Health), and through two specialist NHS ED services in London. Participants were screened using the SCID-5-RV to confirm a current or past diagnosis of AN. Participants with AN were required to have a BMI ≤ 18.5 and recovered participants needed to have a BMI between 19 and 27.

2.2. Materials

The Films Expressions Task (FET) [53] is a facial emotion recognition task, modified to enable concurrent recording of eye movements. In each trial, participants are first presented with an emotion word on-screen. Three images are then presented for 500 ms each, one after another (with a 500 ms blank screen between images; see Figure 1). The height of each image was 15.7° at a viewing distance of 60 cm from the screen. The widths of each image were adjusted to ensure a correct aspect ratio and ranged from 12.4° to 21.4°. Images within each trial present the same actor displaying different emotional expressions (see Figure 2 for an example). Participants were then asked to indicate, as quickly and as accurately as they could, which of the images displayed the emotion word by pressing the corresponding key (1, 2, or 3). There were 53 trials in total (preceded by 3 practice trials). Prior to the task, participants were presented with a sheet listing the target emotion words and their definitions to ensure they were familiar with the words. A full list of the target emotion words is presented in the

Supplementary Materials. Images were from films made in non-English speaking countries to reduce the probability that participants would recognise the actors.

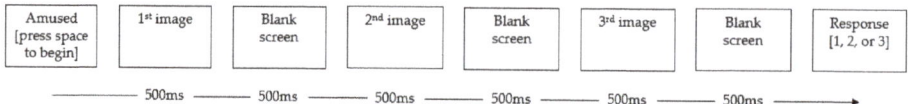

Figure 1. Sequence of events for an example trial of the films expression task.

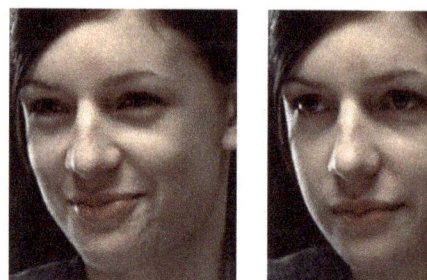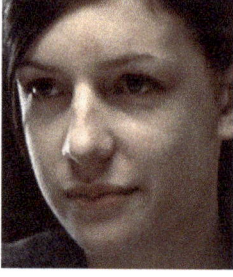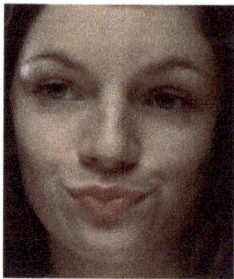

Figure 2. Images from an example trial [amused] of the films expression task.

The FET was chosen due to its depiction of naturalistic facial expressions; its inclusion of a range of both basic and complex emotions; and relatively brief presentation times. Basic and complex emotion trials were presented interleaved in a fixed random order. Foil emotional expressions were selected to be similar to the target emotion in terms of intensity of the expression and perceptual features. Development and validation of the test stimuli is presented in [53]. Dependent measures were: Accuracy (% of trials correct), mean RTs, and time spent looking at the stimuli (as a proportion of presentation time).

The Wechsler Abbreviated Scale of Intelligence, Second Edition (WASI-II) [54] measures verbal intelligence and perceptual reasoning, as well as full-scale IQ. The two subtest version was used (vocabulary and matrix reasoning).

The Autism Diagnostic Observation Schedule–2nd edition (ADOS-2), Module 4 [55] is a standardised semi-structured interview recommended for the assessment of ASD [56]. It includes a range of questions and activities designed to evoke behaviours and cognitions associated with ASD. Interviews were administered by the first author who received ADOS-2 training and met requirements for research reliability for module 4 and also attended reliability meetings throughout the study period. The revised algorithm, which was designed to more closely reflect the DSM-5 criteria for ASD was used for scoring [57]. The algorithm has two subscales: social affect and restrictive and repetitive behaviours, and total scores of 8 or more indicate possible ASD. The ADOS-2 was used in this study to identify participants with low or high ASD traits.

2.3. Questionnaires

The Eating Disorder Examination Questionnaire (EDE-Q) [58] measures severity of ED psychopathology. Global scores are calculated by averaging responses across items, with higher scores indicating more severe symptoms (max 6). HCs with a score of >2.7 were excluded from analyses to ensure those with possible sub-threshold ED symptoms were not included [59]. Cronbach's alpha was 0.93.

The Hospital Anxiety and Depression Scale (HADS) [60] is a 14-item scale with two subscales: anxiety and depression. Subscale scores are interpreted as: normal (0–7), mild (8–10), moderate (11–14), and severe (15–21). Cronbach's alpha was 0.93.

The Liebowitz Social Anxiety Scale (LSAS) [61] has two subscales: fear and avoidance of social situations. A score of 60 has been established as a cut-off indicative of social anxiety disorder (SAD) [62]. Cronbach's alpha was 0.97.

The Social Responsiveness Scale-2nd Edition, adult self-report form (SRS-2) [63] measures symptoms associated with ASD, with higher scores (max 195) indicating more autistic symptoms. There are 5 sub-scales: social awareness, social cognition, social communication, social motivation, and restricted and repetitive interests. Cronbach's alpha was 0.96.

The twenty-item Toronto Alexithymia Scale (TAS-20) [64] has three subscales: difficulty identifying feelings, difficulty describing feelings, and externally oriented thinking. Total scores range from 0 to 100, and cut-offs are as follows: ≤51 = no alexithymia; 52–60 = borderline alexithymia; and ≥61 = alexithymia [65]. Cronbach's alpha was 0.90.

2.4. Procedure

Participants attended a testing session at the Institute of Psychiatry, Psychology & Neuroscience. After written informed consent was obtained, participants completed the FET while their eye movements were recorded using a Tobii TX300 eye-tracker. The desktop mounted eye-tracker has a sampling rate of 300 Hz, a screen resolution of 1920 × 1080, and a diagonal screen size of 23". During tracking, infrared diodes generate reflections on the participant's retinas and corneas. From this reflection the angular rotation of each eye is estimated. A five-point calibration procedure relates this angular rotation to corresponding x and y coordinates on the screen surface. Participants were seated approximately 60 cm from the screen. Stimulus presentation, behavioural data, and eye-tracking data were managed and recorded using custom-written MATLAB software [66].

After the FET, the first author administered the WASI-II and the ADOS-2, and the participant completed the questionnaires. Weight and height measurements were taken to calculate BMI (weight/height^2). Participants were reimbursed £20 for their time.

2.5. Analysis

Histograms and Q-Q plots were inspected to check for normal distributions. Where variables were positively skewed, as was the case for RT and age data, a logarithmic transformation was applied. Homogeneity was assessed using Levene's test. Group differences in psychopathology and demographic information were assessed using one-way ANOVAs and Tukey's post-hoc tests, or Welch's ANOVA with Games-Howell post-hoc tests where the assumption of homogeneity was violated.

Group differences in FET accuracy and RT were assessed with two-way mixed ANOVAs, with the within-subjects factor emotion complexity (basic or complex) and the between-subjects factor group (AN, recovered AN (REC), HC). Although analyses were conducted on log-transformed RT values, medians and interquartile range for the untransformed variable are reported for ease of interpretation, as these are similar to the geometric means. Proportion of time spent looking at faces violated the assumptions of an ANOVA (non-normal distribution, strongly negatively skewed). Therefore, group differences were assessed using the nonparametric Kruskall-Wallis test, and the effects of emotion complexity were analysed using Wilcoxon signed rank tests, with the significance level adjusted for multiple comparisons ($p < 0.01$). Effects of medication on FET outcome measures were examined using independent samples t-tests (or a Mann-Whitney U test in the case of the non-normally distributed time spent looking at faces), comparing those with past or current AN who were on medication to those who were not.

Spearman's correlations were run to examine relationships between emotion recognition performance (the primary outcome measure), demographic variables (age, IQ, BMI), psychopathology scores (EDE-Q, HADS anxiety and depression, LSAS, SRS-2, and TAS-20, ADOS-2 total), and proportion of time spent looking at faces. Variables that showed statistically significant relationships with emotion recognition performance were entered into a hierarchical regression analysis to determine which, if any, explained variance in the outcome measure.

3. Results

3.1. Demographics

In total, 148 participants were recruited (46 AN, 51 REC, 51 HC). Five HCs were subsequently excluded based on their EDE-Q scores and one REC participant was excluded due to a BMI > 27. Due to equipment failure on the day of testing, one AN and one REC participant could not complete the FET and were therefore excluded. Thus, data from 45 participants with AN, 49 REC, and 46 HC were analysed. Eye-tracking data from three HC and one REC participant was of low quality (excessive eye blinks) and was therefore excluded from analyses, however all other data (including FET accuracy and RT) from these participants was retained.

Demographic information and psychopathology scores are presented in Table 1. There were no significant group differences in age, IQ, years of education, or sex.

Table 1. Mean (SD) demographic information and psychopathology scores.

	AN (n = 45)	REC (n = 49)	HC (n = 46)	Test Statistics	p-Value	$\eta p^2/d$
Age (years) [†]	27.04 (8.92)	26.00 (8.10)	23.87 (4.52)	$F_{(2, 85.23)} = 2.16$	0.12	0.02
% female	93.5	98.0	91.1	Fisher's exact test = 2.17	0.31	
BMI	15.75 (1.41) [a]	21.14 (1.91) [b]	21.69 (1.88) [b]	$F_{(2, 136)} = 159.75$	**<0.001**	0.70
Years of education	16.06 (3.07)	16.52 (2.62)	16.63 (2.45)	$F_{(2, 136)} = 0.54$	0.58	0.01
IQ	110.86 (12.29)	110.16 (10.38)	113.78 (7.25)	$F_{(2, 85.30)} = 2.18$	0.12	0.02
Age diagnosed [†]	19.84 (7.39) [a]	16.41 (3.53) [b]	-	$t_{(73.24)} = 2.92$	**0.01**	0.59
Illness length (years)	7.19 (7.88)	5.40 (5.65)	-	$t_{(79.67)} = 1.24$	0.22	0.26
% on psychiatric medication	53.3 [a]	32.7 [b]	-	$\chi^2 = 4.10$	**0.04**	
EDE-Q	3.86 (1.25) [a]	1.81 (1.52) [b]	0.61 (0.58) [c]	$F_{(2, 75.81)} = 125.35$	**<0.001**	0.56
HADS-A	13.56 (4.51) [a]	10.84 (5.11) [b]	5.02 (3.09) [c]	$F_{(2, 87.46)} = 61.90$	**<0.001**	0.40
HADS-D	9.87 (4.40) [a]	5.04 (4.02) [b]	1.54 (1.68) [c]	$F_{(2, 76.50)} = 77.66$	**<0.001**	0.48
LSAS	68.95 (30.78) [a]	57.08 (29.98) [a]	27.91 (18.32) [b]	$F_{(2, 84.80)} = 36.34$	**<0.001**	0.29
SRS-2	82.43 (31.99) [a]	70.04 (31.97) [a]	39.23 (20.18) [b]	$F_{(2, 85.60)} = 34.67$	**<0.001**	0.28
TAS-20	58.16 (13.50) [a]	49.81 (15.08) [b]	37.47 (11.26) [c]	$F_{(2, 136)} = 26.86$	**<0.001**	0.29
ADOS-2						
Total	4.67 (3.94) [a]	4.16 (4.50) [ab]	2.70 (2.52) [b]	$F_{(2, 85.99)} = 4.79$	**0.01**	0.05
SA	4.02 (3.61) [a]	3.71 (3.96) [ab]	2.50 (2.38) [b]	$F_{(2, 86.95)} = 3.48$	**0.04**	0.04
RRB	0.64 (1.00) [a]	0.45 (0.89) [ab]	0.20 (0.58) [b]	$F_{(2, 86.10)} = 3.82$	**0.03**	0.05
% above clinical cut-off	17.8 [a,b]	24.5 [a]	4.3 [b]	$\chi^2 = 7.48$	**0.02**	

ADOS-2: autism diagnostic observation schedule–2nd edition; AN: anorexia nervosa; BMI: body mass index; EDE-Q: eating disorder examination questionnaire; HADS-A: hospital anxiety and depression scale, anxiety subscale; HADS-D: hospital anxiety and depression scale, depression subscale; HC: healthy control; IQ: intelligence quotient; LSAS: Liebowitz social anxiety scale; REC: recovered anorexia nervosa; RRB: restrictive and repetitive behaviors; SA: social affect; SD: standard deviation; SRS-2: social responsiveness scale–2nd edition; TAS-20: twenty-item Toronto alexithymia scale. Different superscripts indicate significant differences between groups, significant p-values are highlighted in bold. [†] Variable was log transformed for analyses, original values are displayed.

3.2. Films Expression Task

Mean emotion recognition accuracy, RTs, and proportion of time spent looking at faces across groups are displayed in Table 2. A 3 (group: AN, REC, HC) × 2 (emotion complexity: basic, complex) mixed ANOVA was computed to examine group differences in emotion recognition accuracy (% correct) for basic and complex emotions. The interaction effect was not significant, though it did reach trend level, $F_{(2, 137)} = 2.43$, $p = 0.09$, $\eta p^2 = 0.03$. The main effect of emotion complexity was significant, $F_{(1, 137)} = 26.65$, $p < 0.001$, $\eta p^2 = 0.16$, indicating accuracy was significantly higher for basic emotions (M = 89.34%, SD = 10.92%) than complex ones (M = 85.44%, SD = 10.19). The main effect of group was not significant, $F_{(2, 132)} = 1.10$, $p = 0.34$, $\eta p^2 = 0.02$. Accuracy (all faces) did not differ between medicated and unmedicated participants $t_{(92)} = 0.42$, $p = 0.67$.

Table 2. Mean (SD) performance and attention during the films expression task.

	AN (n = 45)	REC (n = 49)	HC (n = 46)
Accuracy (% correct)			
Basic emotions	88.25 (11.61)	89.80 (12.88)	89.91 (7.62)
Complex emotions	84.10 (10.79)	84.09 (11.65)	88.18 (7.14)
Reaction time (ms) [†]			
Basic emotions	786.86 (546.32)	668.86 (415.61)	556.61 (352.43)
Complex emotions	875.69 (597.10)	703.59 (518.45)	662.13 (376.79)
Time spent looking at faces (%)			
Basic emotions	95.79 (5.85)	97.60 (2.79)	94.60 (8.23)
Complex emotions	96.54 (5.26)	97.81 (2.64)	94.37 (8.64)

AN: anorexia nervosa; HC: healthy control; REC: recovered anorexia nervosa; SD: standard deviation. [†] Variable was log transformed for analyses, median and IQR (of the untransformed variable) are displayed.

A 3 (group: AN, REC, HC) × 2 (emotion complexity: basic, complex) mixed ANOVA was computed to examine group differences in RTs for basic and complex emotions. The interaction effect was not significant, $F(2, 132) = 0.86$, $p = 0.43$, $\eta p^2 = 0.01$. The main effect of emotion complexity was significant, $F(1, 137) = 60.72$, $p < 0.001$, $\eta p^2 = 0.31$, indicating RTs were significantly shorter for basic emotions (median = 654.14 ms, IQR = 464.68 ms) than complex ones (median = 718.29 ms, IQR = 474.55 ms). The main effect of group was not significant, $F(2, 137) = 2.06$, $p = 0.13$, $\eta p^2 = 0.03$. RTs (all trials) did not differ between medicated and unmedicated participants, $t(92) = -1.03$, $p = 0.31$.

Kruskall-Wallis tests indicated there were no significant differences between groups in the proportion of time spent looking at faces displaying basic emotions, $\chi^2(2) = 4.75$, $p = 0.09$, or complex ones, $\chi^2(2) = 4.61$, $p = 0.10$. Wilcoxon signed-ranks tests indicated that time spent looking at basic versus complex emotions did not significantly differ within either of the three groups (all $p > 0.01$, adjusted significance level for multiple comparisons). Proportion of time spent looking at faces (overall) did not differ between medicated and unmedicated participants, $U = 980.00$, $p = 0.57$.

3.3. Predicting Emotion Recognition Performance

In the whole sample, emotion recognition accuracy was significantly positively associated with the proportion of time spent looking at faces ($r = 0.17$, $p = 0.04$) and IQ ($r = 0.23$, $p = 0.01$), and negatively correlated with TAS-20 ($r = -0.18$, $p = 0.04$) and ADOS-2 scores ($r = -0.17$, $p = 0.04$) (see Supplementary Materials for full table of correlations). To establish whether the relationship between accuracy and attention to faces differed across groups, correlations were run for each of the three groups separately. Proportion of time spent looking at faces significantly correlated with emotion recognition accuracy in the AN group only ($r = 0.34$, $p = 0.02$). However, a linear regression showed that proportion of time spent looking at faces did not significantly predict emotion recognition abilities in those with AN, although the association did reach trend level, $F(1, 42) = 3.36$, $p = 0.07$, adjusted $R^2 = 0.05$. In the whole sample, a hierarchical multiple regression was run to determine if the addition of attention to faces, TAS-20, and ADOS-2 scores would improve the prediction of emotion recognition performance over group membership and IQ. The full model was significant, $R^2 = 0.22$, $F(6, 126) = 5.95$, $p < 0.001$, adjusted $R^2 = 0.18$. Details of each regression model are shown in Table 3. The addition of ADOS-2 scores (model 3) led to a significant increase in R^2 of 0.11, $F(1, 127) = 17.54$, $p < 0.001$. The addition of proportion of time spent looking at faces (model 2) and TAS-20 scores (model 4) did not significantly add to the prediction.

Table 3. Hierarchical regression analysis predicting emotion recognition accuracy from associated demographic variables and psychopathology scores.

	Model 1	Model 2	Model 3	Model 4
IQ	0.22 *	0.23 **	0.17 *	0.15
% of time spent looking at faces		0.17	0.10	0.11
ADOS-2			−0.35 ***	−0.31 ***
TAS-20				−0.14
R^2	0.07	0.10	0.21	0.22

ADOS-2: autism diagnostic observation schedule–2nd edition; IQ: intelligence quotient; TAS-20: twenty-item Toronto Alexithymia Scale. Figures shown are standardized coefficients. Group membership was entered in model 1 but was not significant and not displayed here. * $p < 0.05$; ** $p < 0.01$; *** $p < 0.001$.

3.4. ASD, Emotion Recognition Performance, and Attention to Faces

To further explore the relationship between ASD symptoms and emotion recognition performance, individuals with past or current AN were grouped according to whether they met the clinical cut-off for ASD on the ADOS-2 and compared with HCs. The two HCs who scored above cut-off on the ADOS-2 were excluded, due to their being too few cases to assess group differences. Thus, 44 HC, 20 lifetime AN scoring above the ADOS-2 cut-off (AN + ASD), and 74 lifetime AN scoring below the ADOS-2 cut-off (AN − ASD) were included in analyses.

A 3 (group: AN + ASD, AN − ASD, HC) × 2 (emotion complexity: basic, complex) mixed ANOVA was computed to examine group differences in emotion recognition accuracy (Figure 3). The interaction effect was not significant, though it did reach trend level, $F(2, 135) = 2.70$, $p = 0.07$, $\eta p^2 = 0.04$. The main effect of emotion complexity was significant, $F(1, 135) = 23.13$, $p < 0.001$, $\eta p^2 = 0.15$, indicating accuracy was significantly higher for basic emotions (M = 89.34%, SD = 10.99%) than complex ones (M = 85.49%, SD = 10.22). The main effect of group was also significant, $F(2, 135) = 10.51$, $p < 0.001$, $\eta p^2 = 0.14$, indicating AN + ASD (M = 77.36%, SD = 16.54%) were significantly less accurate at recognising emotions than AN − ASD (M = 87.58, SD = 7.36), and HCs (M = 88.85%, SD = 6.10%), who did not differ from one another. Kruskall-Wallis tests indicated there were no significant differences across groups in the proportion of time spent looking at faces displaying basic emotions $\chi^2(2) = 2.06$, $p = 0.36$, or complex ones, $\chi^2(2) = 2.92$, $p = 0.23$.

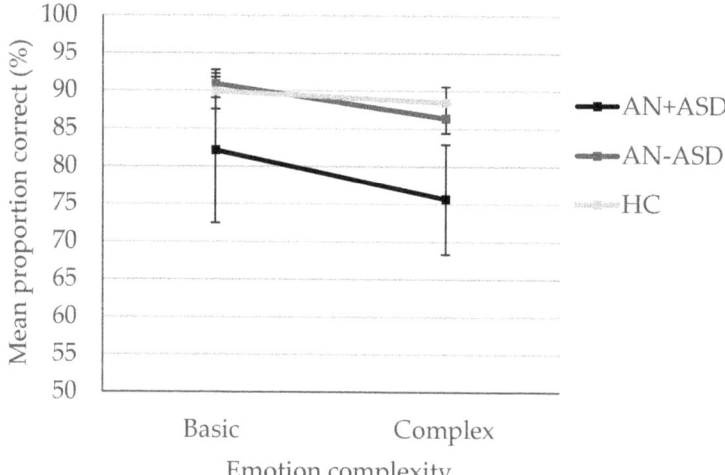

Figure 3. Mean proportion of correct trials on the films expression task. Error bars represent 95% confidence intervals. HC = healthy controls; AN + ASD = lifetime AN, above cut-off on the ADOS-2; AN − ASD = lifetime AN, below cut-off on the ADOS-2.

4. Discussion

The current study aimed to examine emotion recognition abilities in those with acute AN, REC, and HCs. Contrary to our hypotheses, there were no significant differences between groups in basic or complex emotion recognition. Our prediction that emotion recognition abilities would be associated with attention to faces, as well as alexithymia and ASD traits, was partially supported. Emotion recognition accuracy was significantly positively correlated with proportion of time spent looking at faces, and negatively correlated with alexithymia (TAS-20) and autistic features (ADOS-2 scores). However, in regression analyses, only ADOS-2 scores remained a significant predictor of emotion recognition performance while controlling for IQ and group membership. A subsequent analysis demonstrated that considering acute and recovered AN together, those who scored above the clinical cut-off for ASD on the ADOS-2 were significantly less accurate at recognising emotions than those who scored below the ADOS-2 cut off and HCs. These groups did not differ in the proportion of time spent looking at faces, suggesting differences in emotion recognition abilities were not due to differences in attention. Thus, in our sample of adults with a lifetime diagnosis of AN, difficulties in emotion recognition abilities appear to be associated with high ASD traits, rather than a feature of AN.

Our findings suggest that difficulties in emotion recognition are not a feature of the socio-emotional profile hypothesised to contribute to the maintenance of AN [2]. Although our results contrast with studies showing facial emotion recognition difficulties in acute and recovered AN [19,20,29,67], several studies have failed to detect significant differences between groups [23–25,68,69]. It is possible that the different emotion recognition tasks used across studies contribute to the mixed results. The FET was chosen for its relative difficulty; faces are presented for 500 ms only, stimuli are naturalistic facial expressions, and a wide range of complex emotions are included in addition to the six basic emotions. Nonetheless, given that accuracy was relatively high across groups, it may be the case that there were ceiling effects in our sample. This might be due to educational levels or IQ; participants were generally highly educated and mean IQ scores across groups were higher than the population average. Indeed, in the original pilot studies of the FET, distractors were only chosen if they were misidentified as the target emotion less than 30% of the time [53], possibly resulting in the high level of accuracy seen in our sample. It should be noted that the FET has not yet been validated in a normative sample, limiting comparisons with previous literature. However, a recent study using the FET found that individuals with ASD were significantly less accurate at identifying emotions and displayed longer RTs compared to HCs [70]. Mean accuracy in the HC group (87.5% correct) was very similar to that obtained in our sample (88.64%), whereas performance in the ASD group was far lower (70.8%) than in our clinical group (acute AN = 85.2%). Although definitive conclusions cannot be made from cross-study comparisons, this pattern supports intact emotion recognition performance in acute and recovered AN.

Another explanation for the mixed results from emotion recognition studies in AN concern another of our main findings: ASD traits predicted performance rather than ED status. It could be the case that variations in ASD symptoms across study samples contribute to the mixed findings, such that group differences in mean performance may not be apparent in samples with relatively low levels of ASD traits. To further investigate this issue, future studies may benefit from looking beyond group differences in social-cognitive performance. For example, Renwick and colleagues [36] used cluster analysis to explore social- and neuro-cognitive abilities in adults with AN, including measures of set-shifting, central coherence, and theory of mind (ToM). Three clusters emerged: One characterised by average to high social- and neuro-cognitive performance; another showing mixed performance (good set-shifting, average ToM, and poor central coherence and cognitive flexibility); and a final cluster characterised by poor overall performance. The authors propose that the third cluster, which comprised 17% of participants, represented an "ASD-like" cluster. Unfortunately, no diagnostic or self-report measures of ASD were included in the study, so is in not known whether these participants met diagnostic criteria for ASD. Nonetheless, this study demonstrates that distinct sub-groups within the overall diagnosis of AN may exist, potentially with different aetiologies and developmental pathways.

Although our cross-sectional design prevents conclusions regarding the differing developmental pathways that may characterise participants in the current study, recent research presents some interesting hypotheses. For example, individuals with ASD report sensory sensitivities and a limited range of acceptable foods, often from childhood [71,72]. Further, women with ASD report high levels of eating disturbances compared to both men with ASD and neurotypical women, particularly in regards to eating rituals, sensory sensitivity to the taste, smell, and texture of food, and difficulties around eating with others [73]. These difficulties may reinforce food restriction, resulting in energy deficits and a potential trigger for the development of a clinical ED in some individuals with ASD [74]. Another possible pathway through which EDs and ASD may co-occur is via interacting influences of body dissatisfaction and gender identity. There is emerging evidence to suggest that having ASD increases one's chances of experiencing gender dysphoria [75] and rejecting a binary gender identity [76]. In addition, qualitative reports from women with ASD often report conflict between expected feminine roles and their autistic identities [77]. At the same time, transgender individuals are at increased risk of body dissatisfaction and clinical EDs [78,79]. Specifically, restrictive eating and exercise can be a means of achieving a body congruent with one's gender identity [80]. These differing aetiological pathways and maintenance factors for EDs are likely to have important implications for treatment.

The findings from the current study have important clinical implications. In our sample, 17.8% of acute AN and 24.5% of REC scored above the clinical cut-off on the ADOS-2, compared to 4.3% of HCs. Similar findings have been reported previously [69,81]. Interestingly, total scores on the ADOS-2 were significantly higher in acute AN than HCs, while scores in the REC group lay between the two. This pattern of results suggests that although a small proportion of ASD symptoms may be a result of starvation in acute AN, the ADOS-2 algorithm might be robust against picking up false positives. The findings from our recovered group suggest that ASD symptoms may be a stable trait, present before and after the illness in individuals with AN. Consequently, a more personalised approach to treatment in individuals with AN might be required. Treatment modules designed to improve social cognition may not be suitable for the majority of individuals with AN, however, they could prove useful in those with high ASD traits and accompanying emotion recognition difficulties. Interventions such as social skills training groups may be effective in adults and adolescents with ASD, with several studies reporting improvements in social cognition measures, social skills knowledge, and friendship quality [82–86]. In addition, some studies have shown improvements in mental health outcomes, suggesting a relationship between social functioning and wider mental health [87,88]. Whether such interventions might be useful for those with AN and ASD comorbidity is yet to be addressed. Thus far, interventions in AN that have incorporated emotion or social skills training, such as Cognitive Remediation and Emotion Skills Training (CREST) [89] have more heavily emphasised identifying and managing one's own emotions rather than identifying emotions in others. Future treatment protocols may benefit from the inclusion of more extensive social cognition training specifically for those with AN and comorbid ASD.

The current study has a number of strengths. The sample size is one of the largest among eye-tracking studies in individuals with EDs (for a review, see [90]), and it is the first study to measure attention during emotion recognition in both acute and recovered AN. The inclusion of both basic and complex emotions, as well as the use of realistic photo stimuli allowed for a more ecologically valid assessment of emotion recognition abilities. However, several limitations should also be discussed. Most notably, given the short stimuli presentation times (500 ms), our paradigm only provided an assessment of early attentional engagement during emotion recognition. It may be that individuals with AN show differences in attention at later processing stages where attention is under conscious control [91]. This may explain why although attention to faces significantly correlated with emotion recognition accuracy, it did not explain a significant amount of the variance in accuracy in regression analyses. Although our quick presentation times might have replicated the fleeting facial expressions encountered in real life, future studies would benefit from measuring attention over longer periods in order to gain a better understanding of attentional processes in individuals with AN. Further, given the inclusion of both basic and complex emotion words in the FET, it is likely that verbal comprehension abilities explain significant variance in accuracy. Although we assessed associations between full-scale IQ and emotion recognition accuracy, our analyses may have benefited from including verbal IQ instead. Nonetheless, our findings show that individuals with AN have the capacity to process emotions rapidly to the same extent as HCs.

Relatedly, the short stimuli presentation times in the FET prevented a more fine-grained analysis of scan paths across the facial features. Reduced attention to the eyes has been demonstrated in acute AN during free viewing of face images, as well as during real-life social interactions [40,41]. Thus, it could be the case that our measure of overall looking times to faces was too blunt to detect group differences. Another limitation of the current study is the cross-sectional design. It cannot be ruled out that differences in socio-cognitive functioning or psychological resources contributed to the recovery of the recovered AN group. To our knowledge, no study has tested emotion recognition abilities and/or social attention over time in the same group of individuals with AN before and after recovery. Further, it must be noted that although the ADOS-2 is recommended as part of an ASD diagnostic assessment, it does not provide enough information on its own to confer a diagnosis of ASD [56]. Research using developmental measures in addition to assessing current symptoms would be informative in further defining social cognition in the AN+ASD sub-group.

To conclude, the findings of the current study suggest that emotion recognition difficulties are not a feature of the socio-emotional phenotype proposed to characterise AN. Instead, difficulties in emotion recognition appear to only be present in those with high ASD traits, independent of illness state. While it is not known whether this subgroup of individuals meets full diagnostic criteria for ASD, our findings support the notion that AN with and without high ASD traits might be two qualitatively different conditions. Whether these individuals may require different treatment strategies or adaptations to accommodate different communicative styles is a question for future research. Our results also suggest individuals in the acute and recovered stages of AN do not show any differences in attention to faces compared to HCs. However, given the limitations of our study design and the lack of research in this area, future studies should examine attention to individual facial features to expand on our findings.

Supplementary Materials: The following are available online at http://www.mdpi.com/2077-0383/9/4/1057/s1, Table S1: Target emotions in the films expression task; Table S2: Correlations between FET accuracy, time spent looking at faces, and clinical and demographic variables in the full sample.

Author Contributions: Conceptualization, J.K.-G. and K.T.; formal analysis, J.K.-G. and E.J.; funding acquisition, J.K.-G.; investigation, J.K.-G.; methodology, E.L. and J.A.; resources, H.H. and D.M.; software, L.M.; supervision, A.H., D.M. and K.T.; writing—original draft, J.K.-G.; writing—review & editing, L.M., E.J., H.H., A.H., E.L., J.A. and K.T. All authors have read and agreed to the published version of the manuscript.

Funding: J.K. is supported by a doctoral studentship from the Economic and Social Research Council (ESRC) and received research funding from the Psychiatry Research Trust. A.H. is funded by the Medical Research Council (MRC) (MR/S020381/1). K.T. would like to acknowledge MRC-MRF Fund (MR/R004595/1); the Health Foundation, an independent charity committed to bring better health care for people in the UK (1115447); and the Maudsley Charity for their support. The Maudsley Charity is an independent NHS mental health charity which works in partnership with patients and families, clinical care teams and researchers at South London and Maudsley NHS Foundation Trust, the Institute of Psychiatry, Psychology and Neuroscience, King's College London, and community organisations, with a common goal of improving mental health, to support innovation, research and service improvement.

Acknowledgments: The authors would like to thank the participants who took part in the research for their time.

Conflicts of Interest: The authors declare no conflict of interest. The funders had no role in the design of the study; in the collection, analyses, or interpretation of data; in the writing of the manuscript, or in the decision to publish the results.

References

1. American Psychiatric Association. *Diagnostic and Statistical Manual of Mental Disorders*, 5th ed.; American Psychiatric Publishing: Arlington, TX, USA, 2013.
2. Treasure, J.; Schmidt, U. The Cognitive-Interpersonal Maintenance Model of Anorexia Nervosa Revisited: A Summary of the Evidence for Cognitive, Socio-Emotional and Interpersonal Predisposing and Perpetuating Factors. *J. Eat. Disord.* **2013**, *1*, 13. [CrossRef] [PubMed]
3. Lie, S.Ø.; Rø, Ø.; Bang, L. Is Bullying and Teasing Associated with Eating Disorders? A Systematic Review and Meta-Analysis. *Int. J. Eat. Disord.* **2019**, *52*, 497–514. [CrossRef] [PubMed]
4. Cardi, V.; Mallorqui-Bague, N.; Albano, G.; Monteleone, A.M.; Fernandez-Aranda, F.; Treasure, J. Social Difficulties as Risk and Maintaining Factors in Anorexia Nervosa: A Mixed-Method Investigation. *Front. Psychiatry* **2018**, *9*, 12. [CrossRef] [PubMed]
5. Fairburn, C.G.; Cooper, Z.; Doll, H.A.; Welch, S.L. Risk Factors for Anorexia Nervosa: Three Integrated Case-Control Comparisons. *Arch. Gen. Psychiatry* **1999**, *56*, 468–476. [CrossRef]
6. Krug, I.; Penelo, E.; Fernandez-Aranda, F.; Anderluh, M.; Bellodi, L.; Cellini, E.; di Bernardo, M.; Granero, R.; Karwautz, A.; Nacmias, B.; et al. Low Social Interactions in Eating Disorder Patients in Childhood and Adulthood: A Multi-Centre European Case Control Study. *J. Health Psychol.* **2012**, *18*, 26–37. [CrossRef]
7. Westwood, H.; Kerr-Gaffney, J.; Stahl, D.; Tchanturia, K. Alexithymia in Eating Disorders: Systematic Review and Meta-Analyses of Studies Using the Toronto Alexithymia Scale. *J. Psychosom. Res.* **2017**, *99*, 66–81. [CrossRef]
8. Kerr-Gaffney, J.; Harrison, A.; Tchanturia, K. Social Anxiety in the Eating Disorders: A Systematic Review and Meta-Analysis. *Psychol. Med.* **2018**, *48*, 2477–2491. [CrossRef]
9. Rhind, C.; Bonfioli, E.; Hibbs, R.; Goddard, E.; Macdonald, P.; Gowers, S.; Schmidt, U.; Tchanturia, K.; Micali, N.; Treasure, J. An Examination of Autism Spectrum Traits in Adolescents with Anorexia Nervosa and Their Parents. *Mol. Autism* **2014**, *5*, 56. [CrossRef]
10. Winecoff, A.A.; Ngo, L.; Moskovich, A.; Merwin, R.; Zucker, N. The Functional Significance of Shyness in Anorexia Nervosa. *Eur. Eat. Disord. Rev.* **2015**, *23*, 327–332. [CrossRef]
11. Tiller, J.M.; Sloane, G.; Schmidt, U.; Troop, N.; Power, M.; Treasure, J.L. Social Support in Patients with Anorexia Nervosa and Bulimia Nervosa. *Int. J. Eat. Disord.* **1997**, *21*, 31–38. [CrossRef]
12. Patel, K.; Tchanturia, K.; Harrison, A. An Exploration of Social Functioning in Young People with Eating Disorders: A Qualitative Study. *PLoS ONE* **2016**, *11*, e0159910. [CrossRef] [PubMed]
13. Westwood, H.; Lawrence, V.; Fleming, C.; Tchanturia, K. Exploration of Friendship Experiences, before and after Illness Onset in Females with Anorexia Nervosa: A Qualitative Study. *PLoS ONE* **2016**, *11*, e0163528. [CrossRef] [PubMed]
14. Harrison, A.; Mountford, V.A.; Tchanturia, K. Social Anhedonia and Work and Social Functioning in the Acute and Recovered Phases of Eating Disorders. *Psychiatry Res.* **2014**, *218*, 187–194. [CrossRef] [PubMed]
15. Jones, A.; Lindekilde, N.; Lübeck, M.; Clausen, L. The Association between Interpersonal Problems and Treatment Outcome in the Eating Disorders: A Systematic Review. *Nord. J. Psychiatry* **2015**, *9488*, 1–11. [CrossRef] [PubMed]
16. Zipfel, S.; Löwe, B.; Reas, D.L.; Deter, H.-C.; Herzog, W. Long-Term Prognosis in Anorexia Nervosa: Lessons from a 21-Year Follow-up Study. *Lancet* **2000**, *355*, 721–722. [CrossRef]
17. Franko, D.L.; Keshaviah, A.; Eddy, K.T.; Krishna, M.; Davis, M.C.; Keel, P.K.; Herzog, D.B. A Longitudinal Investigation of Mortality in Anorexia Nervosa and Bulimia Nervosa. *Am. J. Psychiatry* **2013**, *170*, 917–925. [CrossRef]
18. Ko, B.C. A Brief Review of Facial Emotion Recognition Based on Visual Information. *Sensors* **2018**, *18*, 401. [CrossRef]
19. Kucharska-Pietura, K.; Nikolaou, V.; Masiak, M.; Treasure, J. The Recognition of Emotion in the Faces and Voice of Anorexia Nervosa. *Int. J. Eat. Disord.* **2004**, *35*, 42–47. [CrossRef]
20. Harrison, A.; Tchanturia, K.; Treasure, J. Attentional Bias, Emotion Recognition, and Emotion Regulation in Anorexia: State or Trait? *Biol. Psychiatry* **2010**, *68*, 755–761. [CrossRef]
21. Jänsch, C.; Harmer, C.; Cooper, M.J. Emotional Processing in Women with Anorexia Nervosa and in Healthy Volunteers. *Eat. Behav.* **2009**, *10*, 184–191. [CrossRef]

22. Russell, T.A.; Schmidt, U.; Doherty, L.; Young, V.; Tchanturia, K. Aspects of Social Cognition in Anorexia Nervosa: Affective and Cognitive Theory of Mind. *Psychiatry Res.* **2009**, *168*, 181–185. [CrossRef] [PubMed]
23. Kessler, H.; Schwarze, M.; Filipic, S.; Traue, H.C.; von Wietersheim, J. Alexithymia and Facial Emotion Recognition in Patients with Eating Disorders. *Int. J. Eat. Disord.* **2006**, *39*, 245–251. [CrossRef] [PubMed]
24. Kim, Y.R.; Eom, J.S.; Yang, J.W.; Kang, J.; Treasure, J. The Impact of Oxytocin on Food Intake and Emotion Recognition in Patients with Eating Disorders: A Double Blind Single Dose within-Subject Cross-over Design. *PLoS ONE* **2015**, *10*, e0137514. [CrossRef]
25. Kucharska, K.; Jeschke, J.; Mafi, R. Intact Social Cognitive Processes in Outpatients with Anorexia Nervosa: A Pilot Study. *Ann. Gen. Psychiatry* **2016**, *15*, 1–6. [CrossRef] [PubMed]
26. Mendlewicz, L.; Linkowski, P.; Bazelmans, C.; Philippot, P. Decoding Emotional Facial Expressions in Depressed and Anorexic Patients. *J. Affect. Disord.* **2005**, *89*, 195–199. [CrossRef] [PubMed]
27. Oldershaw, A.; Hambrook, D.; Stahl, D.; Tchanturia, K.; Treasure, J.; Schmidt, U. The Socio-Emotional Processing Stream in Anorexia Nervosa. *Neurosci. Biobehav. Rev.* **2011**, *35*, 970–988. [CrossRef]
28. Dinkler, L.; Rydberg Dobrescu, S.; Råstam, M.; Gillberg, I.C.; Gillberg, C.; Wentz, E.; Hadjikhani, N. Visual Scanning during Emotion Recognition in Long-Term Recovered Anorexia Nervosa: An Eye-Tracking Study. *Int. J. Eat. Disord.* **2019**, *52*, 691–700. [CrossRef]
29. Oldershaw, A.; Hambrook, D.; Tchanturia, K.; Treasure, J.; Schmidt, U. Emotional Theory of Mind and Emotional Awareness in Recovered Anorexia Nervosa Patients. *Psychosom. Med.* **2010**, *72*, 73–79. [CrossRef]
30. Kanakam, N.; Krug, I.; Raoult, C.; Collier, D.; Treasure, J. Social and Emotional Processing as a Behavioural Endophenotype in Eating Disorders: A Pilot Investigation in Twins. *Eur. Eat. Disord. Rev.* **2013**, *21*, 294–307. [CrossRef]
31. Godart, N.; Radon, L.; Curt, F.; Duclos, J.; Perdereau, F.; Lang, F.; Venisse, J.L.; Halfon, O.; Bizouard, P.; Loas, G.; et al. Mood Disorders in Eating Disorder Patients: Prevalence and Chronology of ONSET. *J. Affect. Disord.* **2015**, *185*, 115–122. [CrossRef]
32. Swinbourne, J.; Touyz, S. The Co-Morbidity of Eating Disorders and Anxiety Disorders: A Review. *Eur. Eat. Disord. Rev.* **2007**, *15*, 215–221. [CrossRef] [PubMed]
33. Westwood, H.; Tchanturia, K. Autism Spectrum Disorder in Anorexia Nervosa: An Updated Literature Review. *Curr. Psychiatry Rep.* **2017**, *19*, 41. [CrossRef] [PubMed]
34. Brewer, R.; Cook, R.; Cardi, V.; Treasure, J.; Bird, G. Emotion Recognition Deficits in Eating Disorders Are Explained by Co-Occurring Alexithymia. *R. Soc. Open Sci.* **2015**, *2*, 140382. [CrossRef] [PubMed]
35. Fujiwara, E.; Kube, V.L.; Rochman, D.; Macrae-Korobkov, A.K.; Peynenburg, V. Visual Attention to Ambiguous Emotional Faces in Eating Disorders: Role of Alexithymia. *Eur. Eat. Disord. Rev.* **2017**, *25*, 451–460. [CrossRef]
36. Renwick, B.; Musiat, P.; Lose, A.; Dejong, H.; Broadbent, H.; Kenyon, M.; Loomes, R.; Watson, C.; Ghelani, S.; Serpell, L.; et al. Neuro- and Social-Cognitive Clustering Highlights Distinct Profiles in Adults with Anorexia Nervosa. *Int. J. Eat. Disord.* **2015**, *48*, 26–34. [CrossRef] [PubMed]
37. Klin, A.; Jones, W.; Schultz, R.; Volkmar, F.; Cohen, D. Visual Fixation Patterns During Viewing of Naturalistic Social Situations as Predictors of Social Competence in Individuals With Autism. *Arch. Gen. Psychiatry* **2002**, *59*, 809. [CrossRef]
38. Klein, J.T.; Shepherd, S.V.; Platt, M.L. Social Attention and the Brain. *Curr. Biol.* **2009**, *19*, R958–R962. [CrossRef]
39. Jones, E.J.H.; Gliga, T.; Bedford, R.; Charman, T.; Johnson, M.H. Developmental Pathways to Autism: A Review of Prospective Studies of Infants at Risk. *Neurosci. Biobehav. Rev.* **2014**, *39*, 1–33. [CrossRef]
40. Watson, K.K.; Werling, D.M.; Zucker, N.L.; Platt, M.L. Altered Social Reward and Attention in Anorexia Nervosa. *Front. Psychol.* **2010**, *1*, 36. [CrossRef]
41. Harrison, A.; Watterson, S.V.; Bennett, S.D. An Experimental Investigation into the Use of Eye-Contact in Social Interactions in Women in the Acute and Recovered Stages of Anorexia Nervosa. *Int. J. Eat. Disord.* **2019**, *52*, 61–70. [CrossRef]
42. Corden, B.; Chilvers, R.; Skuse, D. Avoidance of Emotionally Arousing Stimuli Predicts Social–Perceptual Impairment in Asperger's Syndrome. *Neuropsychologia* **2008**, *46*, 137–147. [CrossRef] [PubMed]
43. Müller, N.; Baumeister, S.; Dziobek, I.; Banaschewski, T.; Poustka, L. Validation of the Movie for the Assessment of Social Cognition in Adolescents with ASD: Fixation Duration and Pupil Dilation as Predictors of Performance. *J. Autism Dev. Disord.* **2016**, *46*, 2831–2844. [CrossRef] [PubMed]

44. Phillipou, A.; Abel, L.A.; Castle, D.J.; Hughes, M.E.; Gurvich, C.; Nibbs, R.G.; Rossell, S.L. Self Perception and Facial Emotion Perception of Others in Anorexia Nervosa. *Front. Psychol.* **2015**, *6*, 1–9. [CrossRef] [PubMed]
45. Pollice, C.; Kaye, W.H.; Greeno, C.G.; Weltzin, T.E. Relationship of Depression, Anxiety, and Obsessionality to State of Illness in Anorexia Nervosa. *Int. J. Eat. Disord.* **1997**, *21*, 367–376. [CrossRef]
46. Attwood, A.S.; Easey, K.E.; Dalili, M.N.; Skinner, A.L.; Woods, A.; Crick, L.; Ilett, E.; Penton-Voak, I.S.; Munafò, M.R. State Anxiety and Emotional Face Recognition in Healthy Volunteers. *R. Soc. Open Sci.* **2017**, *4*, 160855. [CrossRef] [PubMed]
47. Bourke, C.; Douglas, K.; Porter, R. Processing of Facial Emotion Expression in Major Depression: A Review. *Aust. N. Z. J. Psychiatry* **2010**, *44*, 681–696. [CrossRef]
48. Demenescu, L.R.; Kortekaas, R.; den Boer, J.A.; Aleman, A. Impaired Attribution of Emotion to Facial Expressions in Anxiety and Major Depression. *PLoS ONE* **2010**, *5*, e15058. [CrossRef]
49. Hezel, D.M.; McNally, R.J. Theory of Mind Impairments in Social Anxiety Disorder. *Behav. Ther.* **2014**, *45*, 530–540. [CrossRef]
50. Schreiter, S.; Pijnenborg, G.H.M.; Aan Het Rot, M. Empathy in Adults with Clinical or Subclinical Depressive Symptoms. *J. Affect. Disord.* **2013**, *150*, 1–16. [CrossRef]
51. Washburn, D.; Wilson, G.; Roes, M.; Rnic, K.; Harkness, K.L. Theory of Mind in Social Anxiety Disorder, Depression, and Comorbid Conditions. *J. Anxiety Disord.* **2016**, *37*, 71–77. [CrossRef]
52. First, M.B.; Williams, J.B.; Karg, R.S.; Spitzer, R.L. *Structured Clinical Interview for DSM-5 Disorders, Research Version*; American Psychiatric Association: Arlington, TX, USA, 2015.
53. Garrido, L.; Furl, N.; Draganski, B.; Weiskopf, N.; Stevens, J.; Tan, G.C.Y.; Driver, J.; Dolan, R.J.; Duchaine, B. Voxel-Based Morphometry Reveals Reduced Grey Matter Volume in the Temporal Cortex of Developmental Prosopagnosics. *Brain* **2009**, *132*, 3443–3455. [CrossRef] [PubMed]
54. Wechsler, D. *Wechsler Abbreviated Scale of Intelligence, Second Edition (WASI-II)*; NCS Pearson: San Antonio, TX, USA, 2011.
55. Lord, C.; Rutter, M.; Dilavore, P.; Risi, S.; Gotham, K.; Bishop, S. *Autism Diagnostic Observation Schedule, Second Edition (ADOS-2) Modules 1-4*; Western Psychological Services: Los Angeles, CA, USA, 2012.
56. National Institute for Health and Clinical Excellence. *Autism: Recognition, Referral, Diagnosis and Management of Adults on the Autism Spectrum (CG142)*; NICE: London, UK, 2012.
57. Hus, V.; Lord, C. The Autism Diagnostic Observation Schedule, Module 4: Revised Algorithm and Standardized Severity Scores. *J. Autism Dev. Disord.* **2014**, *44*, 1996–2012. [CrossRef] [PubMed]
58. Fairburn, C.G.; Beglin, S.J. Assessment of Eating Disorders: Interview or Self-Report Questionnaire? *Int. J. Eat. Disord.* **1994**, *16*, 363–370. [CrossRef] [PubMed]
59. Lang, K.; Larsson, E.; Mavromara, L.; Simic, M.; Treasure, J.; Tchanturia, K. Diminished Facial Emotion Expression and Associated Clinical Characteristics in Anorexia Nervosa. *Psychiatry Res.* **2016**, *236*, 165–172. [CrossRef] [PubMed]
60. Zigmond, A.S.; Snaith, R.P. The Hospital Anxiety and Depression Scale. *Acta Psychiatr. Scand.* **1983**, *67*, 361–370. [CrossRef] [PubMed]
61. Liebowitz, M.R. Social Phobia. *Mod. Probl. Pharmacopsychiatry* **1987**, *22*, 141–173.
62. Rytwinski, N.K.; Fresco, D.M.; Heimberg, R.G.; Coles, M.E.; Liebowitz, M.R.; Cissell, S.; Stein, M.B.; Hofmann, S.G. Screening for Social Anxiety Disorder with the Self-Report Version of the Liebowitz Social Anxiety Scale. *Depress. Anxiety* **2009**, *26*, 34–38. [CrossRef]
63. Constantino, J.N.; Gruber, C.P. *Social Responsiveness Scale-Second Edition (SRS-2)*; Western Psychological Services: Torrance, CA, USA, 2012.
64. Bagby, R.M.; Parker, J.D.A.; Taylor, G.J. The Twenty-Item Toronto Alexithymia Scale—I. Item Selection and Cross-Validation of the Factor Structure. *J. Psychosom. Res.* **1994**, *38*, 23–32. [CrossRef]
65. Parker, J.D.A.; Taylor, G.J.; Bagby, R.M. Alexithymia and the Processing of Emotional Stimuli: An Experimental Study. *New Trends Exp. Clin. Psychiatry* **1993**, *9*, 9–14.
66. Task Engine. Available online: https://sites.google.com/site/taskenginedoc/ (accessed on 13 February 2020).
67. Tapajóz Pereira De Sampaio, F.; Soneira, S.; Aulicino, A.; Allegri, R.F. Theory of Mind in Eating Disorders and Their Relationship to Clinical Profile. *Eur. Eat. Disord. Rev.* **2013**, *21*, 479–487. [CrossRef]
68. Adenzato, M.; Todisco, P.; Ardito, R.B. Social Cognition in Anorexia Nervosa: Evidence of Preserved Theory of Mind and Impaired Emotional Functioning. *PLoS ONE* **2012**, *7*, e44414. [CrossRef] [PubMed]

69. Bentz, M.; Jepsen, J.R.M.; Pedersen, T.; Bulik, C.M.; Pedersen, L.; Pagsberg, A.K.; Plessen, K.J. Impairment of Social Function in Young Females with Recent-Onset Anorexia Nervosa and Recovered Individuals. *J. Adolesc. Heal.* **2017**, *60*, 23–32. [CrossRef] [PubMed]
70. Loth, E.; Garrido, L.; Ahmad, J.; Watson, E.; Duff, A.; Duchaine, B. Facial Expression Recognition as a Candidate Marker for Autism Spectrum Disorder: How Frequent and Severe Are Deficits? *Mol. Autism* **2018**, *9*, 7. [CrossRef] [PubMed]
71. Marí-Bauset, S.; Zazpe, I.; Mari-Sanchis, A.; Llopis-González, A.; Morales-Suárez-Varela, M. Food Selectivity in Autism Spectrum Disorders. *J. Child Neurol.* **2014**, *29*, 1554–1561. [CrossRef] [PubMed]
72. Sharp, W.G.; Berry, R.C.; McCracken, C.; Nuhu, N.N.; Marvel, E.; Saulnier, C.A.; Klin, A.; Jones, W.; Jaquess, D.L. Feeding Problems and Nutrient Intake in Children with Autism Spectrum Disorders: A Meta-Analysis and Comprehensive Review of the Literature. *J. Autism Dev. Disord.* **2013**, *43*, 2159–2173. [CrossRef]
73. Spek, A.A.; van Rijnsoever, W.; van Laarhoven, L.; Kiep, M. Eating Problems in Men and Women with an Autism Spectrum Disorder. *J. Autism Dev. Disord.* **2019**, 1–8. [CrossRef]
74. Kinnaird, E.; Norton, C.; Stewart, C.; Tchanturia, K. Same Behaviours, Different Reasons: What Do Patients with Co-Occurring Anorexia and Autism Want from Treatment? *Int. Rev. Psychiatry* **2019**, *31*, 308–317. [CrossRef]
75. Strang, J.F.; Kenworthy, L.; Dominska, A.; Sokoloff, J.; Kenealy, L.E.; Berl, M.; Walsh, K.; Menvielle, E.; Slesaransky-Poe, G.; Kim, K.E.; et al. Increased Gender Variance in Autism Spectrum Disorders and Attention Deficit Hyperactivity Disorder. *Arch. Sex. Behav.* **2014**, *43*, 1525–1533. [CrossRef]
76. Kristensen, Z.E.; Broome, M.R. Autistic Traits in an Internet Sample of Gender Variant UK Adults. *Int. J. Transgenderism* **2015**, *16*, 234–245. [CrossRef]
77. Bargiela, S.; Steward, R.; Mandy, W. The Experiences of Late-Diagnosed Women with Autism Spectrum Conditions: An Investigation of the Female Autism Phenotype. *J. Autism Dev. Disord.* **2016**, *46*, 3281–3294. [CrossRef]
78. Diemer, E.W.; Grant, J.D.; Munn-Chernoff, M.A.; Patterson, D.A.; Duncan, A.E. Gender Identity, Sexual Orientation, and Eating-Related Pathology in a National Sample of College Students. *J. Adolesc. Heal.* **2015**, *57*, 144–149. [CrossRef] [PubMed]
79. Jones, B.A.; Haycraft, E.; Bouman, W.P.; Brewin, N.; Claes, L.; Arcelus, J. Risk Factors for Eating Disorder Psychopathology within the Treatment Seeking Transgender Population: The Role of Cross-Sex Hormone Treatment. *Eur. Eat. Disord. Rev.* **2018**, *26*, 120–128. [CrossRef] [PubMed]
80. Couturier, J.; Pindiprolu, B.; Findlay, S.; Johnson, N. Anorexia Nervosa and Gender Dysphoria in Two Adolescents. *Int. J. Eat. Disord.* **2015**, *48*, 151–155. [CrossRef] [PubMed]
81. Sedgewick, F.; Kerr-Gaffney, J.; Leppanen, J.; Tchanturia, K. Anorexia Nervosa, Autism, and the ADOS: How Appropriate Is the New Algorithm in Identifying Cases? *Front. Psychiatry* **2019**, *10*, 1–7. [CrossRef]
82. Hillier, A.; Fish, T.; Cloppert, P.; Beversdorf, D.Q. Outcomes of a Social and Vocational Skills Support Group for Adolescents and Young Adults on the Autism Spectrum. *Focus Autism Other Dev. Disabl.* **2007**, *22*, 107–115. [CrossRef]
83. Kandalaft, M.R.; Didehbani, N.; Krawczyk, D.C.; Allen, T.T.; Chapman, S.B. Virtual Reality Social Cognition Training for Young Adults with High-Functioning Autism. *J. Autism Dev. Disord.* **2013**, *43*, 34–44. [CrossRef]
84. Turner-Brown, L.M.; Perry, T.D.; Dichter, G.S.; Bodfish, J.W.; Penn, D.L. Brief Report: Feasibility of Social Cognition and Interaction Training for Adults with High Functioning Autism. *J. Autism Dev. Disord.* **2008**, *38*, 1777–1784. [CrossRef]
85. Laugeson, E.A.; Frankel, F.; Mogil, C.; Dillon, A.R. Parent-Assisted Social Skills Training to Improve Friendships in Teens with Autism Spectrum Disorders. *J. Autism Dev. Disord.* **2009**, *39*, 596–606. [CrossRef]
86. Schohl, K.A.; Van Hecke, A.V.; Carson, A.M.; Dolan, B.; Karst, J.; Stevens, S. A Replication and Extension of the PEERS Intervention: Examining Effects on Social Skills and Social Anxiety in Adolescents with Autism Spectrum Disorders. *J. Autism Dev. Disord.* **2014**, *44*, 532–545. [CrossRef]
87. Hillier, A.J.; Fish, T.; Siegel, J.H.; Beversdorf, D.Q. Social and Vocational Skills Training Reduces Self-Reported Anxiety and Depression Among Young Adults on the Autism Spectrum. *J. Dev. Phys. Disabil.* **2011**, *23*, 267–276. [CrossRef]

88. Yoo, H.-J.; Bahn, G.; Cho, I.-H.; Kim, E.-K.; Kim, J.-H.; Min, J.-W.; Lee, W.-H.; Seo, J.-S.; Jun, S.-S.; Bong, G.; et al. A Randomized Controlled Trial of the Korean Version of the PEERS Parent-Assisted Social Skills Training Program for Teens With ASD. *Autism Res.* **2014**, *7*, 145–161. [CrossRef] [PubMed]
89. Davies, H.; Fox, J.; Naumann, U.; Treasure, J.; Schmidt, U.; Tchanturia, K. Cognitive Remediation and Emotion Skills Training for Anorexia Nervosa: An Observational Study Using Neuropsychological Outcomes. *Eur. Eat. Disord. Rev.* **2012**, *20*, 211–217. [CrossRef] [PubMed]
90. Kerr-Gaffney, J.; Harrison, A.; Tchanturia, K. Eye-Tracking Research in Eating Disorders: A Systematic Review. *Int. J. Eat. Disord.* **2018**, 3–27. [CrossRef] [PubMed]
91. Bauer, A.; Schneider, S.; Waldorf, M.; Cordes, M.; Huber, T.J.; Braks, K.; Vocks, S. Visual Processing of One's Own Body over the Course of Time: Evidence for the Vigilance-Avoidance Theory in Adolescents with Anorexia Nervosa? *Int. J. Eat. Disord.* **2017**, *50*, 1205–1213. [CrossRef]

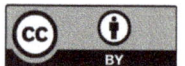

© 2020 by the authors. Licensee MDPI, Basel, Switzerland. This article is an open access article distributed under the terms and conditions of the Creative Commons Attribution (CC BY) license (http://creativecommons.org/licenses/by/4.0/).

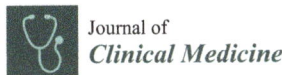

Article

Pragmatic Sensory Screening in Anorexia Nervosa and Associations with Autistic Traits

Emma Kinnaird [1], Yasemin Dandil [1,2], Zhuo Li [1], Katherine Smith [1], Caroline Pimblett [2], Rafiu Agbalaya [2], Catherine Stewart [3] and Kate Tchanturia [1,2,4,*]

[1] King's College London, Department of Psychological Medicine, Institute of Psychology, Psychiatry and Neuroscience, London SE5 8AZ, UK
[2] National Eating Disorders Service, South London and Maudsley NHS Foundation Trust, London BR3 3BX, UK
[3] Child and Adolescent Eating Disorders Service, South London and Maudsley NHS Foundation Trust, London SE5 8AZ, UK
[4] Department of Psychology, Illia State University, Tbilisi 0162, Georgia
* Correspondence: kate.tchanturia@kcl.ac.uk

Received: 10 March 2020; Accepted: 15 April 2020; Published: 20 April 2020

Abstract: Background: Research suggests that people with anorexia nervosa (AN) experience subjective hypersensitivity to external sensations that may require consideration in treatment. These difficulties may be particularly pronounced in people with AN and high autistic traits. The purpose of this pilot study was to explore the use of a brief screening tool to assess sensory sensitivity in individuals receiving treatment for AN, and to assess if self-rated sensitivity in AN is related to autistic traits. Methods: 47 individuals receiving treatment for AN completed a brief sensory screening tool and self-rated their autistic traits. Individuals were also asked to give qualitative feedback on the screening tool. Results: People with AN and high autistic traits rated themselves as more hypersensitive compared to people with AN and low autistic traits. Feedback surrounding the use of the screener was positive. Conclusions: The results of this study suggest that the use of this screener may be beneficial in eating disorder settings to help adjust and calibrate treatment to personal needs, although further research and psychometric evaluation around the clinical use of the screener is required. The finding that people with AN and high autistic traits may experience elevated hypersensitivity also warrants further exploration in future research.

Keywords: anorexia nervosa; eating disorders; sensory sensitivity; autism

1. Introduction

Anorexia nervosa (AN) is an eating disorder (ED) characterised by the persistent restriction of energy intake, an intense fear of weight gain, and disturbance in the evaluation of weight and body shape [1]. With high levels of chronicity in this population and poor treatment response rates, there is an ongoing interest in how existing understandings of AN and related treatment approaches can be adapted [2–4]. One emerging research area is whether people with AN exhibit differences in how they experience their body and its relationship to the environment [5]. Research suggests that AN may be associated with dysregulated sensory processing of external stimuli. Questionnaire-based studies indicate that people with AN experience heightened sensory sensitivity (hypersensitivity) and are more likely to perceive these sensations as aversive, resulting in the attempted avoidance of sensory experiences [6–9]. This sensory profile has been associated with heightened levels of ED symptomatology, emotional dysregulation and body image disturbance, and appears to persist following treatment and weight restoration [7–9]. Sensory experiences, such as lower sensation seeking, are also linked to heightened feelings of self-disgust in this population [6]. It is therefore possible that the core symptom of food restriction in AN may in fact play a role in self-regulating distressing sensory experiences through avoidance. Alternatively, if people with AN have low tolerance of sensory signals, then this may limit their ability to use these sensations to inform their behaviour, or to self-regulate [8].

Whilst questionnaire-based studies consistently suggest hypersensitivity in AN, biological-based findings are more mixed. Recent systematic reviews of taste and smell experiments in this population have identified evidence for both hypersensitivity and hyposensitivity (lowered sensitivity) [10,11]. This apparent discrepancy between subjective and objective measures suggests that sensory dysregulation in AN may not only be driven by potential bottom-up alterations in biological sensitivity, but also by top-down processes in how this information is perceived, interpreted and integrated [5].

Sensory difficulties may be particularly central in understanding the presentation of AN in patients with high autistic traits. Autism is a neurodevelopmental disorder associated with difficulties in social communication, repetitive and/or restrictive behaviours and interests, and sensory problems [1]. Sensory difficulties are very common in autism, with around 95% of autistic adults self-reporting altered sensory processing [12]. Significantly around one in four people with AN present with high levels of autistic traits, and around one in ten people with AN meet criteria for an autism diagnosis [13–15]. Research suggests that autistic traits in AN may be associated with longer illness durations and poorer treatment outcomes, suggesting that treatment adaptations may be required. Recent qualitative research suggests that people with AN and high autistic traits may particularly benefit from adaptations addressing sensory difficulties associated with autism [16–19]. This research indicates that that sensory difficulties in autism may impact AN and its treatment in two key ways: firstly, food-related sensitivities such as an aversion to certain textures may motivate food avoidance [20–22]. Secondly, patients with high autistic traits may find ED service environments aversive: for example, an individual with hypersensitivity to sound may find loud treatment spaces overwhelming [20].

Therefore, people with AN- and people with AN and high autistic traits in particular- may benefit from an assessment of their sensory needs during treatment. For example, if an individual presents with a strong aversion to certain tastes, these could be addressed by working with a dietician to create a meal plan that adapts around these sensitivities. At present, sensory assessments in ED services are typically carried out by a trained occupational therapist. Existing self-report assessments of sensory sensitivity, such as the Adult Sensory Profile, are often lengthy and not always freely available [23]. In this context, clinicians treating this population could benefit from the use of a brief screening tool that assesses potential sensory difficulties. A screening approach could then be used to inform whether a more detailed assessment and treatment adaptations are required.

The aim of the current study was to pilot and explore the use and acceptability of a brief, pragmatic sensory screener in a national ED service. The secondary aim of the study was to explore whether self-rated sensory sensitivities in AN are related to autistic traits.

2. Experimental Section

2.1. Participants

Adult patients with a diagnosis of AN in the South London and Maudsley National Health Service (NHS) Foundation Trust National ED Service completed the measures as part of standard audit data collection in the service. Diagnoses of AN were made by trained clinicians upon admission to the treatment programme. A total of 47 patients completed all of the measures.

2.2. Materials

2.2.1. Clinical and Demographic Information

Information on participant age, diagnosis, duration of ED, and body mass index (BMI) upon admission were taken from patient clinical notes.

2.2.2. Brief Sensory Screener

A copy of the screener is located in the Supplementary Materials for this paper (Table S1). The development of the screener was based on the five basic senses: vision, hearing, smell, taste and touch. Other senses, such as interoception or proprioception, were not included to keep the measure accessible to individuals who may not be familiar with these other modalities. Participants were presented with visual scales for each sensory modality ranging from 0 (hyposensitive) to 10 (hypersensitive), and asked to indicate their sensory level on each scale. A score of 5 indicates no sensory differences. Examples of hyposensitivity and hypersensitivity are given for each modality, with hyposensitivity (under-sensitivity) and hypersensitivity (high sensitivity) defined at the beginning of the screener.

Following an initial pilot of the screener, clinicians and patients suggested that the "touch" modality was overly broad. They suggested that a screening tool for this population could benefit from separating wider domains of touch from food textures. Therefore, the final version includes separate rating scales for touch (with examples based on fabric textures) and texture (with examples based on food textures). A number of participants only completed the first version of the questionnaire, without the separate texture scale. These participants have been included in the current study, with variation in group numbers highlighted in the results.

2.2.3. Item Autism Quotient (AQ-10)

The AQ-10 (adult version) is an autism screening tool recommended for use in adults with suspected high autistic traits [24]. It is a self-report tool consisting of 10 items, with a score of 6 and above indicating that an individual should be considered for a specialist autism assessment. This measure is widely used in this population, including for audit purposes [25,26].

2.2.4. Hospital Anxiety and Depression Scale (HADS)

The HADS is a brief 14-item self-rating measure of anxiety and depression [27]. It consists of a subscale for anxiety, and a subscale for depression, with a score of 11 and above for each subscale indicating moderate to severe symptoms.

2.3. Procedure

Patients admitted to day-patient and inpatient ED services at the South London and Maudsley NHS Foundation Trust routinely complete the AQ-10 and HADS upon admission as part of standard audit data collection. Patients were additionally asked to complete the sensory screener, and to write down any feedback about the screener. This study was carried out as part of a clinical innovation project approved by the Clinical Governance and Audit Committee in South London and Maudsley NHS Trust (032019) in April 2019.

2.4. Analysis

Participants were divided into two groups depending on whether they scored above threshold on the AQ-10. Individuals scoring below threshold were classified as having low autistic traits (LAT), and individuals scoring above threshold were classified as having high autistic traits (HAT). Shapiro-Wilk tests confirmed that the sensory outcomes were normally distributed. Although sample sizes in each group were uneven, Levene's tests suggested that the sample variances were equal on the sensory outcomes. Therefore, independent t-tests were used to compare groups on demographic and clinical characteristics. Categorical variables were compared using the chi square test. Sensory screener data were also analysed using independent t-tests. Cohen's d was used to calculate effect sizes. Across the whole sample, relationships between sensory outcomes and autistic traits, anxiety and depression were explored using a regression analysis. The screener was evaluated using Cronbach's alpha to calculate the internal consistency, and by soliciting written feedback from participants.

3. Results

3.1. Participant Characteristics

A total of 47 participants completed all measures. 30 participants scored below threshold on the AQ-10, forming the LAT group, and 17 participants scored above threshold to form the HAT group. Group clinical and demographic characteristics are summarised in Table 1. There were no significant differences between groups regarding their mean age, illness duration, HADS scores, or sex composition. By design the HAT group had significantly higher AQ-10 scores compared to the LAT group.

Table 1. Summary of group differences on clinical and demographic characteristics.

	LAT (n = 30)	HAT (n = 17)	t-Test (df = 45)	p	d
Age (Years)	30.23 (9.60)	27.76 (10.08)	0.83	0.410	0.25
Sex	96.67% female	88.24% female	$X^2 = 1.29$	0.256	-
AN Subtype	93.33% AN-R 6.67% AN-BP	93.75% AN-R 6.25% AN-BP	$X^2 = 0.03$	0.957	-
Illness duration (Years)	11.08 (8.77)	8.73 (9.32)	0.76	0.451	0.26
BMI	14.41 (2.02)	14.55 (1.67)	−0.23	0.821	0.07
AQ-10	3.60 (1.40)	7.59 (1.12)	−10.02	<0.001	3.04
HADS Anxiety	13.97 (4.70)	13.71 (6.69)	0.015	0.878	0.05
HADS Depression	11.21 (4.69)	11.82 (5.04)	−0.42	0.677	0.13

Group differences are presented as group means, with standard deviations in parentheses. Low autistic traits group (LAT), high autistic traits group (HAT), degrees of freedom (df), anorexia nervosa (AN), restrictive subtype (AN-R), binge-purge subtype (AN-BP), Adult Autism Quotient 10 item (AQ-10), Hospital Anxiety and Depression Scale (HADS), cohen's d (d), chi square (X^2).

3.2. Sensory Screener

Group scores on the sensory screeners are summarised in Table 2. Patients with AN in the HAT group self-rated themselves as significantly more hypersensitive with medium-large effect sizes in the modalities of smell, vision, texture, and total screening scores, compared to LAT patients.

Table 2. Summary of group differences on sensory screening scores.

	LAT (n = 30)	HAT (n = 17)	t-Test (df = 45)	p	d
Taste	5.23 (2.25)	5.91 (2.39)	−0.97	0.337	0.29
Smell	5.67 (2.31)	7.65 (2.57)	−2.71	0.010	0.82
Vision	5.67 (2.30)	7.18 (2.30)	−2.36	0.022	0.72
Sound	6.13 (2.56)	7.18 (3.15)	−1.24	0.223	0.38
Touch	5.60 (2.34)	6.24 (2.86)	−0.82	0.414	0.25
Texture	5.44 (2.12) n = 18	7.31 (2.63) n = 16	−2.29	0.029	0.79
Total Without Texture	28.23 (6.98)	35.06 (9.52)	−2.82	0.007	0.86
Total With Texture	32.94 (8.63) n = 18	41.5 (10.31) n = 16	−2.63	0.013	0.90

Group differences are presented as group means, with standard deviations in parentheses. Abbreviations: low autistic traits group (LAT), high autistic traits group (HAT), degrees of freedom (df).

3.3. Associations with Clinical Variables

A regression analysis was performed using the full sample (n = 47) to explore the associations between sensory outcomes and related clinical variables (autistic traits, anxiety, and depression). Analyses suggested that higher autistic traits were associated with heightened sensitivity in the smell modality only (Table 3). Higher depression scores were associated with lower smell sensitivity. No other significant associations were identified.

Table 3. Regression analysis.

	AQ-10 (B, t, p)	HADS Anxiety (B, t, p)	HADS Depression (B, t, p)
Taste	0.17, 1.05, 0.299	−0.03, −0.35, 0.726	−0.08, −0.92, 0.361
Smell	0.43, 2.57, 0.014	0.10, 1.36, 0.181	−0.25, −2.70, 0.010
Vision	0.22, 1.43, 0.161	−0.01, −0.21, 0.838	0.08, 0.96, 0.343
Sound	0.12, 0.59, 0.559	−0.01, −0.08, 0.938	0.02, 0.16, 0.871
Touch	0.04, 0.24, 0.814	0.03, 0.31, 0.760	−0.00, −0.04, 0.966
Texture	0.34, 1.59, 0.123	−0.02, −0.19, 0.854	−0.13, −1.17, 0.251
Total Without texture	1.10, 1.87, 0.069	0.13, 0.49, 0.624	−0.22, −0.69, 0.496
Total With texture	1.48, 1.67, 0.106	0.13, 0.38, 0.704	−0.45, −0.95, 0.349

Abbreviations: low autistic traits group (LAT), high autistic traits group (HAT), Adult Autism Quotient 10 item (AQ-10), Hospital Anxiety and Depression Scale (HADS), regression coefficient (B), regression t statistic (t), p-value (p).

3.4. Evaluation

Cronbach's Alpha for the scale was 0.72, indicating acceptable internal reliability and that the individual items are measuring the same underlying concept. Across the sample, $n = 9$ (19.15%) of the participants gave feedback on the use of the screener. Feedback was generally positive, including that the form was "clear and easy to follow" and that it gave participants an opportunity to reflect on their sensory experiences. Participants felt that the screener was beneficial in highlighting a need for environmental adaptations:

"It can be very helpful to discover what a particular person likes or dislikes and will help to create an environment comfortable for people who suffer from eating disorders especially during meals."

Negative feedback included changing the formatting and layout of the form to make it clearer, and concerns that only using rating scales did not leave the participants space to fully explore or explain their sensory sensitivities.

4. Discussion

The primary aim of the study was to explore the use and acceptability of a brief, pragmatic sensory screener in a national clinical ED service. This initial pilot study suggests that this screener could potentially be beneficial for use in ED treatment services, with participants generally giving positive feedback and the clinical team finding it helpful to work with this information in the context of treatment. However, further research in larger sample sizes, including an investigation of its psychometric properties, is needed to establish the utility of this screening tool. Potential benefits to this screener identified in this pilot study that could be explored in future research are that it may help both patients and their clinician with awareness, recognition and reflection surrounding sensory difficulties, and their implications for formulation and treatment. The nursing team and dieticians also reported that the tool was quick and easy to administer, and gives useful information that could help make treatment more tailored to individual needs and personalise treatment strategies.

The screener does not provide a detailed exploration of the individual's sensory sensitivities: for example, the single scales for each sensory modality do not capture if someone experiences both hyper- and hyposensitivity in certain situations. Rather, the screener appears to help stimulate thought and discussion around individual sensory needs, and highlights where assessment by an occupational therapist, or using a more detailed sensory measure, could be beneficial. To our knowledge this is the first development of a sensory screening tool specifically for use in ED populations. The piloting of this tool suggests that measures for use in this population could benefit from distinguishing between general sensory sensitivities, and food-specific sensitivities. For example, clinicians and patients recommended that food texture sensitivity be measured independently from general touch/texture sensitivity, and the results indicate that participants did indeed rate themselves differently on these separated modalities.

The secondary aim of the study was to explore whether self-rated sensory sensitivities in AN are related to autistic features, finding that people with AN and high autistic traits scored themselves as more sensitive in the areas of smell, vision, texture, and overall total screening scores, compared to participants with low autistic traits. This is the first study to explore the relationship between self-rated sensory sensitivity and autistic traits in people with AN, and suggests that autistic traits may contribute to hypersensitivity in this condition [6–9]. The results of this study strongly indicate that future research in this area should consider the potential role of autistic traits in study design and analysis. The finding also supports previous qualitative research in this area suggesting that people with AN and high autistic traits may indeed experience elevated sensory difficulties, and reinforces the possibility that this population may benefit from an assessment of their sensory needs during treatment, and subsequent environmental and dietary adaptations as appropriate [20,22].

However, the nature of the relationship between autistic traits, AN, and sensory sensitivities remains unclear. In the current study, people with AN and high autistic traits had higher scores compared to those with low autistic traits. However, the regression analysis suggested that autistic traits predicted elevated sensitivity in the area of smell only. It is possible that autistic traits impact sensory sensitivity in AN through an additional mediating variable, although a strength of this study is that it controlled for the potential confounders of anxiety and depression in the regression analysis. Two prior studies have explored objective experimental measures of smell sensitivity and autistic traits in AN with conflicting results [28,29]. This reflects evidence from previous neuropsychological research in AN which has found a similar lack of agreement between self-report and experimental measures of cognitive flexibility [30]. It is likely that future research in AN could benefit from using both types of approaches. A key advantage of using self-report measures in clinical settings is that clinicians can more easily carry out subjective reports and use this information to tailor treatment approaches, compared to experimental measures which may need additional resources and expertise. Further research in this area is needed to explore associations between self-reported sensory sensitivity and autistic traits in AN, particularly relation to potential underlying mechanisms. Future research could explore mechanisms hypothesised to influence sensory processing in autism in AN to illuminate the relationship between these areas. In particular, sensory processing in autism has been hypothesised to be related to biased central coherence in this population: autistic people are theorised to exhibit a bias towards detail-orientated information processing as opposed to global processing, or seeing the "bigger picture", which may contribute to hypersensitivity [31]. People with AN also exhibit a bias towards detail-orientated processing which has previously been linked to altered visual processing in this condition [32–35]. Further research on sensory processing and autistic traits in AN could consider this as a potential underlying mechanism.

There are a number of limitations to this study. The nature of this pilot and feasibility study meant that the sample size is relatively small, and future studies could benefit from including a higher number of participants. In particular, the current study did not include a healthy control comparison group. Therefore, it cannot draw conclusions surrounding whether people with AN rate their sensory sensitivity levels differently compared to healthy controls. Findings of hypersensitivity in this study therefore reflect people with AN rating themselves as highly sensitive on the screening measure (against a control marker of "no sensory differences"), rather than people with AN rating themselves as highly sensitive in comparison to people without the condition.

In addition, the current study did not include a full evaluation of the psychometric qualities of the screener, although a preliminary assessment does indicate acceptable internal reliability. The sensory screener was designed as a brief, pragmatic measure for use in clinical practice. It was not designed as a research tool, and therefore the goal of the current study was to explore its use and utility, rather than establishing its reliability and validity, or its agreement with other measures of sensory sensitivity. As the findings of the current study suggest that such a screening tool may be clinically beneficial both to patient and clinicians in ED services, future research could further explore the development and psychometric validation of sensory measures and screening in this population. The development of this sensory screener, in particular separating the modality of touch into a non-food example and a food-based "texture" example, suggests that research on the use and development of sensory screening in this population should consider whether sensory difficulties in AN are specific to food-related sensations or more generalised. For clinicians, in addition to the use of screening tools a more detailed assessment of sensory difficulties could consider using other tools, such as the Adult Sensory Profile, or the Swedish Eating Assessment for Autism Spectrum Disorders [23,36]. This assessment explores the presence of eating difficulties associated with autism, including items related to sensory sensitivities.

Finally, the present study does present an initial exploration of the relationship between subjective sensory sensitivity and autistic traits within AN populations, but does so in relation to self-rated autistic traits only. The AQ-10 was used in this study to distinguish people with high autistic traits as it is currently recommended for use in healthcare services for this purpose by UK clinical guidelines [37]. However, the AQ-10 and the original 50-item AQ may lack efficacy in distinguishing autism cases in clinical populations [38–41]. In the current study, that the AQ-10 may lack accuracy is suggested by the fact that participants in the HAT group had a lower, albeit non-significant, duration of illness compared the LAT group, whereas characteristics associated with autism assessed with experimental measures are associated with longer illness durations in AN [17]. Future research in this area should consider exploring sensory sensitivity in individuals with AN only compared to people with AN and a diagnosis of autism, or using gold-standard autism measures such as the Autism Diagnostic Observation Schedule (ADOS) known to be effective in this population [42]. In addition, future explorations of sensory sensitivities in AN and autism could benefit from also including a sample group of autistic people without AN.

In conclusion, the findings of the current study indicate the potential utility of using a brief sensory screener to evaluate subjective sensory sensitivity in individuals accessing ED treatment. In addition, the study suggests that subjective hypersensitivity in AN may be related to autistic traits. Implications for future research and potential clinical adaptations are discussed.

Supplementary Materials: The following are available online at http://www.mdpi.com/2077-0383/9/4/1182/s1, Table S1: Brief Sensory Screener.

Author Contributions: Conceptualization, E.K., K.T. and C.P.; formal analysis, E.K.; investigation, Y.D., Z.L., C.P., K.S. and R.A.; data curation, Y.D. and Z.L.; writing—original draft preparation, E.K.; writing—review and editing, E.K., Y.D., K.S. and K.T.; supervision, K.T. and C.S.; project administration, E.K., Y.D., K.S. and K.T.; funding acquisition, K.T. All authors have read and agreed to the published version of the manuscript.

Funding: K.T. was funded by the MRC-MRF Fund, grant number MR/S020381/1, MR/R004595/1; the Health Foundation (an independent charity committed to bring better health care for people in the UK), grant number AIMS ID 1115447. K.T. additionally received support from the Maudsley Charity, an independent NHS mental health charity which works in partnership with patients and families, clinical care teams and researchers at South London and Maudsley NHS Foundation Trust, the Institute of Psychiatry, Psychology and Neuroscience, King's College London, and community organisations, with a common goal of improving mental health, to support innovation, research and service improvement. E.K. was funded by a Medical Research Council Doctoral Training Partnership studentship, grant number MR/N013700/1.

Acknowledgments: The authors would like to thank the clinical teams working in the National Eating Disorder Service (South London and Maudsley NHS Foundation Trust) for their support with this project.

Conflicts of Interest: The authors declare no conflict of interest.

References

1. American Psychiatric Association. *Diagnostic and Statistical Manual of Mental Disorders*, 5th ed.; American Psychiatric Publishing: Arlington, VA, USA, 2013.
2. Fichter, M.M.; Quadflieg, N.; Hedlund, S. Twelve-year course and outcome predictors of anorexia nervosa. *Int. J. Eat. Disord.* **2006**, *39*, 87–100. [CrossRef] [PubMed]
3. Gowers, S.G.; Clark, A.; Roberts, C.; Griffiths, A.; Edwards, V.; Bryan, C.; Smethurst, N.; Byford, S.; Barrett, B. Clinical effectiveness of treatments for anorexia nervosa in adolescents: Randomised controlled trial. *Br. J. Psychiatry* **2018**, *191*, 427–435. [CrossRef] [PubMed]
4. Wonderlich, S.; Mitchell, J.E.; Crosby, R.D.; Myers, T.C.; Kadlec, K.; LaHaise, K.; Swan-Kremeier, L.; Dokken, J.; Lange, M.; Dinkel, J.; et al. Minimizing and treating chronicity in the eating disorders: A clinical overview. *Int. J. Eat. Disord.* **2012**, *45*, 467–475. [CrossRef] [PubMed]

5. Riva, G.; Dakanalis, A. Altered Processing and Integration of Multisensory Bodily Representations and Signals in Eating Disorders: A Possible Path Toward the Understanding of Their Underlying Causes. *Front. Hum. Neurosci.* **2018**, *12*, 49. [CrossRef]
6. Bell, K.; Coulthard, H.; Wildbur, D. Self-Disgust within Eating Disordered Groups: Associations with Anxiety, Disgust Sensitivity and Sensory Processing. *Eur. Eat. Disord. Rev. J. Eat. Disord. Assoc.* **2017**, *25*, 373–380. [CrossRef]
7. Brand-Gothelf, A.; Parush, S.; Eitan, Y.; Admoni, S.; Gur, E.; Stein, D. Sensory modulation disorder symptoms in anorexia nervosa and bulimia nervosa: A pilot study. *Int. J. Eat. Disord.* **2016**, *49*, 59–68. [CrossRef]
8. Merwin, R.M.; Moskovich, A.A.; Wagner, H.; Ritschel, L.A.; Craighead, L.W.; Zucker, N.L. Emotion regulation difficulties in anorexia nervosa: Relationship to self-perceived sensory sensitivity. *Cogn. Emot.* **2013**, *27*, 441–452. [CrossRef]
9. Zucker, N.L.; Merwin, R.M.; Bulik, C.M.; Moskovich, A.; Wildes, J.E.; Groh, J. Subjective experience of sensation in anorexia nervosa. *Behav. Res. Ther.* **2013**, *51*, 256–265. [CrossRef]
10. Islam, M.A.; Fagundo, A.B.; Arcelus, J.; Aguera, Z.; Jimenez-Murcia, S.; Fernandez-Real, J.M.; Tinahones, F.J.; de la Torre, R.; Botella, C.; Fruhbeck, G.; et al. Olfaction in eating disorders and abnormal eating behavior: A systematic review. *Front. Psychol.* **2015**, *6*. [CrossRef]
11. Kinnaird, E.; Stewart, C.; Tchanturia, K. Taste sensitivity in anorexia nervosa: A systematic review. *Int. J. Eat. Disord.* **2018**. [CrossRef]
12. Crane, L.; Goddard, L.; Pring, L. Sensory processing in adults with autism spectrum disorders. *Autism* **2009**, *13*, 215–228. [CrossRef]
13. Huke, V.; Turk, J.; Saeidi, S.; Kent, A.; Morgan, J.F. Autism Spectrum Disorders in Eating Disorder Populations: A Systematic Review. *Eur. Eat. Disord. Rev.* **2013**, *21*, 345–351. [CrossRef] [PubMed]
14. Westwood, H.; Mandy, W.; Tchanturia, K. Clinical evaluation of autistic symptoms in women with anorexia nervosa. *Mol. Autism* **2017**, *8*. [CrossRef] [PubMed]
15. Westwood, H.; Mandy, W.; Simic, M.; Tchanturia, K. Assessing ASD in Adolescent Females with Anorexia Nervosa using Clinical and Developmental Measures: A Preliminary Investigation. *J. Abnorm. Child Psychol.* **2017**, *46*, 183–192. [CrossRef] [PubMed]
16. Nazar, B.P.; Peynenburg, V.; Rhind, C.; Hibbs, R.; Schmidt, U.; Gowers, S.; Treasure, J. An examination of the clinical outcomes of adolescents and young adults with broad autism spectrum traits and autism spectrum disorder and anorexia nerovsa: A multi-centre study. *Int. J. Eat. Disord.* **2018**, *51*, 174–179. [CrossRef]
17. Saure, E.; Laasonen, M.; Lepisto-Paisley, T.; Mikkola, K.; Algars, M.; Raevuori, A. Characteristics of autism spectrum disorders are associated with longer duration of anorexia nervosa: A systematic review and meta-analysis. *Int. J. Eat. Disord.* **2020**. [CrossRef]
18. Stewart, C.; McEwen, F.S.; Konstantellou, A.; Eisler, I.; Simic, M. Impact of ASD traits on treatment outcomes of eating disorders in girls. *Eur. Eat. Disord. Rev.* **2017**, *25*, 123–128. [CrossRef]
19. Tchanturia, K.; Larsson, E.; Adamson, J. How anorexia nervosa patients with high and low autistic traits respond to group Cognitive Remediation Therapy. *BMC Psychiatry* **2016**, *16*, 334. [CrossRef]
20. Kinnaird, E.; Norton, C.; Stewart, C.; Tchanturia, K. Same behaviours, different reasons: What do patients with co-occurring anorexia and autism want from treatment? *Int. Rev. Psychiatry* **2019**, 1–10. [CrossRef]
21. Kinnaird, E.; Norton, C.; Pimblett, C.; Stewart, C.; Tchanturia, K. Eating as an autistic adult: An exploratory qualitative study. *PLoS ONE* **2019**, *14*, e0221937. [CrossRef]
22. Kinnaird, E.; Norton, C.; Tchanturia, K. Clinicians' views on working with anorexia nervosa and autism spectrum disorder comorbidity: A qualitative study. *BMC Psychiatry* **2017**, *17*, 292. [CrossRef] [PubMed]
23. Brown, C.; Tollefson, N.; Dunn, W.; Cromwell, R.; Filion, D. The Adult Sensory Profile: Measuring Patterns of Sensory Processing. *Am. J. Occup. Ther.* **2001**, *55*, 75–82. [CrossRef] [PubMed]
24. Allison, C.; Auyeung, B.; Baron-Cohen, S. Toward Brief "Red Flags" for Autism Screening: The Short Autism Spectrum Quotient and the Short Quantitative Checklist in 1000 Cases and 3000 Controls. *J. Am. Acad. Child Adolesc. Psychiatry* **2012**, *51*, 202–212. [CrossRef] [PubMed]
25. Tchanturia, K.; Smith, E.; Weineck, F.; Fidanboylu, E.; Kern, N.; Treasure, J.; Cohen, S.B. Exploring autistic traits in anorexia: A clinical study. *Mol. Autism* **2013**, *4*. [CrossRef] [PubMed]
26. Westwood, H.; Eisler, I.; Mandy, W.; Leppanen, J.; Treasure, J.; Tchanturia, K. Using the Autism-Spectrum Quotient to Measure Autistic Traits in Anorexia Nervosa: A Systematic Review and Meta-Analysis. *J. Autism Dev. Disord.* **2016**, *46*, 964–977. [CrossRef]

27. Zigmond, A.S.; Snaith, R.P. The Hospital Anxiety and Depression Scale. *Acta Psychiatr. Scand.* **1983**, *67*, 361–370. [CrossRef]
28. Bentz, M.; Guldberg, J.; Vangkilde, S.; Pedersen, T.; Plessen, K.J.; Jepsen, J.R. Heightened Olfactory Sensitivity in Young Females with Recent-Onset Anorexia Nervosa and Recovered Individuals. *PLoS ONE* **2017**, *12*, e0169183. [CrossRef]
29. Tonacci, A.; Calderoni, S.; Billeci, L.; Maestro, S.; Fantozzi, P.; Ciuccoli, F.; Morales, M.A.; Narzisi, A.; Muratori, F. Autistic traits impact on olfactory processing in adolescent girls with Anorexia Nervosa restricting type. *Psychiatry Res.* **2019**, *274*, 20–26. [CrossRef]
30. Lounes, N.; Khan, G.; Tchanturia, K. Assessment of Cognitive Flexibility in Anorexia Nervosa—Self-Report or Experimental Measure? A Brief Report. *J. Int. Neuropsychol. Soc.* **2011**, *17*, 925–928. [CrossRef]
31. Happé, F.; Frith, U. The Weak Coherence Account: Detail-focused Cognitive Style in Autism Spectrum Disorders. *J. Autism Dev. Disord.* **2006**, *36*, 5–25. [CrossRef]
32. Lang, K.; Lopez, C.; Stahl, D.; Tchanturia, K.; Treasure, J. Central coherence in eating disorders: An updated systematic review and meta-analysis. *World J. Biol. Psychiatry* **2014**, *15*, 586–598. [CrossRef] [PubMed]
33. Lang, K.; Roberts, M.; Harrison, A.; Lopez, C.; Goddard, E.; Khondoker, M.; Treasure, J.; Tchanturia, K. Central Coherence in Eating Disorders: A Synthesis of Studies Using the Rey Osterrieth Complex Figure Test. *PLoS ONE* **2016**, *11*, e0165467. [CrossRef] [PubMed]
34. Madsen, S.K.; Bohon, C.; Feusner, J.D. Visual processing in anorexia nervosa and body dysmorphic disorder: Similarities, differences, and future research directions. *J. Psychiatr. Res.* **2013**, *47*, 1483–1491. [CrossRef] [PubMed]
35. Freeman, R.; Touyz, S.; Sara, G.; Rennie, C.; Gordon, E.; Beumont, P. In the eye of the beholder: Processing body shape information in anorexic and bulimic patients. *Int. J. Eat. Disord.* **1991**, *10*, 709–714. [CrossRef]
36. Karlsson, L.; Rastam, M.; Wentz, E. The SWedish Eating Assessment for Autism spectrum disorders (SWEAA)-Validation of a self-report questionnaire targeting eating disturbances within the autism spectrum. *Res. Dev. Disabil.* **2013**, *34*, 2224–2233. [CrossRef]
37. NICE. Autism Spectrum Disorder in Adults: Diagnosis and Management, Clinical Guideline CG142. Available online: https://www.nice.org.uk/guidance/cg142 (accessed on 6 February 2020).
38. Ashwood, K.L.; Gillan, N.; Horder, J.; Hayward, H.; Woodhouse, E.; McEwen, F.S.; Findon, J.; Eklund, H.; Spain, D.; Wilson, C.E.; et al. Predicting the diagnosis of autism in adults using the Autism-Spectrum Quotient (AQ) questionnaire. *Psychol. Med.* **2016**, *46*, 2595–2604. [CrossRef]
39. Baron-Cohen, S.; Wheelwright, S.; Skinner, R.; Martin, J.; Clubley, E. The Autism-Spectrum Quotient (AQ): Evidence from Asperger syndrome/high-functioning autism, males and females, scientists and mathematicians. *J. Autism Dev. Disord.* **2001**, *31*, 5–17. [CrossRef]
40. Sizoo, B.B.; Horwitz, E.H.; Teunisse, J.P.; Kan, C.C.; Vissers, C.; Forceville, E.J.M.; Van Voorst, A.J.P.; Geurts, H.M. Predictive validity of self-report questionnaires in the assessment of autism spectrum disorders in adults. *Autism* **2015**, *19*, 842–849. [CrossRef]
41. Conner, C.M.; Cramer, R.D.; McGonigle, J.J. Examining the Diagnostic Validity of Autism Measures Among Adults in an Outpatient Clinic Sample. *Autism Adulthood* **2019**, *1*, 60–68. [CrossRef]
42. Sedgewick, F.; Kerr-Gaffney, J.; Leppanen, J.; Tchanturia, K. Anorexia Nervosa, Autism, and the ADOS: How Appropriate Is the New Algorithm in Identifying Cases? *Front. Psychiatry* **2019**, *10*, 507. [CrossRef]

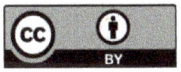

© 2020 by the authors. Licensee MDPI, Basel, Switzerland. This article is an open access article distributed under the terms and conditions of the Creative Commons Attribution (CC BY) license (http://creativecommons.org/licenses/by/4.0/).

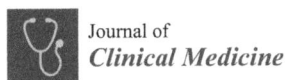

Article

Reduction of High Expressed Emotion and Treatment Outcomes in Anorexia Nervosa—Caregivers' and Adolescents' Perspective

Julia Philipp [1], Stefanie Truttmann [1], Michael Zeiler [1], Claudia Franta [1], Tanja Wittek [1], Gabriele Schöfbeck [1], Michaela Mitterer [1], Dunja Mairhofer [1], Annika Zanko [2], Hartmut Imgart [2], Ellen Auer-Welsbach [3], Janet Treasure [4], Gudrun Wagner [1] and Andreas F. K. Karwautz [1,*]

[1] Eating Disorders Unit, Department of Child and Adolescent Psychiatry, Medical University of Vienna, 1090 Vienna, Austria; julia.philipp@meduniwien.ac.at (J.P.); stefanie.truttmann@meduniwien.ac.at (S.T.); michael.zeiler@meduniwien.ac.at (M.Z.); claudiaparfuss@gmx.at (C.F.); tanja.wittek@meduniwien.ac.at (T.W.); gabriele.schoefbeck@meduniwien.ac.at (G.S.); michaela.mitterer@meduniwien.ac.at (M.M.); dunja.mairhofer@meduniwien.ac.at (D.M.); gudrun.wagner@meduniwien.ac.at (G.W.)
[2] Parkland Clinic, Clinic for Psychosomatic Medicine and Psychotherapy, 34537 Bad Wildungen, Germany; annika.zanko@parkland-klinik.de (A.Z.); hartmut.imgart@parkland-klinik.de (H.I.)
[3] Department for Neurology and Child and Adolescent Psychiatry, 9020 Klagenfurt am Wörthersee, Austria; Ellen.Auer-Welsbach@kabeg.at
[4] Section of Eating Disorders, Department of Psychological Medicine, Institute of Psychiatry, Psychology & Neuroscience, King's College London, London WC2R 2LS, UK; janet.treasure@kcl.ac.uk
* Correspondence: andreas.karwautz@meduniwien.ac.at; Tel.: +43-1-40400-30140

Received: 28 May 2020; Accepted: 22 June 2020; Published: 27 June 2020

Abstract: High expressed emotion (EE) is common in caregivers of patients with anorexia nervosa (AN) and associated with poorer outcome for patients. In this study, we examined the prevalence of high EE in caregivers of adolescents with AN and analyzed predictors for EE using multivariate linear regression models. We further analyzed whether EE is reduced by the "Supporting Carers of Children and Adolescents with Eating Disorders in Austria" (SUCCEAT) intervention using general linear mixed models and whether a reduction of EE predicts patients' outcomes. Caregivers were randomly allocated to the SUCCEAT workshop ($N = 50$) or online intervention ($N = 50$) and compared to a comparison group ($N = 49$). EE and patients' outcomes were assessed at the baseline, post-intervention, and at the 12-month follow-up. Up to 47% of caregivers showed high EE. Lower caregiver skills, higher AN symptom impact, higher levels of depression and motivation to change in caregivers were significant predictors for high EE. EE significantly decreased in the SUCCEAT groups and the comparison group according to the caregivers', but not the patients' perspective. The level of reduction could partially predict subjective improvement and improvement in clinically assessed AN symptoms and body mass index of patients. Implementing interventions for caregivers addressing EE in the treatment of adolescents with AN is strongly recommended.

Keywords: anorexia nervosa; high expressed emotion; children and adolescents; intervention; caregivers

1. Introduction

Expressed emotion (EE) is a concept that describes a set of attitudes and behaviors (e.g., criticism, hostility, warmth, emotional involvement) of relatives towards an ill person. Specifically, the components of EE that have been mainly investigated so far are critical comments/criticism (CC) and emotional overinvolvement (EOI) [1,2]. High EE may represent a maladaptive response to an illness and may contribute to an exacerbation of psychiatric symptoms [2]. EE has been extensively studied in schizophrenia and has been confirmed to be a robust and significant predictor of relapse [3]. High levels of EE have further consistently been associated with treatment outcome, relapse, and treatment dropout in several other psychiatric disorders, including depression, bipolar disorder, anxiety disorders, and also eating disorders (EDs) [1–3].

In the field of EDs, caring for someone with an ED is known to be associated with high EE [1,4,5]. Caregivers often show extreme patterns of emotional reactions [6]. They might respond too intensely and too emotional, be too directive, negative and hostile, and blame the patient (CC), or they can be overprotective, overinvolved, and take over control (EOI). In a systematic review, up to 73.2% of caregivers showed high levels of CC and 89.3% showed high levels of EOI [5]. High EE has been found to be associated with caring for older patients and longer illness duration [4], higher anxiety and depression in caregivers [7], more contact time with the patient [8], higher caregivers' distress [8,9], and less caregiver skills [9]. Other studies revealed no clear association of high EE with the patients' weight or ED psychopathology [1,10], time spent caregiving, and ED severity [9]. Only few studies investigated the ED patients' point of view of EE within the family. Perceived EE in the family assessed by ED patients was reported to be higher than in healthy controls [11]. Patients reported higher EOI for their mothers, but no difference between mothers and fathers for CC [9]. The level of perceived EE from the patients' point of view was independent from age, contact time, and duration of treatment [11]. However, it has consistently been shown that high levels of EE in caregivers, especially in mothers, seem to negatively affect engagement, outcome, and effectiveness of ED treatment [1–3,10,12,13]. Thus, considering EE of caregivers in the patients' treatment seems to be highly relevant.

The key role of interpersonal relationships, particularly, communication and high EE within the family has also been highlighted in the interpersonal maintenance model of anorexia nervosa (AN) [14–16]. EE was related to caregivers' distress. Caregivers' distress was related to patients' distress, which predicted eating disorder symptoms [8]. Interventions based on this model were developed to reduce high EE [17] in order to improve the psychological wellbeing in caregivers and support recovery from the ED in patients [4]. These interventions address misperceptions of EDs and unhelpful reactions to the illness [18] and aim to improve communication skills, reduce negative emotion and build a warm and compassionate family atmosphere [19]. Caregivers learn to use reflective listening and motivational interviewing techniques, reduce confrontation, and be warm, calm, and compassionate.

A meta-analysis showed a moderate-sized reduction of EE in caregivers after participating in such interventions, including workshop-based, online, and self-help interventions [18]. Other recent studies also reported a reduction of high EE following interventions for caregivers [20–22]. However, having investigated the effects of such interventions, the previous literature almost exclusively focused on the parents' perception, while not considering the perception of the patients, although including the patients' perception is recommended and valued to gain additional insight in the family climate of ED patients [1]. One study that included the patients' perspective found that patients did not perceive a change in their caregivers' level of EE after caregivers participated in a specialized intervention [23], while in another study, qualitative improvement in caregivers' EE was mentioned by patients [24].

So far, only few studies have investigated whether a reduction in EE can also improve the patients' treatment outcomes. Two studies reported that an improvement of maternal EE was associated with better ED symptoms at the end of the treatment [10,25]. However, whether the level of reduction in parental EE is associated with the level of reduction in ED symptoms has not been investigated up to now.

SUCCEAT (Supporting Carers of Children and Adolescents with Eating Disorders in Austria) is an intervention for caregivers of adolescents with AN based on the interpersonal maintenance model [14–16] that has already been shown to effectively reduce caregiving burden and increase caregiver skills [26]. This paper presents secondary analyses of the SUCCEAT study, focusing on various aspects of high EE. Firstly, we aimed to examine the prevalence of high EE in a sample of caregivers and whether the level of EE assessed in parents is associated with the level of EE assessed in patients. Secondly, we explored whether different characteristics of caregivers and patients can predict the level of EE. Thirdly, this study aims to investigate whether EE can be reduced by participating in the SUCCEAT intervention and whether a change in assessed parental EE is also perceived by patients. Finally, we aimed to investigate whether a reduction in high EE is associated with patients' outcomes (AN symptoms, body mass index (BMI)).

2. Methods

2.1. Study Design

The SUCCEAT study is a two-arm parallel-group quasi-randomized controlled efficacy trial comparing two types of the SUCCEAT intervention (workshop and online) to a non-randomized control group. This study was conducted between 2014 and 2019. Caregivers of children and adolescents (10–19 years) with typical or atypical AN who received regular inpatient or outpatient treatment according to the National Institute for Health and Care Excellence (NICE) guidelines [27] were included. Caregivers and patients who were not fluent in German or suffered from severe comorbidities (e.g., psychosis) were excluded. For detailed information on the study protocol, see Franta et al. [28]. Written informed consent was obtained from all the participants prior to data collection. The SUCCEAT study protocol and all the informed consent forms were approved by the Ethics Committee of the Medical University of Vienna (#1840/2013). The SUCCEAT study was registered at ClinicalTrials.gov (Identifier: NCT02480907).

2.2. Recruitment and Randomisation

Caregivers of the SUCCEAT intervention group were recruited at the Eating Disorder Unit of the Department of Child and Adolescent Psychiatry at the Medical University of Vienna. If willing to participate, caregivers completed the baseline assessment and were allocated to one of the two intervention arms: workshop (SUCCEAT–WS) or online (SUCCEAT–ONL). The start dates of the groups had been previously fixed. The first block of participants was allocated to the SUCCEAT–WS group, the following block—to the SUCCEAT–ONL group, and so forth. Block sizes of eight participants were planned, however, sizes actually varied due to varying numbers of incoming participants prior to the upcoming group (median group size = 7). Caregivers were informed about the group allocation after they had completed the baseline assessments. Those who declined to participate in the allocated intervention arm were excluded from the study. The procedure slightly differed from the originally planned randomization [28] due to practical reasons, now corresponding to the definition of quasi-randomization [29]. However, there were no systematic differences between the WS and ONL groups at the baseline. Details on the randomization procedure are reported elsewhere [26].

2.3. Interventions

SUCCEAT is an intervention for caregivers of children and adolescents with AN based on the cognitive interpersonal model of maintaining factors for EDs [14–16] with the aim to reduce EE and burden in caregivers and improve caregiver skills. Dysfunctional communication, unhelpful reactions and emotions were addressed to increase communication skills, skills to handle difficult behavior, and strategies to encourage autonomy in patients in order to reduce EE. Additionally, caregivers' burden, wellbeing, and self-care were addressed as burden and psychopathology had been highly correlated with EE. The program was delivered in eight weekly modules as a WS or ONL, designed with the same content and structure and guided by two professional clinicians. Caregivers received weekly handouts, a manual to read more about the topics addressed [30], and a DVD [31] with case examples of unhelpful and helpful communication. A detailed description of the interventions is provided by Franta et al. [28] and Truttmann, Philipp et al. [26].

2.4. Comparison Group

The SUCCEAT groups were compared to a non-randomized comparison group (COMP) of caregivers who received other forms of family treatment within the same time frame at two other facilities: the Department for Neurology and Child and Adolescent Psychiatry, Klagenfurt, Austria (four double sessions of systemic family therapy [32]), and the Parkland Clinic, Clinic for Psychosomatic Medicine and Psychotherapy, Bad Wildungen, Germany (two-day workshop on multi-family therapy based on the Maudsley model of multi-family therapy for AN [33]). Several other inpatient and outpatient units that offer treatment as usual with and without any specialized intervention for caregivers were invited to participate as the control group declined the offer. Therefore, only the two named facilities that already implemented well-established family treatment agreed to participate and served as the COMP group.

2.5. Assessment Measures

Caregivers and patients completed self-report questionnaires at baseline (T0), at post-intervention (T1, approximately 3 months after T0), and at 12-month follow-up (FU) (T2), including the assessment of EE described below.

The Family Questionnaire (FQ [34]) is a self-report questionnaire for caregivers to detect the emotional climate and EE within the family. The 20 questions were answered using a four-point Likert scale providing two subscales of EE in caregivers: "Emotional overinvolvement" (EOI) and "Criticism" (CC). We used the established cut-off values (CC score ≥ 23, EOI score ≥ 27) to define high EE.

The Family Emotional Involvement and Criticism Scale (FEICS [35]) is a self-report questionnaire for children and adolescents to assess perceived EE within the family. Two subscales were calculated ("Emotional Involvement" and "Criticism") using 14 questions that were answered using a four-point Likert scale. For the FEICS scores, no established cut-off values are available.

In addition, self-assessments for caregivers were used to explore predictors of high EE and associations with perceived changes as described below (for details, see Franta et al. [28]).

The General Health Questionnaire (GHQ [36]) was fulfilled by caregivers and used to assess the level of psychological morbidity and distress in caregivers; a higher score indicates higher psychological distress.

The Eating Disorder Symptom Impact Scale (EDSIS [37]) assessed specific caregiving difficulties in caregivers associated with the ED of a child, such as difficulties related to "nutrition", "dysregulated behavior", "guilt", and "social isolation." A higher global score represents higher AN symptom impact in the family reported by caregivers.

The Beck Depression Inventory (BDI-II [38]) measured depression in caregivers; higher scores indicate higher levels of depression.

The State and Trait Anxiety Inventory (STAI [39]) assessed anxiety in caregivers; higher scores indicate higher levels of anxiety.

The Caregiver Skills (CASK) Scale [17] was used to measure self-assessed skills in caregivers (e.g., "insight and acceptance", "emotional intelligence", "frustration tolerance"). A higher total score means more caregiver skills.

The University of Rhode Island Change Assessment Scale (URICA [40]) was used to measure motivation to change in caregivers regarding their own behavior, revealing three scales: "precontemplation", "contemplation", and "action." A lower score on the precontemplation scale and higher scores on the contemplation and action scales represent higher motivation to change in caregivers.

Finally, two more assessments for patients were used as described below.

The Eating Disorder Examination (EDE [41]) is a semi-structured interview with patients reflecting the clinical assessment of ED psychopathology ("restraint", "eating concerns", "weight concerns", "shape concerns"). A higher global score indicates higher ED psychopathology.

The Eating Disorder Inventory-2 (EDI-2 [42]) was completed by the patients and assessed subjective ED symptoms from the patients' perspective (e.g., "drive for thinness", "perfection", "dissatisfaction with the body", etc.). A higher total score indicates more subjective ED symptoms.

Sociodemographic and clinical characteristics of caregivers (sex, age, marital status, highest educational degree, time spent caregiving) and patients (sex, age, AN subtype, BMI percentile, illness duration, type of current treatment) were obtained.

2.6. Statistical Analysis

The statistical analyses were performed using IBM SPSS Statistics 25.0 and R. We first calculated descriptive statistics and compared key sociodemographic and clinical characteristics between caregivers and patients of the SUCCEAT–WS, SUCCEAT–ONL, and the COMP group. We used Chi^2 tests for categorical and ANOVA tests for continuous variables, respectively, and Kruskal–Wallis tests for variables with skewed distribution. We calculated t-tests to analyze differences in CC and EOI scores between a mother and a father and Pearson correlation coefficients to explore associations between CC and EOI obtained from the parents and patients. To analyze predictors for assessed parental and patients' CC and EOI scores at the baseline, we first carried out a series of univariate linear regressions. The following predictors were considered: sex and age of the parent, parental psychological distress and psychopathology (including the GHQ, BDI, and STAI scores), AN symptom impact on the family (EDSIS score), self-reported caregiver skills (CASK score), parental motivation to change (URICA scores), the average time spent caregiving per day (<3 h vs. ≥3 h), the patient's age, treatment type (inpatient vs. outpatient), ED duration in months, BMI percentile (≤1st percentile vs. >1st percentile) and ED symptomatology (EDE and EDI-2 total scores). Variables reaching significance in univariate regressions ($p < 0.05$) were then considered for multivariate regression models using the forward selection method where variables were added to the model of ascending p-values.

In order to analyze the efficacy of the SUCCEAT intervention on EE, we calculated general linear mixed models using the FQ/FEICS scores (CC and EOI) obtained at the baseline, post-intervention, and at 12-month FU as the within factor and the group as the between factor. Firstly, we contrasted the SUCCEAT–WS group to the SUCCEAT–ONL intervention group. Secondly, we tested whether the SUCCEAT intervention (including all WS and ONL participants) differ from participants of the COMP group. Additionally, we performed sensitivity analyses by calculating paired sample t-tests for each group to explore the baseline-to-post-intervention and the baseline-to-12-month FU effect sizes (Cohen's dz). Furthermore, we explored the moderating effect of the patient's treatment type (inpatient vs. outpatient) on the EE outcome by adding a time x treatment type interaction term to the mixed design model.

Further, we explored whether a pre–post change in assessed parental CC and EOI scores corresponds to a change in CC and EOI assessed in the patients by calculating Pearson correlation coefficients.

Finally, we used linear regression analyses to analyze whether the degree of reduction in CC and EOI can predict improvements in ED symptomatology of the patients by using the EDE and EDI-2 change scores as well as the change in the BMI percentile as outcome variables and CC/EOI change scores as predictor variables.

3. Results

3.1. Sample

In total, 149 caregivers (83% mothers, 17% fathers; mean age (SD): 47.2 (4.74) years) provided informed consent and were included in the study. Forty-five percent had a university degree and 77% were married or lived in a partnership. According to their self-reports, the average amount of time spent with their child diagnosed with AN during weekdays was distributed as follows: 0–1 h (10%), 1–3 h (19%), 3–4 h (35%), > 4 h (35%). A total of 50 caregivers were allocated to the SUCCEAT–WS intervention, another 50 caregivers—to the SUCCEAT–ONL intervention, and 49 caregivers were included in the COMP group.

Of the 149 caregivers participating, we obtained data from 144 related patients with AN. The patients were predominantly female (83%) with a mean age of 15.1 years (SD: 1.7). According to ICD-10, most patients were diagnosed with AN restrictive subtype (89%), followed by AN binge/purging subtype (9%) and atypical AN (2%). At the baseline, the median sex-and age-specific BMI percentile was 1%, the average ED duration was 16.6 months (SD: 13.8), 59% received inpatient treatment, and 41% received outpatient treatment of their ED.

Baseline sample characteristics by intervention arm are shown in Table 1. There was a significantly lower proportion of caregivers with university degree in the COMP and patients of caregivers in the COMP had a significantly longer ED duration and higher subjective ED symptomatology scores as measured with EDI-2 and received inpatient treatment more often compared to SUCCEAT groups.

Table 1. Sample characteristics at the baseline (caregivers and eating disorder patients).

	SUCCEAT-WS (N = 50)	SUCCEAT-ONL (N = 50)	COMP (N = 49)	p
Caregivers' characteristics				
Mothers (%)	84.0%	88.0%	75.5%	0.248 [1]
Age (Mean, SD)	46.64 (5.43)	47.72 (4.25)	47.27 (4.48)	0.523 [2]
University degree (%)	60.0%	46.0%	27.7%	0.006 [1]
Married or living in partnership (%)	84.0%	75.0%	70.2%	0.264 [1]
Time spent with the patient during weekdays (%)				
0–1 h/day	6.1%	10.2%	15.2%	0.386 [1]
1–2 h/day	18.4%	22.4%	15.2%	
3–4 h/day	32.7%	42.9%	30.4%	
>4 h/day	42.9%	24.5%	39.1%	
FQ–CC score (Mean, SD)	20.76 (5.96)	21.78 (5.47)	21.82 (5.54)	0.559 [2]
FQ–EOI score (Mean, SD)	26.10 (5.17)	25.44 (4.98)	27.22 (5.05)	0.222 [2]
Patients' characteristics				
Females (%)	90.0%	96.0%	100%	0.061 [1]
Age (Mean, SD)	14.66 (1.91)	15.12 (1.80)	15.43 (1.08)	0.068 [2]
ED diagnosis (%)				
AN restrictive	90.0%	90.0%	87.8%	0.995 [1]
AN binge/purging	8.0%	8.0%	10.2%	
Atypical AN	2.0%	2.0%	2.0%	
ED duration (Mean, SD)	10.41 (7.10)	16.03 (16.05)	23.77 (12.93)	<0.001 [1]
BMI percentile (Median)	1.16	2.74	0.45	0.091 [3]
Inpatient treatment (%)	48.0%	48.0%	81.6%	<0.001 [1]
EDE score (Mean, SD)	3.27 (1.62)	3.32 (1.39)	3.22 (1.36)	0.945 [2]
EDI-2 score (Mean, SD)	67.32 (39.55)	69.62 (38.79)	91.57 (47.35)	0.009 [2]
FEICS–CC score (Mean, SD)	12.15 (4.17)	12.52 (4.44)	13.51 (4.08)	0.272 [2]
FEICS–EOI score (Mean, SD)	23.92 (4.43)	23.53 (4.17)	22.91 (3.94)	0.503 [2]

[1] Chi^2 test; [2] ANOVA test; [3] Kruskal–Wallis test. Abbreviations: AN, anorexia nervosa; CC, criticism; COMP, comparison group; ED, eating disorder; EDE, Eating Disorder Examination Interview, EDI-2, Eating Disorder Inventory-2; EOI, emotional overinvolvement; FEICS, Family Emotional Involvement and Criticism Scale; FQ, Family Questionnaire; ONL, online; SUCCEAT, Supporting Carers of Children and Adolescents with Eating Disorders in Austria; WS, workshop.

Dropout of caregivers in terms of non-completion at one of the FU assessments was 14.8% at the post-intervention assessment (SUCCEAT–WS: 4.0%, SUCCEAT–ONL: 6.0%, COMP: 34.7%) and 29.6% at the 12-month FU assessment (SUCCEAT–WS: 14.0%, SUCCEAT–ONL: 28.0%, COMP: 46.9%). Dropout of patients was 13.9% at the post-intervention assessment (SUCCEAT–WS: 8.3%, SUCCEAT–ONL: 6.1%, COMP: 27.7%) and 35.4% at the 12-month FU assessment (SUCCEAT–WS: 31.2%, SUCCEAT–ONL: 32.7%, COMP: 42.6%). Caregivers and patients who dropped out did not significantly differ from those who completed the study regarding the baseline EE scores (all p-values > 0.200).

3.2. Baseline EE Characteristics

Among the total sample, high CC defined as scores above the pre-defined cut-off in the FQ were observed in 39.2% (95% CI: 31.3; 47.1) and high EOI—in 46.6% (95% CI: 38.5; 54.7) of caregivers. Mean baseline CC and EOI scores obtained from the parents and patients are shown in Table 1. Mothers had slightly higher CC (mean: 21.79, SD: 5.52) and EOI scores (mean: 26.56, SD: 5.18) compared to fathers (CC: mean: 18.87, SD: 5.48; EOI: mean: 24.74, SD: 4.43); however, these differences did not reach statistical significance (CC: $t = 1.613$, $p = 0.109$; EOI: $t = 1.672$, $p = 0.097$).

3.3. Bivariate Correlations between Parents' and Patients' EE Scores

At the baseline, the parental EE scores were not significantly associated with the EE scores obtained from the patients' perspective neither for CC ($r = 0.078$, $p = 0.356$) nor for EOI ($r = 0.115$, $p = 0.171$). This correlation slightly increased at post-intervention (CC: $r = 0.142$, $p = 0.126$; EOI: $r = 0.117$, $p = 0.206$) and 12-month FU (CC: $r = 0.216$, $p = 0.042$; EOI: $r = 0.269$, $p = 0.011$). Considering mothers and fathers separately, we found a strong association between CC scores of fathers and patients at the baseline ($r = 0.509$, $p = 0.009$), while there was no association between CC scores of mothers and patients ($r = 0.006$, $p = 0.946$). No difference between mothers and fathers were found for EOI scores.

3.4. Predictors for EE Scores at the Baseline

Firstly, we explored whether different characteristics of parents and patients are predictive of the EE scores obtained from the parents. In the univariate regression analyses (Table S1 in the electronic Supplementary Materials), we found that the level of parental psychological distress, AN symptom impact, depression, anxiety, caregiver skills, parental motivation to change, and the current treatment setting (inpatient vs. outpatient) of the child were significantly associated with either the CC or EOI score or both. In the multivariate regression model (Table 2), lower caregiver skills, higher level of AN symptom impact, and an outpatient treatment setting were significant predictors for CC with the final model explaining 46.2% of the variance. The parental EOI score was significantly predicted by higher levels of AN symptom impact, higher distress, depression, as well as higher motivation to change and lower caregiving skills with the final model explaining 63.5% of the variance.

We repeated this analysis using the EE scores obtained from the patients' perspective as the outcome variable. In the univariate regression analyses (Table S2 in the electronic Supplementary Materials), ED duration and ED symptomatology as measured with EDE and EDI-2 were significantly associated with CC and parental motivation to change and BMI were significantly associated with EOI. In the multivariate regression model (Table 3), only higher ED symptomatology (EDI-2 score) significantly predicted CC explaining 14.2% of the variance. The EOI score was significantly predicted by lower BMI (<1st BMI percentile) and lower parental motivation to change. However, the final model only explained 8.1% of the variance.

Table 2. Multivariate regression (forward selection method) predicting criticism and emotional overinvolvement (FQ, parents).

Predictor	b(SE)	t (df)	p	R^2	ΔR^2
Outcome: FQ, criticism					
Model 1				0.351	
CASK, total score	−0.240 (0.029)	−8.165 (1,123)	<0.001		
Model 2				0.435	0.084
CASK, total score	−0.171 (0.032)	−5.378	<0.001		
EDSIS, total score	0.127 (0.030)	4.253 (2,122)	<0.001		
Model 3				0.462	0.27
CASK, total score	−0.160 (0.032)	−5.079	<0.001		
EDSIS, total score	0.137 (0.030)	4.624	<0.001		
Treatment type [1]	1.849 (0.755)	2.450 (1,121)	0.016		
Outcome: FQ, emotional overinvolvement					
Model 1				0.500	
EDSIS, total score	0.253 (0.023)	11.035 (1,122)	<0.001		
Model 2				0.567	0.068
EDSIS, total score	0.195 (0.025)	7.741	<0.001		
BDI, total score	0.203 (0.047)	4.354 (2,121)	<0.001		
Model 3				0.601	0.033
EDSIS, total score	0.173 (0.025)	6.863	<0.001		
BDI, total score	0.195 (0.045)	4.320	<0.001		
URICA, contemp.	0.173 (0.055)	3.170 (3,120)	0.002		
Model 4				0.620	0.020
EDSIS, total score	0.154 (0.026)	5.956	<0.001		
BDI, total score	0.160 (0.046)	3.437	0.001		
URICA, contemp.	0.169 (0.054)	3.164	0.002		
CASK, total score	−0.064 (0.026)	−0.2486 (4,119)	0.014		
Model 5				0.635	0.015
EDSIS, total score	0.137 (0.027)	5.119	<0.001		
BDI, total score	0.101 (0.053)	1.916	0.058		
URICA, contemp.	0.162 (0.053)	3.074	0.003		
CASK, total score	−0.061 (0.025)	−2.398	0.018		
GHQ, total score	0.248 (0.113)	2.185 (5,118)	0.031		

[1] 1 = inpatient, 2 = outpatient. Abbreviations: BDI, Beck Depression Inventory; CASK, Caregiver Skills Scale; contemp., contemplation; EDSIS, Eating Disorder Impact Scale; FQ, Family Questionnaire; GHQ, General Health Questionnaire; URICA, University of Rhode Island Change Assessment.

Table 3. Multivariate regression (forward selection method) predicting criticism and emotional overinvolvement (FEICS, patients).

Predictor	b(SE)	t (df)	p	R^2	ΔR^2
Outcome: FEICS, criticism					
Model 1 (final)				0.145	
EDI-2, total score	0.040 (0.009)	4.555 (1,122)	<0.001		
Outcome: FEICS, emotional overinvolvement					
Model 1				0.041	
BMI percentile [1]	−1.681 (0.701)	−2.399 (1,136)	0.018		
Model 2				0.085	0.044
BMI percentile [1]	−2.025 (0.701)	−2.894	0.004		
URICA, precon.	−0.191 (0.074)	−2.563 (2,135)	0.011		

[1] Categorized as follows: 1 ≤ 1st percentile, 2 > 1st percentile. Abbreviations: EDI-2, Eating Disorder Inventory-2; FEICS, Family Emotional Involvement and Criticism Scale; precon., precontemplation; URICA, University of Rhode Island Change Assessment.

3.5. Intervention Outcomes on EE

The change in EE scores by group from the baseline to the post-intervention and the 12-month FU assessment is shown in Figure 1. We first tested whether the SUCCEAT–WS group differs from SUCCEAT–ONL group. We found that the assessed parental CC (F = 7.391, p = 0.001) and EOI scores (F = 45.704, p < 0.001) significantly decreased over time across both groups, but there was no significant time × group interaction effect (CC: F = 0.437, p = 0.782; EOI: F = 0.953, p = 0.435). Considering the patients' perspective, there was no significant main effect of time and group difference neither for CC nor for EOI.

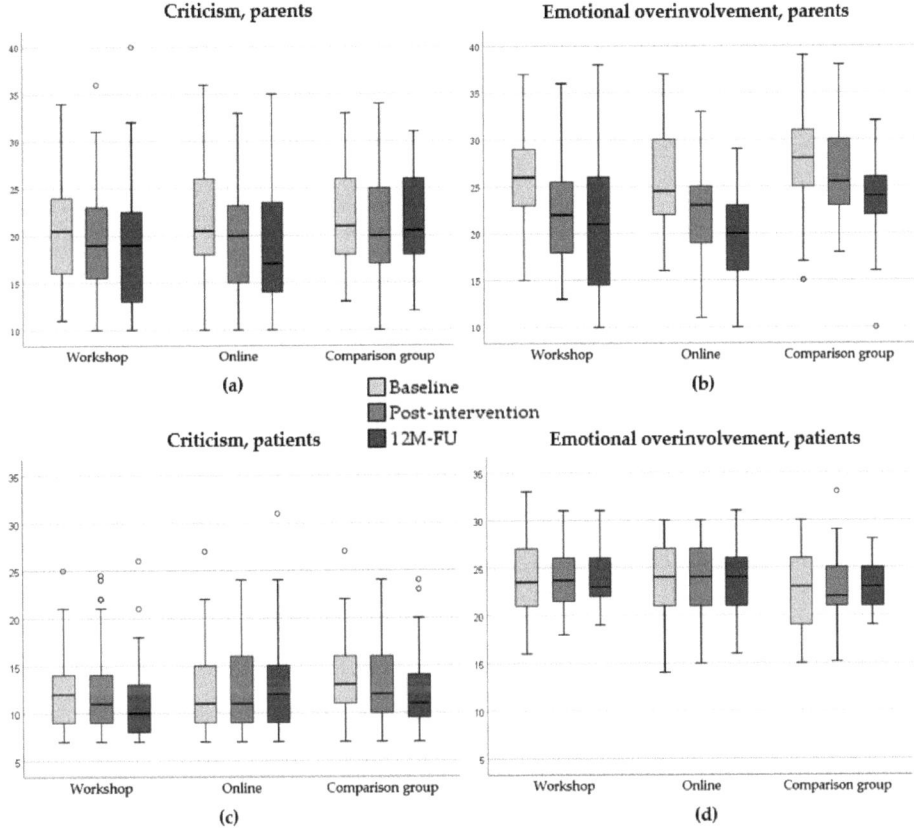

Figure 1. Change of high expressed emotion scores in the SUCCEAT workshop, online, and comparison groups from the baseline (light-grey box) to the post-intervention (mid-grey box) and the 12-month follow-up (dark-grey box) assessment: (**a**) Criticism score (parent perspective), (**b**) Emotional Overinvolvement score (parent perspective), (**c**) Criticism score (patient perspective), (**d**) Emotional Overinvolvement score (patient perspective). The size of the box represents the interquartile range (IQR); the whiskers indicate the minimum/maximum values in case no outliers were observed. Outliers (defined as values > 1.5 × IQR from the 25th quantile and 75th quantile) are depicted as circles. Abbreviations: 12M-FU, 12-month follow-up.

When contrasting the SUCCEAT groups to the COMP group, we found the same pattern of results. The assessed parental CC (F = 5.400, p = 0.005) and EOI scores (F = 36.112, p < 0.001) significantly decreased over time across the groups, but this change was the same for the SUCCEAT and COMP groups (CC: F = 0.089, p = 0.914; EOI: F = 1.612, p = 0.202). Again, no significant effects of time and time x group interaction effects were observed when considering the patients' perspective.

Sensitivity analyses using *t*-tests revealed that for the assessed parental CC, baseline-to-post-intervention reductions were highest for the SUCCEAT–ONL group (dz = 0.44, t = 3.788, p < 0.001) compared to the SUCCEAT–WS (dz = 0.20, t = 1.806, p = 0.077) and COMP groups (dz = 0.32, t = 2.172, p = 0.038). These effects remained stable to the 12-month FU for the SUCCEAT groups (WS: dz = 0.24; ONL: dz = 0.54) and slightly decreased in the COMP group (dz = 0.20). For the assessed parental EOI, baseline-to-post reductions were slightly higher for the SUCCEAT groups (WS: dz = 0.68, t = 5.739, p < 0.001; ONL: dz: 0.76, t = 5.927, p < 0.001) compared to the COMP group (dz = 0.36; t = 2.061, p = 0.048). The effect sizes further increased at the 12-month FU in all the groups (WS: dz = 0.76, ONL: dz = 1.11, COMP: dz = 0.89). Considering the patients' perspective, all effect sizes were close to zero in all the groups.

Further analyses revealed that the type of patients' treatment (inpatient vs. outpatient) was a significant moderator of the intervention outcome. Caregivers of outpatients reported a significantly higher reduction in CC scores than caregivers of inpatients (time x treatment type interaction: F = 4.076, p = 0.018). Regarding EOI, reductions of EOI scores were reported to be faster (from the baseline to post-intervention) in caregivers of outpatients, whereas the reduction was delayed (post-intervention to the 12-month FU) in caregivers of inpatients (time x treatment type interaction: F = 5.011, p = 0.008). This moderator effect was independent of the group.

Figure 2 presents the bivariate correlations between the baseline-to-post-intervention change of parental and patients' CC and EOI scores. In the SUCCEAT group, parental change of CC was moderately associated with the change of CC in patients (r = 0.230, p = 0.031). In the COMP group, this association was not significant (r = 0.209, p = 0.285). For EOI, no significant associations in the change scores were observed (SUCCEAT: r = 0.160, p = 0.137; COMP: r = −0.088, p = 0.655).

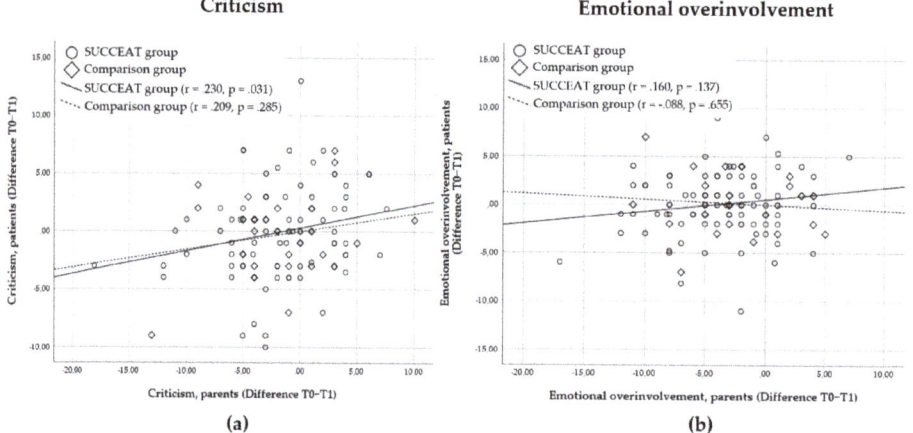

Figure 2. The scatterplot depicting the association (Pearson correlation coefficients) between high expressed emotion change scores (baseline to post-intervention) of parents and patients: (**a**) Criticism change scores; (**b**) Emotional overinvolvement change scores. A significant positive correlation indicates that higher levels of change based on the parents' perspective are associated with higher levels of change based on the perspective of patients.

3.6. Impact of EE Change on the Patient's ED Symptomatology

Table 4 shows whether a reduction in parental or patients' EE scores significantly predicted improvements in ED symptoms (EDE and EDI-2 scores, BMI percentile) for the total sample and separately for inpatients and outpatients. We found that for the total sample, improvements in CC were significantly associated with improvements in ED symptomatology and BMI. On the contrary, reductions in EOI did not significantly predict improvements in ED symptoms.

Table 4. Results of linear regression analyses predicting the change in patient's eating disorder symptoms by the change in high expressed emotion.

	EDE Change Score		EDI-2 Change Score		BMI Perc. Change	
	T0–T1	T0–T2	T0–T1	T0–T2	T0–T1	T0–T2
Change in CC (FQ)	$p = 0.731$	$p = 0.239$	$p = 0.040$	$p = 0.073$	$p = 0.995$	$p = 0.099$
Change in EOI (FQ)	$p = 0.515$	$p = 0.148$	$p = 0.113$	$p = 0.050$	$p = 0.969$	$p = 0.066$
Change in CC (FEICS)	$p = 0.040$	$p = 0.087$	$p = 0.005$	$p < 0.001$	$p = 0.006$	$p = 0.561$
Change in EOI FEICS)	$p = 0.096$	$p = 0.438$	$p = 0.580$	$p = 0.867$	$p = 0.982$	$p = 0.307$

Abbreviations: CC, criticism, EOI, emotional overinvolvement, EDE, Eating Disorder Examination Interview, EDI-2, Eating Disorder Inventory-2, FQ, Family Questionnaire, FEICS, Family Emotional Involvement and Criticism Scale; T0–T1, difference between the baseline and post-intervention scores; T0–T2, difference between the baseline and 12-month FU scores.

4. Discussion

This study explored EE in caregivers and adolescents with AN at the baseline and following a skills training for caregivers, including a long-term FU. In addition, we aimed to investigate whether changes in EE affect patients' outcomes.

Firstly, the caregivers' perspective of EE was analyzed. One third of caregivers showed elevated CC scores and nearly half of the caregivers reported high EOI scores. These prevalence figures are somewhat lower compared to previous studies using the same questionnaire [5,7]. This may be due to older patients (mostly adults) and a longer illness duration in these reports (mostly far longer than one year) compared to our participants (approximately one year). Even though we only observed a tendency that longer illness duration is associated with higher EE scores in this study, this association can be assumed from the literature [4,5,10]. CC and EOI scores tended to be higher for mothers than for fathers, albeit these results did not reach statistical significance due to the small number of fathers included in this study. This is not fully in line with several previous reports describing mothers to be more overinvolved than fathers [5,9,43] and fathers to be more critical than mothers [5,43].

Low perceived caregiver skills, high AN symptom impact on caregivers, and an outpatient treatment setting were significant factors associated with CC, accounting for nearly 50% of the variance. High AN symptom impact on caregivers, depression in caregivers, higher psychological distress, higher motivation to change in caregivers, and less caregiver skills accounted for over 60% of the variance of EOI. Other studies also found associations of high EE with psychological distress or depression [1,43,44]. Caregivers' distress and self-care should therefore be the core elements in interventions for caregivers, beside emotion regulation strategies and communication skills. Less perceived skills were associated with both higher CC and higher EOI. This may reflect that caregivers who feel less competent to deal with ED in the family demonstrate high EE, probably because they feel overwhelmed with this situation. Consequently, one might also assume that enhancing caregivers' skills can have a positive impact on EE. Interestingly, higher motivation to change in parents was associated with higher EOI. This sounds paradoxical. However, caregivers who experience frustration and helplessness when confronted with ED symptoms or associated conflicts more often, which may consequently enhance EE, might also be highly motivated to change their own behavior or aspects of the actual situation. Therefore, it may be of benefit to target motivation to change in interventions for caregivers. Further research is needed to investigate the role of motivation to change in caregivers regarding high EE. Caregivers of outpatients reported higher scores for CC than caregivers of inpatients. It might be assumed that parents of outpatients feel more responsible for an improvement of symptoms compared to inpatients, whereas the responsibility for symptom improvement is delegated to the ED treatment team. This may lead to higher distress and burden in parents of outpatients which may promote more critical comments. Besides, an outpatient treatment setting might induce more situations where high

EE can occur compared to an inpatient setting. In contrast to the literature [43], there was no association with illness severity (patients with lower BMI or higher ED psychopathology). No associations were also found for age of caregivers and age of patients, with only a tendency for caregivers of older patients to report higher EOI scores, in contrast to other studies reporting significantly higher EE in caregivers of older patients [4,5]. This may be because the mean age of patients within those studies was higher than in our sample. As the patient's age and duration of illness often correlate, we assume that including adult patients in the study may lead to a similar result. The time spent caregiving did not play a role in our study regarding EE levels either, in contrast to another study [8]. This study included adult patients and concluded that caring for patients that live in the same household involves more time and leads to higher EE. However, as we only included adolescents, the great majority of whom still lived at home, the time spent caregiving may not play such an important role.

We also explored predictors of high EE based on the patients' perspective. Regarding the patients' point of view on EE, high ED psychopathology was solely associated with CC, whereas a lower BMI and higher motivation to change in caregivers were associated with EOI. Therefore, a somewhat more severe illness (lower BMI and higher ED psychopathology) was correlated with high EE in the family. Moreover, when parents were more motivated to change, the perceived EOI was higher, which is similar to the findings for parents described above. However, our model only accounted for 4% (CC) and 8% (EOI) of the variance. Hence, other factors associated with the patients' perception of EE in the family should be investigated in future research.

Another aim of the study was to explore whether parental and patients' perceptions of EE are correlated. Regarding the total group, there were no significant correlations at the baseline, while the correlations between caregivers and patients slightly increased with time and reached significance at the 12-month FU. It is unclear why parents and patients' perceptions are stronger associated with time, even though the patients' perception of high EE within the family did not decrease like the caregivers' perception did. We assume that either the patients' or the parents' ability to precisely assess the real family climate improves with time, probably due to successful weight restitution or less severe symptoms at T2 or because patients gain valuable insights on family dynamics during their ongoing psychotherapy. However, the low correlations indicate that the parent's and patient's perceptions of EE diverge, which can be targeted in family-based interventions. Interestingly, we found a significant high correlation between the fathers' and patients' perceptions of CC at the baseline and at post-intervention which has to be interpreted with caution due to the low number of fathers included in this study.

We further investigated the efficacy of the SUCCEAT intervention on EE in caregivers. A significant reduction of EE was observed in the SUCCEAT group for the short-term and the long-term FU. This is in line with the literature, showing that EE in caregivers can be reduced after participating in an intervention for caregivers including psychoeducation and skills training [18,20,21,45]. EE was also reduced in the COMP group with no significant difference to the SUCCEAT intervention. That might be because the facilities that recruited participants for the COMP group already implemented specialized family interventions (multi-family therapy [33] or systemic family therapy [32]) also including expressing emotions, conflict management, and communication within the family as the core elements. To note, there were no differences between the three study arms with regard to the majority of caregivers' and patients' sociodemographic and clinical characteristics at the baseline. However, the groups differed with respect to the highest educational degree, ED duration, treatment setting, and subjective ED symptoms with the caregivers of the SUCCEAT group having higher educational levels and the COMP patients having a longer illness duration, higher subjective ED psychopathology, and having been treated in an inpatient setting more often. This should be considered when interpreting the results regarding group differences. Yet, there was no difference for EE scores at the baseline between the three arms. The sensitivity analyses showed that reductions in EOI were generally higher than in CC and that intervention effects remained stable or increased further up to the 12-month FU except for CC in the COMP group where we found a small rebound effect indicating that parents of the COMP group were a bit more critical at the 12-month FU again. Indeed, the current literature suggests that CC is more susceptible to increase again in the long term [43]. Interestingly, the improvement of CC and EOI was stronger in caregivers of outpatients than of inpatients and EOI also improved faster. This might be due to the fact that caregivers of outpatients may have more time and more opportunities to use and practice the communication skills trained in the interventions than caregivers of inpatients.

Unfortunately, no improvements were found when considering the patients' perception of EE within the family. Thus, the patients did not perceive EE to be significantly reduced over time neither in the SUCCEAT nor in the COMP groups. This could be due to several reasons. Firstly, we used questionnaires that measure the same construct, but did not include exactly the same item contents, impeding direct comparisons. The FQ measures subjective CC and EOI towards the patient, whereas the FEICS assesses CC and EOI within the whole family from the patient's point of view, but not specifically towards the parent who completed the FQ. Secondly, in most cases, only one parent (either mother or father) participated in the intervention. It might be the case that the caregivers who did not participate did not change regarding their EE compared to the ones that participated and therefore they may still contribute to a highly negative emotional climate. Thus, if possible, both parents should be encouraged to participate in a caregiver's skills training and be included in further research. Another possible explanation is that parents feel a reduction of EE more intensely, whereas patients do not experience small changes. Rienecke [1] assumed patients with AN to be acutely sensitive to parental EE, so they may have difficulties to experience a change even if the frequency of EE has reduced. In that case, children and adolescents might need more information on EE themselves in order to be more sensitive to notice a change in the family climate [46]. It might be possible to encourage patients themselves to read some chapters of the manual or to watch some parts of the DVD used in the intervention. Another possibility is to arrange one family meeting where this topic can be discussed together or to implement this issue in the patients' therapy.

Although there was no reduction in EE from the patients' point of view, we found a significant association between the perceived change in CC in parents and the perceived change in CC in patients from the baseline to post-intervention in the SUCCEAT group only. However, this correlation was marginal. No such association was observed for EOI. These results were similar to another study [23] that reported a significant reduction of EE in caregivers, no perceived reduction in patients, but a positive correlation between changes in perceived EE between caregivers and patients. Furthermore, patients might experience qualitative improvements in EE as indicated by Goddard et al. [24] which might not have been covered with the questionnaire used in this study.

Finally, we investigated whether reductions in parental or perceived EE affect the outcome of ED pathology and BMI in AN patients. Indeed, improvement in the assessed parental CC was associated with greater changes in subjective ED symptoms. Similarly, greater improvement in CC assessed in patients was associated with greater changes in subjective ED symptoms, clinically assessed ED psychopathology, and BMI. For EOI, no clear association was observed. These results contribute to the literature indicating that a reduction in parental EE is associated with patients' outcomes [10,25]. Although our analyses were explorative, these results indicate that reducing EE through a caregiver skills training can positively affect the ED psychopathology and BMI in patients. These results highlight the benefit and need in a caregiver training in the routine ED treatment.

This study has a couple of strengths. It is the first study investigating whether a change in EE can predict a change in ED psychopathology and BMI in adolescent patients. A long-term outcome was included. Both SUCCEAT groups were uniformly designed and guided by the same two professional clinicians. The study has some limitations, too. The number of fathers included in this study was low. Therefore, the role of fathers and the correlation between patients and both parents as well as between mothers and fathers require further investigation. Furthermore, as ED duration and treatment setting (outpatient or inpatient setting) differ significantly between the three groups at the baseline, results regarding group differences should be interpreted with some caution.

5. Conclusions

Our study confirms that high EE is common in caregivers of adolescent patients with AN. It further highlights that EE can be reduced after interventions for caregivers and that this reduction positively influences patients' outcomes. Our results therefore underline the importance of including a focus on parental EE into the treatment of adolescents with AN. Parental EE was high and was associated with higher distress, higher depression, and a lack of skills. We found that parental EE was significantly reduced after participating in the SUCCEAT intervention or a specialized family intervention and that this reduction remained in the long term. Although the patients' perceptions did not match well with the caregivers' perceptions of EE, there was some evidence that reductions in EE positively affect the patient's treatment course. Altogether, we can strongly recommend to include interventions for caregivers, such as SUCCEAT, into the treatment of adolescents with AN in order to improve the outcome for caregivers and for patients. Patients might further benefit from a conjoint meeting with parents to discuss family climate and to get sensitive to perceive possible changes.

Supplementary Materials: The following are available online at http://www.mdpi.com/2077-0383/9/7/2021/s1: Supplementary Tables S1 and S2.

Author Contributions: Conceptualization, A.F.K.K., J.T., J.P., and G.W.; methodology, C.F., J.P., and M.Z.; formal analysis, M.Z.; investigation, J.P., S.T., A.Z., C.F., and T.W.; resources, H.I., E.A.-W., G.S., M.M., D.M., A.F.K.K., and G.W.; data curation, M.Z.; writing—original draft preparation, J.P.; writing—review and editing, M.Z., A.F.K.K., G.W., and J.P.; visualization, M.Z.; supervision, A.F.K.K. and G.W.; project administration, J.P., S.T., C.F., and T.W.; funding acquisition, A.F.K.K. and G.W. All authors have read and agreed to the published version of the manuscript.

Funding: This research was funded by the Gemeinsame Gesundheitsziele aus dem Rahmen-Pharmavertrag/Pharma Master Agreement (a cooperation between the Austrian pharmaceutical industry and the Austrian social insurance; grant No. 99901002500 given to G.W. and A.K.).

Acknowledgments: We thank all the patients and caregivers who participated, as well as all the staff members that helped to conduct the study.

Conflicts of Interest: J.P. was a coach in the SUCCEAT workshop and online intervention. J.T. co-authored the book that was used as the basis for intervention. The funders had no role in the design of the study; in the collection, analyses, or interpretation of data; in the writing of the manuscript, or in the decision to publish the results.

References

1. Rienecke, R. Expressed Emotion and Eating Disorders: An Updated Review. *Curr. Psychiatry Rev.* **2018**, *14*, 84–98. [CrossRef]
2. Peris, T.S.; Miklowitz, D.J. Parental Expressed Emotion and Youth Psychopathology: New Directions for an Old Construct. *Child Psychiatry Hum. Dev.* **2015**, *46*, 863–873. [CrossRef] [PubMed]
3. Butzlaff, R.L.; Hooley, J.M. Expressed emotion and psychiatric relapse: A meta-analysis. *Arch. Gen. Psychiatry* **1998**, *55*, 547–552. [CrossRef]
4. Zabala, M.J.; Macdonald, P.; Treasure, J. Appraisal of caregiving burden, expressed emotion and psychological distress in families of people with eating disorders: A systematic review. *Eur. Eat. Disord. Rev.* **2009**, *17*, 338–349. [CrossRef]
5. Anastasiadou, D.; Medina-Pradas, C.; Sepulveda, A.R.; Treasure, J. A systematic review of family caregiving in eating disorders. *Eat. Behav.* **2014**, *15*, 464–477. [CrossRef]
6. Treasure, J.; Sepulveda, A.R.; Whitaker, W.; Todd, G.; Lopez, C.; Whitney, J. Collaborative care between professionals and non-professionals in the management of eating disorders: A description of workshops focussed on interpersonal maintaining factors. *Eur. Eat. Disord. Rev.* **2007**, *15*, 24–34. [CrossRef]
7. Kyriacou, O.; Treasure, J.; Schmidt, U. Expressed emotion in eating disorders assessed via self-report: An examination of factors associated with expressed emotion in carers of people with anorexia nervosa in comparison to control families. *Int. J. Eat. Disord.* **2008**, *41*, 37–46. [CrossRef]
8. Goddard, E.; Salerno, L.; Hibbs, R.; Raenker, S.; Naumann, U.; Arcelus, J.; Ayton, A.; Boughton, N.; Connan, F.; Goss, K.; et al. Empirical examination of the interpersonal maintenance model of anorexia nervosa. *Int. J. Eat. Disord.* **2013**, *46*, 867–874. [CrossRef] [PubMed]

9. Rhind, C.; Salerno, L.; Hibbs, R.; Micali, N.; Schmidt, U.; Gowers, S.; Macdonald, P.; Goddard, E.; Todd, G.; Tchanturia, K.; et al. The Objective and Subjective Caregiving Burden and Caregiving Behaviours of Parents of Adolescents with Anorexia Nervosa. *Eur. Eat. Disord. Rev.* **2016**, *24*, 310–319. [CrossRef] [PubMed]
10. Allan, E.; Le Grange, D.; Sawyer, S.M.; McLean, L.A.; Hughes, E.K. Parental Expressed Emotion During Two Forms of Family-Based Treatment for Adolescent Anorexia Nervosa. *Eur. Eat. Disord. Rev.* **2018**, *26*, 46–52. [CrossRef] [PubMed]
11. Di Paola, F.; Faravelli, C.; Ricca, V. Perceived expressed emotion in anorexia nervosa, bulimia nervosa, and binge-eating disorder. *Compr. Psychiatry* **2010**, *51*, 401–405. [CrossRef]
12. Eisler, I.; Simic, M.; Russell, G.F.M.; Dare, C. A randomised controlled treatment trial of two forms of family therapy in adolescent anorexia nervosa: A five-year follow-up. *J. Child Psychol. Psychiatry* **2007**, *48*, 552–560. [CrossRef] [PubMed]
13. Berona, J.; Richmond, R.; Rienecke, R.D. Heterogeneous weight restoration trajectories during partial hospitalization treatment for anorexia nervosa. *Int. J. Eat. Disord.* **2018**, *51*, 914–920. [CrossRef] [PubMed]
14. Schmidt, U.; Treasure, J. Anorexia nervosa: Valued and visible. A cognitive-interpersonal maintenance model and its implications for research and practice. *Br. J. Clin. Psychol.* **2006**, *45*, 343–366. [CrossRef]
15. Treasure, J.; Schmidt, U. The cognitive-interpersonal maintenance model of anorexia nervosa revisited: A summary of the evidence for cognitive, socio-emotional and interpersonal predisposing and perpetuating factors. *J. Eat. Disord.* **2013**, *1*, 13. [CrossRef] [PubMed]
16. Treasure, J.; Willmott, D.; Ambwani, S.; Cardi, V.; Clark Bryan, D.; Rowlands, K.; Schmidt, U. Cognitive Interpersonal Model for Anorexia Nervosa Revisited: The Perpetuating Factors that Contribute to the Development of the Severe and Enduring Illness. *J. Clin. Med.* **2020**, *9*, 630. [CrossRef] [PubMed]
17. Hibbs, R.; Rhind, C.; Salerno, L.; Coco, G.L.; Goddard, E.; Schmidt, U.; Micali, N.; Gowers, S.; Beecham, J.; Macdonald, P.; et al. Development and validation of a scale to measure caregiver skills in eating disorders. *Int. J. Eat. Disord.* **2015**, *48*, 290–297. [CrossRef] [PubMed]
18. Hibbs, R.; Rhind, C.; Leppanen, J.; Treasure, J. Interventions for caregivers of someone with an eating disorder: A meta-analysis. *Int. J. Eat. Disord.* **2015**, *48*, 349–361. [CrossRef] [PubMed]
19. Treasure, J.; Whitaker, W.; Todd, G.; Whitney, J. A description of multiple family workshops for carers of people with anorexia nervosa. *Eur. Eat. Disord. Rev.* **2012**, *20*, e17–e22. [CrossRef]
20. Dimitropoulos, G.; Landers, A.; Freeman, V.; Novick, J.; Schmidt, U.; Olmsted, M. A feasibility study comparing a web-based intervention to a workshop intervention for caregivers of adults with eating disorders. *Eur. Eat. Disord. Rev.* **2019**, *27*, 641–654. [CrossRef]
21. Magill, N.; Rhind, C.; Hibbs, R.; Goddard, E.; Macdonald, P.; Arcelus, J.; Morgan, J.; Beecham, J.; Schmidt, U.; Landau, S.; et al. Two-year Follow-up of a Pragmatic Randomised Controlled Trial Examining the Effect of Adding a Carer's Skill Training Intervention in Inpatients with Anorexia Nervosa. *Eur. Eat. Disord. Rev.* **2015**, *24*. [CrossRef]
22. McEvoy, P.M.; Targowski, K.; McGrath, D.; Carter, O.; Fursland, A.; Fitzgerald, M.; Raykos, B. Efficacy of a brief group intervention for carers of individuals with eating disorders: A randomized control trial. *Int. J. Eat. Disord.* **2019**, *52*, 987–995. [CrossRef] [PubMed]
23. Hoyle, D.; Slater, J.; Williams, C.; Schmidt, U.; Wade, T.D. Evaluation of a web-based skills intervention for carers of people with anorexia nervosa: A randomized controlled trial. *Int. J. Eat. Disord.* **2013**, *46*, 634–638. [CrossRef] [PubMed]
24. Goddard, E.; Macdonald, P.; Treasure, J. An examination of the impact of the Maudsley Collaborative Care skills training workshops on patients with anorexia nervosa: A qualitative study. *Eur. Eat. Disord. Rev.* **2011**, *19*, 150–161. [CrossRef] [PubMed]
25. Moskovich, A.A.; Timko, C.A.; Honeycutt, L.K.; Zucker, N.L.; Merwin, R.M. Change in expressed emotion and treatment outcome in adolescent anorexia nervosa. *Eat. Disord.* **2017**, *25*, 80–91. [CrossRef] [PubMed]
26. Truttmann, S.; Philipp, J.; Zeiler, M.; Franta, C.; Wittek, T.; Merl, E.; Schöfbeck, G.; Koubek, D.; Laczkovics, C.; Imgart, H.; et al. Long-term Efficacy of the Workshop- vs. Online-SUCCEAT (Supporting Carers of Children and Adolescents with Eating Disorders) intervention: A quasi-randomised feasibility trial. *J. Clin. Med.* **2020**, *9*, 1912. [CrossRef]
27. National Guideline Alliance (UK). *Eating Disorders: Recognition and Treatment*; National Institute for Health and Care Excellence: Clinical Guidelines; National Institute for Health and Care Excellence: London, UK, 2017.

28. Franta, C.; Philipp, J.; Waldherr, K.; Truttmann, S.; Merl, E.; Schöfbeck, G.; Koubek, D.; Laczkovics, C.; Imgart, H.; Zanko, A.; et al. Supporting Carers of Children and Adolescents with Eating Disorders in Austria (SUCCEAT): Study protocol for a randomised controlled trial. *Eur. Eat. Disord. Rev.* **2018**, *26*, 447–461. [CrossRef]
29. Higgins, J.; Green, S. Cochrane Handbook for Systematic Reviews of Interventions. Available online: https://handbook-5-1.cochrane.org/ (accessed on 22 May 2020).
30. Treasure, J.; Smith, G.; Crane, A. *Skills-Based Learning for Caring for a Loved One with an Eating Disorder: The New Maudsley Method*; Routledge: London, UK, 2007.
31. The Succeed Foundation. *How to Care for Someone with an Eating Disorder [DVD]*; The Succeed Foundation: London, UK, 2011.
32. Reich, G. Familienbeziehungen und Familientherapie bei Essstörungen. *Prax. Kinderpsychol. Kinderpsychiatr.* **2005**, *54*, 318–336.
33. Imgart, H.; Plassmann, R. Effective factors in multifamily therapy in patients with eating disorders: Critical appraisal and implications for practice. *Neuropsychiatr* **2020**. [CrossRef]
34. Wiedemann, G.; Rayki, O.; Feinstein, E.; Hahlweg, K. The Family Questionnaire: Development and validation of a new self-report scale for assessing expressed emotion. *Psychiatry Res.* **2002**, *109*, 265–279. [CrossRef]
35. Kronmüller, K.-T.; Krummheuer, C.; Topp, F.; Zipfel, S.; Herzog, W.; Hartmann, M. Der Fragebogen zur familiären emotionalen Involviertheit und wahrgenommenen Kritik (FEIWK). *Psychother. Psychosom. Med. Psychol.* **2001**, *51*, 377–383. [CrossRef] [PubMed]
36. Linden, M.; Maier, W.; Achberger, M.; Herr, R.; Helmchen, H.; Benkert, O. Psychological disorders and their treatment in general practice in Germany: Results of a WHO study. *Nervenarzt* **1996**, *67*, 205–215. [PubMed]
37. Sepulveda, A.R.; Whitney, J.; Hankins, M.; Treasure, J. Development and validation of an Eating Disorders Symptom Impact Scale (EDSIS) for carers of people with eating disorders. *Health Qual. Life Outcomes* **2008**, *6*, 28. [CrossRef] [PubMed]
38. Hautzinger, M.; Keller, F.; Kühner, C. *Das Beck Depressionsinventar II*; Harcourt Test Services: Frankfurt, Germany, 2006.
39. Laux, L.; Glanzmann, P.; Schaffner, P.; Spielsberger, C.D. *Das State-Trait-Angstinventar*; Beltz: Weinheim, Germany, 1981.
40. Hasler, G.; Klaghofer, R.; Buddeberg, C. The University of Rhode Island Change Assessment Scale (URICA) psychometric testing of a German version. *PPmP* **2003**, *53*, 406–411. [CrossRef] [PubMed]
41. Hilbert, A.; Tuschen-Caffier, B. *Eating Disorder Examination*; Verlag für Psychotherapie: Münster, Germany, 2006.
42. Rathner, G.; Waldherr, K. Eating Disorder Inventory-2: A German language validation with norms for female and male adolescents. *Z. Klin. Psychol. Psychiatr. Psychother.* **1997**, *45*, 157–182.
43. Schwarte, R.; Timmesfeld, N.; Dempfle, A.; Krei, M.; Egberts, K.; Jaite, C.; Fleischhaker, C.; Wewetzer, C.; Herpertz-Dahlmann, B.; Seitz, J.; et al. Expressed Emotions and Depressive Symptoms in Caregivers of Adolescents with First-Onset Anorexia Nervosa-A Long-Term Investigation over 2.5 Years. *Eur. Eat. Disord. Rev.* **2017**, *25*, 44–51. [CrossRef]
44. Sepulveda, A.R.; Todd, G.; Whitaker, W.; Grover, M.; Stahl, D.; Treasure, J. Expressed emotion in relatives of patients with eating disorders following skills training program. *Int. J. Eat. Disord.* **2010**, *43*, 603–610. [CrossRef]
45. Marcos, Y.; Quiles, M.; Herrera, M.; Sanmartín, R.; Treasure, J. Testing carer skill training programs in Spanish carers of patients with eating disorders. *Psicothema* **2018**, *30*, 295–303. [CrossRef]
46. Giombini, L.; Nesbitt, S.; Kusosa, R.; Fabian, C.; Easter, A.; Tchanturia, K. Adapted emotion skills training group for young people with anorexia nervosa. *Neuropsychiatr* **2020**. [CrossRef]

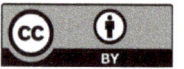

© 2020 by the authors. Licensee MDPI, Basel, Switzerland. This article is an open access article distributed under the terms and conditions of the Creative Commons Attribution (CC BY) license (http://creativecommons.org/licenses/by/4.0/).

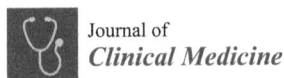

Article

Long-Term Efficacy of the Workshop Vs. Online SUCCEAT (Supporting Carers of Children and Adolescents with Eating Disorders) Intervention for Parents: A Quasi-Randomised Feasibility Trial

Stefanie Truttmann [1,†], Julia Philipp [1,†], Michael Zeiler [1], Claudia Franta [1], Tanja Wittek [1], Elisabeth Merl [1], Gabriele Schöfbeck [1], Doris Koubek [1], Clarissa Laczkovics [1], Hartmut Imgart [2], Annika Zanko [2], Ellen Auer-Welsbach [3], Janet Treasure [4], Andreas F. K. Karwautz [1] and Gudrun Wagner [1,*]

[1] Eating Disorders Unit, Department of Child and Adolescent Psychiatry, Medical University of Vienna, 1090 Vienna, Austria; stefanie.truttmann@meduniwien.ac.at (S.T.); julia.philipp@meduniwien.ac.at (J.P.); michael.zeiler@meduniwien.ac.at (M.Z.); claudiaparfuss@gmx.at (C.F.); tanja.wittek@meduniwien.ac.at (T.W.); elisabeth.merl@outlook.com (E.M.); gabriele.schoefbeck@meduniwien.ac.at (G.S.); praxis@kiju.co.at (D.K.); clarissa.laczkovics@meduniwien.ac.at (C.L.); andreas.karwautz@meduniwien.ac.at (A.F.K.K.)
[2] Parkland Clinic, Clinic for Psychosomatic Medicine and Psychotherapy, 34537 Bad Wildungen, Germany; hartmut.imgart@parkland-klinik.de (H.I.); annika.zanko@parkland-klinik.de (A.Z.)
[3] Department for Neurology and child and adolescents Psychiatry, 9020 Klagenfurt am Wörthersee, Austria; Ellen.Auer-Welsbach@kabeg.at
[4] Section of Eating Disorders, Department of Psychological Medicine, Institute of Psychiatry, Psychology & Neuroscience, King's College London, London WC2R 2LS, UK; janet.treasure@kcl.ac.uk
* Correspondence: gudrun.wagner@meduniwien.ac.at; Tel.: +43-140-4003-0170
† These authors contributed equally to this work.

Received: 6 May 2020; Accepted: 15 June 2020; Published: 18 June 2020

Abstract: Interventions for main carers of adult patients with anorexia nervosa (AN) can reduce the caregiving burden and increase caregiver skills. However, the effectiveness and feasibility for carers of adolescent patients, the optimal form of the intervention and long-term outcomes are largely unknown. We evaluated the efficacy and feasibility of the "Supporting Carers of Children and Adolescents with Eating Disorders in Austria" (SUCCEAT) workshop vs. online intervention. Main caregivers (parents) of adolescent patients with AN were randomly allocated to a workshop ($n = 50$) or online version ($n = 50$). Participants were compared to a non-randomised comparison group ($n = 49$) receiving multi-family or systemic family therapy. Primary (General Health Questionnaire) and secondary outcomes were obtained at baseline, three-month and 12-month follow-up. Adherence was high for workshop and online participants (6.2 and 6.7 sessions completed out of 8). Intention-to-treat analyses revealed significant pre–post reductions in the primary outcome for the workshop ($d = 0.87$ (95%conficence interval (CI): 0.48; 1.26)) and online ($d = 0.65$ (95%CI: 0.31; 0.98)) intervention that were sustained at the 12-month follow-up. There was no significant group difference ($p = 0.473$). Parental psychopathology and burden decreased and caregiver skills increased in all groups; the improvement of caregiver skills was significantly higher in SUCCEAT participants than in the comparison group. Online interventions for parents of adolescents with AN were equally effective as workshops. The improvements remained stable over time.

Keywords: anorexia nervosa; children and adolescents; parents; carers; intervention; workshop; online intervention

1. Introduction

The National Institute for Health and Care Excellence (NICE) Guidelines recommend involving carers in the treatment of adolescent patients with anorexia nervosa (AN) [1]. As AN tends to develop during adolescence, parents usually function as main carers. AN is a life-threatening psychiatric disorder that is often related to a high mortality and a high chronification rate [2]. Furthermore, AN is often associated with lack of insight and low motivation to change in patients. Therefore, the illness can have a serious emotional impact on the whole family, especially the main carer, who usually is a parent. This can cause severe parental distress and lead to enormous burden and relationship problems within the whole family [3–6].

In the cognitive interpersonal model of maintaining factors for eating disorders (ED), Treasure and Schmidt [3] exemplify how interpersonal relationships between caregivers and patients play an important role in the recovery of patients with AN. They illustrate how unhelpful parental reactions, overflowing parental emotions of any kind and dysfunctional parental communication styles may maintain AN symptoms and therefore lead to a vicious circle of dispute, avoidance and misunderstanding, which might worsen the parents' and patients' outcome as a result: It may not only hinder the recovery of the patients but might also lead to clinically relevant anxiety and depression in caregivers themselves [7,8]. Therefore, it is essential to teach main carers, mostly parents, specific skills and communication styles to help them handle difficult situations, in order to break the vicious circle. As confirmed by a meta-analysis of interventions for caregivers of mainly adult patients suffering from AN [9] that are based on the cognitive interpersonal model of maintaining factors for eating disorders (ED) [3,10,11], they can reduce a carer's burden and improve caregiver skills.

Usually, these interventions are delivered as workshop [12,13] or self-help programmes [14–16]. Only a few studies examined online versions, but mainly for carers of adult patients [17–19]. Online interventions have the advantages of flexibility in time and place and may facilitate professional support when face-to-face appointments are not possible or specialists are not available in remote areas. Moreover, participants may experience less anxiety, shame or stigmatization during online counselling [11,20,21]. So far, there is not enough evidence whether online interventions are as effective as face-to-face interventions in the field of ED, especially in terms of carers of adolescent patients [22]. To investigate the efficacy of online interventions seems even more essential regarding the current coronavirus disease 2019 (COVID-19) pandemic, when face-to-face contact should be restricted as much as possible. Although there are still some barriers, such as online privacy and lack of sufficiently free access to mental health service programmes, they offer a lot of opportunities when it comes to the need of high safety [23]. Moreover, online programmes have the potential to provide help for families that may otherwise have difficulties accessing clinical help. However, a recent systematic review [22] reported only eleven studies examining online carer interventions on carer mental health, with two studies focusing on AN [17,18].

Many studies have a short follow-up (FU) period, usually between three [14,18,19] and six months [17]. Long-term outcome was rarely considered in previous research.

The majority of these studies mainly included carers of adult patients [12,14,24]. Evidence for the effectiveness for carers of adolescents is scarce, with only one study focusing solely on adolescents [15]. Comparisons between workshop and online versions are completely missing for carers of adolescent patients. To evaluate interventions for carers of adolescents is essential, as AN tends to start in adolescence and early interventions are known to positively affect its course [1,25]. Many carers of adult patients express a wish to have had early access to such an intervention [13].

Altogether, the effectiveness and feasibility of caregiver interventions for carers of adolescent patients and whether an online version is equally effective and feasible as a face-to-face format is largely unknown. The aim of this study was to compare the feasibility and explore the potential long-term efficacy of "Supporting Carers of Children and Adolescents with Eating Disorders in Austria" (SUCCEAT) programme delivered as a workshop or online programme for carers (usually parents) of adolescent patients. The objective of SUCCEAT is to decrease carers' burden by accrediting them with skills and knowledge, in order to increase their ability to better support their affected children and adolescents [26]. We hypothesise that parents participating in SUCCEAT show a statistically significant reduction of distress, burden and psychiatric symptoms at the post-intervention and at 12-month FU. Furthermore, we aimed to figure out whether the intervention effects are different when delivering the programme via workshops or online modules.

2. Methods

2.1. Study Design

Reporting to this study adheres to the CONSORT (Consolidated Standards of Reporting Trials) guidelines (see online Supplementary Materials "ESM1. Consort checklist"). This is a two-arm parallel group quasi-randomised feasibility trial that was conducted between November 2014 and April 2019. Carers of children and adolescents between 10 and 19 years suffering from AN or atypical AN were eligible to participate in the study. In this study, all main caregivers were parents living in the same household as the patients they cared for. The inclusion criterion for caregivers was German fluency. The inclusion criterion for patients was receipt of treatment as usual, according to NICE guidelines [1]. Participants were excluded if caregivers suffered from a severe mental illness or patients suffered from severe comorbidities at baseline (e.g., psychosis) and if carers lacked Internet access. The SUCCEAT group (workshop/online) was compared to a non-randomised comparison group of carers receiving other forms of family support. Details of the study protocol are published elsewhere [26]. The study was registered at ClinicalTrials.gov (Identifier: NCT02480907).

2.2. Recruitment and Randomisation

The study protocol and the informed consent forms were approved by the Ethical Commission of the Medical University of Vienna (#1840/2013). For each patient, one parent served as main carer and completed the questionnaires. SUCCEAT participants were recruited at the Medical University of Vienna (Department of Child and Adolescent Psychiatry). Patients underwent psychiatric and psychological assessments. If eligible, parents were informed about the study and invited to participate. After providing written informed consent, carers completed the baseline assessments and were allocated to one of the intervention-arms. The practicalities of recruitment (limited number of study participants to be enrolled in a reasonable period of time) meant that we were not able to implement a technically exact randomisation procedure (blockwise in blocks of eight participants) as originally planned and described in the study protocol [26]. Rather, we fixed the start dates of the workshop and online groups in advance and alternately assigned the first block of enrolled participants to the workshop, the next block to the online intervention and so forth. This procedure corresponds to the definition of quasi-randomisation as reported in the Cochrane Handbook for Systematic Reviews (Box 13.4a) [27]. The block sizes slightly varied depending on the number of incoming participants prior to the start of a group (median size = 7). We assumed that the time of enrollment of participants is not systematically related to any participants' characteristics. We tested whether participants allocated to the workshop and online group differed regarding sociodemographic characteristics, clinical characteristics of patients and baseline scores of the outcome questionnaires and found that solely patients of parents assigned to the online group had slightly longer ED duration compared to the workshop group, while there were no other statistically significant differences (see Results section for details). The participants were not informed about the group allocation until baseline assessments were completed. Caregivers who did not want to participate in the intervention to which they were assigned (n = 2 in online group) were excluded. Researchers involved in this study were not blinded to the group allocation.

The comparison group was recruited from the Department for Neurology and Child and Adolescent Psychiatry (Klagenfurt, Austria) and the Parkland Clinic, Clinic for Psychosomatic Medicine and

Psychotherapy (Bad Wildungen, Germany); two clinics specialised in ED treatment. The same procedure for checking eligibility and obtaining informed consent was applied.

2.3. Interventions

SUCCEAT was delivered either via workshop or online. Both intervention arms were designed equally, including 8 weekly modules. The SUCCEAT intervention teaches carers about common emotional and behavioural interactions that may occur when living with a person suffering from anorexia nervosa, such as dysfunctional communication and misattributions. Carers are taught skills to counter these reactions, such as Motivational Interviewing, problem solving, resilience and difficult-behaviour management [5,8]. Caregivers had either face-to-face contact (in the workshops) or had the opportunity to exchange thoughts via an online forum. Two health professionals coached both the workshop and the online intervention. One was a child and adolescent psychiatrist, and the other one was a psychologist and medical doctor in child and adolescent psychiatry training. Both worked in the field of ED treatment and research for several years and were trained in Motivational Interviewing.

2.3.1. Workshop Group

The two healthcare professionals (subsequently referred to as "coaches") delivered these modules in eight weekly sessions. Caregivers received handouts in each session, as well as a comprehensive manual based on a book [28], including detailed information, and a DVD [29] with case examples of caregiver–patient interactions.

2.3.2. Online Group

Caregivers were invited to a face-to-face welcome meeting, where they got to know the coaches and each other. Participants got access to the online programme, the handouts and the manual and were asked to complete one module weekly. They also received the DVD. Once a week, they received written feedback regarding their progress and responses to questions by one of the coaches.

2.3.3. Comparison Group

Comparison-group participants received either four double sessions of systemic family therapy (Klagenfurt, Austria) or multi-family therapy (Bad Wildungen, Germany). Multi-family therapy, based on the Maudsley Model of multi-family therapy for AN, is conducted in a two-day face-to-face workshop delivered by a therapeutic team, including up to 10 families [30].

2.4. Assessments

The parents completed self-report questionnaires at baseline (T0), after the intervention (3-month FU, T1) and at 12-month FU (T2). They rated their own psychopathology and caregiving skills. The evaluation included the following assessments:

The 12-items version of the General Health Questionnaire (GHQ) assesses the level of parental psychological distress [31,32]. Items are rated on a four-point scale (0–3) and are converted to a dichotomous rating ("0" for the two lowest ratings; "1" for the two highest ratings) and summed up to a total score ranging from 0 to 12 (higher scores indicating higher levels of psychological distress).

The Eating Disorder Symptom Impact Scale (EDSIS) assesses specific parental caregiving difficulties for families of people with EDs [33]. A total of 24 items rated on a five-point scale are aggregated to a total score and four sub-scores indicating difficulties in specific areas. Higher scores indicate more difficulties. Subscales comprise difficulties related to "nutrition" (e.g., difficulties preparing meals or arguments during mealtimes), "dysregulated behaviour" (e.g., temper outbursts or lying), feelings of "guilt" (e.g., feelings of having done something wrong) and "social isolation" (e.g., losing friends).

The Symptom Checklist (SCL-90-Revised) [34] consists of 90 items rated on a 5-point scale assessing a broad range of psychopathological symptoms which parents might develop over time while caring for a child with AN (e.g., somatization, obsessive–compulsive behaviour, etc.). For the purpose of this study, only the global severity index (sum score of all items divided by 90; score range: 0–4) was calculated with higher scores, indicating higher levels of psychopathology.

The Beck Depression Inventory (BDI-II) [35,36] comprises 21 items assessing symptoms of parental depression, rated on a four-point scale. Items are aggregated to a total score, with higher scores indicating higher levels of depression.

The State and Trait Anxiety Inventory (STAI) [37], consisting of 40 items rated on a four-point scale, measures two kinds of anxiety. "State-anxiety" is characterised as inner tension and concerns toward future events in carers that vary across time and situations; "trait anxiety" means the tendency of experiencing fear in general. Higher scores indicate higher anxiety.

The Caregiver Skills (CASK) scale [38] measures skills in parents caring for ED patients and included 27 items rated on a visual analogue scale (0–100) which are summed up to the following subscales: "Bigger Picture" (implementing bigger-picture thinking), "Self-Care" (taking care of yourself), "Biting Tongue" (avoiding repetitive, nagging arguments), "Insight and Acceptance" (accepting and managing negative emotions), "Emotional Intelligence" (ability to discuss and manage feelings) and "Frustration Tolerance" (ability to be firm, calm and understanding). Item ratings are aggregated to one total scale and six subscales. Mean scores were calculated for this study, with higher scores indicating higher skill levels.

Furthermore, sociodemographic characteristics of the carers, including gender, age, highest educational degree, marital status and ethnicity, as well as patient characteristics, including gender, age, AN subtype, illness duration, type of current treatment and Body-Mass-Index (BMI), were obtained. Any adverse events reported by the caregivers were recorded during the course of the trial.

2.5. Statistical Analysis

Data analyses were performed with IBM SPSS Statistics 25.0 and R. Differences in sociodemographic and ED-related characteristics of carers and patients between the groups were analysed with t-tests and χ^2-tests. Adherence to the SUCCEAT intervention was explored by calculating the mean number of completed workshop/online sessions and the percentage of carers who have completed more than four sessions. Furthermore, completion of the programme was defined as having completed the last session; full completion was defined as having completed the last session and at least two of the three assessments. Differences in adherence measures between the workshop and online group were explored by using t- and χ^2-tests. Treatment effects of the SUCCEAT interventions were analysed by using a series of general linear mixed models, including outcome scores from the baseline, 3-month and 12-month FU assessments as within-factor and study arm as between-factor. While the main effect of time represents the change of scores across both SUCCEAT study arms, the time x group interaction represents differences in changes between the study arms. Bonferroni-adjusted p-values account for multiple testing when results on questionnaire subscales are presented. Baseline to 3- and 12-month FUs' effect sizes (Cohen's d, including 95% confidence intervals (CI)) were calculated separately by study arm.

Intention-to-treat (ITT) was chosen as the primary analytic strategy. Therefore, participants were analysed within the study arm they were randomised to, regardless of adherence. Missing outcome data were replaced by using the expectation-maximization (EM) method, which is based on maximum-likelihood estimates. Missing data were replaced separately for each outcome variable by using data from other assessment time points (baseline, 3- and 12-month FUs) and study arm as predictors (assuming normal distribution and using 25 iterations). Missing FU data were not significantly related to baseline scores or sociodemographic characteristics. Additionally, a completer analysis was conducted, including only data from carers who completed more than four workshop/online sessions and assessments from all time points. Missing data were not replaced. Thus, this analysis refers to the subgroup of carers highly adherent to both the intervention and assessments.

The same analytic strategy was applied for exploring differences between the SUCCEAT intervention group (including aggregated data from the workshop and online study arm) and the comparison group. As there was no difference in effects between comparison participants recruited from Bad Wildungen and Klagenfurt, data obtained from both sites were analysed in tandem.

3. Results

3.1. Participants

SUCCEAT participants were 102 carers (86% females, mean age: 47.2 years) who were randomised to either the workshop ($n = 50$) or the online ($n = 52$) intervention group. Two participants were excluded post-randomisation because they were not willing to participate in the group they were randomised to, and thus they were not considered in the subsequent analyses. The participants' flow is shown in the consort diagram (Figure 1). Baseline demographic and clinical characteristics of carers and patients are shown in Table 1. No statistically significant differences between participants of the two groups were observed. The only exception was that the AN duration was slightly longer in patients of carers assigned to the online group compared to the workshop group ($p = 0.041$). Furthermore, there were no statistically significant differences between the groups in any outcome variable (GHQ, EDSIS, BDI, STAI, SCL and CASK scores) at baseline, indicating that the quasi-randomisation approach was successful in building two comparable groups. One carer in the workshop group and three carers in the online group discontinued the interventions. Non-completion of the three-month and 12-month FU assessments was 4% and 12% in the workshop group, respectively, and 8% and 28% in the online group. Finally, data from 38 participants of the workshop and 31 participants of the online group were included in the completer analysis.

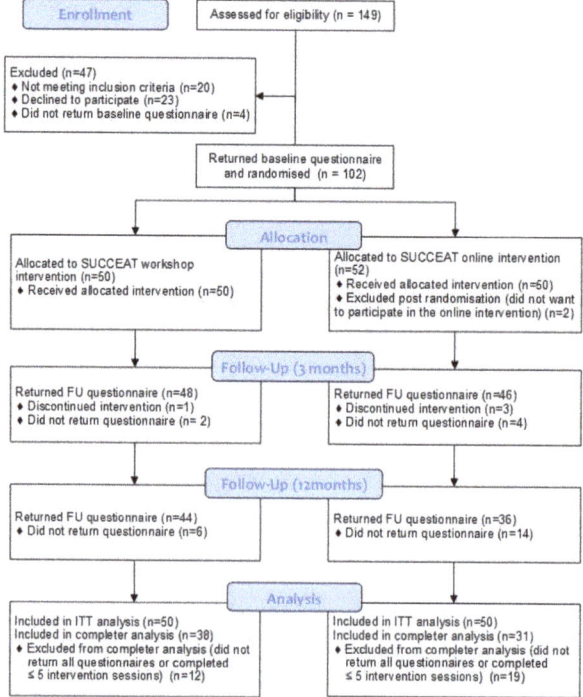

Figure 1. Consort flow diagram. SUCCEAT: Supporting Carers of Children and Adolescents with Eating Disorders in Austria; ITT: Intention-to-treat; FU: Follow-up.

Table 1. Sociodemographic characteristics of the "Supporting Carers of Children and Adolescents with Eating Disorders in Austria" (SUCCEAT) workshop and online group participants and corresponding patients.

	SUCCEAT Workshop Intervention (N = 50)	SUCCEAT Online Intervention (N = 50)	Group Difference Test Statistic (df)	p
Carers (SUCCEAT Participants)				
Females (N, %)	42 (84.0%)	44 (88.0%)	χ^2 (1) = 0.332	0.564
Age (mean, SD)	46.64 (5.43)	47.72 (4.25)	t(98) = 1.108	0.271
Highest educational degree				
university degree (N, %)	30 (60.0%)	23 (46.0%)	χ^2 (2) = 2.885	0.236
A level degree (N, %)	11 (22.0%)	11 (22.0%)		
<A-level degree (N, %)	9 (18.0%)	16 (32.0%)		
Marital status				
single (N, %)	0 (0.0%)	3 (6.3%)	χ^2 (2) = 3.481	0.175
married or living in partnership (N, %)	42 (84.0%)	36 (75.0%)		
divorced or widowed (N, %)	8 (16.0%)	9 (18.8%)		
Ethnicity			χ^2 (1) = 0.000	1.000
Caucasian (N, %)	49 (98%)	49 (98%)		
Asian (N, %)	1 (2%)	1 (2%)		
Patients				
Females (N, %)	45 (90.0%)	48 (96.0%)	χ^2 (1) = 1.382	0.240
Age (mean, SD)	14.66 (1.91)	15.12 (1.80)	t(98) = 1.238	0.219
Eating disorder diagnosis				
Anorexia nervosa—restrictive type (N, %)	45 (90.0%)	45 (90.0%)	χ^2 (2) = 0.000	1.000
Anorexia nervosa—binge/purging type (N, %)	4 (8.0%)	4 (8.0%)		
Atypical anorexia nervosa (N, %)	1 (2.0%)	1 (2.0%)		
Eating disorder duration in months (mean, SD)	10.41 (7.10)	16.03 (16.03)	t(87) = 2.076	0.041
Type of treatment				
Inpatient (N, %)	24 (48.0%)	24 (48.0%)	χ^2 (1) = 0.000	1.000
Outpatients (N, %)	26 (52.0%)	26 (52.0%)		
BMI at baseline (Mean, SD)	15.53 (2.13)	16.36 (2.54)	t(96) = 1.743	0.084

SD: standard deviation; BMI: Body-Mass-Index.

Participants of the comparison group were 49 carers (38 from Bad Wildungen, Germany; 11 from Klagenfurt, Austria) who were recruited over the same time period as the SUCCEAT group and provided consent and completed baseline assessments. The recruitment rate (caregivers who participated in the trial of those approached) was 71%. Statistically significant baseline differences between participants of the SUCCEAT and comparison group were found regarding parental educational degree, AN duration and type of treatment in patients. Participants of the comparison group were significantly less educated ($p = 0.015$) and cared for patients with a longer duration of AN ($p < 0.001$) treated more often in inpatient settings ($p < 0.001$). In the comparison group, non-completion of the three- and 12-month FU assessments was 33% and 55%, respectively, leaving 22 included in the completer analysis.

3.2. Adherence

On average, SUCCEAT workshop participants completed 6.16 (SD: 1.81), and online participants 6.70 (SD 2.19), out of eight sessions, which was not significantly different between the groups (t(98) = 1.344, $p = 0.182$). Completion and full completion rates of the intervention were 72% (workshop) and 70% (online) (Chi^2 (1) = 0.049; $p = 0.826$). Furthermore, the percentage of participants completing more than half of sessions (workshop: 84%, online: 78%) did not differ between the groups (Chi^2 (1) = 0.585, $p = 0.444$). Regarding treatment engagement, 51.1% of workshop and 34.8% of online participants read at least 50% of the manual, and 37.2% of workshop and 43.5% of online participants watched at least 50% of the DVD.

3.3. Primary Outcome

Within groups, the ITT analysis (Table 2) revealed a statistically significant reduction in the carers' burden, as indicated by the GHQ total score across both SUCCEAT interventions (F = 36.252, $p < 0.001$). Baseline-to-post effects sizes were d = 0.87 (95%CI: 0.48; 1.26) in the workshop and d = 0.65

(95%CI: 0.31; 0.98) in the online group. Baseline-to-12-months FU effect sizes were d = 0.81 and 0.98, respectively. Results from the completer analysis (Table S1 in online "ESM2. Supplementary Tables S1–S4") parallel the results of the ITT analysis with a slightly higher baseline-to-12-months FU effect in the online group).

Between-groups changes in GHQ scores across the time points were not significantly different between the SUCCEAT groups (F = 0.752, p = 0.473), thus indicating no difference in the treatment effect for the workshop and online group.

3.4. Secondary Outcomes

Results of the general linear mixed model analyses calculated on an ITT basis are shown in Tables 2 and 3.

ED-related burden: The ITT analysis revealed statistically significant reductions in caregivers' burden related to AN symptomatology across SUCCEAT interventions, which was persistent to 12-month FU. Effect sizes were highest for the EDSIS nutrition subscale (large effects), whereby effect sizes for the other subscales were in the low-to-medium range. There was no statistically significant difference between the workshop and online group for the EDSIS total score or subscales.

Psychopathology: Carers' general psychopathology, as measured with the SCL-90 R, was significantly reduced over time, across both SUCCEAT intervention-arms, while there was no statistically significant time × group interaction effect in the ITT analysis. Significant long-term reductions in symptom levels were also observed for depression and anxiety scores across both SUCCEAT groups.

Caregiver skills: From baseline to three- and 12-month FUs, caregiver skills as measured with the CASK significantly increased across both SUCCEAT intervention-arms, while there was no statistically significant time × group interaction in the total and any of CASK subscales (Table 3). Effect sizes were medium to high.

Results of the completer analyses for secondary outcome measures (Tables S1 and S2 in "ESM2. Supplementary Tables S1–S4") were largely congruent with results of the ITT analyses, but with two exceptions: For the SCL-90-R score, the completer analysis revealed higher reductions in the online compared to the workshop group (F = 4.467, p = 0.014). Furthermore, the statistically significant interaction effect for the "Emotional Intelligence" subscale of the CASK observed in the ITT analysis was not found in the completer analysis.

Relation to comparison group: As indicated by the statistically significant main effects of the group in the ITT analysis (Table S3 in "ESM2. Supplementary Tables S1–S4"), carers of the comparison group receiving either multi-family therapy or systemic family therapy generally scored higher across all time points in all burden and psychopathology measures than participants of the SUCCEAT groups. Baseline to three-month FU effect sizes were slightly higher in SUCCEAT participants, as compared to participants from the comparison group. However, the time × group interaction did not reach statistical significance for any outcome measure, except for the CASK total score, where caregiver skills increased significantly more in SUCCEAT participants, as compared to participants of the comparison group (F = 5.570, p = 0.004). Considering data from completers only (Table S4 in "ESM2. Supplementary Tables S1–S4"), only statistically significant main effects of time were observed.

3.5. Adverse Events

No harms were reported by any caregiver, and no patient died during the trial.

Table 2. Means (SDs) and results of the mixed-effects model repeated measures ANOVA for outcomes of the SUCCEAT workshop vs. SUCCEAT online intervention regarding caregiving burden and psychopathology (intention-to-treat analysis).

	Mean (SD)				ANOVA (F, p)			Cohen's d (95% CI Lower; Upper)		
	Baseline (T0)	3M FU (T1)	12M FU (T2)		Group	Time	Time × Group	T0-T1		T0-T2
GHQ Total Score [a]										
SUCCEAT Workshop	4.41 (3.15)	1.84 (2.74)	1.94 (1.39)		0.065 (0.800)	36.252 (<0.001)	0.752 (0.473)	0.87 (0.48; 1.26)		0.81 (0.42; 1.21)
SUCCEAT Online	4.33 (3.76)	2.14 (2.92)	1.39 (2.18)					0.65 (0.31; 0.98)		0.98 (0.50; 1.39)
EDSIS Total Score										
SUCCEAT Workshop	33.32 (15.02)	22.59 (13.24)	20.28 (16.29)		2.421 (0.123)	57.005 (<0.001)	0.166 (0.847)	0.75 (0.50; 1.00)		0.83 (0.54; 1.12)
SUCCEAT Online	29.11 (12.70)	19.83 (11.82)	16.60 (11.41)					0.76 (0.42; 1.09)		1.04 (0.60; 1.47)
EDSIS Nutrition [b]										
SUCCEAT Workshop	16.61 (7.34)	10.09 (5.78)	8.09 (6.28)		1.983 (0.162)	99.430 (<0.001)	0.747 (0.475)	0.96 (0.69; 1.22)		1.24 (0.91; 1.56)
SUCCEAT Online	14.38 (6.31)	8.83 (5.83)	7.24 (5.03)					0.91 (0.58; 1.24)		1.24 (0.80; 1.69)
EDSIS Guilt [b]										
SUCCEAT Workshop	7.80 (4.75)	5.52 (3.96)	5.17 (4.75)		1.547 (0.217)	19.856 (<0.001)	0.534 (0.587)	0.52 (0.22; 0.81)		0.55 (0.26; 0.85)
SUCCEAT Online	6.51 (4.23)	5.06 (3.52)	4.33 (3.63)					0.37 (0.08; 0.66)		0.55 (0.19; 0.91)
EDSIS Dysregulated Behavior [b]										
SUCCEAT Workshop	6.02 (4.96)	4.51 (4.21)	4.53 (4.29)		0.167 (0.683)	9.651 (<0.001)	0.197 (0.821)	0.32 (0.12; 0.52)		0.32 (0.05; 0.59)
SUCCEAT Online	5.64 (3.93)	4.50 (3.36)	4.07 (3.74)					0.31 (0.03; 0.59)		0.41 (0.08; 0.74)
EDSIS Social Isolation [b]										
SUCCEAT Workshop	2.87 (2.60)	2.48 (2.72)	2.49 (3.17)		5.971 (0.016)	7.190 (0.001)	2.698 (0.070)	0.14 (−0.16; 0.45)		0.12 (−0.19; 0.45)
SUCCEAT Online	2.64 (2.82)	1.43 (1.95)	0.96 (1.50)					0.50 (0.12; 0.87)		0.73 (0.31; 1.15)
SCL 90-R Total Mean Score										
SUCCEAT Workshop	0.42 (0.36)	0.24 (0.26)	0.33 (0.37)		0.003 (0.953)	12.864 (<0.001)	2.261 (0.107)	0.53 (0.32; 0.75)		0.25 (−0.02; 0.54)
SUCCEAT Online	0.43 (0.42)	0.31 (0.36)	0.26 (0.26)					0.29 (0.03; 0.54)		0.45 (0.12; 0.78)
BDI Total Score										
SUCCEAT Workshop	11.60 (7.01)	6.45 (5.43)	6.80 (6.24)		0.155 (0.694)	25.946 (<0.001)	2.394 (0.094)	0.80 (0.52; 1.08)		0.72 (0.33; 1.12)
SUCCEAT Online	10.11 (7.03)	7.72 (8.18)	5.74 (5.97)					0.31 (0.04; 0.58)		0.67 (0.30; 1.03)

Table 2. Cont.

	Mean (SD)			ANOVA (F, p)			Cohen's d (95% CI Lower; Upper)	
	Baseline (T0)	3M FU (T1)	12M FU (T2)	Group	Time	Time × Group	T0-T1	T0-T2
STAI State Score [c]								
SUCCEAT Workshop	49.44 (10.14)	39.80 (10.16)	37.85 (10.31)	0.060 (0.807)	42.972 (<0.001)	3.312 (0.039)	0.95 (0.57; 1.33)	1.13 (0.73; 1.54)
SUCCEAT Online	45.98 (11.16)	41.84 (12.17)	37.99 (10.31)				0.35 (0.06; 0.65)	0.74 (0.40; 1.08)
STAI Trait Score [c]								
SUCCEAT Workshop	41.73 (8.61)	37.86 (8.62)	36.16 (9.65)	<0.001 (0.987)	22.651 (<0.001)	0.169 (0.845)	0.45 (0.22; 0.68)	0.61 (0.29; 0.92)
SUCCEAT Online	41.25 (10.15)	38.01 (10.57)	36.56 (9.50)				0.31 (0.10; 0.52)	0.48 (0.20; 0.75)

[a] Primary outcome; [b] p-values for these subscales are tested against a Bonferroni-adjusted significance level of 0.0125; [c] p-values for these subscales are tested against a Bonferroni-adjusted significance level of 0.025.

Table 3. Means (SDs) and results of the mixed-effects model repeated measures ANOVA for outcomes of the SUCCEAT workshop vs. SUCCEAT online intervention regarding caregiver skills (intention-to-treat analysis).

	Mean (SD)			ANOVA (F, p)			Cohen's d (95% CI Lower; Upper)	
	Baseline (T0)	3M FU (T1)	12M FU (T2)	Group	Time	Time × Group	T0–T1	T0–T2
CASK Total Score								
SUCCEAT Workshop	64.64 (15.34)	75.33 (13.68)	79.53 (15.25)	0.202 (0.654)	51.351 (<0.001)	0.636 (0.530)	0.73 (0.40; 1.05)	0.97 (0.56; 1.38)
SUCCEAT Online	65.20 (13.74)	74.08 (12.63)	77.01 (12.87)				0.67 (0.35; 0.99)	0.89 (0.55; 1.22)
CASK Bigger Picture [a]								
SUCCEAT Workshop	71.01 (17.63)	79.14 (13.68)	83.98 (15.38)	0.530 (0.468)	23.631 (<0.001)	1.420 (0.244)	0.51 (0.19; 0.83)	0.78 (0.36; 1.21)
SUCCEAT Online	71.27 (14.22)	78.60 (12.54)	79.28 (13.80)				0.54 (0.21; 0.88)	0.57 (0.24; 0.90)
CASK Selfcare [a]								
SUCCEAT Workshop	57.23 (18.00)	71.23 (17.00)	76.37 (20.19)	0.222 (0.638)	59.621 (<0.001)	0.012 (0.988)	0.80 (0.44; 1.16)	1.00 (0.60; 1.39)
SUCCEAT Online	58.33 (19.05)	72.86 (14.69)	77.57 (15.28)				0.84 (0.53; 1.14)	1.11 (0.70; 1.52)
CASK Biting Tongue [a]								
SUCCEAT Workshop	53.73 (20.44)	72.20 (17.13)	78.40 (19.11)	0.178 (0.674)	90.700 (<0.001)	0.465 (0.629)	0.97 (0.64; 1.30)	1.25 (0.84; 1.64)
SUCCEAT Online	57.03 (22.07)	72.56 (16.78)	78.69 (15.78)				0.78 (0.46; 1.10)	1.10 (0.74; 1.45)
CASK Insight and Acceptance [a]								
SUCCEAT Workshop	68.67 (20.27)	77.94 (17.99)	82.11 (18.29)	0.005 (0.944)	32.987 (<0.001)	<0.001 (1.000)	0.48 (0.23; 0.74)	0.69 (0.39; 1.00)
SUCCEAT Online	68.50 (19.23)	77.76 (14.57)	81.85 (13.21)				0.54 (0.21; 0.86)	0.79 (0.43; 1.16)
CASK Emotional Intelligence [a]								
SUCCEAT Workshop	66.10 (19.03)	74.54 (16.66)	75.40 (17.07)	2.652 (0.107)	6.804 (0.001)	1.606 (0.203)	0.47 (0.15; 0.80)	0.51 (0.13; 0.90)
SUCCEAT Online	65.36 (17.64)	67.59 (18.50)	69.20 (18.59)				0.12 (−0.18; 0.42)	0.21 (−0.10; 0.52)
CASK Frustration Tolerance [a]								
SUCCEAT Workshop	64.45 (16.40)	73.85 (15.02)	78.13 (15.36)	0.045 (0.833)	37.927 (<0.001)	0.347 (0.707)	0.60 (0.26; 0.93)	0.93 (0.51; 1.35)
SUCCEAT Online	64.88 (16.36)	73.90 (14.31)	75.84 (13.87)				0.58 (0.26; 0.91)	0.81 (0.44; 1.19)

[a] p-values for these subscales are tested against a Bonferroni-adjusted significance level of 0.008.

4. Discussion

We evaluated the efficacy of the SUCCEAT programme for carers of adolescents with AN and focused on a potential difference between using a workshop or online format for delivering the content. Within both groups, the primary outcome and all secondary outcomes improved. Caregivers reported a statistically significant reduction in distress, burden, anxiety and depression, as well as a statistically significant increase in caregiver skills. These improvements were maintained to the one-year FU. Our study, therefore, confirms that interventions for caregivers of adolescents patients with AN based on the cognitive interpersonal model [3,10,11] are (1) effective for caregivers of an adolescent population and (2) independent from the type of intervention (workshop or online).

Adherence of SUCCEAT was high. Completion rates of SUCCEAT were high (70–72%) compared to a systematic review of online interventions for patients with ED and carers with a range of 18.4–95.5% [39]. Full completion was as high as completion, indicating that participants who completed the intervention also completed at least one of the FU assessments. Thus, compliance to participate in the assessments was high. However, compared to other guided interventions for caregivers of adult patients with ED based on the same theoretical framework as SUCCEAT, the adherence was similar [17–19,24], but higher than in other reports investigating self-help material [15,16]. "Overcoming Anorexia Online", which was investigated in different studies [17–19,24], seems comparable to the concept of SUCCEAT, as it is also designed as an interactive, multi-media intervention consisting of eight modules that were presented offline or online, mostly with additional guidance that usually was provided by specialised clinicians. On the contrary, adherence of SUCCEAT was better than in studies investigating self-help with guidance from less-experienced coaches [15,16]. Even though the content was similar in all these approaches, a more diversified, structured and professionally guided presentation, as it was offered in SUCCEAT, may have positively influenced engagement. Moreover, adherence in the online intervention may have been facilitated by the welcome meeting with the coaches and other carers, as personal contact with the coaches may improve the commitment to complete the intervention. Furthermore, patients received treatment at the same facilities where the interventions were offered, enabling a conjoint case-management that may enhance the compliance in caregivers. Interestingly, the results of the ITT and completer analysis are similar, indicating that the programme effects were robust across high- and less-compliant participants.

Furthermore, a higher proportion of workshop participants read at least half of the manual, compared to the online participants. This difference may be explained by the fact that online participants already had to read all of the information at the online platform and thus may not be willing to spend even more time reading additional contents, whereas workshop participants were offered a face-to-face presentation of the material and may have been more willing to read the additional information. Otherwise, more online participants watched more than half of the DVD, as compared to the workshop participants. This may be due to the fact that communication skills could easily and concretely be demonstrated in the workshops by the coaches, but not so much online. Therefore, online participants probably had to harken back to the DVD more often. However, to what extent the additional material was used was left to the parents. Parents were regularly encouraged to gather more information on specific topics if they felt the need to, but the focus was clearly on the participation of the workshop or the online programme. However, not reading the whole manual and not watching the whole DVD might not be clinically relevant, as the topics in the additional material are fully covered within the workshops or online modules. Anyway, the engagement to read the manual and watch the DVD was better in SUCCEAT than in a previous study using self-help material [15], even though the manual and the DVD were the only materials offered in that specific study.

Carers' distress (GHQ) was reduced significantly over the course of the SUCCEAT intervention. Furthermore, psychiatric symptoms (anxiety and depression) in caregivers decreased. ED specific burden also significantly decreased with the largest effects on the "Nutrition" subscale. This could be due to the fact, that the items of this subscale (e.g., difficulties preparing meals, tension during mealtimes, etc.) were intensively addressed in the SUCCEAT intervention. Caregivers of ED patients are known to report a lack of support especially with meal-times [40]. Therefore, this is an important topic to address, as situations around meal-times are clearly associated with high frustration and extreme emotional reactions in caregivers. Skills and communication techniques that aim to improve meal-times and associated situations were repeatedly demonstrated in the workshop and the online programme of SUCCEAT. In addition, this information was also considered in detail on the DVD, which included specific scenarios of unhelpful and helpful communication between patients and carers, especially around meal-times. Reducing the burden and improving skills in that domain may support a better outcome of the affected patient by improving confidence in caregivers to support their children and adolescents, especially in these fundamental everyday situations.

Moreover, statistically significant improvements in all domains of caregiver skills was found, which seems unique for the SUCCEAT intervention. It is assumed that stabilising the mental health of caregivers and improving their skills may positively affect patients' outcomes as well [3,10,11,16]. Emotional regulation or positive communication may support recovery in patients with ED, and therefore, interventions that increase caregiving skills in carers, are seen as an important add-on in patients' treatment.

In summary, the SUCCEAT intervention revealed remarkably high effect sizes in both groups, as compared to prior studies [9,15,16,19]. In SUCCEAT, highly structured material with guidance from professional coaches was used. In previous studies, carers specifically reported a lack of information from professional healthcare workers and emphasised the wish for contact with clinicians [40,41]. Naturally, participants of the workshop group could ask questions as often as they wanted and received individual feedback from the professional coaches during the workshop sessions. Likewise, participants of the online arm had the possibility to write as many messages to the coach as they wanted while working through the online sessions, even though they only received one message from the coach per week, meaning that they also had multiple options to contact the coach. Both SUCCEAT intervention arms were delivered and guided by the same two coaches trained in Motivational Interviewing and with a high level of experience in the field of adolescent EDs, which has previously found to moderate outcome [22]. Guidance from experienced clinicians may contribute to higher effect sizes [17,24].

The SUCCEAT workshop and online formats appeared to be equally effective, although the study did not have sufficient power to detect moderately sized between-group effects. There already is evidence that online interventions can support recovery from ED and prevent chronicity in patients [39,42,43] and can reduce burden and increase skills in carers of adult patients with ED [17–19]. This study adds to the literature that online interventions are also effective for carers of adolescent patients with ED. Online interventions are promising in terms of effectiveness and also acceptability [22]. They are of great benefit, as they are transregional, highly flexible, widely accessible at any time and delivered with minimal resources. Even coaches when responding via email can provide support with high flexibility. Online programmes have the potential to provide information for carers that may otherwise experience difficulties to access help or to contact clinicians. This is even more important in times of the current COVID-19 pandemic, when professionals' face-to-face support is partially restricted in highly affected areas. As a result of associated uncertainty, ED symptoms, anxiety and burden within the whole family might increase [44]. Thus, as there are limited possibilities to contact clinicians face-to-face, online interventions like SUCCEAT may actually gain importance.

Caregiver skills increased more in the SUCCEAT group than in the comparison group, indicating that the main target of the SUCCEAT intervention (increasing skills on how to care for adolescents with an AN) was reached. Every content obtained in the subscales was intensively and repeatedly addressed in the SUCCEAT intervention. Whereas the topics of some subscales of the CASK were part of multi-family or systemic family therapy as well (e.g., 'Emotional Intelligence' or 'Insight and Acceptance'), most seem to be approached more deeply in SUCCEAT (e.g., "Self-Care"), and some seem unique for the SUCCEAT intervention (e.g., "Bigger Picture") [30,45]. Besides, the SUCCEAT intervention offers more time to develop and strengthen these skills. Moreover, carers may benefit from the opportunity to participate in this programme without the presence of the patients, in contrast to carers of the comparison group, where patients were included in the family treatment. However, this group difference must be interpreted with caution, considering the baseline differences between SUCCEAT and comparison group participants. Moreover, there were no further statistically significant differences between SUCCEAT and the active comparison group for the primary and other secondary outcomes measures. Regarding baseline data, the comparison group showed higher scores for burden and psychopathology measures, which may be due to longer illness duration or more severe courses.

This study has several strengths: This is the first study to compare the efficacy of a workshop- and online-based intervention for carers of adolescents suffering from AN, including long-term outcomes. A core strength of this study is the usage of the same design in both interventions, containing eight modules with the same content delivered within the same time frame. Both had access to clinical guidance (either in the workshops or via weekly online messages) and the possibility to exchange personal experiences with other carers (either in the workshops or via online forum). Furthermore, the coaches were the same in both groups. We found high fidelity to the intervention in that carer skills improved, and adherence was good.

This study also has some limitations: We included carers of AN patients only. More work is needed to investigate the effects of interventions for carers of adolescent patients with bulimia nervosa and binge-eating disorder. We could not compare the efficacy of SUCCEAT to a randomised control group. Other inpatient and outpatient psychiatric facilities that have been asked to recruit control-group participants with treatment-as-usual declined. Consequently, only two units that already implemented specialised family interventions (multi-family or systemic family therapy) in their routine ED treatment concept participated. Therefore, we could only compare the efficacy of SUCCEAT to these well-established treatments, rather than to caregivers without receiving any such intervention. Moreover, the participants of the comparison group were recruited from different facilities partially located in a different country (Germany) from the SUCCEAT participants. Although the core principles of ED treatment should be comparable across all facilities involved, slight differences in treatment approaches cannot be ruled out. Besides, a direct comparison between the groups may be further impeded by different numbers of intervention sessions and baseline differences between participants of the SUCCEAT and comparison groups. Furthermore, dropout at FU assessments was higher in the comparison group than in the SUCCEAT group. The three-months dropout might have been lower for the SUCCEAT groups because the three-month assessments were conducted shortly after the SUCCEAT intervention was finished, whereas the assessment was not temporally correlated with the end of the family intervention in the comparison group. For the differences regarding the dropout rates at the 12-month FU, we assume that the participants who already filled out two assessment batteries might also be more willing to complete the final FU assessment. These differences have to be taken into account when comparing the SUCCEAT group to the comparison group. Nevertheless, the current study provides a rough estimation of the effects of SUCCEAT compared to other well-established caregiver interventions. Further research is needed, including a randomised control group and larger group sizes in all arms, to confirm the effectiveness of SUCCEAT. Data on patient outcomes are needed to investigate whether the reduction of burden and improvement of skills in caregivers positively influences ED outcomes as well.

5. Conclusions

This study provides support for the efficacy of SUCCEAT, an intervention for carers of adolescents with AN, reducing carer's burden, distress and psychopathology and improving caregiver skills with high adherence and long-lasting medium-to-high effects underpinning its clinical relevance. SUCCEAT can easily be delivered and disseminated. Both the workshop and the online version can be integrated into clinical routine care of inpatient and outpatient adolescents with AN, as an adjunct to the treatment. Guidance by trained professionals and conjoint case-management at the same facility seem important for the efficacy and adherence of the intervention.

Supplementary Materials: The following are available online at http://www.mdpi.com/2077-0383/9/6/1912/s1, ESM1. Consort checklist and ESM2. Table S1: Means (SDs) and results of the repeated measures ANOVA for outcomes of the SUCCEAT workshop vs. SUCCEAT online intervention regarding caregiving burden and psychopathology (completer analysis), Table S2: Means (SDs) and results of the repeated measures ANOVA for outcomes of the SUCCEAT workshop vs. SUCCEAT online intervention group regarding caregiver skills (completer analysis), Table S3: Results of the mixed-methods ANOVA comparing the SUCCEAT intervention ($n = 100$) and the comparison group ($n = 49$) (intention-to-treat analysis), Table S4: Results of the mixed-methods ANOVA comparing the SUCCEAT intervention and the comparison group (completer analysis).

Author Contributions: Conceptualization, A.F.K.K., J.T., J.P. and G.W.; methodology, C.F., J.P. and M.Z.; formal analysis, M.Z.; investigation, J.P., E.M., S.T., A.Z., C.F. and T.W.; resources, H.I., E.A.-W., G.S., D.K., C.L., A.F.K.K. and G.W.; data curation, M.Z.; writing—original draft preparation, S.T. and J.P.; writing—review and editing, J.P., S.T., M.Z., J.T., A.F.K.K. and G.W.; visualization, M.Z.; supervision, A.F.K.K. and G.W.; project administration, J.P., S.T., C.F. and T.W.; funding acquisition, A.F.K.K. and G.W. All authors have read and agreed to the published version of the manuscript.

Funding: This research was funded by "Gemeinsame Gesundheitsziele aus dem Rahmen-Pharmavertrag/Pharma Master Agreement" (cooperation between the Austrian pharmaceutical industry and the Austrian social insurance; Grant 99901002500, given to A.K. and G.W.).

Acknowledgments: We want to thank all the staff members that helped to conduct the study, as well as all patients and their caregivers who agreed to participate.

Conflicts of Interest: J.T. is co-author of the book used in the SUCCEAT intervention and was part of the team that developed the DVD. J.P. and E.M. provided coaching in the workshops and online intervention. The funders had no role in the design of the study; in the collection, analyses or interpretation of data; in the writing of the manuscript; or in the decision to publish the results.

References

1. National Guideline Alliance (UK). *Eating Disorders: Recognition and Treatment*; National Institute for Health and Care Excellence: Clinical Guidelines; National Institute for Health and Care Excellence (UK): London, UK, 2017.
2. Herpertz-Dahlmann, B.; van Elburg, A.; Castro-Fornieles, J.; Schmidt, U. ESCAP Expert Paper: New developments in the diagnosis and treatment of adolescent anorexia nervosa—A European perspective. *Eur. Child Adolesc. Psychiatry* **2015**, *24*, 1153–1167. [CrossRef] [PubMed]
3. Schmidt, U.; Treasure, J. Anorexia nervosa: Valued and visible. A cognitive-interpersonal maintenance model and its implications for research and practice. *Br. J. Clin. Psychol.* **2006**, *45*, 343–366. [CrossRef] [PubMed]
4. Zabala, M.J.; Macdonald, P.; Treasure, J. Appraisal of caregiving burden, expressed emotion and psychological distress in families of people with eating disorders: A systematic review. *Eur. Eat. Disord. Rev.* **2009**, *17*, 338–349. [CrossRef] [PubMed]
5. Treasure, J.; Whitaker, W.; Todd, G.; Whitney, J. A description of multiple family workshops for carers of people with anorexia nervosa. *Eur. Eat. Disord. Rev.* **2012**, *20*, e17–e22. [CrossRef]
6. Rhind, C.; Salerno, L.; Hibbs, R.; Micali, N.; Schmidt, U.; Gowers, S.; Macdonald, P.; Goddard, E.; Todd, G.; Tchanturia, K.; et al. The Objective and Subjective Caregiving Burden and Caregiving Behaviours of Parents of Adolescents with Anorexia Nervosa. *Eur. Eat. Disord. Rev.* **2016**, *24*. [CrossRef]
7. Kyriacou, O.; Treasure, J.; Schmidt, U. Understanding how parents cope with living with someone with anorexia nervosa: Modelling the factors that are associated with carer distress. *Int. J. Eat. Disord.* **2008**, *41*, 233–242. [CrossRef]
8. Anastasiadou, D.; Medina-Pradas, C.; Sepulveda, A.R.; Treasure, J. A systematic review of family caregiving in eating disorders. *Eat. Behav.* **2014**, *15*, 464–477. [CrossRef]
9. Hibbs, R.; Rhind, C.; Leppanen, J.; Treasure, J. Interventions for caregivers of someone with an eating disorder: A meta-analysis. *Int. J. Eat. Disord.* **2015**, *48*, 349–361. [CrossRef]
10. Treasure, J.; Schmidt, U. The cognitive-interpersonal maintenance model of anorexia nervosa revisited: A summary of the evidence for cognitive, socio-emotional and interpersonal predisposing and perpetuating factors. *J. Eat. Disord.* **2013**, *1*, 13. [CrossRef]
11. Treasure, J.; Willmott, D.; Ambwani, S.; Cardi, V.; Clark Bryan, D.; Rowlands, K.; Schmidt, U. Cognitive Interpersonal Model for Anorexia Nervosa Revisited: The Perpetuating Factors that Contribute to the Development of the Severe and Enduring Illness. *J. Clin. Med.* **2020**, *9*. [CrossRef]

12. Whitney, J.; Murphy, T.; Landau, S.; Gavan, K.; Todd, G.; Whitaker, W.; Treasure, J. A practical comparison of two types of family intervention: An exploratory RCT of family day workshops and individual family work as a supplement to inpatient care for adults with anorexia nervosa. *Eur. Eat. Disord. Rev. J. Eat. Disord. Assoc.* **2012**, *20*, 142–150. [CrossRef] [PubMed]
13. Sepulveda, A.R.; Lopez, C.; Todd, G.; Whitaker, W.; Treasure, J. An examination of the impact of "the Maudsley eating disorder collaborative care skills workshops" on the well being of carers: A pilot study. *Soc. Psychiatry Psychiatr. Epidemiol.* **2008**, *43*, 584–591. [CrossRef] [PubMed]
14. Goddard, E.; Macdonald, P.; Sepulveda, A.R.; Naumann, U.; Landau, S.; Schmidt, U.; Treasure, J. Cognitive interpersonal maintenance model of eating disorders: Intervention for carers. *Br. J. Psychiatry* **2011**, *199*, 225–231. [CrossRef] [PubMed]
15. Hodsoll, J.; Rhind, C.; Micali, N.; Hibbs, R.; Goddard, E.; Nazar, B.P.; Schmidt, U.; Gowers, S.; Macdonald, P.; Todd, G.; et al. A Pilot, Multicentre Pragmatic Randomised Trial to Explore the Impact of Carer Skills Training on Carer and Patient Behaviours: Testing the Cognitive Interpersonal Model in Adolescent Anorexia Nervosa. *Eur. Eat. Disord. Rev. J. Eat. Disord. Assoc.* **2017**, *25*, 551–561. [CrossRef] [PubMed]
16. Hibbs, R.; Magill, N.; Goddard, E.; Rhind, C.; Raenker, S.; Macdonald, P.; Todd, G.; Arcelus, J.; Morgan, J.; Beecham, J.; et al. Clinical effectiveness of a skills training intervention for caregivers in improving patient and caregiver health following in-patient treatment for severe anorexia nervosa: Pragmatic randomised controlled trial. *BJPsych Open* **2015**, *1*, 56–66. [CrossRef]
17. Grover, M.; Naumann, U.; Mohammad-Dar, L.; Glennon, D.; Ringwood, S.; Eisler, I.; Williams, C.; Treasure, J.; Schmidt, U. A randomized controlled trial of an Internet-based cognitive-behavioural skills package for carers of people with anorexia nervosa. *Psychol. Med.* **2011**, *41*, 2581–2591. [CrossRef]
18. Hoyle, D.; Slater, J.; Williams, C.; Schmidt, U.; Wade, T.D. Evaluation of a web-based skills intervention for carers of people with anorexia nervosa: A randomized controlled trial. *Int. J. Eat. Disord.* **2013**, *46*, 634–638. [CrossRef]
19. Dimitropoulos, G.; Landers, A.; Freeman, V.; Novick, J.; Schmidt, U.; Olmsted, M. A feasibility study comparing a web-based intervention to a workshop intervention for caregivers of adults with eating disorders. *Eur. Eat. Disord. Rev.* **2019**, *27*, 641–654. [CrossRef]
20. Amichai-Hamburger, Y.; Vinitzky, G. Social network use and personality. *Comput. Hum. Behav.* **2010**, *26*, 1289–1295. [CrossRef]
21. Titov, N.; Hadjistavropoulos, H.D.; Nielssen, O.; Mohr, D.C.; Andersson, G.; Dear, B.F. From Research to Practice: Ten Lessons in Delivering Digital Mental Health Services. *J. Clin. Med.* **2019**, *8*, 1239. [CrossRef]
22. Spencer, L.; Potterton, R.; Allen, K.; Musiat, P.; Schmidt, U. Internet-Based Interventions for Carers of Individuals With Psychiatric Disorders, Neurological Disorders, or Brain Injuries: Systematic Review. *J. Med. Internet Res.* **2019**, *21*, e10876. [CrossRef] [PubMed]
23. Taylor, C.B.; Fitzsimmons-Craft, E.E.; Graham, A.K. Digital technology can revolutionize mental health services delivery: The COVID-19 crisis as a catalyst for change. *Int. J. Eat. Disord.* **2020**. [CrossRef] [PubMed]
24. Grover, M.; Williams, C.; Eisler, I.; Fairbairn, P.; McCloskey, C.; Smith, G.; Treasure, J.; Schmidt, U. An off-line pilot evaluation of a web-based systemic cognitive-behavioral intervention for carers of people with anorexia nervosa. *Int. J. Eat. Disord.* **2011**, *44*, 708–715. [CrossRef] [PubMed]
25. Zipfel, S.; Giel, K.E.; Bulik, C.M.; Hay, P.; Schmidt, U. Anorexia nervosa: Aetiology, assessment, and treatment. *Lancet Psychiatry* **2015**, *2*, 1099–1111. [CrossRef]
26. Franta, C.; Philipp, J.; Waldherr, K.; Truttmann, S.; Merl, E.; Schöfbeck, G.; Koubek, D.; Laczkovics, C.; Imgart, H.; Zanko, A.; et al. Supporting Carers of Children and Adolescents with Eating Disorders in Austria (SUCCEAT): Study protocol for a randomised controlled trial. *Eur. Eat. Disord. Rev.* **2018**, *26*, 447–461. [CrossRef]
27. Higgins, J.; Green, S. Cochrane Handbook for Systematic Reviews of Interventions. Available online: https://handbook-5-1.cochrane.org/ (accessed on 29 April 2020).
28. Treasure, J.; Smith, G.; Crane, A. *Skills-Based Learning for Caring for a Loved One with an Eating Disorder: The New Maudsley Method*; Routledge: London, UK, 2007; pp. 1–245. [CrossRef]
29. The Succeed Foundation. *How to Care for Someone with an Eating Disorder*; Learn the techniques designed by one of the world's top eating disorder researchers; The Succeed Foundation: London, UK, 2011; (DVD).
30. Imgart, H.; Plassmann, R. [Effective factors in multifamily therapy in patients with eating disorders: Critical appraisal and implications for practice]. *Neuropsychiatr. Klin. Diagn. Ther. Rehabil.* **2020**. [CrossRef]

31. Linden, M.; Maier, W.; Achberger, M.; Herr, R.; Helmchen, H.; Benkert, O. Psychische erkrankungen und ihre behandlung in allgemeinarztpraxen in Deutschland: Ergebnisse aus einer studie der Weltgesundheitsorganisation (WHO). [Psychological disorders and their treatment in general practice in Germany: Results of a WHO study.]. *Nervenarzt* **1996**, *67*, 205–215.
32. Goldberg, D.P.; Gater, R.; Sartorius, N.; Ustun, T.B.; Piccinelli, M.; Gureje, O.; Rutter, C. The validity of two versions of the GHQ in the WHO study of mental illness in general health care. *Psychol. Med.* **1997**, *27*, 191–197. [CrossRef]
33. Sepulveda, A.R.; Whitney, J.; Hankins, M.; Treasure, J. Development and validation of an Eating Disorders Symptom Impact Scale (EDSIS) for carers of people with eating disorders. *Health Qual. Life Outcomes* **2008**, *6*, 28. [CrossRef]
34. Franke, G.H. *Die Symptom-Checkliste von Derogatis (SCL-90-R)—Deutsche*; Version 2; Beltz: Göttingen, Germany, 2002.
35. Hautzinger, M.; Keller, F.; Kühner, C. *Beck Depressions Inventar, 2. Auflage (BDI-II)*; Pearson: Hallbergmoos, Germany, 2006.
36. Kühner, C.; Bürger, C.; Keller, F.; Hautzinger, M. Reliabilität und Validität des revidierten Beck-Depressionsinventars (BDI-II). *Nervenarzt* **2007**, *78*, 651–656. [CrossRef]
37. Laux, L.; Glanzmann, P.; Schaffner, P.; Spielsberger, C.D. *STAI—Das State-Trait-Angstinventar*, 1st ed.; Beltz: Weinheim, Germany, 1981.
38. Hibbs, R.; Rhind, C.; Salerno, L.; Lo Coco, G.; Goddard, E.; Schmidt, U.; Micali, N.; Gowers, S.; Beecham, J.; Macdonald, P.; et al. Development and validation of a scale to measure caregiver skills in eating disorders. *Int. J. Eat. Disord.* **2015**, *48*, 290–297. [CrossRef] [PubMed]
39. Schlegl, S.; Bürger, C.; Schmidt, L.; Herbst, N.; Voderholzer, U. The potential of technology-based psychological interventions for anorexia and bulimia nervosa: A systematic review and recommendations for future research. *J. Med. Internet Res.* **2015**, *17*, e85. [CrossRef] [PubMed]
40. Haigh, R.; Treasure, J. Investigating the needs of carers in the area of eating disorders: Development of the Carers' Needs Assessment Measure (CANAM). *Eur. Eat. Disord. Rev.* **2003**, *11*, 125–141. [CrossRef]
41. Yim, S.H.; Spencer, L.; Gordon, G.; Allen, K.; Musiat, P.; Schmidt, U. Eating disorder sufferers' and carers' views on online self-help programmes. *Eur. J. Public Health* **2019**. (submitted).
42. Wagner, G.; Penelo, E.; Wanner, C.; Gwinner, P.; Trofaier, M.-L.; Imgart, H.; Waldherr, K.; Wöber-Bingöl, C.; Karwautz, A.F.K. Internet-delivered cognitive-behavioural therapy v. conventional guided self-help for bulimia nervosa: Long-term evaluation of a randomised controlled trial. *Br. J. Psychiatry J. Ment. Sci.* **2013**, *202*, 135–141. [CrossRef] [PubMed]
43. Yim, S.H.; Schmidt, U. Self-Help Treatment of Eating Disorders. *Psychiatr. Clin.* **2019**, *42*, 231–241. [CrossRef]
44. Fernández-Aranda, F.; Casas, M.; Claes, L.; Bryan, D.C.; Favaro, A.; Granero, R.; Gudiol, C.; Jiménez-Murcia, S.; Karwautz, A.; Grange, D.L.; et al. COVID-19 and implications for eating disorders. *Eur. Eat. Disord. Rev.* **2020**, *28*, 239–245. [CrossRef]
45. Reich, G. Familienbeziehungen und Familientherapie bei Essstörungen. *Prax. Kinderpsychol. Kinderpsychiatr.* **2005**, *54*, 318–336.

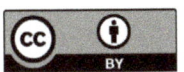

© 2020 by the authors. Licensee MDPI, Basel, Switzerland. This article is an open access article distributed under the terms and conditions of the Creative Commons Attribution (CC BY) license (http://creativecommons.org/licenses/by/4.0/).

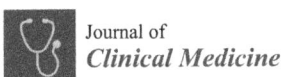

Article

Outcomes of an Accelerated Inpatient Refeeding Protocol in 103 Extremely Underweight Adults with Anorexia Nervosa at a Specialized Clinic in Prien, Germany

Thorsten Koerner [1], Verena Haas [2], Julia Heese [1], Matislava Karacic [1], Elmar Ngo [1], Christoph U. Correll [2,3,4], Ulrich Voderholzer [1,5,*] and Ulrich Cuntz [1,6]

1. Schön Clinic Roseneck; Am Roseneck 6, 83209 Prien am Chiemsee, Germany; thkoerner@schoen-klinik.de (T.K.); jheese@schoen-klinik.de (J.H.); mkaracic@schoen-klinik.de (M.K.); engo@schoen-klinik.de (E.N.); UCuntz@schoen-klinik.de (U.C.)
2. Clinic for Psychiatry, Psychosomatics and Psychotherapy of childhood and adolescence, Charité – University Berlin, corporate member of Free University Berlin, Humboldt-University Berlin, and Berlin Institute of Health, 13353 Berlin, Germany; verena.haas@charite.de (V.H.); christoph.correll@charite.de (C.U.C.)
3. Department of Psychiatry and Molecular medicine, Donald and Barbara Zucker School of Medicine at Hofstra/Northwell, Hempstead, NY 11549, USA
4. Department of Psychiatry, the Zucker Hillside Hospital, Glen Oaks, NY 11004, USA
5. Department of Psychiatry and Psychotherapy, Ludwig-Maximilians-Universität München (LMU), 80336 München, Germany
6. Research program for the evaluation of psychotherapy in complex therapeutic settings, PMU Paracelsus Medical University Salzburg, 5020 Salzburg, Austria
* Correspondence: uvoderholzer@schoen-klinik.de

Received: 17 March 2020; Accepted: 13 May 2020; Published: 19 May 2020

Abstract: Background: In mildly to moderately malnourished adolescent patients with anorexia nervosa (AN), accelerated refeeding protocols using higher initial calory supply coupled with phosphate supplements were not associated with a higher incidence of refeeding syndrome (RS). It is unclear whether this is also a feasible approach for extremely malnourished, adult AN patients. Methods: Outcomes of a clinical refeeding protocol involving a targeted initial intake of ≥2000 kcal/day, routine supplementation of phosphate and thiamine as well as close medical monitoring, were evaluated. A retrospective chart review including AN patients with a body mass index (BMI) <13 kg/m^2 was conducted, to describe changes in weight, BMI, and laboratory parameters (phosphate, creatine kinase, hematocrit, sodium, liver enzymes, and blood count) over four weeks. Results: In 103 female patients (age, mean ± standard deviation (SD) = 23.8 ± 5.3 years), BMI between admission and follow-up increased from 11.5 ± 0.9 to 13.1 ± 1.1 kg/m^2 and total weight gain within the first four weeks was 4.2 ± 2.0 kg (mean, SD). Laboratory parameter monitoring indicated no case of RS, but continuous normalization of blood parameters. Conclusions: Combined with close medical monitoring and electrolyte supplementation, accelerated refeeding may also be applied to achieve medical stabilization in extremely underweight adults with AN without increasing the risk of RS.

Keywords: anorexia nervosa; caloric intake; refeeding syndrome; refeeding protocol

1. Introduction: Refeeding and Refeeding Syndrome

Refeeding syndrome (RS) is a sudden, threatening deterioration in the general physical condition of a cachectic patient undergoing refeeding, especially in the first two to three weeks of refeeding following a prolonged period of hunger. RS has been scientifically described, among other conditions, in prisoners of war after the Second World War [1,2] and later in the refeeding of predominantly older underweight patients and patients with tumor cachexia [3,4]. Characteristic features of RS are fluid shifts and electrolyte fluctuations, which can occur as a result of endocrine and metabolic changes resulting from the onset of refeeding. At the center of RS are hypophosphatemia, hyponatremia, disturbed glucose metabolism, and insufficient thiamine supply [5]. Drastic malnutrition is associated with depleted intracellular phosphate stores. Initially, refeeding causes a change from a catabolic to anabolic metabolism, and concomitant hyperparathyroidism may contribute to the development of hypophosphatemia [6]. This process can lead to a critical drop in the intracellular concentration of adenosine triphosphate (ATP) and thus in the energy supply of the cells [7]. Clinical consequences range from severe organ dysfunction and rhabdomyolysis to seizures, delirium, coma, and death. The definition of RS is not clear-cut, and so there are no clear prevalence figures for RS in patients with anorexia nervosa (AN). In adult AN patients, the incidence of hypophosphatemia during refeeding is reported to range from 0%–80% [8,9]. Appropriate control of energy intake, as well as monitoring and adequate supplementation of electrolytes, are essential in the early stages of refeeding to avoid complications [10].

Due to the fear of serious medical complications related to RS, "start low, go slow" approaches (e.g., starting at 1200 kcal/d and increasing by 200 calories every other day) have been practiced for a long time in the refeeding of patients with AN. In practice, this approach leads initially to a hypocaloric diet and the maintenance of severe energy deficiency and to additional weight loss, which, in some cases, can lead to pronounced hypoglycemia with subsequent organ damage, as well as to longer hospital stays. In adolescent patients with AN, higher initial weight gain has been linked with a higher likelihood of remission by the end of treatment [11].

There is currently no consensus regarding the adequate initial energy supply during the refeeding of AN patients, which leads to inconsistent procedures. A scientific basis for the very restrictive dietary guidelines for the initial caloric intake in severely underweight adult patients is still missing, and presumably, the initial BMI [12] or the expression of cachexia is a predictor of RS [13]. Study protocols, in which an initially higher caloric intake was compared with a low-caloric diet [14] or with high energy intake in the first week and a gradual reduction of energy supply [15], showed no difference in the occurrence of components of RS, but larger and faster weight gain with the higher-caloric refeeding approach. In addition, a review of 22 studies by Garber et al. [16] showed that in mildly to moderately malnourished AN patients a low initial energy intake was too conservative and that higher initial energy levels were not associated with an increased risk of RS, as long as electrolytes, water balance, and cardiovascular parameters were closely monitored and controlled; however, most studies included in the review were conducted in adolescents. For extremely underweight adult patients, there are currently only a few studies examining higher caloric refeeding, and therefore no commonly accepted, reliable recommendations regarding the value and safety of accelerated refeeding strategies exist. In a recent study on 119 adults with AN, higher initial caloric refeeding (i.e., 1500 instead of 1000 kcal/d) was described to provide additional nourishment, to medically stabilize patients, and to prevent RS [17]. The authors concluded that future research is needed to examine whether higher-calorie intakes (i.e., 2000 kcal/d), similar to those studied in adolescent patients, may also be beneficial to treat adult patients.

This retrospective study aimed to describe (i) a clinical, high-caloric refeeding protocol established in a specialist ward of a psychosomatic clinic, targeting an initial intake of 2000 kcal/d and the accompanying essential medical measures; (ii) the outcomes of this approach regarding changes in weight and selected blood parameters to reflect physiological status and risk of RS.

2. Methods

2.1. Design and Population

The 24-bed ward featured in this study admitted patients with a diagnosis of anorexia nervosa who are at least 18 years old and who, due to their underweight, excessive exercising and/or vomiting and/or medical complications, require intensive medical and therapeutic surveillance.

For this retrospective chart review, patient data from all consecutive admissions were included if they fulfilled the following inclusion criteria:

- Age > 18 years; no upper age limit was defined as an inclusion criterion.
- Treated at a 24-bed unit for extremely underweight patients with 6 surveillance beds at Schön Klinik Roseneck, Rosenheim, Germany, between 1/1/2016 and 12/31/2018 (oral nutrition, no forced feeding or medication, no tube feeding, and all meals accompanied).
- Main diagnosis of AN (restrictive, active, and atypical AN).
- BMI ≤ 13 kg/m^2.
- Retention period of ≥28 days, as RS and related phenomena, are expected in this time window.
- Availability of laboratory data: five measurements from the time of admission until day 28.

Exclusion criteria were age <18 years, treatment at the institution outside of the time window, a BMI > 13 kg/m^2, and other eating disorder diagnoses, such as bulimia nervosa and binge eating disorders.

2.2. Ethical Approval

All procedures performed in studies involving human participants were in accordance with the ethical standards of the institutional review board of the Ludwig Maximilian Universität (LMU) Munich and with the 1964 Helsinki declaration and its later amendments or comparable ethical standards. According to the guidelines by the institutional review board of the LMU Munich, retrospective studies conducted on already available, anonymized data are exempt from requiring ethics approval.

2.3. Routine, Clinical Management of Meals, and Refeeding

All patients received three meals with an average total energy content of 2000 kcal per day from day 1 after admission to the ward, divided into three main meals with a choice between vegetarian and non-vegetarian menus. The caloric intake was adjusted and increased according to weight development to aim for an increase in body weight of 700–1000 g/week. The criterion for sufficient food intake was weight gain, which should be at least 100 g per day. If the agreed amount of food intake for weight gain could not be achieved, the portion size of one or more main meals was increased, and up to three snacks between meals were added. In addition, liquid food was offered to substitute for energy losses in case a part of the meals could not be eaten. All meals were therapeutically accompanied by a nurse or therapist in a 1:6 group supervision. Patient adherence to dietary intake was supported through daily therapeutic contacts and medical rounds. Patients ate their meals in a stable group setting and supported each other. Peer pressure may play an important role. In weekly eating protocol sessions, patients reviewed their progress and committed to new goals related to food avoidance, fears, and counteractive behavior. Patients did not receive nasogastric feeding since the normalization of eating behavior is a common therapeutic goal. All patients were prescribed 2000 kcal/d (three meals) starting from the day of admission. The average caloric value (data provided by the caterer and controlled in samples) for the non-vegetarian menu was 743, 717, and 704 (total 2164) kcal for breakfast, lunch, and dinner; and 743, 737, and 683 (total: 2162) for the vegetarian option. If patients did not finish their meal (50%–99% eaten) they were asked to drink 1 supplemental drink (400 kcal, Fresubin 200 mL with 2 kcal/mL). If patients ate less than 50% of their respective meal, they were asked to replace the missed-out calories by drinking 2 supplemental drinks (2 × 400 kcal). The group setting and the support from experienced therapists were considered essential for compliance with dietary adherence. Contingency measures were often necessary to regulate excessive exercising and slow weight gain. During the first 28 days, it was rare that patients required more than 2000 kcal/d but many patients received liquid food to replace unfinished meals. Patients reduced their calorie consumption by limiting their physical activity. Contingency contracts and video surveillance with 24/7 nursing staff presence as well as very moderate exercise therapy play an important role in normalizing movement behavior.

During the first 4 weeks, which was the observation period in this study, most patients gained sufficient weight with 2000 kcal/d spread over three meals. This was supported by restricting their physical activity and exercising. In individual cases, an energy intake of more than 4000 kcal was necessary to ensure sufficient weight gain. All patients participated in an intensive therapeutic program adapted to the special needs of the severely underweight women and suitable for therapeutically addressing the considerable anxieties and resistance associated with weight gain. This included daily individual cognitive behavioral therapy (CBT) sessions and medical rounds, accompanied meals, participation in group therapy (twice weekly problem-solving group, Cognitive Remediation Therapy (CRT), and art therapy, and daily morning and evening rounds with the nursing staff).

Daily documentation occurred for clinical and therapeutic observations and nursing contacts as well as weight measurement and comments on the accompanied meals. Physical examination including neurological assessment and vital signs was a standard procedure at admission and brief daily medical check during rounds. The SUSS (Sit up, squat, stand) test, as specified by the British Royal College of Psychiatrists MARSIPAN (Management of Really Sick Patients with AN) workgroup, assessed physical performance. It was used at admission and during rounds to follow up on physical performance. Patients used wheelchairs during the first weeks on the ward if their weight is below 13 kg/m^2. A normal result of the SUSS test plus a BMI of 13 kg/m^2 and above show that a wheelchair was no longer necessary.

As part of the routine refeeding protocol: weight was monitored daily in underwear (Scale: Seca Model Nr. 6357021004). Height was measured at admission. Blood work was performed at least once a week including blood count (without white blood cell differential), electrolytes (sodium, potassium, phosphate, and chloride), transaminases, gamma-glutamyl-transferase (γ-GT), creatine kinase, creatinine, and urea. Further investigations included continuous monitoring of vital signs (electrocardiogram (ECG), heart rate, and blood pressure), hematocrit (<25%) and weight progression, routine clinical examination including neurological assessment and vital signs, SUSS test, sonography, and bioelectrical impedance analysis to assess edema status. Phosphate (612 mg to 1224 mg/d) and thiamine (200 mg/d) were supplemented routinely for two weeks and phosphate thereafter if needed. In some patients, the administration of diuretics was necessary at times when either the severity of the edema was subjectively too stressful or the heart rate per minute exceeded the systolic blood pressure in mmHg.

2.4. Data Assessment

The American Society of Parental and Enteral Nutrition developed consensus guidelines for the following diagnostic criteria for RS [18]: (i) a decrease of serum phosphorus, potassium, and/or magnesium levels by 10%–20% (mild RS), 20%–30% (moderate RS), or >30% and/or organ dysfunction resulting from a decrease in any of these and/or due to thiamin deficiency (severe RS) (ii) and occurring within 5 days of reinitiating or substantially increasing energy provision. These ASPEN criteria did not appear suitable to us for assessing the risk of the patients we treat in our unit: phosphate and thiamine were routinely supplemented and it was therefore unlikely that such a deficiency will occur in the context of malnutrition. Potassium was controlled even more closely (possibly several times a day), because of the risk of cardiac arrhythmia. If a drop in serum potassium occurred, potassium, as well as magnesium, were supplemented. In this respect, we chose not to adhere to these guidelines, and to report on a broad range of blood parameters to cover as many of the risks associated with re-nutrition as it was possible using our retrospective data from routine treatment.

The following criteria were used to define a case of RS:

- Critical deterioration of the general condition (e.g., severe edema, pericardial effusion, and weakness).
- Critical drop of serum phosphate to values <0.75 mmol/L.
- Increase in creatine kinase to >1000 U/L.
- Decrease of hematocrit to <25%.

- Decrease of serum sodium to <125 mmol/L.
- For the assessment of the clinical condition, the following laboratory parameters were also used:
    - Aspartate aminotransferase (GOT) (>35 U/L) and alanine aminotransferase (GPT) (>35 U/L) for estimation of liver cell damage.
    - Leukocytes (<3.98 G/L), hemoglobin (<11.2 g/L), and thrombocytes (<182 G/L) for the assessment of bone marrow function.

The following data were collected on admission and weekly thereafter for 4 weeks in clinical care and are presented in this study: body weight, height, BMI, and blood work (creatin kinase, phosphate, sodium, GOT, GPT, leucocytes, hematocrit, hemoglobin, and thrombocytes).

The following cut-off values were used to define pathological blood values: creatin kinase, >170 U/L; phosphate, <0.75 mmol/L; sodium, <12 mmol/L; GOT, GPT >35 U/L; leucocytes, <3.98 G/L, hemoglobin, <25%; thrombocytes, <182 G/L.

2.5. Statistical Analysis

All data were examined with the Shapiro–Wilk test for normal distribution and presented as mean ± standard deviation (normally distributed data) or as median and 25th/75th percentile (non-normally distributed data). For the change of BMI, weight, laboratory values over time, a paired samples t-test (for normally distributed differences), or a non-parametric, related samples Wilcoxon test (difference not normally distributed) was chosen. To assess how pathological laboratory values developed over time, the change in the percentage of pathological values in the total sample was treated as a categorical variable (pathological: y/n) and examined at the beginning and after 4 weeks using the two-sided Fisher's Exact Test (https://www.graphpad.com/quickcalcs/contingency1.cfm). The Fisher's Exact Test (Fisher–Yates test, exact chi-square test) is a significant test for independence in contingency tables. In contrast to the Chi-square independence test, however, it does not impose any requirements on the sample size and provides reliable results even with a small number of observations per cell.

A two-sided p-value <0.05 was considered statistically significant. Statistical analyses were performed by using SPSS version 21.0 for Windows (IBM Corp., Armonk, NY, USA).

3. Results

Between 01/01/2016 and 12/31/2018, 335 patients were admitted to the 24-bed unit for extremely underweight patients at Schön Klinik Roseneck in Rosenheim, Germany within a 120-bed hospital for psychosomatic medicine and psychotherapy. Of these 335 patients, 181 had a main diagnosis of AN, and 161 had a BMI <13 kg/m^2 as well as a length of stay ≥28 days, with 43 of these (27.3%) discontinuing therapy in the first four weeks. None of these 43 patients had refeeding syndrome. A total of 103 patients with a BMI <13 kg/m^2, a stay of ≥4 weeks, and available laboratory data per the inclusion criteria were included in this study. These 103 patients had complete data sets, i.e., the laboratory values were available weekly (+− 2 days) for all measurement times. Most of the patients with incomplete data sets were discharged or transferred before the end of the 28 days, mostly due to lack of motivation—in none of these cases was a transfer necessary due to critical deterioration of the general condition. All participants were female and aged 23.8 ± 5.3 (range = 18–47) years. No males in the weight range <13 kg/m^2 were admitted in the observation period.

The weekly change in weight and BMI is shown in Table 1. The weight of the female patients increased during four weeks by an average of 1.0 ± 0.5 kg/week, and by a total of 4.2 ± 2.0 kg over four weeks (mean, SD). This weight change corresponds to a total increase of 1.6 ± 0.8 BMI units in four weeks (p = 0.001). None of the patients experienced a critical deterioration of their physical condition, and all patients improved their performance level with weight gain (sit up, squat, stand (SUSS) test score as specified by the MARSIPAN workgroup (32).

Table 1. Weekly change in weight and body mass index.

	Weight	BMI		Weight	BMI
Week 1	31.5 ± 3.6 (23.5–40.1)	11.5 ± 0.9 (9.5–13.0)	Week 1–2	1.3 (0.6/3.0) *** (−2.2–8.4)	0.5 (0.2/1.1) *** (−0.8–3.4)
Week 2	33.4 ± 3.7 (24.0–41.5)	12.3 ± 1.1 (9.7–15.2)	Week 2–3	0.8 ± 0.9 *** (−1.2–3.4)	0.3 (0.1/0.5) *** (−0.5–1.4)
Week 3	34.2 ± 3.6 (26.0–41.5)	12.6 ± 1.1 (9.8–15.9)	Week 3–4	0.7 ± 0.7 *** (−0.8–2.8)	0.2 (0.1/0.4) *** (−0.4–1.2)
Week 4	35.0 ± 3.5 (26.5–42.0)	12.8 ± 1.1 (10.0–16.1)	Week 4–5	0.8 (0.4/1.1) *** (−1.4–1.9)	0.3 (0.1/0.5) *** (−0.5–0.8)
Week 5	35.7 ± 3.4 (27.8–43.9)	13.1 ± 1.1 (10.0–16.9)	Week 1–5	4.0 (2.9/5.0) *** (−2.5–9.7)	1.4 (1.1/1.9) *** (−0.8–4.1)

***, $p < 0.001$; t-test for normally distributed data are presented as mean (SD), and for non-normally distributed data as median (25/75 percentile) using a Wilcoxon test. change; BMI: body mass index; data in parenthesis are ranges.

The weight gain was highest in the first week with an average of 1.9 ± 2.0 kg, leveling off to 0.7–0.8 kg/week in the following three weeks. The maximum increase observed in the first week was 8.4 kg, which was mostly due to rehydration (traceable by hematocrit decrease). In 20 patients (19%), the weekly weight gain in the first week was between 0.1 and 0.6 kg, in 13 (13%) between 0.7 and 1.0 kg, in 22 (21%) between 1.1 and 2.0 kg, in 24 (23%) between 2.1 and 4.0 kg, and in 13 (13%) >4.0 kg. In 11 patients (11%) a weight stagnation or weight loss was recorded in the first week, and this group had a mean weight loss of 0.7 kg (max. 2.2 kg to min. 0 kg).

All patients received 200 mg thiamine daily for the first four weeks and 612–1024 mg phosphate daily for the first two weeks. With this supplementation, serum phosphate levels increased during the observation period (Table 2, Figure 1). On admission, 7 (6.2%) of the 103 subjects had hypophosphatemia with values <0.75 mmol/L, and one subject had a critical value <0.5 mmol/L. After one week, only five patients had slightly decreased serum phosphate levels (<0.75 mmol/L) and after two weeks only three patients.

The decrease in the mean creatine kinase values during the observation period of the first four weeks of treatment clearly shows that the increase in energy intake and the consecutive significant weight gain right at the beginning of treatment was not associated with an increased risk of rhabdomyolysis (Table 2, Figure 1). Strongly elevated values for creatine kinase (>1000 U/L) were only observed in one patient at intake with 9941 U/L, which completely normalized within fourteen days with adequate nutrition and phosphate substitution.

While critical hyponatremia with values <125 mmol/L also occurred only on admission in one patient, the initially already low average value for hematocrit fell from 37% to 35% after fourteen days, and then slowly rose again to 36% after four weeks. Accordingly, up to three (different) patients with their hematocrit fell below the critical value of 25% at the first three measurement points. After four weeks, the values in two patients were still below the critical value. In parallel to the increase in weight, the transaminases, which were strongly elevated at admission, decreased significantly. Further, 54 (51.9%) of the patients had elevated GOT and 62 patients (59.6%) had elevated GPT > 35 U/L at admission, only 12 patients (11.5%) still had elevated values of GOT after four weeks, and the number of pathological values for GPT did not change on average during the four weeks being still $n = 61$ (59.2%).

Similarly, the rapid refeeding led to a highly significant increase in thrombocytes and leukocytes (Figure 1, Table 2), while the hemoglobin, in parallel to the hematocrit, dropped from an initial average of 12.5 ± 1.76 g/dL to 11.5 ± 1.69 g/dL in the third week, and stabilized at 11.6 ± 1.5 g/dL by week 4.

Table 2. Laboratory values at admission (T1) and after four weeks (T5), Mean and SD for 103 pt.

	CK	Phos	Sodium	GOT	GPT	Leuco	Haematocrit	Hb	Pla
cut off	>170 U/L	<0.75 mmol/L	<125 mmol/L	>35 U/L	>35 U/L	<3.98 G/L	<25 %	<11.2 g/L	<182 G/L
At admission	222 ± 974	1.15 ± 0.29	138.7 ± 4.7	67.9 ± 117.8	85.6 ± 121.9	4.1 ± 1.8	37.0 ± 5.0	12.5 ± 1.8	242 ± 81
	(27–9941)	(0.46–1.92)	(112.0–152.0)	(15.3–1078.0)	(8.3–742.0)	(1.1–14.0)	(22.9–44.7)	(7.5–15.6)	(45–494)
After four weeks	75 ± 54 ***	1.34 ± 0.18 ***	141.3 ± 2.7 ***	25.9 ± 8.0 ***	42.3 ± 21.6 ***	4.8 ± 1.8 ***	36.1 4.2 **	11.6 ± 1.5 ***	300 ± 92 ***
	(22–374)	(0.94–1.88)	(133.0–148.0)	(12.7–53.0)	(10.7–133.0)	(1.6–12.8)	(23.0–42.0)	(6.6–14.3)	(185–849)
pathologic at admission	19 (103)	7 (103)	7 (103)	54 (103)	62 (103)	54 (103)	23 (103)	21 (103)	21 (103)
	18.4%	6.8%	6.8%	52.4%	60.2%	52.4%	22.3%	20.4%	20.4%
pathologic after four weeks	6 (103)	0 (103)	0 (103)	12 (103)	61 (103)	37 (101)	22 (101)	36 (101)	0 (101)
	5.8% *	0% *	0% *	11.7% ***	59.2%	36.6% *	21.8%	35.6% *	(0%) ***

The T-test was used for normally distributed differences in blood values between two measurement points. A Wilcoxon test was used for non-normally distributed differences. For the percentage change in the proportion of pathological blood values, the two-sided Fischer's exact test was used * $p < 0.05$; ** $p < 0.01$;*** . $p < 0.001$; data in parenthesis are ranges. Abbreviations: CK: creatine kinase; Phos: inorganic phosphate; GOT: aspartate aminotransferase; GPT: alanine aminotransferase; Leuco: leukocytes; Hb: hemoglobin; Pla: platelets; SD, standard deviation.

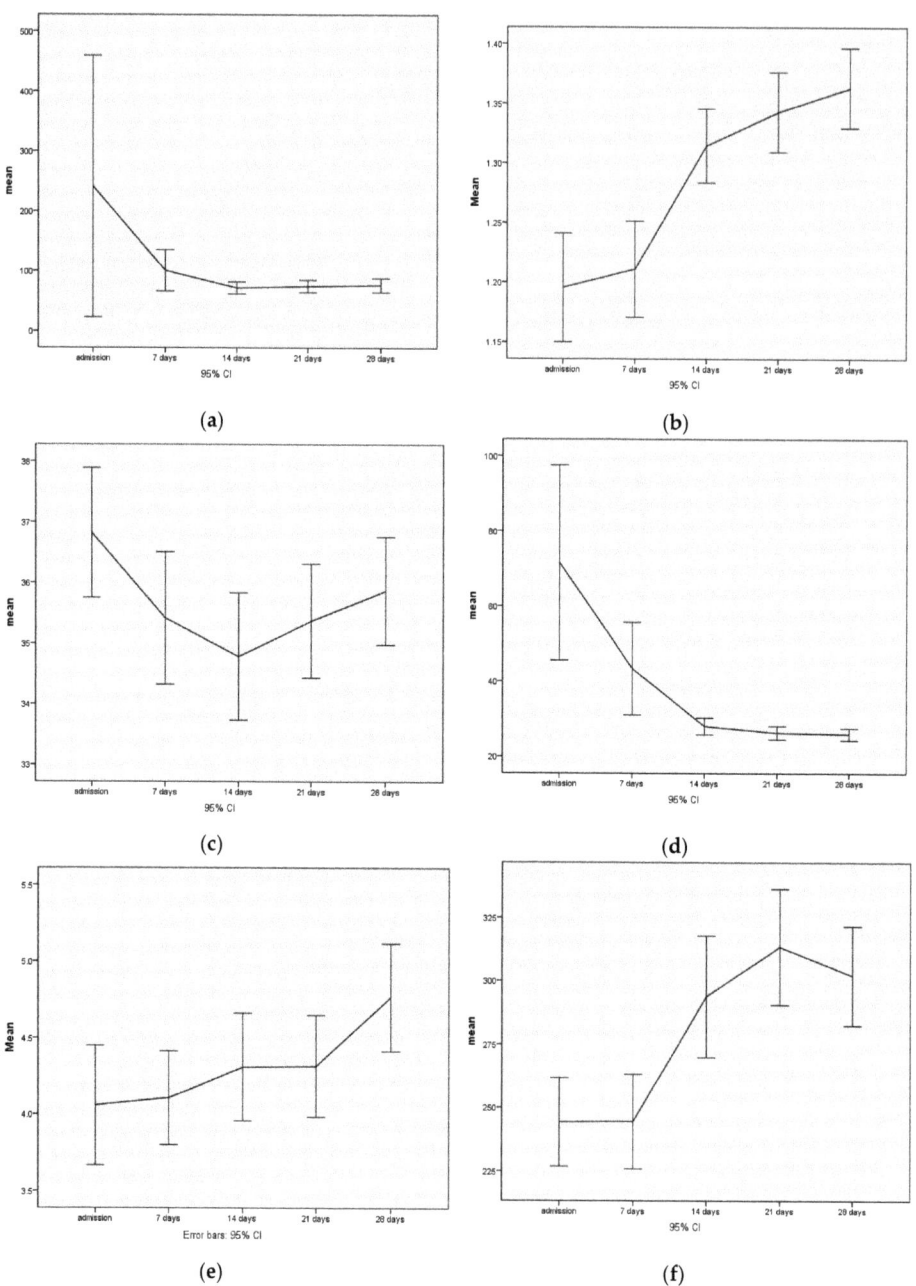

Figure 1. The course of creatine kinase (CK), inorganic phosphate (Phos) × 100, hematocrit (HK), and aspartate aminotransferase (GOT) leukocytes and platelets over four weeks with F-values of the measurement repeatability analysis. T1 to T5 (T1 intake, followed by weekly intervals of the laboratory survey). (**a**) Creatin kinase (F 2,3 df 4, p 0.056.); (**b**) Phosphate (F 23,9, df 4, p 0.000); (**c**) Hematocrit (F 12,3 df 4, p 0.000); (**d**) GOT (F 13,8 df 4, p 0.000); (**e**) Leucocytes (F 8,9, df 4, p 0.000); (**f**) Platelets (F 19,8, df 4 p 0.000.). T1, admission; T5, 28 days after admission.

4. Discussion

In the sample of 103 adult and severely malnourished patients with AN described here, an oral refeeding protocol with 2000 kcal/d as an initial target and weight-development-adapted increases in energy intake was applied. On average, the patients' body weight increased by more than 1040 g per week over four weeks and hypophosphatemia could be avoided with phosphate substitution. With this accelerated refeeding protocol, no case of refeeding syndrome (RS) was observed.

4.1. Physiological Effects of the Refeeding Protocol in the Present Study

Hyperhydration was common among the patients during the first four weeks of refeeding. This was self-limiting in most cases with only a small number of patients requiring oral diuretics. The initially low average hematocrit value fell significantly within the first fourteen days as a sign of hyperhydration, only to rise slowly thereafter; however, sodium levels remained stable or increased slightly on average, so that the cause of hyperhydration is unlikely to be inadequate vasopressin release or polydipsia. There is no indication that the drop in hematocrit could be avoided with slower refeeding. Hyperhydration could lead to cardiac problems, including myocardial dystrophy that has been associated with malnutrition [14]. In the present sample, the decrease in hematocrit was transient and clinically manageable without cardiac complications. A significant decrease in transaminases was observed as a sign of improvement in general body condition associated with weight gain. The increase in transaminases is considered a sign of the autolysis of body cells associated with the lack of energy [19]. In this respect, the decrease in transaminases can be seen as a sign of improved cellular energy supply. The bone marrow can transform gelatinously [20] when the patient is severely underweight over a prolonged period, thus significantly limiting hematopoiesis. The significant increase in platelets and leukocytes can be seen as a sign of bone marrow recovery and hematopoiesis. On the other hand, hemoglobin did not increase during the observation period, which can be explained by the slower erythropoiesis and the simultaneous hyperhydration with a decrease of hematocrit.

4.2. Previously Described Refeeding Protocols and Outcomes in Moderately Malnourished Adolescents with AN

Up till now, initial higher-caloric refeeding was mostly assessed in mildly to moderately malnourished adolescents. For example, in a group of 129 adolescent AN patients (mean intake BMI: 15.9 kg/m^2), Smith et al. found no case of refeeding syndrome with an initial energy intake of 1585 kcal/d and a rapid increase in energy intake to 3626 kcal/d by day 14 after hospital intake [14]. In that study, phosphate levels were monitored and, if necessary, corrected, which was the case in 75% of the patients. BMI increased by 0.6 BMI units per week over a time of 15 days. Madden et al. [19] also developed a high caloric refeeding protocol for adolescents: in 78 AN patients (78% expected body weight, no BMI information), initial caloric intake started with 2400 kcal/d on days 0–3 by continuous (24 h) nasogastric tube feeding, the weight increased by 2.5 kg in the first week, and by 5.1 kg 2.5 weeks after intake. Using this protocol, none of the patients receiving prophylactic phosphate supplementation developed hypophosphatemia, hypoglycemia, or other signs of RS. In contrast, one of the few case descriptions in the literature of RS refers to a 15-year-old adolescent with a BMI of 11.6 kg/m^2, low phosphate (0.78 mmol/L), and low glucose (2.6 mmol/L). With phosphate administration, the phosphate level of this patient remained low, and with an energy administration of only 800 kcal/d and a slow increase to 1000 kcal/d after 6 days, an RS developed with severe impairment of the mental state up to delirium [20].

4.3. Previously Described Refeeding Protocols and Outcomes in Severely Malnourished, Adults with AN

Gaudiani et al. [9] prescribed 990 kcal/d at the beginning with an increase to 2000 kcal/d after 19 days in 25 adults with AN (mean BMI at admission 13.1 kg/m^2), resulting in a BMI increase of 0.5 BMI units per week over a time of 19 days. Hypoglycemia occurred in 44% of patients, 76% showed abnormal liver function, 45% developed hypophosphatemia, and 92% developed hypothermia [9]. The observed complications by Gaudiani may have been due to initial low caloric intake (hypoglycemia and consecutive liver dysfunction) and less proactive phosphate substitution (hypophosphatemia). Hofer et al. [21] reported on 65 adults with AN (mean BMI at intake 13.7 kg/m^2) who were refed at 437 kcal/d with an initial increase to 1506 kcal/d, leading to an increase of 0.3 BMI units per week over a time of three weeks. This strategy was associated with severe hypokalemia in two patients, but no patient developed hypophosphatemia (due to phosphate supplementation). In 10.5% of patients, the following medical complications occurred: pretibial edema (n = 4), organ dysfunction as mild and transient pancreatitis, transient stage 2 renal failure, and urinary tract infection (n = 3). In two patients with already existing heart failure at admission with an echocardiographic ejection fraction of 40%, the malnutrition increased the severity of the existing disease. In a recent retrospective, observational study by Matthews et al. with 119 adult AN patients, higher caloric refeeding (group 1: baseline BMI of 17.2 kg/m^2 and intake of 1500 kcal/d vs. group 2: baseline BMI of 14.9 kg/m^2 and intake of 1000 kcal/d) along with close medical monitoring stabilized the patients and prevented RS. Our findings are in line with these results, and firstly, extend to an even more malnourished group of patients and second, to higher initial caloric intake.

4.4. Relevance of the Findings with Respect to Current Guideline Recommendations

Given these data, it is important to question the recommendations of the current guidelines for the management of AN. The German S3 guideline refers to the U.S.–American studies in adolescents, which recommend faster re-nutrition, but with the remark that at the time of the guideline update no comparable studies from the German-speaking countries and in adults were available. Other guidelines, however, seem to be based on older studies in which the paradigm shift towards faster refeeding had not yet become apparent. For example, the current guidelines for adults with AN (Table 3) recommend a consistently low energy intake, which does not allow for adequate weight gain.

Table 3. Current, national refeeding guidelines for malnourished patients with anorexia nervosa.

Guidelines	Age	Recommended Energy Intake
Australia and New Zealand	adult	1400 kcal/d [22]
Europe [23]	adult	start at 10, slowly increase to 15 kcal/kg/d (Day 1–3)
United Kingdom: Royal College of Psychiatrists [24]	adult	10–20 kcal/kg/d
United Kingdom: MARSIPAN [25]	adult	5–20 kcal/kg/d
American Psychiatric Association/American Dietetic Association [26]	adult	30–40 kcal/kg/d (1000–1600 kcal/d)
United Kingdom: Junior MARSIPAN [27]	<18 years	20 kcal/kg/d

Recent data implies that combined with close medical monitoring, a more accelerated approach appears to be safe, minimize complications, prevent mortality, and to reduce the length of stay in hospitals for patients with AN; however, as long as there is still not sufficient evidence-based data to support a new, general recommendation for severely malnourished, adult patients, nutritional rehabilitation must remain tailored to the individual patient.

There is still a need for systematic research to finally answer the question, which initial refeeding strategy for managing severe malnutrition should be the first-line treatment for AN patients. Further studies are needed that allow a detailed analysis of energy intake, weight change, and any associated complications. The approach presented in the current analysis appears promising and, to our knowledge, unique in this form in adults concerning faster and at the same time safe refeeding.

The strength of the present study is the large sample size and the uniform medical and therapeutic care under the largely standardized medication and diagnostics. One of the methodological limitations is that this is not a randomized patient selection, but a naturalistic setting in a single clinic. A randomized controlled trial (RCT) comparing "slow or regular" versus "fast" refeeding would be the next step to provide evidence for changing refeeding guidelines. We analyzed data from a consecutive cohort of extremely underweight patients. For such patients, inclusion in an RCT might be problematic for ethical reasons. With the chosen procedure, there was no evidence of critical deterioration of the physical condition, on the contrary, a consolidation of critical health status due to the rapid increase in weight was observed. Another limitation of the study is that the individual energy intake of the patients as well as adherence to the dietary recommendations and frequency of contingency measures were not objectively recorded and could only be given with a description of the general refeeding protocol that was as accurate as possible. On the other hand, an exact and objective recording of the energy intake of patients with AN is difficult to achieve, even under controlled conditions, and the comparatively high and rapid initial weight gain proves that correspondingly high energy intake must have taken place. Even though low blood glucose levels and thus hypoglycemia have been reported during refeeding in patients with AN, data on blood glucose levels is not included in the manuscript. To our experience hypoglycemia does not occur if the patients are sufficiently nourished, however, we cannot be sure that there were periods of hypoglycemia in the patient cohort described in our study.

Key messages:

(1) There are few evidence-based high caloric refeeding protocols for severely malnourished adult AN patients.
(2) In the present study, a rapid initial weight restoration strategy targeting oral energy intake of 2000 kcal/d from day one of treatment resulted in an average weight gain of 1040 g/week over four weeks. Combined with close medical monitoring and supplementation of phosphate and thiamine, this accelerated refeeding strategy was not associated with refeeding complications in severely malnourished adult AN patients.
(3) To derive safe and commonly accepted guidelines, further and prospective studies comparing different refeeding regimes are required.
(4) Following previous recommendations [18], the findings of the present study do not constitute medical advice. While the acknowledgment of the accelerated refeeding protocol presented in this study may assist in rethinking models of nutritional management of adult, severely malnourished AN patients, the judgment of the treating professional about the choice of an adequate refeeding strategy for an individual patient should prevail.

5. Conclusions

In summary, data from this naturalistic study indicate that the rapid refeeding strategy described here was effective and safe and that RS was not a consequence of more rapid refeeding. Future studies should further assess the efficacy and safety of rapid refeeding protocols in adults with AN who are severely underweight.

Author Contributions: Conceptualization: U.C., T.K., and U.V.; methodology: U.C. and V.H.; validation: V.H.; formal analysis, U.C., J.H., M.K.; Investigation, U.C., U.V., T.K., J.H., M.K., and E.N.; resources: U.C., and U.V.; data curation, U.C., J.H., and M.K.; writing—original draft preparation, T.K., U.C., V.H., and E.N.; writing—review and editing, U.V., V.H., C.U.C., and T.K.; visualization, U.C.; supervision, U.C. and U.V.; project administration: T.K. All authors have read and agreed to the published version of the manuscript.

Conflicts of Interest: The authors declare no conflict of interest.

References

1. Keys, A. Human starvation and its consequences. *J. Am. Diet. Assoc.* **1946**, *22*, 582–587. [PubMed]
2. Schnitker, M.A.; Mattman, P.E.; Bliss, T.L. A clinical study of malnutrition in Japanese prisoners of war. *Ann. Intern. Med.* **1951**, *35*, 69–96. [CrossRef] [PubMed]
3. Apovian, C.M.; McMahon, M.M.; Bistrian, B.R. Guidelines for refeeding the marasmic patient. *Crit. Care Med.* **1990**, *18*, 1030–1033. [CrossRef] [PubMed]
4. Vaszar, L.T.; Culpepper-Morgan, J.A.; Winter, S.M. Refeeding syndrome induced by cautious enteral alimentation of a moderately malnourished patient. *Gastroenterologist* **1998**, *6*, 79–81.
5. Solomon, S.M.; Kirby, D.F. The refeeding syndrome: A review. *JPEN J. Parenter. Enter. Nutr.* **1990**, *14*, 90–97. [CrossRef]

6. Cumming, A.D.; Farquhar, J.R.; Bouchier, I.A.D. Refeeding Hypophosphatemia in Anorexia-Nervosa and Alcoholism. *Brit. Med. J.* **1987**, *295*, 490–491. [CrossRef]
7. Gourley, D.R.H. The Role of Adenosine Triphosphate in the Transport of Phosphate in the Human Erythrocyte. *Arch. Biochem. Biophys.* **1952**, *40*, 1–12. [CrossRef]
8. Friedli, N.; Stanga, Z.; Sobotka, L.; Culkin, A.; Kondrup, J.; Laviano, A.; Mueller, B.; Schuetz, P. Revisiting the refeeding syndrome: Results of a systematic review. *Nutrition* **2017**, *35*, 151–160. [CrossRef]
9. Gaudiani, J.L.; Sabel, A.L.; Mascolo, M.; Mehler, P.S. Severe anorexia nervosa: Outcomes from a medical stabilization unit. *Int. J. Eat. Disord.* **2012**, *45*, 85–92. [CrossRef]
10. Hilbert, A.; Hoek, H.W.; Schmidt, R. Evidence-based clinical guidelines for eating disorders: International comparison. *Curr. Opin. Psychiatry* **2017**, *30*, 423–437. [CrossRef]
11. Le Grange, D.; Accurso, E.C.; Lock, J.; Agras, S.; Bryson, S.W. Early weight gain predicts outcome in two treatments for adolescent anorexia nervosa. *Int. J. Eat. Disord.* **2014**, *47*, 124–129. [CrossRef] [PubMed]
12. Lund, B.C.; Hernandez, E.R.; Yates, W.R.; Mitchell, J.R.; McKee, P.A.; Johnson, C.L. Rate of Inpatient Weight Restoration Predicts Outcome in Anorexia Nervosa. *Int. J. Eat. Disord.* **2009**, *42*, 301–305. [CrossRef] [PubMed]
13. Redgrave, G.W.; Coughlin, J.W.; Schreyer, C.C.; Martin, L.M.; Leonpacher, A.K.; Seide, M.; Verdi, A.M.; Pletch, A.; Guarda, A.S. Refeeding and weight restoration outcomes in anorexia nervosa: Challenging current guidelines. *Int. J. Eat. Disord.* **2015**, *48*, 866–873. [CrossRef] [PubMed]
14. Smith, K.; Lesser, J.; Brandenburg, B.; Lesser, A.; Cici, J.; Juenneman, R.; Beadle, A.; Eckhardt, S.; Lantz, E.; Lock, J.; et al. Outcomes of an inpatient refeeding protocol in youth with Anorexia Nervosa and atypical Anorexia Nervosa at Children's Hospitals and Clinics of Minnesota. *J. Eat. Disord.* **2016**, *4*, 35. [CrossRef]
15. Pettersson, C.; Tubic, B.; Svedlund, A.; Magnusson, P.; Ellegard, L.; Swolin-Eide, D.; Forslund, H.B. Description of an intensive nutrition therapy in hospitalized adolescents with anorexia nervosa. *Eat. Behav.* **2016**, *21*, 172–178. [CrossRef]
16. Garber, A.K.; Sawyer, S.M.; Golden, N.H.; Guarda, A.S.; Katzman, D.K.; Kohn, M.R.; Le Grange, D.; Madden, S.; Whitelaw, M.; Redgrave, G.W. A systematic review of approaches to refeeding in patients with anorexia nervosa. *Int. J. Eat. Disord.* **2016**, *49*, 293–310. [CrossRef]
17. Matthews, K.; Hill, J.; Jeffrey, S.; Patterson, S.; Davis, A.; Ward, W.; Palmer, M.; Capra, S. A Higher-Calorie Refeeding Protocol Does Not Increase Adverse Outcomes in Adult Patients with Eating Disorders. *J. Acad. Nutr. Diet.* **2018**, *118*, 1450–1463. [CrossRef]
18. da Silva, J.S.V.; Seres, D.S.; Sabino, K.; Adams, S.C.; Berdahl, G.J.; Citty, S.W.; Cober, M.P.; Evans, D.C.; Greaves, J.R.; Gura, K.M.; et al. ASPEN Consensus Recommendations for Refeeding Syndrome. *Nutr. Clin. Pr.* **2020**, *35*, 178–195. [CrossRef]
19. Madden, S.; Miskovic-Wheatley, J.; Clarke, S.; Touyz, S.; Hay, P.; Kohn, M.R. Outcomes of a rapid refeeding protocol in Adolescent Anorexia Nervosa. *J. Eat. Disord.* **2015**, *3*, 8. [CrossRef]
20. Norris, M.L.; Pinhas, L.; Nadeau, P.O.; Katzman, D.K. Delirium and refeeding syndrome in anorexia nervosa. *Int. J. Eat. Disord.* **2012**, *45*, 439–442. [CrossRef]
21. Hofer, M.; Pozzi, A.; Joray, M.; Ott, R.; Hahni, F.; Leuenberger, M.; von Kanel, R.; Stanga, Z. Safe refeeding management of anorexia nervosa inpatients: An evidence-based protocol. *Nutrition* **2014**, *30*, 524–530. [CrossRef] [PubMed]
22. Hay, P.; Chinn, D.; Forbes, D.; Madden, S.; Newton, R.; Sugenor, L.; Touyz, S.; Ward, W.; Royal, A.; Royal Australian and New Zealand College of Psychiatrists. Royal Australian and New Zealand College of Psychiatrists clinical practice guidelines for the treatment of eating disorders. *Aust. N Z J Psychiatry* **2014**, *48*, 977–1008. [CrossRef] [PubMed]
23. Stanga, Z.; Brunner, A.; Leuenberger, M.; Grimble, R.F.; Shenkin, A.; Allison, S.P.; Lobo, D.N. Nutrition in clinical practice-the refeeding syndrome: Illustrative cases and guidelines for prevention and treatment. *Eur. J. Clin. Nutr.* **2008**, *62*, 687–694. [CrossRef] [PubMed]
24. Guidelines for the Nutritional Management of Anorexia Nervosa. Available online: https://cdn.ymaws.com/www.feast-ed.org/resource/resmgr/Docs/Meal_Plans/Guidelines_nutritional_AN_cr.pdf (accessed on 29 July 2019).
25. Robinson, P.; Jones, W.R. Management of really sick patients with anorexia nervosa. *Bjpsych Adv.* **2018**, *24*, 20–32. [CrossRef]

26. Practice Guideline for the Treatment of Patients with Eating Disorders Third edition. Available online: https://psychiatryonline.org/pb/assets/raw/sitewide/practice_guidelines/guidelines/eatingdisorders.pdf (accessed on 24 April 2020).
27. Junior MARSIPAN: Management of Really Sick Patients under 18 with Aanorexia Nervosa. Available online: https://www.rcpsych.ac.uk/docs/default-source/improving-care/better-mh-policy/college-reports/college-report-cr168.pdf (accessed on 31 July 2019).

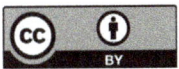

© 2020 by the authors. Licensee MDPI, Basel, Switzerland. This article is an open access article distributed under the terms and conditions of the Creative Commons Attribution (CC BY) license (http://creativecommons.org/licenses/by/4.0/).

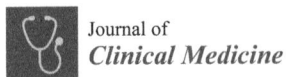

Article

Does ADHD Symptomatology Influence Treatment Outcome and Dropout Risk in Eating Disorders? A Longitudinal Study

Giulia Testa [1,2,†], Isabel Baenas [1,2,†], Cristina Vintró-Alcaraz [1,2], Roser Granero [1,3], Zaida Agüera [1,2,4], Isabel Sánchez [1,2], Nadine Riesco [1,2], Susana Jiménez-Murcia [1,2,5] and Fernando Fernández-Aranda [1,2,5,*]

[1] Ciber Physiopathology, Obesity and Nutrition (CIBERObn), Instituto de Salud Carlos III, 08907 Barcelona, Spain; gtesta@idibell.cat (G.T.); ibaenas@bellvitgehospital.cat (I.B.); cvintro@bellvitgehospital.cat (C.V.-A.); Roser.Granero@uab.cat (R.G.); zaguera@bellvitgehospital.cat (Z.A.); isasanchez@bellvitgehospital.cat (I.S.); nriesco@bellvitgehospital.cat (N.R.); sjimenez@bellvitgehospital.cat (S.J.-M.)
[2] Department of Psychiatry, Bellvitge University Hospital-IDIBELL, 08907 Barcelona, Spain
[3] Department of Psychobiology and Methodology of Health Sciences, Universitat Autònoma de Barcelona, 08193 Barcelona, Spain
[4] Department of Public Health, Mental Health and Maternal-Child Nursing, School of Nursing, University of Barcelona, 08907 Barcelona, Spain
[5] Department of Clinical Sciences, School of Medicine, University of Barcelona, 08907 Barcelona, Spain
* Correspondence: ffernandez@bellvitgehospital.cat
† Share first authorship.

Received: 4 June 2020; Accepted: 15 July 2020; Published: 20 July 2020

Abstract: Attention-deficit/hyperactivity disorder (ADHD) and its symptoms have been shown to be present in patients with eating disorders (EDs) and are associated with increased psychopathology and more dysfunctional personality traits. This study aimed to assess if the presence of ADHD symptoms in patients with EDs affects their short and long-term therapy outcome. A total of 136 consecutively treated ED patients were considered in this study. Baseline pre-treatment evaluation included the Adult ADHD Self-Report Scale (ASRS v1.1) for ADHD symptoms and the assessment of eating symptomatology using the Eating Disorders Inventory (EDI-2). Treatment outcome was evaluated in terms of ED symptoms after cognitive behavioral therapy (CBT) and dropout rate during treatment. Furthermore, we evaluated ED symptoms in treatment completers after a follow-up of 8 years on average. Path analyses assessed the potential mediational role of the EDI-2 total score in the relationship between ADHD and treatment outcome. Results showed that baseline symptoms of ADHD indirectly affected treatment outcome after CBT; the ASRS positive screening was related to higher eating symptomatology (standardized coefficient B = 0.41, $p = 0.001$, 95% CI: 0.26 to 0.55), and the presence of high ED levels contributed to the increase of dropout (B = 0.15, $p = 0.041$, 95% CI: 0.03 to 0.33) and a worse treatment outcome (B = 0.18, $p = 0.041$, 95% CI: 0.01 to 0.35). No direct effect was found between the ASRS positive screening with the risk of dropout (B = −0.08, $p = 0.375$) and worse treatment outcome (B = −0.07, $p = 0.414$). These results suggest the relevance of identifying specific treatment approaches for patients with ADHD symptoms and severe eating symptomatology.

Keywords: attention-deficit/hyperactivity disorder; ADHD; eating disorders; longitudinal; treatment outcome; dropout

1. Introduction

Attention-deficit/hyperactivity disorder (ADHD), which is characterized by symptoms of impulsivity, hyperactivity and inattention, has been described in relation to several psychiatric disorders including eating disorders (EDs) [1–4]. Accordingly, a higher prevalence of ADHD symptoms in EDs has been reported in many studies, in comparison with the general population [4–10]. Likewise, ADHD has been related with increased risk of disordered eating in childhood and adulthood [11–14], obesity [15] and behavioral addictions [16,17].

From a neurobiological perspective, a recent study examined the genetic factors common to both disorders and observed a stronger genetic association between ADHD and binge-eating behaviors [18]. From a clinical view, ADHD symptoms in ED were associated with higher ED symptomatology [19], specifically binge ED subtypes, with greater psychopathology [19–21], and increased levels of motor and cognitive impulsivity [22,23], as well as impulsive personality traits [24,25].

Despite the evidence linking ADHD and EDs, there is a lack of studies investigating whether ADHD symptoms may impact treatment response in patients with EDs, both in terms of treatment adherence (i.e., dropout rate) and outcome. To the best of our knowledge, there is only one previous study in female patients with EDs reporting higher ADHD symptoms at baseline as a predictor of non-recovery from eating-related symptomatology one year after treatment, especially for patients with loss of control overeating, bingeing and purging [26]. However, a high dropout rate (61%) was shown in that study, highlighting the need for future studies examining the impact of ADHD symptoms over dropout rate in EDs treatment.

The first aim of the present study was to evaluate if the initial presence of ADHD symptomatology impacts the therapy outcome after a cognitive behavioral therapy (CBT) treatment for EDs and dropout rate during treatment. The second aim was to analyze whether the baseline ADHD symptomatology had an impact on long-term therapy outcome (after eight years on average). Furthermore, we assessed the influence of EDs severity over the relationship between ADHD symptoms and treatment results.

2. Materials and Methods

2.1. Participants

The initial sample was comprised of 191 adult women diagnosed with an ED and presented for treatment to the Eating Disorder Unit within the Department of Psychiatry at Bellvitge University Hospital (HUB) (Barcelona, Spain) from 16 April 2009 to 31 January 2011. The baseline data of the initial sample was previously reported by Fernández-Aranda et al. (2013). Patients were diagnosed according to the DSM-IV-TR criteria [27], and diagnoses were reanalyzed and recodified post hoc using the DSM-5 criteria [28]. In the present study, we analyzed this sample of patients following a CBT treatment and after a longer follow-up (mean = 8.81 years; SD = 1.5). To that end, clinical records and an online shared medical network were analyzed retrospectively throughout the region of Catalonia (Spain). Thirty-three patients who did not start treatment were excluded from the original sample ($n = 191$); however, neither online nor paper clinical records were available for 22 out of 158 patients who started treatment. Thus, a final sample of 136 patients was included in the principal analysis. There were no baseline differences between patients who were included in this study and those who were not. Sixty-four participants included in the final sample did not complete treatment sessions (dropout) whereas 72 patients out of 136 completed the treatment (see flowchart; Figure 1).

2.2. Assessment

Adult ADHD Self-Report Scale (ASRS-v1.1) [29]: The ASRS-v1.1 is a self-administered scale designed to screen ADHD in the adult population (aged 18 years and older). It comprises 6 items that are consistent with the DSM-IV-TR [27] criteria and address the manifestation of ADHD in adults; the first 4 questions examine the inattention component of ADHD, and the final 2, the hyperactivity component. Each item is assessed using a 5-point Likert scale (0–4). The total score ranges between 0 and 24, with the cut-off being set at 12. The Spanish validation reported good psychometric properties [30]. Internal consistency in the sample analyzed in this work was good (Cronbach's alpha $\alpha = 0.77$).

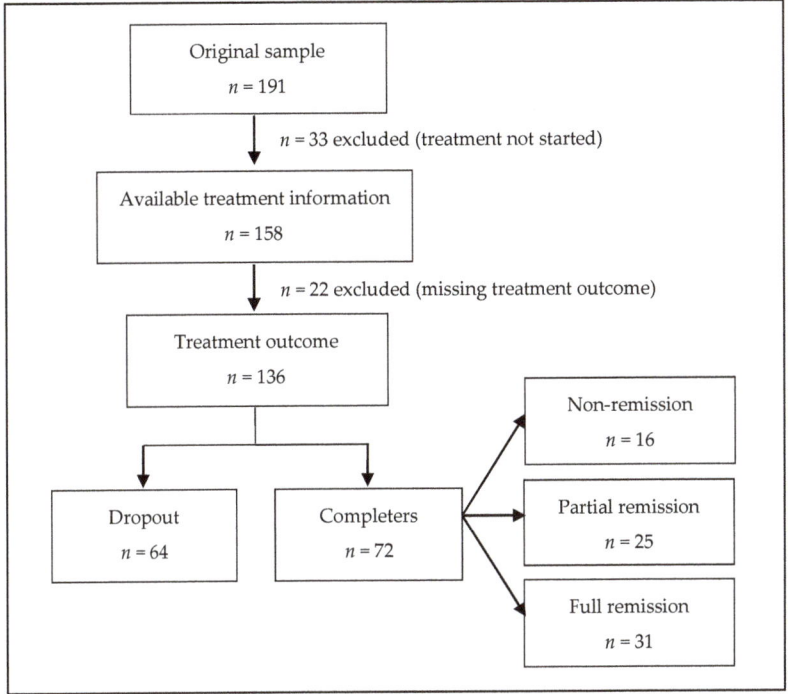

Figure 1. Flow chart for the sampling procedure.

Eating Disorders Inventory-2 (EDI-2) [31]: This self-report questionnaire consists of 91 items, answered on a 6-point Likert scale, that assess different cognitive and behavioral characteristics related to ED. The EDI-2 provides standardized subscale scores as well as a global measure of ED severity, which can be obtained based on the sum of all the items. A Spanish version of this questionnaire [32] has been validated and it obtained excellent psychometrical properties as an external global measure of ED severity. Internal consistency for the total score in this study was good (Cronbach's alpha $\alpha = 0.85$).

2.3. Treatment

As described elsewhere [33,34], all patients received cognitive behavioral therapy (CBT) at HUB, which was carried out by clinical psychology experts in the field. The CBT group therapy intervention for bulimia nervosa (BN), binge eating disorder (BED) and other specified feeding or eating disorders (OSFED) consisted of 16 weekly outpatient sessions lasting 90 minutes each and a follow-up period of about two years' duration that was carried out in a group format. Patients with BN first received six sessions of psychoeducational brief group therapy to offer information and psychoeducation about the negative consequences of BN. Patients diagnosed with anorexia nervosa (AN) completed a day hospital treatment program, which included two daily group CBT sessions during an average of 3 months. If they were severely underweight (IMC < 15 kg/m^2), they were offered an in-patient treatment with a maximum duration of three months. Patients with AN also had a two-year follow-up period with individual/group sessions. The goals of the treatment were to train patients to implement CBT strategies to reduce eating symptoms and to enable patients to acquire good healthy habits.

Patients were re-evaluated at discharge and categorized into the following three categories: full remission, partial remission and non-remission. According to DSM-5 criteria [28], the definition of full remission is a total absence of symptoms meeting diagnostic criteria for at least 4 consecutive weeks; partial remission is defined as a substantial symptomatic improvement but with residual symptoms; and patients who present poor outcomes are defined as non-remission. These categories were previously used to assess treatment outcome in threshold ED in other published studies [33,34]. Voluntary treatment discontinuation was categorized as dropout (i.e., not attending treatment for at least three consecutive sessions).

2.4. Follow-Up

A longitudinal follow-up of the patients was collected during an average period of 8.8 years (SD = 1.5), from the end of the first contact made in our unit to April 2020. This first contact coincided with the assessment using the ASRS screening questionnaire. By searching through centralized Catalonian clinical records and an online shared medical network, we assessed clinical evolution of all ED patients over the time, in terms of symptomatological remission (categorized as positive follow-up) or clinical non-remission of eating symptomatology (categorized as negative follow-up). From the total sample, clinical records were available for 123 patients, while 13 patients were missing (10.5% attrition rate).

2.5. Ethics

The present study was carried out in accordance with the latest version of the Declaration of Helsinki. The Bellvitge University Hospital Clinical Research Ethics Committee approved the study and signed informed consent was previously obtained from all participants.

2.6. Statistical Analyses

Stata16 for Windows was used to carry out statistical analyses [35]. A comparison between the groups defined by the risk of dropout during the CBT (yes/no) and the classification of the therapy outcome (full/partial remission versus dropout/non-remission) was done with a chi-square test (χ^2).

Survival function (Kaplan–Meier product-limit estimator) modeled the rate of dropout during the therapy. This procedure is usually used to describe the probability of the patients "living/surviving" for a certain amount of time after one concrete intervention [36]. In this study, "surviving" was defined for patients without dropout after the beginning of the CBT.

Path analyses assessed the potential mediational role of the ED severity level (EDI-2 total score) in the relationship between ADHD and treatment outcome (i.e., therapy outcome after a CBT treatment and dropout rate during treatment). This procedure was defined in this work as a case of structural equation modeling (SEM), with the maximum-likelihood estimation method of parameter estimation, adjusting by the covariates participants' age and the duration of the ED. The goodness-of-fit was evaluated using a standard statistical test, and it was considered adequate fitting for [37]: non-significant result ($p > 0.05$) in the χ^2 test, root mean square error of approximation (RMSEA) < 0.08, Bentler's comparative fit index (CFI) > 0.90, Tucker–Lewis Index (TLI) > 0.90 and standardized root mean square residual (SRMR) < 0.10. In this study, the relatively low sample size and the high correlations between the EDI-2 scores did not allow the SEM to be included in all the EDI-2 subscales registered for the participants (goodness-of-fit was not achieved).

3. Results

3.1. Characteristics of the Sample

No statistical differences between participants selected for the study and those excluded were found for marital status ($\chi^2 = 0.07$, $p = 0.982$), education level ($\chi^2 = 1.03$, $p = 0.317$), socioeconomic status ($\chi^2 = 2.67$, $p = 0.446$), age ($T = 1.04$, $p = 0.300$), duration of the eating problems ($T = 0.62$, $p = 0.535$), onset of the ED ($T = 0.70$, $p = 0.487$), ED-symptom levels ($T = 0.52$, $p = 0.603$) and ADHD-symptom levels ($T = 0.74$, $p = 0.462$).

Table 1 shows the descriptive for the sociodemographic and clinical variables of the final sample included in the study. All participants were women, with a mean age of 28.7 years (SD = 9.6), most were single (66.9%) and had achieved a secondary education level (61.0%). The number of patients within the ASRS positive screening group was $n = 46$ (point prevalence estimate equal to 33.8%). Regarding CBT outcomes, the dropout rate in the total sample was 47.0%, non-remission was registered for 11.8%, partial remission for 18.4% and full remission for 22.8%. Within the completers subsample ($n = 72$), non-remission was registered for 22.2% of the participants, partial remission for 34.7% and full remission for 43.1%.

Table 1. Descriptive for the sample ($n = 136$).

Sociodemographic		n	%	Therapy Outcomes	n	%
Marital	Single	91	66.9%	Total sample ($n = 136$)		
	Married/Partner	34	25.0%	Dropout	64	47.0%
	Divorced/Separated	11	8.1%	Non-remission	16	11.8%
Education	Primary	32	23.5%	Partial remission	25	18.4%
	Secondary	83	61.0%	Full remission	31	22.8%
	University	21	15.5%	Completers subsample ($n = 72$)		
Age and ED severity level		Mean	SD	Non-remission	16	22.2%
Chronological age (years)		28.74	9.59	Partial remission	25	34.7%
EDI-2 total score		97.91	44.52	Full remission	31	43.1%
ADHD (ASRS screening)		n	%			
Positive screening		46	33.8%			
Negative screening		90	66.2%			

Note. SD: standard deviation.

Table 2 includes the correlation matrix (Pearson correlation coefficients, R) between the ADHD level (measured through the ASRS scales) with the ED symptom level (EDI-2 scales). Due the strong relationship between the significance test for the correlation model and the sample size (high coefficients estimated in low samples sizes tend to show non-significance, while low coefficients tend to show significance obtained in samples with a large number of participants), Table 2 shows in bold the coefficients with an effect size that is in the moderate-mild ($|R| > 0.24$) to high-large range ($|R| > 0.37$). While moderate to high correlations were found between most EDI-2 scales, low correlation was found between ASRS inattention with hyperactive scores ($R = 0.166$). ASRS inattention positively correlated with all the EDI-2 scales, except for maturity fears, perfectionism and impulse regulation. ASRS hyperactivity also positively correlated with drive for thinness, body dissatisfaction, interoceptive awareness, impulse regulation and total. ASRS total correlated with all the EDI-2 scales (except for perfectionism), achieving the highest R-coefficient with the EDI-2 total ($R = 0.497$).

Table 2. Correlation matrix for the Adult ADHD Self-Report Scale (ASRS) and Eating Disorders Inventory (EDI-2) scores ($n = 136$).

		2	3	4	5	6	7	8	9	10	11	12	13	14	15
1.	ASRS: inattention	0.166	0.882 †	0.252 †	0.356 †	0.384 †	0.287 †	0.287 †	0.425 †	0.183	0.033	0.220	0.312 †	0.419 †	0.420 †
2.	ASRS: hyperactive	—	0.609 †	0.372 †	0.282 †	0.341 †	0.226	0.086	0.207	0.214	0.116	0.336 †	0.210	0.149	0.342 †
3.	ASRS: total		—	0.379 †	0.419 †	0.474 †	0.337 †	0.267	0.438 †	0.246 †	0.078	0.337 †	0.346 †	0.402 †	0.497 †
4.	EDI-2: Drive.thinness			—	0.622 †	0.582 †	0.367 †	0.341	0.483 †	0.297 †	0.339 †	0.364 †	0.628 †	0.440 †	0.720 †
5.	EDI-2: Body.dissatisf.				—	0.503 †	0.483 †	0.383	0.596 †	0.283 †	0.211	0.429 †	0.506 †	0.457 †	0.751 †
6.	EDI-2: Interoc.awar.					—	0.508 †	0.500	0.700 †	0.371 †	0.305 †	0.604 †	0.666 †	0.637 †	0.838 †
7.	EDI-2: Bulimia						—	0.238	0.430 †	0.032	0.056	0.385 †	0.486 †	0.262 †	0.562 †
8.	EDI-2: Interp.distrust							—	0.561 †	0.306 †	0.168	0.347 †	0.385 †	0.697 †	0.626 †
9.	EDI-2: Ineffectiveness								—	0.503 †	0.296 †	0.568 †	0.650 †	0.749 †	0.865 †
10.	EDI-2: Maturity fears									—	0.277 †	0.366 †	0.279 †	0.496 †	0.549 †
11.	EDI-2: Perfectionism										—	0.331 †	0.314 †	0.299 †	0.438 †
12.	EDI-2: Impulse.regul.											—	0.541 †	0.576 †	0.717 †
13.	EDI-2: Ascetic												—	0.503 †	0.768 †
14.	EDI-2: Social.insec.													—	0.790 †
15.	EDI-2: Total score														—

Note. † Correlation with effect size in the moderate-mild ($|R| > 0.24$) to high-large range ($|R| > 0.37$).

The ADHD level was not directly related to the short-term therapy outcomes in the study; the prevalence of the ASRS positive screening score was statistically equal for completers and dropouts, as well as for participants with partial remission and full remission versus those with dropout and non-remission (Table 3). No association was found even when stratified by the diagnostic subtype (Supplementary Table S1). Regarding data registered after the follow-up, neither was there any statistical association found between the ASRS positive screening with therapy outcome.

Table 3. Description of ADHD measures within the groups defined by the short term therapy outcomes ($n = 136$) and the follow-up ($n = 123$).

Treatment Outcome	Completers ($n = 72$)		Dropout ($n = 64$)		p
ADHD screening (+); n-%	25	34.7%	21	32.8%	0.814
Short-term therapy outcome	Full/partial remission ($n = 56$)		Dropout/non-remission ($n = 80$)		p
ADHD screening (+); n-%	21	37.5%	25	31.3%	0.448
Outcome at follow-up	Remission ($n = 87$)		Non-remission ($n = 36$)		p
ADHD screening (+); n-%	29	33.3%	12	33.3%	1.00

Figure 2 includes the cumulate survival function for the time to dropout. The higher proportion of dropouts was registered during the two weeks after the beginning of the treatment (12.1% for the total sample), followed by the next two weeks (at the end of the first month 24.1% had followed). No statistical contribution was found between ASRS score with the rate to dropout (log rank test = 0.01, $p = 0.995$).

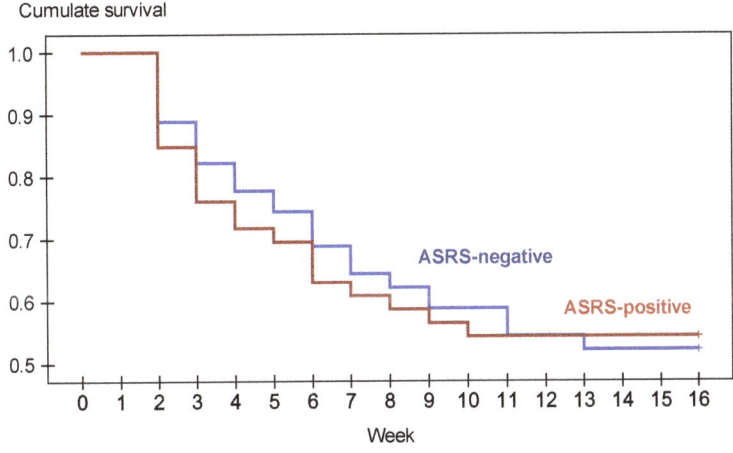

Figure 2. Survival function for dropout ($n = 136$).

Supplementary Table S2 includes the associations between the ADHD levels (registered in the ASRS inattention, hyperactivity and total score) and the ED symptom levels (registered in the EDI-2 scores) with the treatment outcomes (during therapy, at short-term and in the follow-up). No statistical differences were found comparing the mean scores in the ASRS and the EDI-2 between the groups of the study.

3.2. Path Analysis

Figure 3 shows the results of the SEM assessing the mediational link of the ED severity into the relationship between ADHD and the CBT outcomes. Goodness of fit was achieved for both models (risk of dropout: $\chi^2 = 0.807$ ($p = 0.848$), RMSEA = 0.001, CFI = 0.999, TLI = 0.998, SRMR = 0.015;

better CBT outcome: $\chi^2 = 0.029$ ($p = 0.864$), RMSEA = 0.001, CFI = 0.999, TLI = 0.998, SRMR = 0.004). These results confirmed the indirect effect of ADHD on the therapy outcome; being in the ASRS positive screening group is related to higher ED severity (higher EDI-2 total), and this worse ED level contributed to the increase in the risk of dropout and a worse treatment outcome.

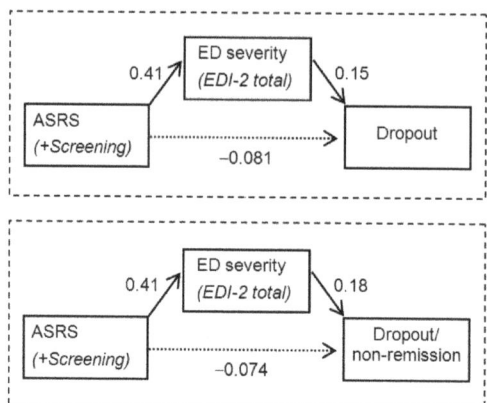

Figure 3. Path-diagrams: standardized coefficients in the SEM for the short-term therapy outcome ($n = 136$). Continuous line: significant coefficient. Dash line: non-significant coefficient. Results adjusted by age and duration of the ED.

Figure 4 shows the results of the SEM adding the patients' state at the end of the follow-up (adequate fitting was achieved: $\chi^2 = 0.519$ ($p = 0.771$), RMSEA = 0.001, CFI = 0.999, TLI = 0.998, SRMR = 0.016). This new model indicates that the ADHD screening score was not related (through a direct or indirect link) to the clinical condition measured in the follow-up.

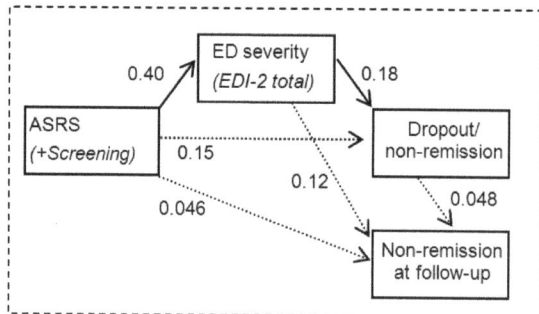

Figure 4. Path-diagrams: standardized coefficients in the SEM for the follow-up ($n = 123$). Continuous line: significant coefficient. Dash line: non-significant coefficient. Results adjusted by age and duration of the ED.

4. Discussion

This study investigated whether the presence of ADHD symptoms in patients with EDs may impact treatment outcome and dropout for EDs. The second aim was to examine the influence of EDs severity on the relationship between ADHD symptoms and treatment outcome/dropout rate. Finally, a long-term follow-up was included to assess the effect of ADHD symptoms at baseline on the clinical evolution of EDs.

ADHD screening at baseline did not directly predict treatment outcome or dropout rate in patients attending a CBT for EDs. However, our results highlighted that the severity of eating symptomatology mediates the relation between ADHD and treatment outcome/dropout rate. Specifically, positive screening for ADHD symptoms was directly associated with the severity of EDI-2, which in turn is related to a higher dropout rate and a worse treatment outcome, in terms of dropout during treatment and non-remission of ED symptomatology.

The only previous study investigating the effect of ADHD over treatment for ED suggested that patients with higher ADHD symptoms presented a higher risk of poor post-treatment outcome, although the impact of ED severity on this relation was not assessed [26]. Interestingly, a high dropout from treatment was also reported in that study (61%), further suggesting the importance of taking into account dropout as a negative outcome of ED treatment. Considering that patients with ADHD tend to act impulsively, they may be more likely to abandon treatment, although limited information has been reported linking the effect of ADHD symptomatology in the treatment of comorbid psychopathology, in terms of dropout. These studies were mostly focused on substance use disorder (SUD), such as tobacco [38] or cocaine [39–41]. When SUD and ADHD are co-morbid, some factors seem to increase the risk of dropout, including: disruptive behaviors related to ADHD [40], cognitive deficit (e.g., executive dysfunctions) and the type of substance of abuse [41]. Concerning EDs, this is the first study suggesting that higher severity of EDs and co-occurring ADHD symptoms increase the risk of dropout.

In spite of the higher proportion of dropouts registered within the first two weeks of treatment, the ASRS score does not differ between early or later dropout, suggesting that ADHD symptoms may increase the dropout rate at different stages of treatment. Furthermore, we included a longer follow-up of the majority of the patients, showing that positive screening for ADHD symptoms at baseline did not affect the longer terms evolution of EDs. This is the first retrospective study which allows the evaluation of the impact of ADHD symptoms on EDs with a longitudinal follow-up of roughly 8 years.

This study must be interpreted in light of its limitations. First, a self-reporting instrument was used to measure the frequency of adult ADHD symptoms, which may lead to an overestimation of this symptomatology. Therefore, future studies should focus on EDs patients with comorbidity with ADHD, not only taking into account ADHD symptomatology. Furthermore, comorbidity with others psychiatric disorders often associated with EDs (e.g., anxiety, depression) should be addressed by future studies in larger samples. Second, only female EDs patients were included in this study, so further studies would benefit from including male population as men report a higher prevalence of ADHD in adult life [42]. Third, it would have been advisable to have objective measures available after the follow-up. Finally, the retrospective nature of the design should be considered.

In conclusion, the present findings suggest a higher risk for dropout of treatment (i.e., CBT for EDs) and worse treatment outcomes in patients with more severe ED-symptoms, and an indirect effect of ADHD symptomatology on the treatment outcomes mediated by the ED severity levels. This was the first study to examine the effect of ADHD over the risk of dropout in patients treated for EDs, suggesting the relevance of identifying specific treatment approaches for patients with greater degrees of ADHD symptoms and severe EDs.

Supplementary Materials: The following are available online at http://www.mdpi.com/2077-0383/9/7/2305/s1, Table S1: Description of ADHD measures within the groups defined by the short-term therapy outcome ($n = 136$), Table S2: Description of ADHD measures within the groups defined by the short term therapy outcomes ($n = 136$) and the follow-up ($n = 123$).

Author Contributions: G.T., I.B. and C.V.-A. contributed to the conceptualization and writing of the present study; S.J.-M. and F.F.-A. supervised the study; R.G. performed the formal analysis; Z.A., I.B., I.S. and N.R. aided with data collection and also with the interpretation of data; G.T. and I.B. shared first authorship. All authors have read and agreed to the published version of the manuscript.

Funding: This work was partially supported by Instituto de Salud Carlos III (PI17/01167) and Generalitat de Catalunya (PERIS/SLT006/17/00246). CIBERObn and CIBERSAM are both initiatives of ISCIII Spain. C.V.-A. was supported by a FPU grant (FPU16/01453) from Ministerio de Educación, Cultura y Deporte (Spain). I.B. was partially supported by a Post-Residency Grant from the Research Committee of the University Hospital of Bellvitge

(HUB; Barcelona, Spain) 2019–2020. The funders had no role in the study design, data collection and analysis, decision to publish or preparation of the manuscript.

Acknowledgments: We thank the CERCA Programme/Generalitat de Catalunya for institutional support.

Conflicts of Interest: The authors declare no conflict of interest.

References

1. Bleck, J.; DeBate, R.D. Exploring the co-morbidity of attention-deficit/hyperactivity disorder with eating disorders and disordered eating behaviors in a nationally representative community-based sample. *Eat. Behav.* **2013**, *14*, 390–393. [CrossRef] [PubMed]
2. Mikami, A.Y.; Hinshaw, S.P.; Patterson, K.A.; Lee, J.C. Eating Pathology Among Adolescent Girls With Attention-Deficit/Hyperactivity Disorder. *J. Abnorm. Psychol.* **2008**, *117*, 225–235. [CrossRef]
3. Mikami, A.Y.; Hinshaw, S.P.; Arnold, L.E.; Hoza, B.; Hechtman, L.; Newcorn, J.H.; Abikoff, H.B. Bulimia nervosa symptoms in the multimodal treatment study of children with ADHD. *Int. J. Eat. Disord.* **2010**, *43*, 248–259. [CrossRef]
4. Nazar, B.P.; Pinna, C.M.D.S.; Coutinho, G.; Segenreich, D.; Duchesne, M.; Appolinario, J.C.; Mattos, P. Review of literature of attention-deficit/hyperactivity disorder with comorbid eating disorders. *Rev. Bras. Psiquiatr.* **2008**, *30*, 384–389. [CrossRef]
5. Blinder, B.J.; Cumella, E.J.; Sanathara, V.A. Psychiatric comorbidities of female inpatients with eating disorders. *Psychosom. Med.* **2006**, *68*, 454–462. [CrossRef]
6. Farber, S.K. The Comorbidity of Eating Disorders and Attention-Deficit Hyperactivity Disorder. *Eat. Disord.* **2009**, *18*, 81–89. [CrossRef] [PubMed]
7. Stulz, N.; Hepp, U.; Gächter, C.; Martin-Soelch, C.; Spindler, A.; Milos, G. The severity of ADHD and eating disorder symptoms: A correlational study. *BMC Psychiatry* **2013**, *13*, 44. [CrossRef] [PubMed]
8. Svedlund, N.E.; Norring, C.; Ginsberg, Y.; von Hausswolff-Juhlin, Y. Symptoms of Attention Deficit Hyperactivity Disorder (ADHD) among adult eating disorder patients. *BMC Psychiatry* **2017**, *17*, 19. [CrossRef]
9. Wentz, E.; Lacey, J.H.; Waller, G.; Råstam, M.; Turk, J.; Gillberg, C. Childhood onset neuropsychiatric disorders in adult eating disorder patients. *Eur. Child. Adolesc. Psychiatry* **2005**, *14*, 431–437. [CrossRef]
10. Yates, W.R.; Lund, B.C.; Johnson, C.; Mitchell, J.; McKee, P. Attention-deficit hyperactivity symptoms and disorder in eating disorder inpatients. *Int. J. Eat. Disord.* **2009**, *42*, 375–378. [CrossRef]
11. Reinblatt, S.P.; Leoutsakos, J.-M.S.; Mahone, E.M.; Forrester, S.; Wilcox, H.C.; Riddle, M.A. Association between binge eating and attention-deficit/hyperactivity disorder in two pediatric community mental health clinics. *Int. J. Eat. Disord.* **2015**, *48*, 505–511. [CrossRef] [PubMed]
12. Levin, R.L.; Rawana, J.S. Attention-deficit/hyperactivity disorder and eating disorders across the lifespan: A systematic review of the literature. *Clin. Psychol. Rev.* **2016**, *50*, 22–36. [CrossRef] [PubMed]
13. Sonneville, K.R.; Calzo, J.P.; Horton, N.J.; Field, A.E.; Crosby, R.D.; Solmi, F.; Micali, N. Childhood hyperactivity/inattention and eating disturbances predict binge eating in adolescence. *Psychol. Med.* **2015**, *45*, 2511–2520. [CrossRef] [PubMed]
14. Nazar, B.P.; de Sousa Pinna, C.M.; Suwwan, R.; Duchesne, M.; Freitas, S.R.; Sergeant, J.; Mattos, P. ADHD Rate in Obese Women With Binge Eating and Bulimic Behaviors From a Weight-Loss Clinic. *J. Atten. Disord.* **2016**, *20*, 610–616. [CrossRef]
15. Sepúlveda, A.R.; Solano, S.; Blanco, M.; Lacruz, T.; Veiga, O. Feasibility, acceptability, and effectiveness of a multidisciplinary intervention in childhood obesity from primary care: Nutrition, physical activity, emotional regulation, and family. *Eur. Eat. Disord. Rev.* **2020**, *28*, 184–198. [CrossRef]
16. Mestre-Bach, G.; Steward, T.; Potenza, M.N.; Granero, R.; Fernández-Aranda, F.; Mena-Moreno, T.; Magaña, P.; Vintró-Alcaraz, C.; del Pino-Gutiérrez, A.; Menchón, J.M.; et al. The Role of ADHD Symptomatology and Emotion Dysregulation in Gambling Disorder. *J. Atten. Disord.* **2019**, 108705471989437. [CrossRef]
17. Aymamí, N.; Jiménez-Murcia, S.; Granero, R.; Ramos-Quiroga, J.A.; Fernández-Aranda, F.; Claes, L.; Sauvaget, A.; Grall-Bronnec, M.; Gómez-Peña, M.; Savvidou, L.G.; et al. Clinical, Psychopathological, and Personality Characteristics Associated with ADHD among Individuals Seeking Treatment for Gambling Disorder. *Res. Artic. Clin.* **2015**. [CrossRef]

18. Yao, S.; Kuja-Halkola, R.; Martin, J.; Lu, Y.; Lichtenstein, P.; Hübel, C.; Almqvist, C.; Magnusson, P.K.; Bulik, C.M.; Larsson, H.; et al. Associations Between Attention-Deficit/Hyperactivity Disorder and Various Eating Disorders: A Swedish Nationwide Population Study Using Multiple Genetically Informative Approaches. *Biol. Psychiatry* **2019**, *86*, 577–586. [CrossRef]
19. Fernández-Aranda, F.; Agüera, Z.; Castro, R.; Jiménez-Murcia, S.; Ramos-Quiroga, J.A.; Bosch, R.; Fagundo, A.B.; Granero, R.; Penelo, E.; Claes, L.; et al. ADHD symptomatology in eating disorders: A secondary psychopathological measure of severity? *BMC Psychiatry* **2013**, *13*, 166. [CrossRef]
20. Barkley, R.A.; Murphy, K.; Kwasnik, D. Psychological adjustment and adaptive impairments in young adults with ADHD. *J. Atten. Disord.* **1996**, *1*, 41–54. [CrossRef]
21. Schredl, M.; Alm, B.; Sobanski, E. Sleep quality in adult patients with attention deficit hyperactivity disorder (ADHD). *Eur. Arch. Psychiatry Clin. Neurosci.* **2007**, *257*, 164–168. [CrossRef]
22. Malloy-Diniz, L.; Fuentes, D.; Leite, W.B.; Correa, H.; Bechara, A. Impulsive behavior in adults with attention deficit/hyperactivity disorder: Characterization of attentional, motor and cognitive impulsiveness. *J. Int. Neuropsychol. Soc. JINS* **2007**. [CrossRef]
23. Scheres, A.; Lee, A.; Sumiya, M. Temporal reward discounting and ADHD: Task and symptom specific effects. *J. Neural. Transm.* **2008**, *115*, 221–226. [CrossRef] [PubMed]
24. Donfrancesco, R.; Di Trani, M.; Porfirio, M.C.; Giana, G.; Miano, S.; Andriola, E. Might the temperament be a bias in clinical study on attention-deficit hyperactivity disorder (ADHD)?: Novelty Seeking dimension as a core feature of ADHD. *Psychiatry Res.* **2015**, *227*, 333–338. [CrossRef] [PubMed]
25. Valko, L.; Doehnert, M.; Müller, U.C.; Schneider, G.; Albrecht, B.; Drechsler, R.; Maechler, M.; Steinhausen, H.C.; Brandeis, D. Differences in neurophysiological markers of inhibitory and temporal processing deficits in children and adults with ADHD. *J. Psychophysiol.* **2009**, *23*, 235–246. [CrossRef]
26. Svedlund, N.E.; Norring, C.; Ginsberg, Y.; von Hausswolff-Juhlin, Y. Are treatment results for eating disorders affected by ADHD symptoms? A one-year follow-up of adult females. *Eur. Eat. Disord. Rev.* **2018**, *26*, 337–345. [CrossRef]
27. American Psychiatric Association. *Diagnostic and Statistical Manual of Mental Disorders*, 4th ed.; American Psychiatric Association: Washington, DC, USA, 2000.
28. APA American Psychiatric Association. *Diagnostic and Statistical Manual of Mental Disorders*, 5th ed.; American Psychiatric Association: Washington, DC, USA, 2013.
29. Kessler, R.C.; Adler, L.; Ames, M.; Demler, O.; Faraone, S.; Hiripi, E.; Howes, M.J.; Jin, R.; Secnik, K.; Spencer, T.; et al. The World Health Organization adult ADHD self-report scale (ASRS): A short screening scale for use in the general population. *Psychol. Med.* **2005**, *35*, 245–256. [CrossRef] [PubMed]
30. Ramos-Quiroga, J.A.; Daigre, C.; Valero, S.; Bosch, R.; Gómez-Barros, N.; Nogueira, M.; Palomar, G.; Roncero, C.; Casas, M. Validation of the Spanish version of the attention deficit hyperactivity disorder adult screening scale (ASRS v. 1.1): A novel scoring strategy. *Rev. Neurol.* **2009**, *48*, 449–452. [CrossRef] [PubMed]
31. Garner, D.M. *Inventario de Trastornos de la Conducta Alimentaria (EDI-2)-Manual*; TEA: Madrid, Spain, 1998.
32. Corral, S.; González, M.; Pereña, J.; Seisdedos, N. *Adaptación española del Inventario de trastornos de la conducta alimentaria, Inventario de Trastornos de la Conducta Alimentaria*; TEA: Madrid, Spain, 1998.
33. Agüera, Z.; Sánchez, I.; Granero, R.; Riesco, N.; Steward, T.; Martín-Romera, V.; Jiménez-Murcia, S.; Romero, X.; Caroleo, M.; Segura-García, C.; et al. Short-Term Treatment Outcomes and Dropout Risk in Men and Women with Eating Disorders. *Eur. Eat. Disord. Rev.* **2017**, *25*, 293–301. [CrossRef] [PubMed]
34. Riesco, N.; Agüera, Z.; Granero, R.; Jiménez-Murcia, S.; Menchón, J.M.; Fernández-Aranda, F. Other Specified Feeding or Eating Disorders (OSFED): Clinical heterogeneity and cognitive-behavioral therapy outcome. *Eur. Psychiatry* **2018**, *54*, 109–116. [CrossRef]
35. *StataCorp Stata Statistical Software*, Release 16; StataCorp LLC: College Station, TX, USA, 2019.
36. Singer, J.D.; Willett, J.B.; Willett, J.B. *Applied Longitudinal Data Analysis: Modeling Change and Event Occurrence*; Oxford University Press: New York, NY, USA, 2003.
37. Barrett, P. Structural equation modelling: Adjudging model fit. *Pers. Individ. Dif.* **2007**, *42*, 815–824. [CrossRef]
38. Bidwell, L.C.; Karoly, H.C.; Hutchison, K.E.; Bryan, A.D. ADHD symptoms impact smoking outcomes and withdrawal in response to Varenicline treatment for smoking cessation. *Drug Alcohol Depend.* **2017**, *179*, 18–24. [CrossRef] [PubMed]

39. Carroll, K.M.; Rounsaville, B.J. History and significance of childhood attention deficit disorder in treatment-seeking cocaine abusers. *Compr. Psychiatry* **1993**, *34*, 75–82. [CrossRef]
40. Sullivan, M.A.; Rudnik-Levin, F. Attention Deficit/Hyperactivity Disorder and Substance Abuse. *Ann. N. Y. Acad. Sci.* **2006**, *931*, 251–270. [CrossRef]
41. Van Emmerik-van Oortmerssen, K.; Blankers, M.; Vedel, E.; Kramer, F.; Goudriaan, A.E.; van den Brink, W.; Schoevers, R.A. Prediction of drop-out and outcome in integrated cognitive behavioral therapy for ADHD and SUD: Results from a randomized clinical trial. *Addict. Behav.* **2020**, *103*, 106228. [CrossRef] [PubMed]
42. Faraone, S.V.; Biederman, J. What is the prevalence of adult ADHD? Results of a population screen of 966 adults. *J. Atten. Disord.* **2005**, *9*, 384–391. [CrossRef] [PubMed]

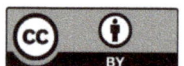

© 2020 by the authors. Licensee MDPI, Basel, Switzerland. This article is an open access article distributed under the terms and conditions of the Creative Commons Attribution (CC BY) license (http://creativecommons.org/licenses/by/4.0/).

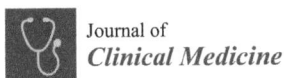

Article

Validity of Virtual Reality Body Exposure to Elicit Fear of Gaining Weight, Body Anxiety and Body-Related Attentional Bias in Patients with Anorexia Nervosa

Bruno Porras-Garcia [1], Marta Ferrer-Garcia [1], Eduardo Serrano-Troncoso [2], Marta Carulla-Roig [2], Pau Soto-Usera [2], Helena Miquel-Nabau [1], Nazilla Shojaeian [1], Isabel de la Montaña Santos-Carrasco [3], Bianca Borszewski [3], Marina Díaz-Marsá [3], Isabel Sánchez-Díaz [4], Fernando Fernández-Aranda [4] and José Gutiérrez-Maldonado [1,*]

[1] Department of Clinical Psychology and Psychobiology, University of Barcelona, Passeig de la Vall d'Hebron 171, 08035 Barcelona, Spain; brporras@ub.edu (B.P.-G.); martaferrerg@ub.edu (M.F.-G.); helena.mn29@gmail.com (H.M.-N.); nazila.shojaeian@gmail.com (N.S.)

[2] Department of Child and Adolescent Psychiatry and Psychology, Hospital Sant Joan de Déu of Barcelona; Passeig de Sant Joan de Déu, 2, 08950 Esplugues de Llobregat, Spain; eserrano@sjdhospitalbarcelona.org (E.S.-T.); mcarulla@sjdhospitalbarcelona.org (M.C.-R.); psoto@sjdhospitalbarcelona.org (P.S.-U.)

[3] Department of Psychiatry and Mental Health, Hospital Clínico San Carlos, Madrid, Calle del Prof Martín Lagos, s/n, 28040 Madrid, Spain; isabelmsc.is@gmail.com (I.d.l.M.S.-C.); biancbor@ucm.es (B.B.); marinadiaz.marsa@salud.madrid.org (M.D.-M.)

[4] Department of Psychiatry and Mental Health, Hospital Universitario de Bellvitge- IDIBELL and CIBEROBN, Barcelona; Carrer Feixa Llarga s/n, 08907 Hospitalet del Llobregat, Spain; isasanchez@bellvitgehospital.cat (I.S.-D.); ffernandez@bellvitgehospital.cat (F.F.-A.)

* Correspondence: jgutierrezm@ub.edu

Received: 28 August 2020; Accepted: 2 October 2020; Published: 5 October 2020

Abstract: Fear of gaining weight (FGW), body image disturbances, associated anxiety and body-related attentional bias are the core symptoms of anorexia nervosa (AN) and play critical roles in its development and maintenance. The aim of the current study is to evaluate the usefulness of virtual reality-based body exposure software for the assessment of important body-related cognitive and emotional responses in AN. Thirty female patients with AN, one of them subclinical, and 43 healthy college women, 25 with low body dissatisfaction (BD) and 18 with high BD, owned a virtual body that had their silhouette and body mass index. Full-body illusion (FBI) over the virtual body was induced using both visuo-motor and visuo-tactile stimulation. Once the FBI was induced, the FBI itself, FGW, body anxiety and body-related attentional bias toward weight-related and non-weight-related body areas were assessed. One-way analyses of covariance (ANCOVA), controlling for age, showed that AN patients reported higher FGW, body anxiety and body-related attentional bias than healthy controls. Unexpectedly, patients with AN reported significantly lower FBI levels than healthy participants. Finally, Pearson correlations showed significant relationships between visual analog scales and body-related attentional bias measures, compared to other eating disorder measures. These results provide evidence about the usefulness of virtual reality-based body exposure to elicit FGW and other body-related disturbances in AN patients. Thus, it may be a suitable intervention for reducing these emotional responses and for easing weight recovery.

Keywords: anorexia nervosa; virtual reality; fear of gaining weight; body anxiety; body image disturbances; body-related attentional bias

1. Introduction

Anorexia nervosa (AN) is considered one of the most serious eating disorders (ED), affecting women worldwide [1]. Although the age of onset of AN is established at around 14 to 19 years old [2,3], this condition has been progressively diagnosed in younger patients [4,5], making early preventive interventions in AN a public health priority.

According to the Diagnostic and Statistical Manual of Mental Disorders, 5th Edition [6], individuals with AN show severe restriction of food intake that leads to a significantly low body weight. In addition, they usually feel an intense fear of gaining weight (FGW) and disturbances in the way they experience their body weight and shape, also referred to as body image disturbances [7]. Greater FGW has also been related to more severe ED symptoms [8,9], and it is considered as one of the strongest predictors of ED symptomatology (e.g., dietary restraint and compulsive exercise) in AN patients [10]. In fact, it has been suggested that AN patients are more susceptible to learning fear associations than healthy individuals [11] (Strober, 2004); for instance, they are more likely to develop an intense FGW after starting a low-fat diet. Another psychopathological model has highlighted the importance of the anxiety symptomatology that AN patients usually experience as a direct reinforcement of their fears and behaviors [12]. The subjective feelings of tension, worried thoughts and physical changes that AN patients present are sometimes focused on their own body or toward specific body areas (i.e., weight-related body areas), a phenomenon known as body anxiety [13]. Previous studies have suggested that the core fears in AN (such as FGW) elicit high anxiety levels, which, in turn, lead to a progressive increase in ritualistic eating- and activity-related behaviors (e.g., the initiation of noncaloric diets or doing intense physical exercise). Over time, this allows the reinforcement of undereating and other dysfunctional behavioral disturbances [12].

Other theories have focused on the study of the mechanisms underlying the information processing biases typically found among individuals with EDs: biases in memory, interpretation and attention of body-related information, which, in turn, influence and maintain body image disturbances and ED symptomatology [14,15]. Among these cognitive biases, the dysfunctional role of attention has received increasing consideration over the last decades. Previous research suggests that ED patients pay more attention to disorder-relevant information (e.g., food- and body-related stimuli) than to other sorts of information [16,17]. Furthermore, dysfunctional body-related attention presumably maintains body image disturbances by processing only body information that is consistent with dysfunctional cognitive schema content (such as my thighs or stomach are getting fatter), while schema-inconsistent information tends to be visually neglected [16]. When considering patients with AN, body-related attentional bias seems to be especially pronounced in restrictive-type AN patients [18].

Therefore, these body-related constructs and underlying cognitive mechanisms may play a critical differential role in the development and maintenance of AN symptomatology. Consequently, the implementation of specific, tailored interventions targeting them is needed in AN.

Mirror exposure therapy aims to decrease body- and weight-related fears and is used to improve cognitive behavioral therapy (CBT) [19]. Several studies support the use of mirror exposure therapy to reduce body image disturbances in ED patients [20,21] and high body-dissatisfied individuals [22,23]. However, mirror exposure therapy frequently elicits a highly negative initial reaction in patients [24], which increases the probability of treatment rejection and the risk of dropout [25]. Furthermore, mirror exposure therapy is usually conducted in controlled settings (e.g., a laboratory or therapist's office), and the generalization of positive changes learned during exposure is impaired [26].

These limitations can be overcome by the application of virtual reality (VR) techniques. For instance, VR technology is proposed as a good complement to in vivo exposure, especially in the initial stages of the intervention, since it is perceived as safer by participants and reduces the rates of withdrawal [27]. In addition, although VR is also conducted in a controlled setting, it allows researchers to create real-size 3D simulations of participants' bodies with their physical characteristics and place them in immersive environments that reproduce real life situations related to their body image concerns (e.g., a dressing room, a beach or a bathroom), thus enhancing the generalization of positive results [26,28]. Another advantage of using VR is that it allows certain stimuli or environments to be manipulated in ways that may not be possible in mirror exposure therapy. For instance, it allows patients with AN to increase/decrease the weight (or the body mass index (BMI)) of the virtual avatar until it reaches a target weight, thus helping to confront their core fears (i.e., the fear of gaining weight).

VR technology has evolved notably over the last few years. For instance, the newest VR systems can achieve a full-body motion tracking that captures the individual's body silhouette and movements using a head-mounted display, VR controllers and a series of body trackers that can be attached to different body areas (e.g., the feet and the waist). These technological advances have allowed the development of countless applications for improving health-related problems in a new transdisciplinary research field known as embodied medicine or embodied technology (for an extensive review, see [29,30]). This paradigm allows individuals to perceive and feel a virtual body as their real body by activating predicting neurological brain circuits to elicit the feelings of ownership over a virtual avatar [29,30]. Specifically, the subjective experience in which individuals feel an artificial body to be their own is known as full-body illusion (FBI) [31]. To accomplish this, different types of information (visual, acoustic, proprioceptive and vestibular) must be combined into multisensory representations [32].

One of the most widely studied and best-known paradigms for eliciting feelings of ownership over a specific body area is the rubber hand illusion [33], in which the participant's nonvisible real hand is synchronously touched by the experimenter while the participants see the same touches delivered to a fake rubber hand. Following the rubber hand illusion paradigm, a previous study found that ED patients tend to experience a stronger illusion over a fake hand than healthy individuals [34]. Alternatively, a large number of studies have investigated the effects of the FBI on the whole body to assess body image disturbances, for a review, see [28], finding that the perception of body size and weight may be changed in nonclinical samples [35–38] and ED patients [39–41]. Specifically, among AN patients, Keizer et al. [39] found that owning a skinny virtual body significantly reduced the perceived body size in AN patients, as well as in healthy participants. These results were later replicated by two case report studies, which showed that VR embodiment-based techniques (e.g., using a visuo-tactile stimulation procedure) allowed the modification of body image disturbances either in the short term [40] or over several sessions [41].

Curiously, while most body exposure-based therapies, such as mirror exposure therapy, focus on treating body image disturbances, little information is available about the use of body exposure techniques, with or without VR, to treat FGW. Levinson, Rapp and Riley [42] proposed an imaginal exposure procedure that consisted of five sessions in which the patient had to visualize her own weight gain and the possible associated adverse consequences. The authors reported a clinically significant change in ED symptomatology from pretherapy to one-month follow-up and a steady increase in weight throughout the exposure sessions, which was maintained at follow-up. Imaginal exposure therapy directly targeting the FGW seems to be an interesting approach in AN treatments. However, its effectiveness must be explored in controlled clinical studies. Furthermore, imagery exposure may have some significant limitations—for example, difficulty in achieving or maintaining visualization and the risk of avoidance of the most feared stimulus during visualization. These limitations can be overcome by the application of VR techniques that do not rely on the patient's visualization ability and reduce the possibility of avoidance behaviors. Therefore, VR exposure therapy provides a useful approach to targeting FGW [41].

The aim of the current study was to assess the usefulness of a VR-based body exposure software to elicit FGW and other important body-related cognitive and emotional responses, such as body anxiety or body-related attentional bias among patients with AN. Specifically, the objective was to assess levels of FBI, body anxiety, FGW and body-related attentional bias when healthy women with high and low body dissatisfaction (BD) and AN patients owned a virtual body (VB) with their real silhouette and body mass index (BMI). In addition, the relationship between FGW, body anxiety and body-related attentional bias experienced during VR exposure and ED measures, collected prior to entering the VR, were assessed. Based on previous research, it was expected that: (i) AN patients would report higher levels of FBI, body anxiety and FGW than healthy women when they owned their real-size VB; (ii) AN patients would show higher body-related attentional bias, specifically in weight-related body areas, than healthy participants; (iii) healthy women with high BD would show higher FBI, body anxiety, FGW and body-related attentional bias than women with low BD; (iv) and there would be positive relationships between the measures assessed during VR exposure and the ED measures.

2. Materials and Methods

2.1. Participants

Forty-three female college students from the University of Barcelona, Spain and 30 AN female patients from different ED units in Barcelona participated in the study. College women were recruited through campus flyers and advertisements in social network groups. The exclusion criteria were a self-reported diagnosis of a current ED, a body mass index (BMI) of less than 17 (moderate thinness) or over 30 (obesity, according to the World Health Organization, 2004) or a self-reported current severe mental disorder diagnosis (e.g., schizophrenia or bipolar disorder).

The inclusion criteria were patients with a primary diagnosis of AN (DSM-5 criteria) over 13 years of age with a BMI < 19. Furthermore, one subsyndromal patient who met all anorexia criteria but two was also included. Visual deficits that prevent exposure, epilepsy, pregnancy and clinical cardiac arrhythmia were considered exclusion criteria for the nonclinical and clinical samples.

Nineteen adolescents with AN were diagnosed at the ED Unit of Hospital Sant Joan de Déu of Barcelona, while 11 adults with AN were diagnosed at the ED Unit of Bellvitge Hospital and Hospital Clínico San Carlos of Madrid, Spain. All patients underwent a day-patient treatment for adolescents and young adults with ED. This was an intensive day-patient treatment program conducted at the ED Unit in 11-h periods, with permission to sleep at home.

2.2. Measures

2.2.1. ED Symptomatology Measures

- BMI = weight (in kilograms)/ height (in m)^2.
- Eating Disorder Inventory (EDI-3) [43]. The EDI-3 is a self-reported inventory consisting of 12 scales and 91 items, in which the answers are provided on a 6-point Likert scale. In the current study, only the 10-item body dissatisfaction scale (EDI-BD) and 7-item drive for thinness (EDI-DT) scales were used. EDI-BD measures body dissatisfaction with the whole body and specific body parts. EDI-DT measures the desire to be thinner, concern with dieting, preoccupation with weight and FGW. The Spanish version of the EDI-3 has robust validity indices and good internal consistency, with a Cronbach's alpha ranging from 0.74 to 0.96 [44]. In the current study, Cronbach's alphas for the clinical samples were 0.76 for the EDI-BD scale and 0.84 for EDI-DT. Cronbach's alpha values for both scales were 0.77 to 0.79 in the nonclinical sample.
- Physical Appearance State and Trait Anxiety Scale (PASTAS) [13]. The PASTAS is a self-reported questionnaire that assesses body anxiety, understood as the subjective feelings of tension, worried thoughts and physical changes that patients and participants feel about their body or toward specific parts of their body. The PASTAS comprises two self-report scales measuring weight-related and non-weight-related anxiety. In this study, the weight scale (W) with 8 items was used. The questionnaire presents good reliability, with a Cronbach's alpha between 0.82 and 0.92 and good test-retest ($r = 0.87$) and convergent validity indices for the W scale ($r = 0.74$ EDI-BD and $r = 0.62$ EDI-DT) [13].
- Body Image Assessment Scale-Body Dimensions (BIAS-BD) [45]. The BIAS-BD was used to assess body image disturbances in this study. The BIAS is a figural drawing scale questionnaire, which presents the physical anthropometric dimensions of adult women in a series of human silhouettes. Participants selected the one that was perceived as their body size (perceived

silhouette) and the one they desired to have (desired body size). Then, according to their BMI, the real silhouette was also selected. The scale allows researchers to estimate the participant's body dissatisfaction (discrepancy between perceived and ideal body size) and body distortion (discrepancy between perceived and real body size). This scale shows good psychometric properties, such as good test-retest reliability (r = 0.86) with data collection before and after a two-week interval and good concurrent validity (r = 0.76) after comparing participants' perceived actual body size and self-reported BMI [45].

- Body Appreciation Scale (BAS) [46], translated by Jáuregui-Lobera and Bolaños-Ríos [47]. The BAS consists of 12 items assessing a positive attitude towards one's body on a 5-point Likert scale. It presents good internal consistency, with a Cronbach's alpha of 0.908 [47].

2.2.2. Body-Related Attentional Bias

Weight-related body parts (W-AOIs or areas of interest) were chosen based on the weight scale of body items from the PASTAS questionnaire [13] and drawn onto a picture of a female avatar in a frontal view. Body parts included in the W-AOIs were the legs, thighs, buttocks, hips, stomach (abdomen) and waist. After the separation of the W-AOIs, the remaining body parts (head, neck, chest, shoulders, arms and feet) were labeled as non-weight-related body parts (NW-AOIs) (Figure 1).

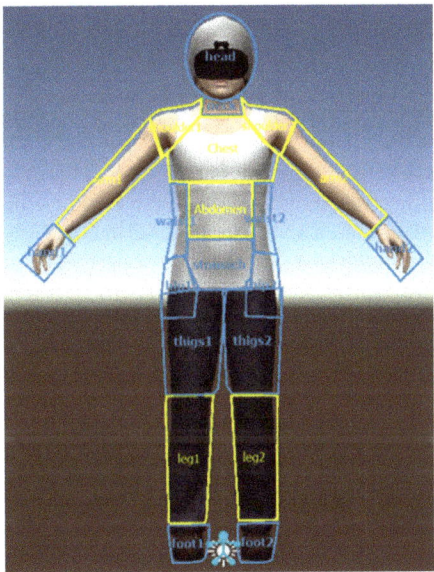

Figure 1. Weight-related and non-weight-related areas of interest on the female virtual avatar.

Participants' selective visual attention was measured using the complete fixation time and number of fixations on the areas of interest (AOIs). Visual fixation was defined by Jacob and Karn [48] as the visual act of maintaining one's gaze on a single location for a minimum duration, usually 100–200 ms. In this study, a duration of 100 ms was considered. Previous studies focusing on body-related attention used these specific gaze-behavioral measures, provided by eye-tracking (ET) technology, as reliable and continuous measures of attention allocation toward specific body areas [18,49–52].

2.2.3. Visual Analog Scales (VAS)

- Full-body illusion (FBI) was assessed by means of a VAS estimating the intensity of the illusion from 0 to 100. "On a scale of 0 to 100, indicate to what extent you felt that the virtual body was your own body, where 0 is not at all and 100 is completely."
- FGW and anxiety related to the whole body were assessed on a VAS from 0 to 100. "On a scale of 0 to 100, indicate the level of anxiety toward your body that you are feeling at this moment, where 0 is not at all and 100 is a lot." "On a scale of 0 to 100, indicate to what extent you are afraid of gaining weight at this moment, where 0 is not at all and 100 is a lot."

2.3. Hardware and Software Features

All participants were exposed to an immersive virtual scenario using a VR HTC-VIVE head-mounted display (HMD HTC VIVE, HTC Corporation, New Taipei City, Taiwan). In addition to the two controllers that HTC-VIVE usually provides, three additional body trackers were used to achieve full-body motion tracking. The VR trackers and headsets were connected to a computer with a powerful graphics card (Nvidia RTX 2080, Nvidia Corporation, Santa Clara, CA, USA) to run VR environments fluently.

HMD FOVE-Eye Tracking (FOVE, Inc., Torrance, CA, USA) was used to detect and register eye movements. The headset uses the incorporated position and orientation eye-tracking systems. The FOVE display has 2560*1440 pixels and creates 70 frames per second. Infrared eye-tracking sensors create 120 frames per second, with an accuracy level of less than 1 degree. FOVE setup 0.16.0 (FOVE, Inc., Torrance, CA, USA) and Unity 3D 3.0.0 (Unity Technologies, San Francisco, CA, USA) were used to create the virtual simulations. The virtual avatars were created using the software Blender 2.78. The virtual environment consisted of a room with a large mirror on the front wall. The mirror was large enough to reflect every limb of the body and was placed 1.5 m in front of the participants. A young female avatar wearing a basic white t-shirt with blue jeans and black trainers was created. The avatar also wore a swim cap to avoid any influence of hairstyle and an HMD, like the participants.

2.4. Procedure

This study was approved by the ethics committee of the University of Barcelona (Institutional review board IRB00003099), and all sessions were conducted at the ED units of each hospital. Furthermore, all AN patients were previously informed about the nature of the study by the clinicians responsible for their care at each ED unit. All participants signed the informed consent after being informed about the study, the data confidentiality and the possibility of withdrawing from the study at any point without consequences. When participants were under 18, informed consent was also signed by their legal guardians. Additionally, confidentiality was ensured by assigning a different identification code to each participant. Patients were previously diagnosed by senior trained clinical psychologists and psychiatrists using nonstructured clinical interviews and applying the DSM-5 criteria strictly. The Mini International Neuropsychiatric Interview (MINI) [53] was also conducted at two of the ED units. The assessment was carried out by trained clinical psychologists who had previous experience with the latest version of the MINI.

Before the start of the assessment session, each participant was measured to calculate their BMI, and the researchers asked questions in relation to the inclusion and exclusion criteria. In the ED units, the clinicians responsible for the patients were contacted to complete the identification form for the study, with information about current BMI, AN subtype diagnosis and previous history of the disorder, and to confirm that the inclusion and exclusion criteria were fulfilled.

All the participants underwent the same procedure. Firstly, the virtual avatar was generated by taking frontal and lateral photos of the participant and creating an avatar whose silhouette matched the pictures by adjusting the body parts (shoulders, arms, chest, waist, stomach, hip, thighs and legs) to the photographs. In the meantime, a second researcher administered the paper-based questionnaires.

Next, the FBI was induced using two procedures: visuo-motor and visuo-tactile stimulation. Visuo-motor stimulation consisted of synchronizing the movement of the participants and the avatar using motion capture sensors placed on the hands, feet and waist. Once inside the virtual environment, all participants could observe themselves in the first-person perspective and look at themselves in a mirror (in the third-person perspective). The movements were carried out in a structured way, and the procedure lasted one and a half minutes. The visuo-tactile stimulation consisted of synchronizing the participants' visual and tactile stimulation. When participants were touched with one of the HTC-VIVE controllers on different areas of the body (upper and lower limbs and stomach), they saw (in first and third person) how their avatars were touched in the same areas at the same time by a virtual controller. The visuo-tactile stimulation lasted one and a half minutes and was always performed by a female experimenter. Once the FBI was induced, the three VAS examining the intensity of the FBI, body-related anxiety and the FGW were assessed.

Finally, to assess the body-related attentional bias, a calibration and recording procedure was conducted using VR HMD-FOVE-Eye Tracking. The participants' gaze was tracked while they were asked to observe their virtual body in the mirror for 30 s (a similar recording time to that used in other studies) [50,54,55]. During the process, and as a cover story, the participant was told to remain still and avoid abrupt head movements while the virtual avatar position was being recalibrated.

2.5. Statistical Analysis

Ogama (Open Gaze Mouse Analyzer) software (Freie Universität, Berlin, Germany) was used to transform ET raw data into suitable quantitative data. The sum of the visual fixation times of each of the subjects was estimated using the complete fixation time and the number of fixations on the AOIs. This was achieved by summing up separate complete fixation times and the number of fixations displayed on W-AOIs vs. on NW-AOIs. Additional data transformation was conducted by calculating the difference between weight-related and non-weight-related AOIs (e.g., complete fixation time (W-AOIs: 1615 ms − NW-AOIs: 1505 ms = 110 ms)). Therefore, a positive outcome would mean that the participant looked at weight-related body parts longer than at non-weight-related body parts, while a negative outcome would mean the opposite.

Likewise, healthy women were divided into high vs. low BD levels using the median score of the EDI-BD as a cut-off point ($_{Me}$ BD = 8).

One-way analyses of covariance (ANCOVA) were run to determine if there were differences in all measures, including ED measures assessed prior to entering the VR environment, VR-VASs and ET measures between participants with high and low BD and AN patients. Given the age differences between ED and healthy participants, this variable was controlled and introduced as a covariable in the analyses. Analyses of ET measures were conducted for the groups of AOIs (e.g., the difference between W-AOIs and NW-AOIs) and for single W-AOIs (e.g., arms, shoulders and chest, etc.).

There was homogeneity of the regression slopes as the interaction terms were not statistically significant ($p > 0.05$) for any of the measures. The other assumptions were partially met. There was homogeneity of the variances, as assessed by Levene's test, in almost all measures except for BMI, EDI-BD, EDI-DT and BIAS-BD. In addition, data were not normally distributed in all the variables assessed by the Kolmogorov–Smirnov test. However, it was decided to conduct the analyses regardless, as ANCOVA is considered a robust test, even in the case of deviation from normality [56]. Finally, a few outliers were detected in some measures, as assessed by inspection of a boxplot. Statistical analyses were conducted with and without the outliers. Since the results did not differ significantly, it was decided to include them in the analyses.

Finally, Pearson correlations were run to assess the relationship between ED measures, VASs and body-related attentional bias measures in the overall sample. They were also conducted separately among healthy participants with low and high BD and patients with AN. All the analyses were conducted with the statistical software IBM SPSS Statistics v.24 (IBM Corp. Released 2016. Armonk, NY, USA).

3. Results

The demographic and clinical information of healthy controls and AN patients are summarized here. The healthy control sample consisted of 43 healthy college women (M_{age} = 21.12, SD = 1.56 and age range: 18–23 years and M_{BMI} = 21.94, SD = 2.53 and BMI range: 17.12–27.82), with 25 women with low BD and 18 women with high BD. The clinical sample consisted of 30 AN female patients (M_{age} = 17.73 and SD = 4.60 and M_{BMI} =17.55 and SD =1.07), with 19 adolescents (age range: 13–17 years and BMI range: 16.06–18.94 kg/m^2) and 11 adults (age range: 18–32 years and BMI range: 13.96–18.98). Of the adolescent AN patients, 18 were diagnosed with restrictive AN (AN-R) and the other one with purgative AN (AN-P). Three adolescent patients presented comorbidities with anxiety disorders: two presented mood-related disorders, and one presented both anxiety and mood-related disorders. Eight patients received pharmacological treatment: two with antidepressants, three with anxiolytics and three with a combination of antidepressants and anxiolytics.

Six of the adult patients were diagnosed with the AN-P subtype and five with the AN-R subtype. In addition, two adult patients presented comorbidities with borderline personality disorder, one presented borderline personality disorder and post-traumatic stress disorder and one presented a major depressive disorder. Five adult patients were receiving pharmacological treatment: one with antidepressants, one with anxiolytics and antidepressants and three with antidepressants or anxiolytics combined with antipsychotics.

All the descriptive results are summarized in Table 1, including ED measures assessed prior to entering the VR environment, VASs assessed within the VR environment and body-related attentional bias measures.

Table 1. Adjusted for age and unadjusted descriptive results. Mean (M), standard deviation (SD) and standard error (SE).

	Women with Low BD (n= 25)		Women with High BD (n= 18)		AN Patients (n = 30)	
	Unadjusted	Adjusted	Unadjusted	Adjusted	Unadjusted	Adjusted
	M (SD)	M (SE)	M (SD)	M (SE)	M (SD)	M (SE)
BMI	21.65 (2.39)	21.60 (.42)	22.38 (2.75)	22.32 (.53)	17.55 (1.07)	17.63 (0.40)
EDI-3-DT	1.88 (1.76)	2.41 (1.07)	4.89 (4.39)	5.57 (1.27)	19.23 (7.43)	18.38 (1.03)
EDI-3-BD	4.04 (1.44)	4.53 (1.32)	14.61 (6.30)	15.26 (1.56)	24.03 (10.03)	23.23 (1.27)
PASTAS	5.04 (3.77)	5.80 (1.09)	8.56 (4.77)	9.70 (1.38)	17.20 (7.18)	15.95 (1.05)
BIAS-Body distortion	9.60 (13.06)	9.93 (3.59)	18.13 (13.76)	18.61 (4.51)	39.17 (21.45)	38.63 (3.43)
BIAS-Body dissatisfaction	7.40 (9.90)	7.53 (4.02)	14.37 (19.56)	14.56 (5.07)	36.83 (24.62)	36.62 (3.86)
BAS	52.32 (5.29)	51.82 (1.57)	42.06 (7.54)	41.32 (1.98)	29.43 (9.30)	30.24 (1.51)
VAS-FBI	65.72 (23.25)	67.94 (5.05)	54.94 (19.20)	58.24 (6.38)	46.18 (29.50)	42.15 (4.86)
VAS-A	15.20 (19.12)	17.44 (5.15)	26.25 (22.97)	29.60 (6.51)	40.00 (31.15)	35.34 (4.95)
VAS-FGW	22.88 (28.80)	25.12 (5.84)	51.88 (26.39)	55.21 (7.38)	79.82 (27.70)	72.86 (5.62)
Complete fixation time (in ms) *	−2858 (10,589)	−4492 (1732)	965 (7578)	−1079 (2055)	6899 (7457)	10,198 (2014)
Number of fixations *	2.20 (15.80)	−0.45 (2.96)	5.20 (15.49)	1.90 (3.51)	22.00 (12.99)	27.25 (3.41)

Note: body mass index (BMI); Eating Disorder Inventory (EDI-3) drive for thinness (DT) and body dissatisfaction (BD) scales; Physical Appearance State and Trait Anxiety Scale (PASTAS); Body Image Assessment Test (BIAS); Body Appreciation Scale (BAS) and visual analog scales (VAS) of full body illusion (FBI), body anxiety (A) and fear of gaining weight (FGW). AN = Anorexia Nervosa. Complete fixation time in milliseconds (ms). * For eye-tracking (ET) measures, the clinical sample was comprised of 19 adolescents and 5 adults with AN.

3.1. Eating Disorder Measures Assessed Prior to Entering the VR Environment

As Table 1 shows, patients with AN reported higher levels of BD, a drive for thinness, body anxiety and body image disturbances (including body distortion and BD assessed with BIAS and EDI questionnaires, respectively) than healthy participants. Patients with AN also had lower BMI and showed lower body appreciation than healthy participants.

After adjusting for age, the ANCOVA analyses showed group differences on all ED measures. Specifically, the results showed significant group differences in BMI ($F(2,67) = 29.035$, $p < 0.001$, partial $\eta^2 = 0.464$); drive for thinness ($F(2,69) = 56.775$, $p < 0.001$, partial $\eta^2 = 0.622$); BD ($F(2,69) = 49.101$, $p < 0.001$, partial $\eta^2 = 0.587$); body anxiety ($F(2,67) = 20.600$, $p < 0.001$, partial $\eta^2 = 0.381$); body image disturbances (including body distortion: $F(2,67) = 15.703$, $p < 0.001$, partial $\eta^2 = 0.319$ and BD: $F(2,67) = 12,968$, $p < 0.001$, partial $\eta^2 = 0.279$, as assessed with the BIAS-BD questionnaire) and body appreciation ($F(2,67) = 45.426$, $p < 0.001$). Post-hoc analyses revealed that there were significant differences ($p < 0.05$) between patients with AN and women with high and low BD in all ED measures.

3.2. VASs of Full-Body Illusion, Body Anxiety and Fear of Gaining Weight

Once in the VR environment, and according to the VASs, AN patients reported lower values of FBI than healthy participants. Additionally, AN patients reported higher levels of body anxiety and FGW, while owning their real-size VB, than healthy participants. Women with high BD also reported higher body anxiety and FGW, as well as lower levels of FBI than women with low BD (see Table 1).

To clarify whether these differences between patients with AN and women with high and low BD were, indeed, significant, one-way ANCOVAs were run. After controlling for age, the results reported significant group differences in FBI levels ($F(2,68) = 6.252$, $p = 0.003$, partial $\eta^2 = 0.157$); FGW ($F(2,67) = 16,670$, $p < 0.001$, partial $\eta^2 = 0.332$) and marginally significant differences in body anxiety ($F(2,67) = 3.077$, $p = 0.053$, partial $\eta^2 = 0.084$). Effect sizes according to Cohen (1988) were medium in body anxiety, high in FBI and very high in FGW. Post-hoc analyses revealed significant differences ($p < 0.05$) between patients with AN and women with low BD in FBI and FGW VASs and marginally significant differences ($p = 0.057$) in VAS-A (see Table 2). In addition, there were also significant differences between women with high BD and low BD (see Table 2).

Table 2. Post-hoc analyses (pairwise comparison) between AN patients and women with high and low BD.

Measures	AN Patients vs. Women with Low BD			AN Patients vs. Women with High BD			Women with High vs. Low BD		
	MD	p	95% CI	MD	p	95% CI	MD	p	95% CI
VAS-FBI	−25.79	0.002	(−43.72, −7.86)	−16.10	0.179	(−36.73, 4.53)	−9.69	0.672	(−29.08, 9.70)
VAS-A	17,89	0.057	(−0.39, 36.18)	5,74	0.896	(−15.30, 26.78)	12,15	0.408	(−7.62, 31.93)
VAS-FGW	47.74	<0.001	(68.48, 27.00)	17.64	0.221	(−6.21, 41.51)	30.09	0.005	(7.66, 52.52)
Complete fixation time (in ms) *	14,722	<0.001	(7626, 21,818)	11,317	0.002	(3590, 19,045)	3404	0.568	(−2904, 9712)
Number of fixations *	27.70	<0.001	(15.66, 39.74)	25.35	<0.001	(12.24, 38.45)	2.35	0.787	(−8.34, 13.05)

Note: Mean differences (MD), p-values and 95% confidence intervals (CI) stated for each group comparison. ms = milliseconds. * For ET measures, the clinical sample was comprised of 19 adolescents and 5 adults with AN.

3.3. Body-Related Attentional Bias Measures

The descriptive results of both ET measures revealed that AN patients spent more time looking at and showed a higher number of fixations on weight-related AOIs than on non-weight-related AOIs, as indicated by a positive outcome in both ET measures. In contrast, women with high BD spent a similar time and number of fixations looking at weight- and non-weight-related AOIs. Finally, women with low BD showed a tendency to spend more time looking at NW-AOIs and a similar number of fixations on weight- and non-weight-related AOIs (see Table 1).

The one-way ANCOVA results showed statistically significant group differences in the complete fixation time ($F(2,63) = 13.114$, $p < 0.001$, partial $\eta^2 = 0.294$) and the number of fixations ($F(2,63) = 17.107$, $p < 0.001$, partial $\eta^2 = 0.352$) after controlling for age. Post-hoc analyses revealed that these differences were statically significant ($p < 0.05$) between patients with AN and women with high and low BD in both attentional bias measures (see Table 2). Finally, there were no significant differences ($p > 0.05$) between women with high and low BD.

One-way ANCOVAs were also run to assess the group differences at single W-related AOIs. After controlling for age, the results showed statistically significant group differences ($p < 0.05$) for the thighs (complete fixation time: $F(2,63) = 7707$, $p = 0.001$, partial $\eta 2 = 0.197$ and number of fixations: $F(2,63) = 10.573$, $p < 0.001$, partial $\eta 2 = 0.251$); hips (number of fixations: $F(2,63) = 4663$, $p < 0.013$, partial $\eta 2 = 0.129$) and stomach (complete fixation time: $F(2,63) = 5239$, $p = 0.008$, partial $\eta 2 = 0.143$ and number of fixations: $F(2,63) = 7078$, $p = 0.002$, partial $\eta 2 = 0.183$). Post-hoc analyses revealed that patients with AN spent significantly more time looking and showed higher numbers of fixations on the stomach, hips and, particularly, the thighs in contrast to women with low and high BD (Figure 2). No significant differences were found between women with high and low BD for any of the single AOIs.

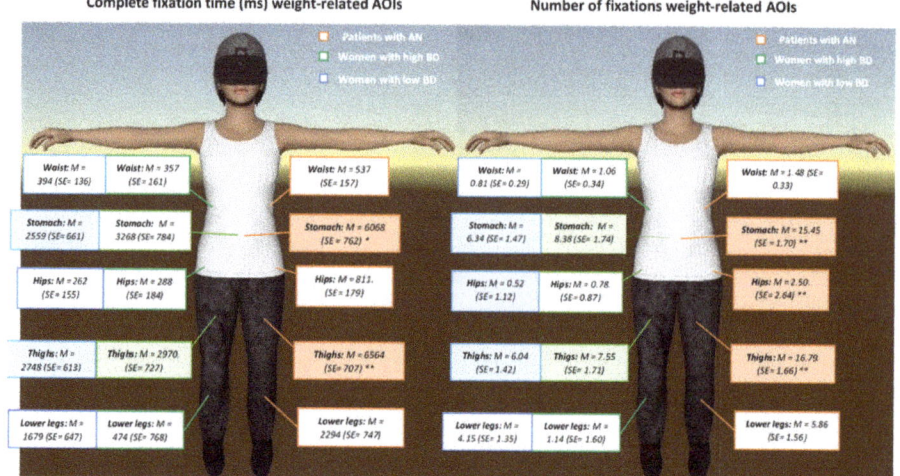

Figure 2. Differences between patients with Anorexia Nervosa (AN) and women with high and low body dissatisfaction (BD) (means and standard errors) in the complete fixation time (in milliseconds; ms) and the number of fixations on individual weight-related areas of interest (AOIs). Post-hoc analyses: ** $p < 0.01$ and * $p < 0.05$.

3.4. Pearson Correlations

According to multiple Pearson correlations, the results showed statistically significant moderate or large positive correlations between VAS-A and VAS-FGQ and all ED measures ($p < 0.05$), which were significantly larger for VAS-FGW (see Table 3). There were also moderate or large positive correlations between VAS-A/FGW and the BMI and BAS scale. Furthermore, VAS-FBI negatively correlated ($p < 0.05$) with the VAS-FGW, EDI-DT, EDI-BD, BAS and BIAS-BD measures, with moderate correlations (Cohen, 1988). There was a moderate positive correlation between the VAS-FBI and BAS. Finally, there were significant moderate positive correlations between the body-related attentional bias measures and the EDI-DT, EDI-BD and PASTAS (only for the number of fixations (NF)) scales, while there were moderate negative correlations between the body-related attentional bias measures and the BMI and BAS.

Multiple Pearson correlations were conducted separately for women with low and high BD and for patients with AN. The results among women with low BD showed that, overall, the previously reported positive and negative correlations between the VASs/attentional bias measures and other ED measures were not significant, with the exception of the VAS-FGW and PASTAS/BAS (see Table 4). Similar results were found among women with high BD, in which there were statistically significant positive/negative correlations between the VAS-FGW and BMI, EDI-DT, PASTAS and BAS (See Table 5). Finally, among patients with AN, there were statistically significant and similar positive and negative correlations to those previously reported for the entire clinical and nonclinical samples (see Table 6).

Table 3. Correlations between eating disorder (ED) measures and virtual reality (VR) body exposure responses in the entire sample.

	VAS-FBI	VAS-A	VAS-FGW	CFT	NF
VAS-FBI					
VAS-A	−0.16				
VAS-FGW	−0.24 *	0.70 **			
CFT	−0.21	0.16	0.35 **		
NF	−0.28	1.18	0.42 **	0.91 **	
BMI	0.23	−0.22	−0.38 **	−0.38 **	−0.43 **
EDI-DT	−0.37 **	0.55 **	0.72 **	0.32 **	0.41 **
EDI-BD	−0.30 **	0.53 **	0.73 **	0.35 **	0.40 **
PASTAS	−0.22	0.60 **	0.80 **	0.22	0.32 **
BIAS-Body distortion	−0.43 **	0.38 **	0.56 **	0.16	0.21
BIAS-Body dissatisfaction	−0.38 **	0.28 *	0.50 **	0.19	0.23
BAS	0.34 **	−0.58 **	−0.77 **	−0.32 **	−0.40 **

* = *p*-values < 0.005 or ** = *p*-values < 0.001. NOTE: CFT = complete fixation time. NF = number of fixations.

Table 4. Correlations between ED measures and VR body exposure responses in healthy participants with low BD.

	VAS-FBI	VAS-A	VAS-FGW	CFT	NF
VAS-FBI					
VAS-A	−0.028				
VAS-FGW	−0.209	0.778 **			
CFT	−0.290	−0.097	0.205		
NF	−0.255	0.064	0.402 *	0.938 **	1.00
BMI	−0.020	0.071	−0.013	−0.277	−0.243
EDI-DT	−0.268	0.279	0.325	0.235	0.246
EDI-BD	−0.045	0.153	0.172	0.316	0.336
PASTAS	−0.057	0.728 **	0.686 **	−0.045	0.015
BIAS-Body distortion	−0.147	0.142	−0.085	−0.155	−0.199
BIAS- Body dissatisfaction	0.239	0.195	−0.041	−0.149	−0.099
BAS	−0.201	−0.503 *	−0.593 **	−0.214	−0.322

* = *p*-values < 0.05 or ** = *p*-values < 0.01. NOTE: CFT = complete fixation time. NF = number of fixations.

Table 5. Correlations between ED measures and VR body exposure responses in healthy participants with high BD.

	VAS-FBI	VAS-A	VAS-FGW	CFT	NF
VAS-FBI					
VAS-A	0.173				
VAS-FGW	0.282	0.710 **			
CFT	0.300	0.040	0.017		
NF	0.433	0.183	0.006	0.876 **	
BMI	0.170	−0.045	0.016	−0.096	0.009
EDI-DT	0.086	0.271	0.519 *	−0.241	−0.281
EDI-BD	0.035	0.452	0.546 *	0.071	0.132
PASTAS	0.077	0.719 **	0.753 **	0.030	0.057
BIAS-Body distortion	−0.103	0.171	0.377	0.041	−0.143
BIAS-Body dissatisfaction	−0.108	−0.246	0.048	0.040	−0.093
BAS	−0.162	−0.350	−0.674 **	0.053	0.099

* = *p*-values < 0.05 or ** = *p*-values < 0.01. NOTE: CFT = complete fixation time. NF = number of fixations.

Table 6. Correlations between ED measures and VR body exposure responses in patients with AN.

	VAS-FBI	VAS-A	VAS-FGW	CFT	NF
VAS-FBI					
VAS-A	−0.093				
VAS-FGW	−0.031	0.563 **			
CFT	−0.057	−0.187	−0.191		
NF	−0.064	−0.317	−0.340	0.862 **	
BMI	0.042	0.116	0.059	0.141	0.149
EDI-DT	−0.290	0.562 **	0.620 **	−0.326	−0.263
EDI-BD	−0.107	0.442 *	0.594 **	−0.211	−0.206
PASTAS	0.014	0.399 *	0.675 **	−0.527 *'	−0.472 *
BIAS-Body distortion	−0.425 *	0.216	0.458 *	−0.280	−0.220
BIAS-Body dissatisfaction	−0.436 *	0.163	0.396 *	−0.164	−0.172
BAS	0.351	−0.550 **	−0.564**	0.377	0.321

* = p-values < 0.05 or ** = p-values < 0.01. NOTE: CFT = complete fixation time. NF = number of fixations.

Surprisingly, some of the strongest significant negative correlations were found in FBI levels and body image disturbance measures only among patients with AN. To explain these preliminary results, it was hypothesized that the individuals with higher body image disturbance (i.e., body distortion/body dissatisfaction) levels were those who experienced lower FBI levels once they owned their real-size virtual body. Thus, it was decided to conduct predictive post-hoc linear regression analyses. The results showed that having higher body distortion levels statistically significantly predicted experiencing lower FBI levels ($F(1,29) = 6.160$, $p = 0.019$), accounting for 18% of the explained variability in FBI levels only among patients with AN. This relationship between body distortion and FBI levels was not significant among women with high and low BD ($p > 0.05$). Similarly, experiencing higher BD levels significantly predicted experiencing lower FBI levels ($F(1, 29) = 6.561$, $p = 0.016$), which accounted for 19% of the explained variability in FBI levels only among patients with AN. Again, the relationship between body distortion and FBI levels was not significant among women with high and low BD ($p > 0.05$).

4. Discussion

The current study aimed to provide initial evidence of the usefulness of VR body exposure to elicit FGW, body anxiety and body-related attentional bias in patients with AN. For this purpose, we assessed whether there were significant differences in the levels of FBI, body anxiety, FGW and body-related attentional bias when AN patients and healthy women with high and low BD owned a virtual body with their real silhouette and body mass index (BMI). As expected, patients with AN showed higher levels of FGW, body anxiety and body-related attentional bias than healthy controls when they owned their real-size VB. Unexpectedly, patients with AN reported significantly lower levels of FBI than women with low BD. Furthermore, no significant differences were found between healthy women with high and low BD on FBI, body anxiety or body-related attentional bias. The only significant group differences were observed in the levels of FGW reported.

Furthermore, the relationship between the ED measures assessed prior to entering the VR and the responses produced during VR exposure was also assessed. As expected, there were positive relationships between some measures assessed by VR body exposure (e.g., body anxiety and FGW) software and other ED measures assessed previously. This relation was particularly strong among patients with AN. Hence, the participants and patients with higher ED symptomatology were also those who experienced higher levels of FGW, body anxiety and attentional bias during exposure. Additionally, significant negative relationships were found among FBI and body image disturbance measures, including body distortion and BD, only among patients with AN.

According to the measures assessed during the VR body exposure, patients with AN reported significantly higher FGW and body anxiety levels than women with high and low BD, with high effect sizes. Specifically, the FGW was the variable that best distinguished between AN patients and women with low BD and between women with high and low BD. Relatedly, the FGW during VR body exposure was the measure that had the largest significant correlations with the ED measures assessed before exposure, such as BD, drive for thinness, body anxiety, BMI and body appreciation. Similar tendencies were observed not only among patients with AN but, also, among women with high BD. These results support the increasing evidence in favor of the critical role that the FGW might display not only in AN [6,8–10] but, also, in healthy women with body concerns. Indeed, several studies have reported high prevalence of FGW among adult women [2,57] and young women between 16 to 25 years old [58].

Unexpectedly, patients with AN reported significantly lower FBI levels than healthy participants with low BD. Our results seem to contradict previous research that found that ED patients tend to experience a stronger illusion than healthy individuals [34]. However, those studies induced the feeling of ownership in one hand only, following the rubber hand illusion paradigm [33]. In the current study, the illusion of ownership was induced over a whole virtual body, which suggests that other body-related factors (e.g., body image disturbances) could influence these results as well. For instance, several patients with AN described their virtual body as being slimmer than their real body, while healthy women with high and low BD did not report such a phenomenon. Accordingly, there was a significant negative relationship between FBI and body image disturbances only among patients with AN, while this relationship was not significant among women with high and low BD. After further analyses, it was found that AN patients with higher body distortion and body dissatisfaction levels experienced lower FBI levels once they owned their real-size virtual body. These results provide preliminary evidence about the influence that body image disturbances have on FBI over the whole body among patients with AN. Accordingly, two interesting questions should be considered. Firstly, would these low FBI levels increase during a body exposure treatment, for instance, over several sessions? Secondly, if this were the case, would a continuous increase in FBI levels produce a change in body image disturbances in the participants or the other way around? Unfortunately, it is not possible to answer either question, since there is a lack of studies in which FBI levels were assessed over several sessions with AN patients. In fact, to the best of our knowledge, only one study has assessed FBI over a short period among healthy participants, finding that, after a synchronous visuo-motor embodiment procedure, FBI levels remained high after 30 and 55 s of synchronous or no movement [59].

Regarding body-related attentional bias measures, our results agree with previous studies that suggest that women with EDs tend to pay more attention to self-defined unattractive body areas, while healthy participants tend to show more general scanning behavior, covering the whole body [17,54,60,61]. While most of the studies assessing body-related attention have been conducted with adults, little information is available about body-related attention in youths. Therefore, our results also support studies that assessed body-related attentional bias among adolescents with EDs and showed that adolescents with AN and Bulimia Nervosa spent more time on self-reported unattractive body parts [18,62]. For instance, Bauer et al. [18] found that dysfunctional body-related attention was more marked among adolescents with AN-R than among healthy individuals and other ED patients (e.g., patients with AN-binge eating/purging subtype or Bulimia Nervosa). Since almost all our patients were diagnosed with an AN-R subtype, this study reinforced the evidence of dysfunctional body-related attention among adolescents with AN-R. When single W-related AOIs were considered, we observed that all individuals paid more attention to the thighs, stomach and lower legs. The W-AOIs that best distinguished between patients with AN and women with high and low BD were the thighs, the stomach, and the hips (only in number of fixations). This suggests that these areas might be particularly salient for patients with AN.

Nevertheless, some key methodological differences between the current study and other studies that assess body-related attentional bias should be mentioned. As described before, some previous studies used a similar free-viewing, single-body paradigm but measured the attentional bias towards self-reported attractive vs. unattractive body areas. This is a successful, well-established methodology to define the areas of interest [16,17]. Although self-reported unattractive body areas among individuals with EDs could indeed be areas related with weight, the evidence for attentional bias towards specific weight-related body areas could not be clearly established, since there might be weight-related body areas in both the self-reported attractive and unattractive body parts. In this study and in previous studies conducted by our group, a different methodology was used to define the areas of interest, in which an individual's gazing behavior was analyzed using the same definition of areas of interest for all participants e.g., weight- vs. non-weight-related body areas [50,51]. These areas of interest were defined based on well-established questionnaires that assess the same body image construct, such as the weight-related scale of the PASTAS.

Finally, no differences in body-related attentional bias were found between women with high and low BD. Women with high BD tended to pay more attention to W-related AOIs, while women with low BD showed the opposite visual tendency toward NW-related AOIs. None of these tendencies showed a clear attentional bias to weight- or non-weight-related AOIs. However, overall, both groups showed more general scanning behavior, covering the whole body. These results are in-line with a previous study conducted in our group [50] in which women with high and low BD showed similar attentional patterns toward their own virtual bodies. This previous study was conducted with a previous version of the virtual simulation. Although the results obtained were very similar, some technical improvements that were made to the current version of the simulation should be considered. For instance, a more precise method could be used to create the avatar (by taking a frontal and lateral photo and incorporating the BMI information of each participant), and the full-body tracking system could be improved to conduct a visual-motor stimulation.

Some limitations should be considered in the current study. For instance, most of the patients with AN were adolescents (19 out of 30), while the healthy women were college students between 18 and 22 years old. Although the potential effect of age between groups was controlled in this study by ANCOVAs, these statistical analyses could not control the effect that age might play within each group and, particularly, in the more heterogeneous AN sample. Future studies should try to overcome this important bias and replicate the current study with age-balanced samples.

Regarding the assessment, no screening questionnaires or structured clinical interviews were used properly to assess the presence of EDs or other mental disorders among the healthy participants. Furthermore, to diagnosticate the clinical sample, a MINI diagnostic interview was used in two of the three ED units, while, at the last ED unit, senior trained clinical psychologists and psychiatrists conducted nonstructured clinical interviews following thoroughly the DSM-5 criteria.

FBI and FGW were assessed using a VAS; even though VASs are usually considered as a valid measure to assess this sort of construct (for instance, FGW among patients with AN [63]), they should be complemented with evidence-based questionnaires. For instance, the embodiment questionnaire [64] might offer a more accurate assessment of the FBI based on the location of the body, the ownership illusion, the motor agency and the general appearance. One of the reasons for using the VAS was to assess the FBI while patients and participants were owning their real-size virtual bodies. It was important to assess the FBI levels directly in the VR environment and not later, since this bodily illusion might have been reduced once the participants left the VR (after the ET assessment task), and the results might have been affected as a consequence. However, since several questionnaires were already used in the current research, it was decided not to extend the assessment sessions (which lasted approximately 1h) any further and to refrain from applying larger tests. Future studies might try to implement evidence-based questionnaires that assess these two measures. Finally, in the current study, the average levels of BD among women labeled as "high BD" were very similar to in a previous study conducted by our group [50], corresponding to medium-to-high BD levels among nonclinical Spanish women [44]. Thus, it would have been necessary to recruit participants with higher levels of BD to provide a more exhaustive distinction of the BD levels among women with high and low BD. Relatedly, the suitability of using the median as an "artificial categorization" of a continuous variable—in this study, BD—could have some limitations. These could affect the statistical power and accuracy of the estimated relations and reduce the observed relations among the variables [65].

Some limitations in the VR software should also be considered. Although several improvements were implemented (e.g., the avatar sharing the same silhouette and BMI as the participant), the general appearance of the virtual body (clothes and skin color, etc.) was not exactly that of the individuals. The latest VR studies allow the simulation of an exact 3D biometric avatar with all the individual's features [66] using 3D body scans. This sort of technology might notably enhance the realism of VR embodiment-based techniques and, consequently, improve VR studies on body-related issues and EDs. The current study used two separate HMDs: one for conducting the visuo-tactile and visuo-motor FBI procedures (HTC-VIVE) and the other to record the body-related attentional bias measures (FOVE-VR). Having two separate devices might have reduced the FBI levels when the participants had to change from one HMD to the other. This limitation could have been overcome by using the new generation of VR HMD with ET devices all-in-one (e.g., the HTC VIVE-Pro Eye, which has a complete full-body tracking system and can be used to elicit FBI over the virtual body and measure gaze patterns).

The implications of VR embodiment-based techniques might be critical to improving evidence-based therapies in AN, such as body exposure-based techniques. For instance, instead of exposing a patient with AN to food or to her current body image, as has been done so far, what would be the result of exposing her to her core fear, i.e., weight gain? Patients with AN associate weight gain with negative consequences, and food avoidance prevents them from learning that maintaining a normal weight does not lead to such catastrophic consequences [67]. Consequently, focusing on the primary conditioned stimulus (weight gain) rather than on the secondary ones, such as eating, may be an effective strategy. As has been reported, VR embodiment-based techniques are a successful way to change body image disturbances in patients with AN [39–41]. We propose going one step further. First, we could allow the patient with AN to experience the illusion of ownership of a virtual body that reproduces their real-size silhouette, with their specific physical particularities and their exact BMI. Then, we could apply progressive increases in weight (or an increase in the BMI) of the virtual avatar, until it reaches a healthy BMI.

Furthermore, the combination of VR and ET technologies to assess body-related attentional bias might lead to new possibilities in coming years. For instance, it might improve some of the current limitations of research conducted with fixed ET, such as the lack of external validity [68]. In other words, combining ET and VR might enable the reproduction of more ecological environments, such as bathrooms and dressing rooms, to assess patient's gaze patterns while they own their real-size virtual avatars in each session or before and after the therapy.

To sum up, our results show that, while owning their real-size virtual body, patients with AN reported significantly higher FGW and body anxiety levels than women with low BD, with high effect sizes. Specifically, FGW was the variable that best distinguished between AN patients and healthy participants and between healthy participants with high and low BD. Unexpectedly, patients with AN reported significantly lower FBI levels than healthy participants with low BD. After post-hoc analyses, it was found that body image disturbances influence FBI levels among patients with AN. Furthermore, our results suggest that the patients with AN showed a body-related attentional bias. Specifically, they spent more time and looked more frequently at the weight-related body areas (e.g., thighs, stomach and hips) than healthy women. Finally, these results provide evidence about the usefulness of VR-based body exposure to elicit FGW and other body-related disturbances in AN patients. Thus, it may be a suitable intervention for reducing these emotional responses and for easing weight recovery.

Author Contributions: Conceptualization, B.P.-G., M.F.-G., M.D.-M., I.S.-D.; F.F.-A. and J.G.-M; validation, B.P.-G., M.C.-R., P.S.-U., H.M.-N., I.d.l.M.S.-C. and B.B.; formal analysis, B.P.-G.; investigation, B.P.-G., H.M.-N., N.S., I.d.l.M.S.-C. and B.B.; resources, E.S.-T., M.C.-R., P.S.-U., M.D.-M., I.S.-D.; F.F.-A. and J.G.-M.; data curation, B.P.-G., writing—original draft preparation, B.P.-G., writing—review and editing, B.P.-G., M.F.-G., N.S. and J.G.-M.; visualization, B.P.-G. and M.F.-G.; supervision M.F.-G. and J.G.-M.; project coordinator; J.G.-M. and funding acquisition, J.G.-M. All authors have read and agreed to the published version of the manuscript.

Funding: This study was funded by the Spanish Ministry of Science and Innovation (Ministerio de Ciencia e Innovación, Spain/Project PID2019-108657RB-I00: Modification of attentional bias, with virtual reality, for improving anorexia nervosa treatment and Project PSI2015-70389-R: Development of virtual reality-based exposure techniques for improving anorexia nervosa treatment) and by AGAUR, Generalitat de Catalunya, 2017SGR1693.

Acknowledgments: CIBEROBN is an initiative of Instituto Carlos III (Spain).

Conflicts of Interest: The authors declare no conflict of interest. The funders had no role in the design of the study; in the collection, analyses or interpretation of data; in the writing of the manuscript or in the decision to publish the results.

References

1. Hoek, H.W. Review of the worldwide epidemiology of eating disorders. *Curr. Opin. Psychiatry* **2016**, *29*, 336–339. [CrossRef] [PubMed]
2. Micali, N.; Hagberg, K.W.; Petersen, I.; Treasure, J.L. The incidence of eating disorders in the UK in 2000–2009: Findings from the General Practice Research Database. *BMJ Open* **2013**, *3*. [CrossRef] [PubMed]
3. Herpertz-Dahlmann, B. A1dolescent Eating Disorders: Definitions, Symptomatology, Epidemiology and Comorbidity. *Child. Adolesc. Psychiatr. Clin. N. Am.* **2009**, *24*, 177–196. [CrossRef] [PubMed]
4. Favaro, A.; Caregaro, L.; Tenconi, E.; Bosello, R.; Santonastaso, P. Time trends in age at onset of anorexia nervosa and bulimia nervosa. *J. Clin. Psychiatry* **2009**, *70*, 1715–1721. [CrossRef]
5. Nicholls, D.E.; Lynn, R.; Viner, R.M. Childhood eating disorders: British national surveillance study. *Br. J. Psychiatry* **2011**, *198*, 295–301. [CrossRef]
6. American Psychiatric Association. *Diagnostic and Statistical Manual of Mental Disorders*, 5th ed.; American Psychiatric Association: Arlington, VA, USA, 2013.
7. Legenbauer, T.; Thiemann, P.; Vocks, S. Body image disturbance in children and adolescents with eating disorders: Current evidence and future directions. *Z. Kinder. Jugendpsychiatr. Psychother.* **2014**, *42*, 51–59. [CrossRef]
8. Carter, J.C.; Bewell-Weiss, C.V. Nonfat phobic anorexia nervosa: Clinical characteristics and response to inpatient treatment. *Int. J. Eat. Disord.* **2011**, *44*, 220–224. [CrossRef]
9. Calugi, S.; El Ghoch, M.; Conti, M.; Dalle Grave, R. Preoccupation with shape or weight, fear of weight gain, feeling fat and treatment outcomes in patients with anorexia nervosa: A longitudinal study. *Behav. Res. Ther.* **2018**, *105*, 63–68. [CrossRef]
10. Linardon, J.; Phillipou, A.; Castle, D.; Newton, R.; Harrison, P.; Cistullo, L.L.; Griffiths, S.; Hindle, A.; Brennan, L. The relative associations of shape and weight over-evaluation, preoccupation, dissatisfaction, and fear of weight gain with measures of psychopathology: An extension study in individuals with anorexia nervosa. *Eat. Behav.* **2018**, *29*, 54–58. [CrossRef]
11. Strober, M. Pathologic Fear Conditioning and Anorexia Nervosa: On the Search for Novel Paradigms. *Int. J. Eat. Disord.* **2004**, *35*, 504–508. [CrossRef]
12. Steinglass, J.E.; Sysko, R.; Glasofer, D.; Albano, A.M.; Simpson, H.B.; Walsh, B.T. Rationale for the application of exposure and response prevention to the treatment of anorexia nervosa. *Int. J. Eat. Disord.* **2011**, *44*, 134–141. [CrossRef] [PubMed]
13. Reed, D.L.; Thompson, J.K.; Brannick, M.T.; Sacco, W.P. Development and validation of the physical appearance state and trait anxiety scale (PASTAS). *J. Anxiety Disord.* **1991**, *5*, 323–332. [CrossRef]
14. Williamson, D.A.; White, M.A.; York-Crowe, E.; Stewart, T.M. Cognitive-behavioral theories of eating disorders. *Behav. Modif.* **2004**, *28*, 711–738. [CrossRef] [PubMed]
15. Lee, M.; Shafran, R. Information processing biases in eating disorders. *Clin. Psychol. Rev.* **2004**, *24*, 215–238. [CrossRef] [PubMed]
16. Rodgers, R.F.; DuBois, R.H. Cognitive biases to appearance-related stimuli in body dissatisfaction: A systematic review. *Clin. Psychol. Rev.* **2016**, *46*, 1–11. [CrossRef]
17. Kerr-Gaffney, J.; Harrison, A.; Tchanturia, K. Eye-tracking research in eating disorders: A systematic review. *Int. J. Eat. Disord.* **2019**, *52*, 3–27. [CrossRef]
18. Bauer, A.; Schneider, S.; Waldorf, M.; Braks, K.; Huber, T.J.; Adolph, D.; Vocks, S. Selective Visual Attention Towards Oneself and Associated State Body Satisfaction: An Eye-Tracking Study in Adolescents with Different Types of Eating Disorders. *J. Abnorm. Child. Psychol.* **2017**, *45*, 1647–1661. [CrossRef]

19. Forrest, L.N.; Jones, P.J.; Ortiz, S.N.; Smith, A.R. Core psychopathology in anorexia nervosa and bulimia nervosa: A network analysis. *Int. J. Eat. Disord.* **2018**, *51*, 668–679. [CrossRef]
20. Hildebrandt, T.; Loeb, K.; Troupe, S.; Delinsky, S. Adjunctive mirror exposure for eating disorders: A randomized controlled pilot study. *Behav. Res. Ther.* **2012**, *50*, 797–804. [CrossRef]
21. Key, A.; George, C.L.; Beattie, D.; Stammers, K.; Lacey, H.; Waller, G. Body image treatment within an inpatient program for anorexia nervosa: The role of mirror exposure in the desensitization process. *Int. J. Eat. Disord.* **2002**, *31*, 185–190. [CrossRef]
22. Moreno-Domínguez, S.; Rodríguez-Ruiz, S.; Fernández-Santaella, M.C.; Jansen, A.; Tuschen-Caffier, B. Pure versus guided mirror exposure to reduce body dissatisfaction: A preliminary study with university women. *Body Image* **2012**, *9*, 285–288. [CrossRef] [PubMed]
23. Jansen, A.; Voorwinde, V.; Hoebink, Y.; Rekkers, M.; Martijn, C.; Mulkens, S. Mirror exposure to increase body satisfaction: Should we guide the focus of attention towards positively or negatively evaluated body parts? *J. Behav. Ther. Exp. Psychiatry* **2016**, *50*, 90–96. [CrossRef] [PubMed]
24. Vocks, S.; Legenbauer, T.; Wächter, A.; Wucherer, M.; Kosfelder, J. What happens in the course of body exposure? Emotional, cognitive, and physiological reactions to mirror confrontation in eating disorders. *J. Psychosom. Res.* **2007**, *62*, 231–239. [CrossRef] [PubMed]
25. Delinsky, S.S.; Wilson, G.T. Mirror exposure for the treatment of body image disturbance. *Int. J. Eat. Disord.* **2006**, *39*, 108–116. [CrossRef]
26. Gutiérrez-Maldonado, J.; Wiederhold, B.K.; Riva, G. Future directions: How virtual reality can further improve the assessment and treatment of eating disorders and obesity. *Cyberpsychol. Behav. Soc. Netw.* **2016**, *19*, 148–153. [CrossRef]
27. Garcia-Palacios, A.; Botella, C.; Hoffman, H.; Fabregat, S. Comparing acceptance and refusal rates of virtual reality exposure vs. in vivo exposure by patients with specific phobias. *Cyberpsychol. Behav.* **2007**, *10*, 722–724. [CrossRef]
28. Gutiérrez-Maldonado, J.; Ferrer-García, M.; Dakanalis, A.; Riva, G. Virtual reality: Applications to eating disorders. In *The Oxford Handbook of Eating Disorders*; Oxford University Press: Oxford, UK, 2018.
29. Riva, G.; Serino, S.; Di Lernia, D.; Pavone, E.F.; Dakanalis, A. Embodied medicine: Mens sana in corpore virtuale sano. *Front. Hum. Neurosci.* **2017**, *11*, 120. [CrossRef]
30. Riva, G.; Wiederhold, B.K.; Mantovani, F. Neuroscience of Virtual Reality: From Virtual Exposure to Embodied Medicine. *Cyberpsychol. Behav. Soc. Netw.* **2019**, *22*, 82–96. [CrossRef]
31. Maselli, A.; Slater, M. The building blocks of the full body ownership illusion. *Front. Hum. Neurosci.* **2013**, *7*, 83. [CrossRef]
32. Piryankova, I.V.; Wong, H.Y.; Linkenauger, S.A.; Stinson, C.; Longo, M.R.; Bülthoff, H.H.; Mohler, B.J. Owning an overweight or underweight body: Distinguishing the physical, experienced and virtual body. *PLoS ONE* **2014**, *9*, e103428.
33. Botvinick, M.; Cohen, J. Rubber hands 'feel' touch that eyes see. *Nature* **1998**, *391*, 756. [CrossRef] [PubMed]
34. Eshkevari, E.; Rieger, E.; Longo, M.R.; Haggard, P.; Treasure, J. Increased plasticity of the bodily self in eating disorders. *Psychol. Med.* **2012**, *42*, 819–828. [CrossRef] [PubMed]
35. Serino, S.; Pedroli, E.; Keizer, A.; Triberti, S.; Dakanalis, A.; Pallavicini, F.; Chirico, A.; Riva, G. Virtual reality body swapping: A tool for modifying the allocentric memory of the body. *Cyberpsychol. Behav. Soc. Netw.* **2016**, *19*, 127–133. [CrossRef] [PubMed]
36. Preston, C.; Ehrsson, H.H. Illusory changes in body size modulate body satisfaction in a way that is related to non-clinical eating disorder psychopathology. *PLoS ONE* **2014**, *9*, e85773.
37. Preston, C.; Ehrsson, H.H. Illusory obesity triggers body dissatisfaction responses in the insula and anterior cingulate cortex. *Cereb. Cortex* **2016**, *26*, 4450–4460. [CrossRef]
38. Porras Garcia, B.; Ferrer Garcia, M.; Olszewska, A.; Yilmaz, L.; González Ibañez, C.; Gracia Blanes, M.; Gültekin, G.; Serrano Troncoso, E.; Gutiérrez Maldonado, J. Is this my own body? Changing the perceptual and affective body image experience among college students using a new virtual reality embodiment-based technique. *J. Clin. Med.* **2019**, *8*, 925. [CrossRef]
39. Keizer, A.; Van Elburg, A.; Helms, R.; Dijkerman, H.C. A virtual reality full body illusion improves body image disturbance in anorexia nervosa. *PLoS ONE* **2016**, *11*, e0163921. [CrossRef]
40. Serino, S.; Polli, N.; Riva, G. From avatars to body swapping: The use of virtual reality for assessing and treating body-size distortion in individuals with anorexia. *J. Clin. Psychol.* **2019**, *75*, 313–322. [CrossRef]

41. Porras-Garcia, B.; Serrano-Troncoso, E.; Carulla-Roig, M.; Soto-Usera, P.; Ferrer-Garcia, M.; Figueras-Puigderrajols, N.; Yilmaz, L.; Onur Sen, Y.; Shojaeian, N.; Gutiérrez-Maldonado, J. Virtual Reality Body Exposure Therapy for Anorexia Nervosa. A Case Report with Follow-Up Results. *Front. Psychol.* **2020**, *11*, 956. [CrossRef]
42. Levinson, C.A.; Rapp, J.; Riley, E.N. Addressing the fear of fat: Extending imaginal exposure therapy for anxiety disorders to anorexia nervosa. *Eat. Weight Disord. Stud. Anorex. Bulim. Obes.* **2014**, *19*, 521–524. [CrossRef]
43. Garner, D. *Eating Disorder Inventory-3: Professional Manual*; Psychological Assessment Resources: Lutz, FL, USA, 2004.
44. Elosua, P.; López-Jaúregui, A.; Sánchez-Sánchez, F. *EDI-3, Inventario de Trastornos de la Conducta Alimentaria-3, Manual*; Tea Ediciones: Madrid, Spain, 2010.
45. Gardner, R.M.; Jappe, L.M.; Gardner, L. Development and validation of a new figural drawing scale for body-image assessment: The BIAS-BD. *J. Clin. Psychol.* **2009**, *65*, 113–122. [CrossRef] [PubMed]
46. Avalos, L.; Tylka, T.L.; Wood-Barcalow, N. The body appreciation scale: Development and psychometric evaluation. *Body Image* **2005**, *2*, 285–297. [CrossRef] [PubMed]
47. Lobera, I.J.; Ríos, P.B. Spanish Version of the Body Appreciation Scale (BAS) for Adolescents. *Span. J. Psychol.* **2011**, *14*, 411–420. [CrossRef] [PubMed]
48. Jacob, R.J.K.; Karn, K.S. Eye Tracking in Human-Computer Interaction and Usability Research. Ready to Deliver the Promises. In *The Mind's Eye: Cognitive and Applied Aspects of Eye Movement Research*; Elsevier: Amsterdam, The Netherlands, 2003; pp. 573–605.
49. Jiang, M.Y.W.; Vartanian, L.R. A review of existing measures of attentional biases in body image and eating disorders research. *Aust. J. Psychol.* **2018**, *70*, 3–17. [CrossRef]
50. Porras-Garcia, B.; Ferrer-Garcia, M.; Ghita, A.; Moreno, M.; López-Jiménez, L.; Vallvé-Romeu, A.; Serrano-Troncoso, E.; Gutiérrez-Maldonado, J. The influence of gender and body dissatisfaction on body-related attentional bias: An eye-tracking and virtual reality study. *Int. J. Eat. Disord.* **2019**, *52*, 181–1190. [CrossRef]
51. Porras-Garcia, B.; Ferrer-Garcia, M.; Yilmaz, L.; Sen, Y.O.; Olszewska, A.; Ghita, A.; Serrano-Troncoso, E.; Treasure, J.; Gutiérrez-Maldonado, J. Body-related attentional bias as mediator of the relationship between body mass index and body dissatisfaction. *Eur. Eat. Disord. Rev.* **2020**. [CrossRef]
52. Porras-Garcia, B.; Exposito-Sanz, E.; Ferrer-Garcia, M.; Castillero-Mimenza, O.; Gutiérrez-Maldonado, J. Body-Related Attentional Bias among Men with High and Low Muscularity Dissatisfaction. *J. Clin. Med.* **2020**, *9*, 1736. [CrossRef]
53. Sheehan, D.V.; Lecrubier, Y.; Sheehan, K.H.; Amorim, P.; Janavs, J.; Weiller, E.; Dunbar, G.C. The Mini-International Neuropsychiatric Interview (MINI): The development and validation of a structured diagnostic psychiatric interview for DSM-IV and ICD-10. *J. Clin. Psychiatry* **1998**, *9*, 1736.
54. Jansen, A.; Nederkoorn, C.; Mulkens, S. Selective visual attention for ugly and beautiful body parts in eating disorders. *Behav. Res. Ther.* **2005**, *50*, 90–96. [CrossRef]
55. Roefs, A.; Jansen, A.; Moresi, S.; Willems, P.; van Grootel, S.; van der Borgh, A. Looking good. BMI, attractiveness bias and visual attention. *Appetite* **2008**, *51*, 552–555. [CrossRef]
56. Schminder, E.; Ziegler, M.; Danay, E.; Beyer, L.; Bühner, M. Is it really robust? Reinvestigating the robustness of ANOVA against violations of the normal distribution. *Methodology* **2010**, *6*, 147–151. [CrossRef]
57. Gagne, D.A.; Von Holle, A.; Brownley, K.A.; Runfola, C.D.; Hofmeier, S.; Branch, K.E.; Bulik, C.M. Eating disorder symptoms and weight and shape concerns in a large web-based convenience sample of women ages 50 and above: Results of the gender and body image (GABI) study. *Int. J. Eat. Disord.* **2012**, *45*, 832–844. [CrossRef] [PubMed]
58. Slof-Op 't Landt, M.C.T.; van Furth, E.F.; van Beijsterveldt, C.E.M.; Bartels, M.; Willemsen, G.; de Geus, E.J.; Ligthart, L.; Boomsma, D.I. Prevalence of dieting and fear of weight gain across ages: A community sample from adolescents to the elderly. *Int. J. Public Health* **2017**, *62*, 911–919. [CrossRef] [PubMed]
59. Keenaghan, S.; Bowles, L.; Crawford, G.; Thurlbeck, S.; Kentridge, R.W.; Cowie, D. My body until proven otherwise: Exploring the time course of the full body illusion. *Conscious. Cogn.* **2020**, *78*, 102882. [CrossRef] [PubMed]
60. Freeman, R.; Touyz, S.; Sara, G.; Rennie, C.; Gordon, E.; Beumont, P. In the eye of the beholder: Processing body shape information in anorexic and bulimic patients. *Int. J. Eat. Disord.* **1991**, *10*, 709–714. [CrossRef]

61. Tuschen-Caffier, B.; Bender, C.; Caffier, D.; Klenner, K.; Braks, K.; Svaldi, J. Selective visual attention during mirror exposure in anorexia and bulimia nervosa. *PLoS ONE* **2015**, *10*, e0145886. [CrossRef] [PubMed]
62. Heinrich, H.; Moll, G.H.; Horndasch, S.; Hönig, F.; Nöth, E.; Kratz, O.; Holczinger, A. "Looks do matter"—Visual attentional biases in adolescent girls with eating disorders viewing body images. *Psychiatry Res.* **2012**, *198*, 321–323.
63. Rushford, N. Fear of gaining weight: Its validity as a visual analogue scale in anorexia nervosa. *Eur. Eat. Disord. Rev.* **2006**, *14*, 104–110. [CrossRef]
64. Gonzalez-Franco, M.; Peck, T.C. Avatar embodiment. Towards a standardized questionnaire. *Front. Robot. AI* **2018**, *5*, 74. [CrossRef]
65. MacCallum, R.C.; Zhang, S.; Preacher, K.J.; Rucker, D.D. On the practice of dichotomization of quantitative variables. *Psychol. Methods* **2002**, *7*, 19–40. [CrossRef]
66. Mölbert, S.C.; Thaler, A.; Mohler, B.J.; Streuber, S.; Romero, J.; Black, M.J.; Zipfel, S.; Karnath, H.O.; Giel, K.E. Assessing body image in anorexia nervosa using biometric self-avatars in virtual reality: Attitudinal components rather than visual body size estimation are distorted. *Psychol. Med.* **2018**, *48*, 642–653. [CrossRef] [PubMed]
67. Murray, S.B.; Loeb, K.L.; Le Grange, D. Dissecting the core fear in anorexia nervosa: Can we optimize treatment mechanisms? *JAMA Psychiatry* **2016**, *73*, 891–892. [CrossRef] [PubMed]
68. Kredel, R.; Vater, C.; Klostermann, A.; Hossner, E.J. Eye-tracking technology and the dynamics of natural gaze behavior in sports: A systematic review of 40 years of research. *Front. Psychol.* **2017**, *8*, 1845. [CrossRef] [PubMed]

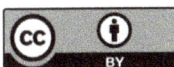

© 2020 by the authors. Licensee MDPI, Basel, Switzerland. This article is an open access article distributed under the terms and conditions of the Creative Commons Attribution (CC BY) license (http://creativecommons.org/licenses/by/4.0/).

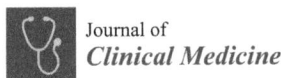

Review

Cognitive Interpersonal Model for Anorexia Nervosa Revisited: The Perpetuating Factors that Contribute to the Development of the Severe and Enduring Illness

Janet Treasure [1,†], Daniel Willmott [1,†,*], Suman Ambwani [2], Valentina Cardi [1], Danielle Clark Bryan [1], Katie Rowlands [1] and Ulrike Schmidt [1]

1. Section of Eating Disorders, Department of Psychological Medicine, Institute of Psychiatry, Psychology and Neuroscience, King's College London, SE5 8AF London, UK; janet.treasure@kcl.ac.uk (J.T.); valentina.cardi@kcl.ac.uk (V.C.); danielle.clarkbryan@kcl.ac.uk (D.C.B.); katie.rowlands@kcl.ac.uk (K.R.); ulrike.schmidt@kcl.ac.uk (U.S.)
2. Department of Psychology, Dickinson College, Carlisle, PA17013, USA; ambwanis@dickinson.edu
* Correspondence: daniel.p.willmott@kcl.ac.uk
† These authors equally contributed to this work.

Received: 30 January 2020; Accepted: 25 February 2020; Published: 27 February 2020

Abstract: The cognitive interpersonal model was outlined initially in 2006 in a paper describing the valued and visible aspects of anorexia nervosa (Schmidt and Treasure, 2006). In 2013, we summarised many of the cognitive and emotional traits underpinning the model (Treasure and Schmidt, 2013). In this paper, we describe in more detail the perpetuating aspects of the model, which include the inter- and intrapersonal related consequences of isolation, depression, and chronic stress that accumulate in the severe and enduring stage of the illness. Since we developed the model, we have been using it to frame research and development at the Maudsley. We have developed and tested interventions for both patients and close others, refining the model through iterative cycles of model/intervention development in line with the Medical Research Council (MRC) framework for complex interventions. For example, we have defined the consequences of living with the illness on close others (including medical professionals) and characterised the intense emotional reactions and behaviours that follow. For the individual with an eating disorder, these counter-reactions can allow the eating disorder to become entrenched. In addition, the consequent chronic stress from starvation and social pain set in motion processes such as depression, neuroprogression, and neuroadaptation. Thus, anorexia nervosa develops a life of its own that is resistant to treatment. In this paper, we describe the underpinnings of the model and how this can be targeted into treatment.

Keywords: anorexia nervosa; cognitive interpersonal model; severe enduring

1. Introduction

The Medical Research Council has described a framework for the process of development of complex interventions [1]. This involves a procedure in which treatments targeting risk or maintaining factors for an illness are fine-tuned following feedback from proof of concept, feasibility, and pilot studies, including both quantitative and qualitative outcomes. Furthermore, within UK health care research conducted in the National Health Service (NHS), a strong emphasis is placed upon the involvement of patients, carers, and the public to co-design interventions and services. We have used this combined approach to design interventions and services for people with anorexia nervosa (AN).

The first iteration of the cognitive interpersonal model for AN outlined core valued and visible maintaining factors of the illness (Figure 1) [2]; the visible aspects of the disorder elicit deep concern from close others, which is in stark contrast to the egosyntonic nature of the illness, where the sufferer values certain aspects of the illness and does not identify themselves as 'sick'. In the next iteration of the model, we outlined the underpinning neuroscience, the interaction between vulnerability traits and eating disorder behaviours, and how this serves to strengthen the hold of the disorder, allowing it over time to develop a life of its own [3]. Indeed, individuals with a persistent form of the illness often state that they want to change but cannot do so. Examples of interactions between vulnerability traits and eating disorder behaviours include personality traits such as conscientiousness and introversion [4], which can predispose to disordered eating [5] and allow eating disorder habits to become fixed. Furthermore, recent genetic findings reported on correlations between polygenic risk scores, not only with other "brain" disorders, but also with "metabolic" traits related to growth, size, lipids, and insulin sensitivity [6]. Thus, a possible hypothesis is that homeostatic forces maintaining energy balance might be weaker in terms of increasing appetite and stronger in terms of a foraging or over active response to "food shortage". This argument has been developed in more detail in an evolutionary-based model of AN and might benefit from further exploration [7].

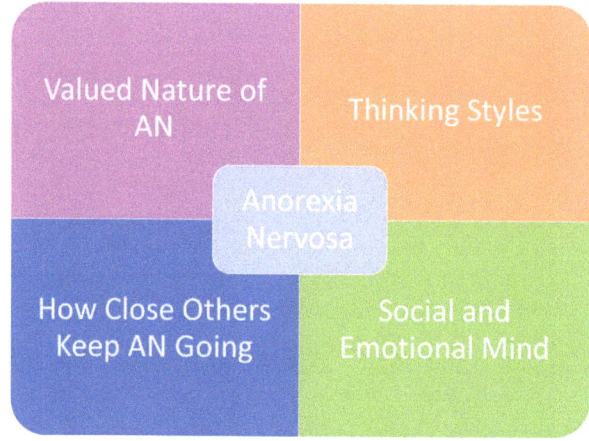

Figure 1. The cognitive–interpersonal maintenance model of anorexia nervosa.

2. Staging Models of Anorexia Nervosa: the Enhanced Cognitive Interpersonal Maintenance Model

This next iteration of the model describes in more detail the development of the severe and enduring form of AN [8]. Current diagnostic procedures do not account for clinical features such as illness trajectory, severity, and co-morbidity, which may impact on the effectiveness of current treatments. The maintenance model of severe and enduring AN consists of three components (Figure 2). The first domain includes the interpersonal consequences of AN. These arise in part because of the impact of chronic starvation on social cognition and the reaction of others to the illness. The next domain relates to the behavioural consequences of AN. Neuroadaptation and habits develop as a consequence of repeated behaviours. Moreover, feeding experiences can increase aversive learning towards food. The third domain relates to the chronic stress response, which may relate to a genetic predisposition to susceptibility, early adversity, or be a secondary response to chronic starvation.

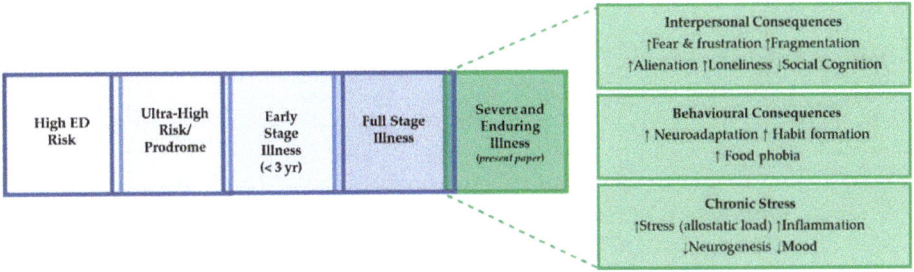

Figure 2. Severe and enduring anorexia nervosa: a maintenance model.

In this paper, we consider in more depth these three domains that contribute to the development of the severe enduring form of illness.

3. Social Risk and Maintaining Factors

Difficulties with interpersonal relationships predispose to the development of AN and are also secondary consequences of the disorder, contributing to the perseverance of the illness.

Social anxiety is a common precursor of eating disorders [9]. In some cases, this is part of the autistic spectrum profile of symptoms that has been observed [10,11], and problems with social cognition may form part of the genetic liability. For example, the offspring of mothers with a history of an eating disorder had anomalies in social cognition during childhood [12]. This familial association suggests that problems in social cognition may be an endophenotype that increases the risk of developing an ED. In addition, adverse social experiences during development such as childhood maltreatment [13], insecure attachment [14], or teasing, bullying, or social exclusion [15] can shape interpersonal relationships and disrupt normal identity development, potentially by increasing the salience of competitive patterns of interaction that can fuel striving for perfection and greater internalisation of beauty ideals as a standard to define the self [16].

Furthermore, people with AN are more likely to report early maladaptive schema (pervasive negative themes regarding the self and one's relationship with others [17]) and difficulties in emotion regulation, with a greater use of dysfunctional interpersonal emotion regulation strategies [18,19]. Problems in emotion regulation may play a key role in maintaining the symptoms of AN [20]. Thus, an interaction between social vulnerability traits, risks within the interpersonal environment, and dysfunctional emotion processing can predispose to the development of AN, a "social–emotional disorder" [21].

Problems in social cognition also can arise as secondary consequences of starvation. Anomalies in social cognition are most pronounced in the acute phase of illness and are less marked after recovery [22]. The anomalies include deficits in nonverbal emotional expression [23,24], an inability to provide a spontaneous social narrative and to identify the social salience of stimuli [25], a sensitivity to threat [26], to social comparison [27], misalignments in social reciprocity [28], and the avoidance or suppression of emotions, particularly to avoid conflict [19]. Impairments in nonverbal communication and a lack of reciprocation of warmth elicits the "uncanny valley" aversive response in others [29–31]. This can lead to social exclusion and isolation, which is a defining facet of the illness [32].

3.1. Interpersonal Reactions to Living with Anorexia Nervosa

A mental health professional with lived experience of AN used one word to epitomize the illness: "isolation" [32]. However, family members are usually closely involved in the evolution of AN, which commonly has its onset in early adolescence. Close others can encourage help seeking in the early phase of the illness, which in turn may have a favourable effect on the prognosis. Nevertheless, the individual's resistance to the need for treatment can make negotiating this transition difficult. The disruption of family functioning, work, and social adjustment varies accordingly with the developmental age, mood, and other clinical features. Many patients with a chronic form of illness remain dependent on their families or the state during their lifetime [33].

The anxiety engendered by the overt "ill state" and the frustration caused by the resistance to implement the obvious solution "to eat" fuels a profound and mixed emotional reaction in both professionals (nurses on inpatient units) [34] and families [35]. Lack of insight into the illness is particularly pronounced in restrictive AN and persists during and after treatment [36,37]. Critical, hostile, overprotective, and controlling behaviours can develop as counter reactions [38,39]. Family members may appease and collude with eating disorder behaviours, becoming organised around eating disorder rules (accommodating to the illness) and ignoring or covering up for the negative consequences of the behaviours (inadvertently enabling the illness) [40].

These diverse reactions can cause divisions amongst family members. Some family members shoulder an overly high burden, whilst others become disempowered and disengaged. Aspects of the caregiving experience are summarised in systematic reviews [35]. High perceived burden and low caregiving efficacy are common and are associated with clinical levels of depression and anxiety. In addition, the societal reaction to the illness (including interactions with services) can be problematic.

Carers' own practical and emotional reactions to the illness can cause harm to the family unit as relationship ruptures occur in response to accommodating and enabling behaviours [41] or divergent forms of reactive expressed emotion develop. Siblings can be drawn into caregiving, develop their own problems, or leave home prematurely as their needs may be neglected [42,43]. Thus, a vicious circle of escalating interpersonal stress can develop.

The protracted course of the illness and the entanglement between eating and social function means that close others have the potential to remediate these difficulties. Therefore, it is important that carers and close others are involved across the lifespan and not excluded from the treatment process. Clinicians explain this exclusion through concerns around confidentiality, but this is considered a misinterpretation of the law [44].

3.2. Targeting Stressful Interpersonal Reactions

A hypothesis that follows from the cognitive interpersonal model is that the toxic consequences that accrue from the isolation and loneliness of an eating disorder can be ameliorated by skills training for family members or close others across the lifespan [45]. Improving the interpersonal environment often begins at home. Close others are highly motivated to help but are often uncertain of what they can do. Materials coproduced with carers and patients have been developed to illustrate these problems [39] and provide a curriculum for workshops to help carers provide effective support.

These materials explain how the patients' primary and secondary difficulties in social cognition make relationships difficult. For example, the reduced facial expressivity of eating disorder patients [23,24] makes it hard for others to appreciate their level of terror or show appreciation of the carers' distress. AN patients appear to be impervious to the impact of their behaviours on other people. This lack of concern for others appears in the domain of caregiving when others are distressed at their lack of insight and unwillingness to accept the sick role. It also can be evident in treatment facilities where overt demonstration and discussion of eating disorder behaviours can trigger distress in their peers.

The three basic elements of carer skill-sharing interventions include:

(1) Psychoeducation about the illness and framing patient presentation within the cognitive–interpersonal model, highlighting predisposing, precipitating, and perpetuating factors.

(2) Information about how carers might be able to moderate and mould the energy and insight from their own emotional reactions to foster a calm, compassionate, and collaborative context (a life skill that they can role model to the person with the eating disorder).

(3) Introduction to effective support and behaviour change skills such as motivational interviewing, the use of risk-taking experiments, and exposure to fear [46].

Interventions based on this model have been delivered in a range of different formats including workshops and guided self-help interventions with individual or group support. An improved understanding about the illness reduces carer distress and burden [35,45,47,48]. Several studies have found that augmenting treatment with these resources for carers reduces both carer and service burden [49–51]. Often this has involved a 'train the trainer' approach whereby carers and patients deliver these interventions. Pépin and King [52] tested the workshops in a pilot study in Australia, finding participation led to reductions in carer distress and burden and helped them to modify their emotional reactions to the illness. Psychoeducational carer workshops reduce carer psychological distress and burden, yet when collaborative carer skills are taught as well, there are secondary effects on alleviating patients' anxiety and depression [53].

Treatment for individuals with AN based on the cognitive interpersonal model, the Maudsley Model of Anorexia Treatment for Adults (MANTRA) [54,55], also includes a section for carers. Carers are encouraged to cultivate their own emotional and social intelligence by examining the relevant modules for patients so that they can role model these skills to their loved ones. It is helpful if both parties externalise the illness and understand how the AN voice can trap everyone into spirals of confusion. A compassionate, mutually supportive family environment is essential as it is inevitable that miscues and mistakes will happen, but these can be reframed as being valuable opportunities of learning.

4. Behavioural Consequences of Anorexia Nervosa

The repeated patterns of behaviour that underpin the development of AN, such as avoiding high caloric, highly palatable foods, becomes habitual. Initially, these behaviours are initiated to achieve a specific goal and are reinforced as they are positively rewarding. With daily repetition, the actions become automatic and entrenched until they are activated with no conscious effort in response to a stimulus or cue [56]. A recent cognitive neuroscience model of AN proposes that habitual behaviours are mediated within dorsal frontostriatal circuits [57–59]. In line with this, techniques from habit reversal therapy with inpatients led to significant reductions in eating disorder symptoms and self-reported habit strengths [60]. These preliminary findings could be used to augment or guide developments in treatment for those with severe and enduring difficulties.

In addition, fear and/or disgust responses to food represents a key challenge to weight restoration [61]. People with AN show reduced extinction of fear learning but increased fear generalisation and reinstatement, which may contribute to the strength of these fear learning networks [62]. These fears may originate from adverse experiences relating to food and body shape during sensitive periods of development [63]. Furthermore, these could be iatrogenically aggravated by coercive treatment experiences such as nasogastric feeding under restraint. A qualitative study with nurses identified that power battles over 'punitive' feeding causes patients great anguish and can rupture the therapeutic alliance [64]. These interactions may be overlooked as a complicating feature within family-based treatment [65]. Interestingly, in adolescence, reduced extinction of fears appears to be more pronounced with co-morbid depression [66].

Exposure is the standard treatment for fear learning. The underlying mechanism involves developing new learning to the threatening stimulus (as opposed to habituation to anxiety) and updating the fear pathways in the brain [67,68]. There are some caveats in applying this treatment to AN. First, one of the feared consequences, weight gain, is an expected and necessary consequence of refeeding. Furthermore, with fluid fluxes and other aspects of metabolic instability during this phase, a "lack of control of weight" can maintain AN cognitions. Moreover, it is probable that neurogenesis is reduced as a sequelae of the chronic stress of AN, reducing the effectiveness of exposure. A variety of techniques have been used to facilitate this learning. These include positive mood induction [69], the addition of cycloserine to consolidate learning [70,71], and virtual reality [72].

Other training approaches developed to target risk factors show some promise in proof-of-concept studies. These include cognitive remediation approaches that focus on cultivating a flexible, big picture style of thinking [73], cognitive skills training for social avoidance [74], and go/no-go inhibition training [75], which may be of value for the binge–purge form of the illness. Food-related attention bias modification training is also being investigated as an add-on intervention for AN, following directions from anxiety disorder research [76,77].

5. Chronic Stress Response: Co-Morbidity with Depression and Anxiety

Another maintaining factor in the model is the impact of chronic starvation leading to anhedonia and accentuating existing co-morbidities. Emotional distress is common as both a predisposition and a secondary consequence that perpetuates the illness [20,78,79]. This emotional distress may occur due to a shared genetic predisposition [6]; developmental trauma [80], with emotional abuse (e.g., bullying) playing a central role [81]; or as a feature of starvation [82].

Depressive symptomatology may follow a persistent trajectory over the lifetime, independently from eating disorder symptoms [83,84]. Approximately 50% of patients with AN report a minimum of one episode of a mood disorder during their lifetime [85,86]. Depression, anxiety, and interpersonal sensitivity are central nodes in a network analysis of symptoms [87] with key bridging roles [81]. The symptom profile differs somewhat from that of unipolar depression in that somatic features such as loss of energy and reduced activation are less pronounced, whereas cognitive features such as negative views of the self are higher [88]. Indeed, the chance of recovery is reduced in people who developed AN after they had experienced depression [89]. In addition, the long-term outcomes of patients with AN complicated with mood comorbidity were reduced [90]. Consequently, psychological well-being, positive supportive relationships, hope, identity, meaning, and purpose are important markers of recovery [91,92].

Anxiety traits are also linked to eating disorders. Obsessive–compulsive personality traits, obsessive–compulsive disorders, and anxiety [9,93,94] often present in childhood prior to the onset of AN. In addition, there is a strong familial association with these traits [95,96]. The strongest polygenic risk correlations from genome wide association studies (GWAS) of AN is shared with OCD [97], whereas correlations with neuroticism, depression, and anxiety are half the size [6]. In a network analysis of eating disorder and anxiety traits, avoidance of social eating was the strongest bridge node, with eating symptoms and low self-confidence being the strongest bridge node with anxiety traits [98].

In a longitudinal study, the neural correlates of disordered eating and obsessive–compulsive disorder at age 14 included an increase in grey matter volume in the orbitofrontal cortex, the right dorsolateral prefrontal cortex, and the ventral striatum [99]. However, people with a chronic illness had a decrease in grey matter in the cerebellum and the mesencephalon, specifically the substantia nigra and ventral tegmental area [100]. Hippocampal volume is particularly reduced [101–103] which is associated with anxiety and depression [102] and correlated with raised cortisol [104]. Patients in the later stage of AN have increased ventral striatal activation to body image cues than patients in the early stage of illness [105,106].

The chronic stress profile associated with enduring AN [107] is similar to that found in treatment resistant depression [108] and with the 'ecophenotype' associated with childhood maltreatment [109]. This chronic stress response includes hyperactivity of the hypothalamic pituitary adrenal (HPA) axis [101,110–112], activation of the immune system [113,114], and anomalies in the microbiome [115,116]. There is a widespread reduction in brain volume, which is possibly secondary to reduced neurogenesis [117], which may be the most marked in the hippocampus [118] and associated with raised cortisol levels [104]. This broad stress response reduces resilience [119] and may be accompanied by reduced mesolimbic dopamine function, anhedonia, and lack of motivation [120]. Thus, a sizeable proportion of patients could be classified as fulfilling the criteria of treatment-resistant depression.

Treatment-Resistant Depression and other Co-Morbidities as Maintaining Factors: Implications for Treatment

Treatments targeting nutritional recovery are less effective for improving mood [49,50,79,121–123]. Therefore, it is possible that strategies used for treatment-resistant depression might be of benefit for people with severe enduring AN. Proof-of-concept studies of neuromodulation such as deep brain stimulation [124] and repetitive transcranial magnetic stimulation have shown potential [125–127]. Interestingly, the trajectory of symptom change following these neuromodulation techniques shows differences to that found with more traditional eating disorder treatment, in that an improvement in mood is the main initial effect, whereas improvements in eating disorder psychopathology follow later [125,126,128].

Interest in pharmacological approaches is starting to increase, as summarised in a recent review [129]. There is mixed evidence for the use of antipsychotic medications to treat AN [130], although a recent multicenter outpatient study of olanzapine found small positive effects on agitation and weight gain (albeit with no difference in rates of hospitalisation) [131]. The field may need to consider using drugs that have been shown to have benefit in OCD. For example, high doses of Selective Serotonin Reuptake Inhibitors (SSRIs), exposure, and response treatment are effective for people in the later stages of OCD [132], which has also been recently conceptualized within a staging framework [133]. In addition, there is interest in pharmacological approaches that are being used for treatment-resistant depression, such as ketamine and psilocybin [134]. Interestingly, ketamine showed some promise in a small series of studies in the 1990s [135]. A pilot study of the effects of ketamine on mood and eating disorder cognitions in people with severe and enduring AN is registered on the Australia New Zealand Clinical Trial Registry (anzctr.org.au, ACTRN12618001393246p) and additionally, a psilocybin trial for AN is currently registered (ClinicalTrials.gov, NCT04052568). Therefore, we echo the call by Franko and colleagues [90] to consider using a combined approach to target both mood and eating disorder symptoms, with clear characterization of the patient group.

Although not the topic of this paper, given the similarities between staging models for other psychiatric disorders [8], it may be of interest to look at the other end of the trajectory, the ultra-high risk (UHR) group, and consider whether there might be interventions that could be matched to this stage and provide primary or secondary prevention approaches. The first step is to define the UHR phenotype, which may include traits such as behavioural inhibition, perfectionism, early symptoms of OCD, or social–emotional difficulties.

6. Conclusions

In this latest iteration of the cognitive interpersonal model, we have described treatments targeting modifiable elements. Increasing social connection through encouraging a collaborative inclusive approach towards recovery, by increasing the knowledge and skills of family members, decreases the need for high-intensity care (day or inpatient) and reduces carer burden and patient isolation [49–51,136]. Treatment using MANTRA focuses on both inter and intrapersonal model elements [55,56]. Augmenting treatment through digital technology is showing potential [137]. Finally, we are borrowing approaches that show promise in other domains of psychiatry in which a chronic stress response has led to the illness having a life of its own. Neuromodulation techniques are encouraging, and new pharmacological approaches are in progress. Services may need to implement broader clinical assessment skills to more accurately stage the illness to personalise treatments to match patient's needs and preferences.

However, it is too early for this model to be ossified. The field of eating disorders has been starved of resources for research, and so the evidence is limited. Nevertheless, we think that by using this framework in order to identify targets and by using high-quality randomised controlled trials, we will be able to develop more effective treatments through an iterative process.

Author Contributions: Conceptualization, J.T.; writing—original draft preparation, J.T. and D.W.; writing and editing, J.T. and D.W.; reviewing manuscript, S.A., D.C.B., V.C., K.R. and U.S. All authors have read and agreed to the published version of the manuscript.

Funding: This manuscript was funded through the NIHR-HTA program (project reference number 14/68/09).

Acknowledgments: VC, JT and US acknowledge financial support from the National Institute for Health Research (NIHR) Specialist Biomedical Research Centre for Mental Health award to the South London and Maudsley NHS

Foundation Trust and the Institute of Psychiatry, King's College London. US is supported by an NIHR Senior Investigator Award.

Conflicts of Interest: The authors declare no conflicts of interest.

References

1. Craig, P.; Dieppe, P.; Macintyre, S.; Michie, S.; Nazareth, I.; Petticrew, M. Developing and evaluating complex interventions: The new Medical Research Council guidance. *BMJ* **2008**, *337*, a1655. [CrossRef] [PubMed]
2. Schmidt, U.; Treasure, J. Anorexia nervosa: Valued and visible. A cognitive-interpersonal maintenance model and its implications for research and practice. *Br. J. Clin. Psychol.* **2006**, *45*, 343–366. [CrossRef] [PubMed]
3. Treasure, J.; Schmidt, U. The cognitive-interpersonal maintenance model of anorexia nervosa revisited: A summary of the evidence for cognitive, socio-emotional and interpersonal predisposing and perpetuating factors. *J. Eat. Disord.* **2013**, *1*, 13. [CrossRef]
4. Farstad, S.M.; McGeown, L.M.; von Ranson, K.M. Eating disorders and personality, 2004–2016: A systematic review and meta-analysis. *Clin. Psychol. Rev.* **2016**, *46*, 91–105. [CrossRef]
5. Miller, J.L.; Schmidt, L.A.; Vaillancourt, T.; McDougall, P.; Laliberte, M. Neuroticism and introversion: A risky combination for disordered eating among a non-clinical sample of undergraduate women. *Eat. Behav.* **2006**, *7*, 69–78. [CrossRef]
6. Watson, H.J.; Yilmaz, Z.; Thornton, L.M.; Hübel, C.; Coleman, J.R.; Gaspar, H.A.; Medland, S.E. Genome-wide association study identifies eight risk loci and implicates metabo-psychiatric origins for anorexia nervosa. *Nat. Genet.* **2019**, *51*, 1207–1214. [CrossRef]
7. Guisinger, S. Adapted to flee famine: Adding an evolutionary perspective on anorexia nervosa. *Psychol. Rev.* **2003**, *110*, 745. [CrossRef]
8. Treasure, J.; Stein, D.; Maguire, S. Has the time come for a staging model to map the course of eating disorders from high risk to severe enduring illness? An examination of the evidence. *Early Interv. Psychiatry* **2015**, *9*, 173–184. [CrossRef]
9. Goddard, E.; Treasure, J. Anxiety and social-emotional processing in eating disorders: Examination of family trios. *Cogn. Ther. Res.* **2013**, *37*, 890–904. [CrossRef]
10. Rhind, C.; Bonfioli, E.; Hibbs, R.; Goddard, E.; Macdonald, P.; Gowers, S.; Treasure, J. An examination of autism spectrum traits in adolescents with anorexia nervosa and their parents. *Mol. Autism* **2014**, *5*, 56. [CrossRef]
11. Nielsen, S.; Anckarsäter, H.; Gillberg, C.; Gillberg, C.; Råstam, M.; Wentz, E. Effects of autism spectrum disorders on outcome in teenage-onset anorexia nervosa evaluated by the Morgan-Russell outcome assessment schedule: A controlled community-based study. *Mol. Autism* **2015**, *6*, 14. [CrossRef] [PubMed]
12. Kothari, R.; Barona, M.; Treasure, J.O.; Micali, N. Social cognition in children at familial high-risk of developing an eating disorder. *Front. Behav. Neurosc.* **2015**, *9*, 208. [CrossRef] [PubMed]
13. Johnson, J.G.; Cohen, P.; Kasen, S.; Brook, J.S. Childhood adversities associated with risk for eating disorders or weight problems during adolescence or early adulthood. *Am. J. Psychiatry* **2002**, *159*, 394–400. [CrossRef] [PubMed]
14. Jewell, T.; Collyer, H.; Gardner, T.; Tchanturia, K.; Simic, M.; Fonagy, P.; Eisler, I. Attachment and mentalization and their association with child and adolescent eating pathology: A systematic review. *Int. J. Eat. Disord.* **2016**, *49*, 354–373. [CrossRef]
15. Cardi, V.; Tchanturia, K.; Treasure, J. Premorbid and illness-related social difficulties in eating disorders: An overview of the literature and treatment developments. *Curr. Neuropharmacol.* **2018**, *16*, 1122–1130. [CrossRef]
16. Vartanian, L.R.; Hayward, L.E.; Smyth, J.M.; Paxton, S.J.; Touyz, S.W. Risk and resiliency factors related to body dissatisfaction and disordered eating: The identity disruption model. *Int. J. Eat. Disord.* **2018**, *51*, 322–330. [CrossRef]
17. Young, J.E.; Klosko, J.S.; Weishaar, M.E. *Schema Therapy: A Practitioner's Guide*; Guilford Press: New York, NY, USA, 2003.

18. Arcelus, J.; Haslam, M.; Farrow, C.; Meyer, C. The role of interpersonal functioning in the maintenance of eating psychopathology: A systematic review and testable model. *Clin. Psychol. Rev.* **2013**, *33*, 156–167. [CrossRef]
19. Oldershaw, A.; Lavender, T.; Sallis, H.; Stahl, D.; Schmidt, U. Emotion generation and regulation in anorexia nervosa: A systematic review and meta-analysis of self-report data. *Clin. Psychol. Rev.* **2015**, *39*, 83–95. [CrossRef]
20. Engel, S.G.; Wonderlich, S.A.; Crosby, R.D.; Mitchell, J.E.; Crow, S.; Peterson, C.B.; Gordon, K.H. The role of affect in the maintenance of anorexia nervosa: Evidence from a naturalistic assessment of momentary behaviors and emotion. *J. Abnorm. Psychol.* **2013**, *122*, 709. [CrossRef]
21. Rapee, R.M.; Oar, E.L.; Johnco, C.J.; Forbes, M.K.; Fardouly, J.; Magson, N.R.; Richardson, C.E. Adolescent development and risk for the onset of social-emotional disorders: A review and conceptual model. *Behav. Res. Ther.* **2019**, *123*, 103501. [CrossRef]
22. Caglar-Nazali, H.P.; Corfield, F.; Cardi, V.; Ambwani, S.; Leppanen, J.; Olabintan, O.; Micali, N. A systematic review and meta-analysis of 'Systems for Social Processes' in eating disorders. *Neurosci. Biobehav. Rev.* **2014**, *42*, 55–92. [CrossRef] [PubMed]
23. Cardi, V.; Corfield, F.; Leppanen, J.; Rhind, C.; Deriziotis, S.; Hadjimichalis, A.; Treasure, J. Emotional processing, recognition, empathy and evoked facial expression in eating disorders: An experimental study to map deficits in social cognition. *PLoS ONE* **2015**, *10*, e0133827. [CrossRef] [PubMed]
24. Davies, H.; Wolz, I.; Leppanen, J.; Fernandez-Aranda, F.; Schmidt, U.; Tchanturia, K. Facial expression to emotional stimuli in non-psychotic disorders: A systematic review and meta-analysis. *Neurosci. Biobehav. Rev.* **2016**, *64*, 252–271. [CrossRef] [PubMed]
25. Oldershaw, A.; DeJong, H.; Hambrook, D.; Schmidt, U. Social attribution in anorexia nervosa. *Eur. Eat. Disord. Rev.* **2018**, *26*, 197–206. [CrossRef]
26. Cardi, V.; Di Matteo, R.; Corfield, F.; Treasure, J. Social reward and rejection sensitivity in eating disorders: An investigation of attentional bias and early experiences. *World J. Biol. Psychiatry* **2013**, *14*, 622–633. [CrossRef]
27. Cardi, V.; Di Matteo, R.; Gilbert, P.; Treasure, J. Rank perception and self-evaluation in eating disorders. *Int. J. Eat. Disord.* **2014**, *47*, 543–552. [CrossRef]
28. Ambwani, S.; Berenson, K.R.; Simms, L.; Li, A.; Corfield, F.; Treasure, J. Seeing things differently: An experimental investigation of social cognition and interpersonal behavior in anorexia nervosa. *Int. J. Eat. Disord.* **2016**, *49*, 499–506. [CrossRef]
29. Szczurek, L.; Monin, B.; Gross, J.J. The Stranger Effect: The Rejection of Affective Deviants. *Psychol. Sci.* **2012**, *23*, 1105–1111. [CrossRef]
30. Hess, U.; Fischer, A. Emotional Mimicry as Social Regulation. *Personal. Soc. Psychol. Rev.* **2013**, *17*, 142–157. [CrossRef]
31. Schneider, K.G.; Hempel, R.J.; Lynch, T.R. That "poker face" just might lose you the game! the impact of expressive suppression and mimicry on sensitivity to facial expressions of emotion. *Emotion* **2013**, *13*, 852–866. [CrossRef]
32. McKnight, R.; Boughton, N. Anorexia Nervosa. *Br. Med. J.* **2014**, *22*, 1–9. [CrossRef] [PubMed]
33. Hjern, A.; Lindberg, L.; Lindblad, F. Outcome and prognostic factors for adolescent female in-patients with anorexia nervosa: 9-to 4-year follow-up. *Br. J. Psychiatry* **2006**, *189*, 428–432. [CrossRef] [PubMed]
34. Treasure, J.; Crane, A.; McKnight, R.; Buchanan, E.; Wolfe, M. First do no harm: Iatrogenic maintaining factors in anorexia nervosa. *Eur. Eat. Disord. Rev.* **2011**, *19*, 296–302. [CrossRef] [PubMed]
35. Anastasiadou, D.; Medina-Pradas, C.; Sepulveda, A.R.; Treasure, J. A systematic review of family caregiving in eating disorders. *Eat. Behav.* **2014**, *15*, 464–477. [CrossRef]
36. Konstantakopoulos, G.; Tchanturia, K.; Surguladze, S.A.; David, A.S. Insight in eating disorders: Clinical and cognitive correlates. *Psychol. Med.* **2011**, *41*, 1951–1961. [CrossRef]
37. Gorwood, P.; Duriez, P.; Lengvenyte, A.; Guillaume, S.; Criquillion, S. Clinical insight in anorexia nervosa: Associated and predictive factors. *Psychiatry Res.* **2019**, *281*, 112561. [CrossRef]
38. Treasure, J.; Schmidt, U.; Macdonald, P. (Eds.) *The Clinician's Guide to Collaborative Caring in Eating Disorders: The New Maudsley Method*; Routledge: London, UK, 2009.
39. Treasure, J.; Smith, G.; Crane, A. *Skills-Based Caring for a Loved One With an Eating Disorder: The New Maudsley Method*; Routledge: London, UK, 2016.

40. Sepulveda, A.R.; Kyriacou, O.; Treasure, J. Development and validation of the accommodation and enabling scale for eating disorders (AESED) for caregivers in eating disorders. *BMC Health Serv. Res.* **2009**, *9*, 171. [CrossRef]
41. Salerno, L.; Rhind, C.; Hibbs, R.; Micali, N.; Schmidt, U.; Gowers, S.; Treasure, J. An examination of the impact of care giving styles (accommodation and skilful communication and support) on the one year outcome of adolescent anorexia nervosa: Testing the assumptions of the cognitive interpersonal model in anorexia nervosa. *J. Affect. Disord.* **2016**, *191*, 230–236. [CrossRef]
42. Dimitropoulos, G.; Klopfer, K.; Lazar, L.; Schacter, R. Caring for a sibling with anorexia nervosa: A qualitative study. *Eur. Eat. Disord. Rev. Prof. J. Eat. Disord. Assoc.* **2009**, *17*, 350–365. [CrossRef]
43. Dimitropoulos, G.; Freeman, V.E.; Bellai, K.; Olmsted, M. Inpatients with severe anorexia nervosa and their siblings: Non-shared experiences and family functioning. *Eur. Eat. Disord. Rev.* **2013**, *21*, 284–293. [CrossRef]
44. House of Commons Health Committee. *Suicide Prevention: Interim Report. Fourth Report of Session*; House of Commons: London, UK, 2016.
45. Treasure, J.; Nazar, B.P. Interventions for the carers of patients with eating disorders. *Curr. Psychiatry Rep.* **2016**, *18*, 16. [CrossRef] [PubMed]
46. Langley, J.; Treasure, J.; Todd, G. *Caring for a Loved One with an Eating Disorder: The New Maudsley Skills-Based Training Manual*; Routledge: London, UK, 2018.
47. Treasure, J.; Murphy, T.; Szmukler, T.; Todd, G.; Gavan, K.; Joyce, J. The experience of caregiving for severe mental illness: A comparison between anorexia nervosa and psychosis. *Soc. Psychiatry Psychiatr. Epidemiol.* **2001**, *36*, 343–347. [CrossRef]
48. Magill, N.; Rhind, C.; Hibbs, R.; Goddard, E.; Macdonald, P.; Arcelus, J.; Treasure, J. Two-year follow-up of a pragmatic randomised controlled trial examining the effect of adding a carer's skill training intervention in inpatients with anorexia nervosa. *Eur. Eat. Disord. Rev.* **2016**, *24*, 122–130. [CrossRef] [PubMed]
49. Hibbs, R.; Magill, N.; Goddard, E.; Rhind, C.; Raenker, S.; Macdonald, P.; Schmidt, U. Clinical effectiveness of a skills training intervention for caregivers in improving patient and caregiver health following in-patient treatment for severe anorexia nervosa: Pragmatic randomised controlled trial. *BJPsych Open* **2015**, *1*, 56–66. [CrossRef] [PubMed]
50. Hodsoll, J.; Rhind, C.; Micali, N.; Hibbs, R.; Goddard, E.; Nazar, B.P.; Landau, S. A pilot, multicentre pragmatic randomised trial to explore the impact of carer skills training on carer and patient behaviours: Testing the cognitive interpersonal model in adolescent anorexia nervosa. *Eur. Eat. Disord. Rev.* **2017**, *25*, 551–561. [CrossRef]
51. Adamson, J.; Cardi, V.; Kan, C.; Harrison, A.; Macdonald, P.; Treasure, J. Evaluation of a novel transition support intervention in an adult eating disorders service: ECHOMANTRA. *Int. Rev. Psychiatry* **2019**, *31*, 382–390. [CrossRef]
52. Pépin, G.; King, R. Collaborative care skills training workshops: Helping carers cope with eating disorders from the UK to Australia. *Soc. Psychiatry Psychiatr. Epidemiol.* **2013**, *48*, 805–812. [CrossRef]
53. Quiles, M.Y.; Quiles, S.M.; Escolano, H.M.; Sanmartín, R.; Treasure, J. Testing carer skill training programs in Spanish carers of patients with eating disorders. *Psicothema* **2018**, *30*, 295.
54. Schmidt, U.; Wade, T.D.; Treasure, J. The Maudsley Model of Anorexia Nervosa Treatment for Adults (MANTRA): Development, key features, and preliminary evidence. *J. Cog. Psychother.* **2014**, *28*, 48–71. [CrossRef]
55. Schmidt, U.; Startup, H.; Treasure, J. *A Cognitive-Interpersonal Therapy Workbook for Treating Anorexia Nervosa: The Maudsley Model*; Routledge: London, UK, 2018.
56. Walsh, B.T. The enigmatic persistence of anorexia nervosa. *Am. J. Psychiatry* **2013**, *170*, 477–484. [CrossRef]
57. Steinglass, J.E.; Walsh, B.T. Neurobiological model of the persistence of anorexia nervosa. *J. Eat. Disord.* **2016**, *4*, 19. [CrossRef] [PubMed]
58. Uniacke, B.; Walsh, B.T.; Foerde, K.; Steinglass, J. The role of habits in anorexia nervosa: Where we are and where to go from here? *Curr. Psychiatry Rep.* **2018**, *20*, 61. [CrossRef] [PubMed]
59. Steinglass, J.E.; Berner, L.A.; Attia, E. Cognitive neuroscience of eating disorders. *Psychiatr. Clin.* **2019**, *42*, 75–91. [CrossRef] [PubMed]
60. Steinglass, J.E.; Glasofer, D.R.; Walsh, E.; Guzman, G.; Peterson, C.B.; Walsh, B.T.; Wonderlich, S.A. Targeting habits in anorexia nervosa: A proof-of-concept randomized trial. *Psychol. Med.* **2018**, *48*, 2584–2591. [CrossRef]

61. Levinson, C.A.; Brosof, L.C.; Ma, J.; Fewell, L.; Lenze, E.J. Fear of food prospectively predicts drive for thinness in an eating disorder sample recently discharged from intensive treatment. *Eat. Behav.* **2017**, *27*, 45–51. [CrossRef]
62. Lambert, E.; Purves, K.; McGregor, T.; Treasure, J.; Cardi, V. Fear conditioning in women with a lifetime diagnosis of anorexia nervosa and healthy controls. In Preparation.
63. Cardi, V.; Leppanen, J.; Mataix-Cols, D.; Campbell, I.C.; Treasure, J. A case series to investigate food-related fear learning and extinction using in vivo food exposure in anorexia nervosa: A clinical application of the inhibitory learning framework. *Eur. Eat. Disord. Rev.* **2019**, *27*, 173–181. [CrossRef]
64. Ramjan, L.M. Nurses and the 'therapeutic relationship': Caring for adolescents with anorexia nervosa. *J. Adv. Nurs.* **2004**, *45*, 495–503. [CrossRef]
65. Kimber, M.; McTavish, J.R.; Couturier, J.; Le Grange, D.; Lock, J.; MacMillan, H.L. Identifying and responding to child maltreatment when delivering family-based treatment—A qualitative study. *Int. J. Eat. Disord.* **2019**, *52*, 292–298. [CrossRef]
66. Den, M.L.; Graham, B.M.; Newall, C.; Richardson, R. Teens that fear screams: A comparison of fear conditioning, extinction, and reinstatement in adolescents and adults. *Dev. Psychobiol.* **2015**, *57*, 818–832. [CrossRef]
67. Koskina, A.; Campbell, I.C.; Schmidt, U. Exposure therapy in eating disorders revisited. *Neurosci. Biobehav. Rev.* **2013**, *37*, 193–208. [CrossRef]
68. Murray, S.B.; Treanor, M.; Liao, B.; Loeb, K.L.; Griffiths, S.; Le Grange, D. Extinction theory & anorexia nervosa: Deepening therapeutic mechanisms. *Behav. Res. Ther.* **2016**, *87*, 1–10. [PubMed]
69. Cardi, V.; Esposito, M.; Clarke, A.; Schifano, S.; Treasure, J. The impact of induced positive mood on symptomatic behaviour in eating disorders. An experimental, AB/BA crossover design testing a multimodal presentation during a test-meal. *Appetite* **2015**, *87*, 192–198. [CrossRef] [PubMed]
70. Steinglass, J.; Sysko, R.; Schebendach, J.; Broft, A.; Strober, M.; Walsh, B.T. The application of exposure therapy and D-cycloserine to the treatment of anorexia nervosa: A preliminary trial. *J. Psychiatr. Pract.* **2007**, *13*, 238. [CrossRef]
71. Levinson, C.A.; Rodebaugh, T.L.; Fewell, L.; Kass, A.E.; Riley, E.N.; Stark, L.; Lenze, E.J. D-Cycloserine facilitation of exposure therapy improves weight regain in patients with anorexia nervosa: A pilot randomized controlled trial. *J. Clin. Psychiatry* **2015**, *76*, e787. [CrossRef]
72. Cardi, V.; Krug, I.; Perpiñá, C.; Mataix-Cols, D.; Roncero, M.; Treasure, J. The use of a nonimmersive virtual reality programme in anorexia nervosa: A single case-report. *Eur. Eat. Disord. Rev.* **2012**, *20*, 240–245. [CrossRef]
73. Tchanturia, K.; Davies, H.; Reeder, C.; Wykes, T. Cognitive Remediation Therapy for AN Therapist Manual. 2010. Available online: http://www.katetchanturia.com/publications/c1y51 (accessed on 26 February 2020).
74. Cardi, V.; Esposito, M.; Bird, G.; Rhind, C.; Yiend, J.; Schifano, S.; Treasure, J. A preliminary investigation of a novel training to target cognitive biases towards negative social stimuli in Anorexia Nervosa. *J. Affect. Disord.* **2015**, *188*, 188–193. [CrossRef]
75. Turton, R.; Nazar, B.P.; Burgess, E.E.; Lawrence, N.S.; Cardi, V.; Treasure, J.; Hirsch, C.R. To go or not to go: A proof of concept study testing food-specific inhibition training for women with eating and weight disorders. *Eur. Eat. Disord. Rev.* **2018**, *26*, 11–21. [CrossRef]
76. Werthmann, J.; Simic, M.; Konstantellou, A.; Mansfield, P.; Mercado, D.; van Ens, W.; Schmidt, U. Same, same but different: Attention bias for food cues in adults and adolescents with anorexia nervosa. *Int. J. Eat. Disord.* **2019**, *52*, 681–690. [CrossRef]
77. Mercado, D.; Schmidt, U.; O'Daly, O.; Campbell, I.; Werthmann, J. Food related attention bias modification training for anorexia nervosa and its potential underpinning mechanisms. *J. Eat. Disord.* **2020**, *8*, 1. [CrossRef]
78. Wildes, J.E.; Marcus, M.D.; Bright, A.C.; Dapelo, M.M. Emotion and eating disorder symptoms in patients with anorexia nervosa: An experimental study. *Int. J. Eat. Disord.* **2012**, *45*, 876–882. [CrossRef]
79. Rodgers, R.F.; Paxton, S.J. The impact of indicated prevention and early intervention on co-morbid eating disorder and depressive symptoms: A systematic review. *J. Eat. Disord.* **2014**, *2*, 30. [CrossRef] [PubMed]
80. Molendijk, M.L.; Hoek, H.W.; Brewerton, T.D.; Elzinga, B.M. Childhood maltreatment and eating disorder pathology: A systematic review and dose-response meta-analysis. *Psychol. Med.* **2017**, *47*, 1402–1416. [CrossRef] [PubMed]

81. Monteleone, A.M.; Mereu, A.; Cascino, G.; Criscuolo, M.; Castiglioni, M.C.; Pellegrino, F.; Zanna, V. Re-conceptualization of anorexia nervosa psychopathology: A network analysis study in adolescents with short duration of the illness. *Int. J. Eat. Disord.* **2019**, *52*, 1263–1273. [CrossRef] [PubMed]
82. Sauro, C.L.; Ravaldi, C.; Cabras, P.L.; Faravelli, C.; Ricca, V. Stress, hypothalamic-pituitary-adrenal axis and eating disorders. *Neuropsychobiology* **2008**, *57*, 95–115. [CrossRef] [PubMed]
83. Chua, Y.W.; Lewis, G.; Easter, A.; Lewis, G.; Solmi, F. Eighteen-year trajectories of depressive symptoms in mothers with a lifetime eating disorder: Findings from the ALSPAC cohort. *Br. J. Psychiatry* **2019**, *14*, 1–7. [CrossRef]
84. Tomba, E.; Tecuta, L.; Crocetti, E.; Squarcio, F.; Tomei, G. Residual eating disorder symptoms and clinical features in remitted and recovered eating disorder patients: A systematic review with meta-analysis. *Int. J. Eat. Disord.* **2019**, *52*, 759–776. [CrossRef]
85. Godart, N.; Radon, L.; Curt, F.; Duclos, J.; Perdereau, F.; Lang, F.; Corcos, M. Mood disorders in eating disorder patients: Prevalence and chronology of ONSET. *J. Affect. Disord.* **2015**, *185*, 115–122. [CrossRef]
86. Dobrescu, S.R.; Dinkler, L.; Gillberg, C.; Råstam, M.; Gillberg, C.; Wentz, E. Anorexia nervosa: 30-year outcome. *Br. J. Psychiatry* **2019**, *22*, 1–8. [CrossRef]
87. Solmi, M.; Collantoni, E.; Meneguzzo, P.; Tenconi, E.; Favaro, A. Network analysis of specific psychopathology and psychiatric symptoms in patients with anorexia nervosa. *Eur. Eat. Disord. Rev.* **2019**, *27*, 24–33. [CrossRef]
88. Voderholzer, U.; Hessler-Kaufmann, J.B.; Lustig, L.; Läge, D. Comparing severity and qualitative facets of depression between eating disorders and depressive disorders: Analysis of routine data. *J. Affect. Disord.* **2019**, *257*, 758–764. [CrossRef]
89. Keski-Rahkonen, A.; Raevuori, A.; Bulik, C.M.; Hoek, H.W.; Rissanen, A.; Kaprio, J. Factors associated with recovery from anorexia nervosa: A population-based study. *Int. J. Eat. Disord.* **2014**, *47*, 117–123. [CrossRef] [PubMed]
90. Franko, D.L.; Tabri, N.; Keshaviah, A.; Murray, H.B.; Herzog, D.B.; Thomas, J.J.; Eddy, K.T. Predictors of long-term recovery in anorexia nervosa and bulimia nervosa: Data from a 22-year longitudinal study. *J. Psychiatr. Res.* **2018**, *96*, 183–188. [CrossRef] [PubMed]
91. Duncan, T.K.; Sebar, B.; Lee, J. Reclamation of power and self: A meta-synthesis exploring the process of recovery from anorexia nervosa. *Adv. Eat. Disord. Theory Res. Pract.* **2015**, *3*, 177–190. [CrossRef]
92. de Vos, J.A.; LaMarre, A.; Radstaak, M.; Bijkerk, C.A.; Bohlmeijer, E.T.; Westerhof, G.J. Identifying fundamental criteria for eating disorder recovery: A systematic review and qualitative meta-analysis. *J. Eat. Disord.* **2017**, *5*, 34. [CrossRef]
93. Measelle, J.R.; Stice, E.; Hogansen, J.M. Developmental trajectories of co-occurring depressive, eating, antisocial, and substance abuse problems in female adolescents. *J. Abnorm. Psychol.* **2006**, *115*, 524. [CrossRef]
94. Degortes, D.; Zanetti, T.; Tenconi, E.; Santonastaso, P.; Favaro, A. Childhood obsessive–compulsive traits in anorexia nervosa patients, their unaffected sisters and healthy controls: A retrospective study. *Eur. Eat. Disord. Rev.* **2014**, *22*, 237–242. [CrossRef]
95. Lilenfeld, L.R.; Kaye, W.H.; Greeno, C.G.; Merikangas, K.R.; Plotnicov, K.; Pollice, C.; Nagy, L. A controlled family study of anorexia nervosa and bulimia nervosa: Psychiatric disorders in first-degree relatives and effects of proband comorbidity. *Arch. Gen. Psychiatry* **1998**, *55*, 603–610. [CrossRef]
96. Cederlöf, M.; Thornton, L.M.; Baker, J.; Lichtenstein, P.; Larsson, H.; Rück, C.; Mataix-Cols, D. Etiological overlap between obsessive-compulsive disorder and anorexia nervosa: A longitudinal cohort, multigenerational family and twin study. *World Psychiatry* **2015**, *14*, 333–338. [CrossRef]
97. Yilmaz, Z.; Halvorsen, M.; Bryois, J.; Yu, D.; Thornton, L.M.; Zerwas, S.; Erdman, L. Examination of the shared genetic basis of anorexia nervosa and obsessive–compulsive disorder. *Mol. Psychiatry* **2018**. [CrossRef]
98. Forrest, L.N.; Jones, P.J.; Ortiz, S.N.; Smith, A.R. Core psychopathology in anorexia nervosa and bulimia nervosa: A network analysis. *Int. J. Eat. Disord.* **2018**, *51*, 668–679. [CrossRef]
99. Montigny, C.; Castellanos-Ryan, N.; Whelan, R.; Banaschewski, T.; Barker, G.J.; Büchel, C.; Nees, F. A phenotypic structure and neural correlates of compulsive behaviors in adolescents. *PLoS ONE* **2013**, *8*, e80151. [CrossRef] [PubMed]
100. Fonville, L.; Giampietro, V.; Williams, S.C.R.; Simmons, A.; Tchanturia, K. Alterations in brain structure in adults with anorexia nervosa and the impact of illness duration. *Psychol. Med.* **2014**, *44*, 1965–1975. [CrossRef]

101. Connan, F.; Treasure, J. Stress, eating and neurobiology. In *Neurobiology in the Treatment of Eating Disorders*; Wiley: Chichester, UK, 1998; pp. 211–236.
102. Myrvang, A.D.; Vangberg, T.R.; Stedal, K.; Rø, Ø.; Endestad, T.; Rosenvinge, J.H.; Aslaksen, P.M. Hippocampal subfields in adolescent anorexia nervosa. *Psychiatry Res. Neuroimaging* **2018**, *282*, 24–30. [CrossRef] [PubMed]
103. Nickel, K.; Joos, A.; Tebartz van Elst, L.; Matthis, J.; Holovics, L.; Endres, D.; Maier, S. Recovery of cortical volume and thickness after remission from acute anorexia nervosa. *Int. J. Eat. Disord.* **2018**, *51*, 1056–1069. [CrossRef]
104. Chui, H.T.; Christensen, B.K.; Zipursky, R.B.; Richards, B.A.; Hanratty, M.K.; Kabani, N.J.; Katzman, D.K. Cognitive function and brain structure in females with a history of adolescent-onset anorexia nervosa. *Paediatrics* **2008**, *122*, e426–e437. [CrossRef] [PubMed]
105. Fladung, A.K.; Grön, G.; Grammer, K.; Herrnberger, B.; Schilly, E.; Grasteit, S.; von Wietersheim, J. A neural signature of anorexia nervosa in the ventral striatal reward system. *Am. J. Psychiatry* **2009**, *167*, 206–212. [CrossRef]
106. Fladung, A.K.; Schulze, U.M.E.; Schöll, F.; Bauer, K.; Grön, G. Role of the ventral striatum in developing anorexia nervosa. *Transl. Psychiatry* **2013**, *3*, e315. [CrossRef]
107. Chami, R.; Treasure, J. *The Neurobiology of Trauma and Eating Disorders. Trauma-Informed Approaches to Eating Disorders*; Springer Publishing Company: New York, NY, USA, 2018.
108. Akil, H.; Gordon, J.; Hen, R.; Javitch, J.; Mayberg, H.; McEwen, B.; Nestler, E.J. Treatment resistant depression: A multi-scale, systems biology approach. *Neurosci. Biobehav. Rev.* **2018**, *84*, 272–288. [CrossRef]
109. Teicher, M.H.; Samson, J.A. Childhood maltreatment and psychopathology: A case for ecophenotypic variants as clinically and neurobiologically distinct subtypes. *Am. J. Psychiatry* **2013**, *170*, 1114–1133. [CrossRef]
110. Putignano, P.; Dubini, A.; Toja, P.; Invitti, C.; Bonfanti, S.; Redaelli, G.; Cavagnini, F. Salivary cortisol measurement in normal-weight, obese and anorexic women: Comparison with plasma cortisol. *Eur. J. Endocrinol.* **2001**, *145*, 165–171. [CrossRef]
111. Misra, M.; Klibanski, A. Endocrine consequences of anorexia nervosa. *Lancet Diabetes Endocrinol.* **2014**, *2*, 581–592. [CrossRef]
112. Chami, R.; Monteleone, A.M.; Treasure, J.; Monteleone, P. Stress hormones and eating disorders. *Mol. Cell. Endocrinol.* **2018**, *497*, 110349. [CrossRef] [PubMed]
113. Dalton, B.; Campbell, I.; Chung, R.; Breen, G.; Schmidt, U.; Himmerich, H. Inflammatory Markers in Anorexia Nervosa: An Exploratory Study. *Nutrients* **2018**, *10*, 1573. [CrossRef]
114. Dalton, B.; Leppanen, J.; Campbell, I.C.; Chung, R.; Breen, G.; Schmidt, U.; Himmerich, H. A longitudinal analysis of cytokines in anorexia nervosa. *Brain Behav. Immun.* **2019**. [CrossRef]
115. Herpertz-Dahlmann, B.; Seitz, J.; Baines, J. Food matters: How the microbiome and gut–brain interaction might impact the development and course of anorexia nervosa. *Eur. Child Adolesc. Psychiatry* **2017**, *26*, 1031–1041. [CrossRef]
116. Seitz, J.; Trinh, S.; Herpertz-Dahlmann, B. The microbiome and eating disorders. *Psychiatr. Clin.* **2019**, *42*, 93–103. [CrossRef]
117. Barona, M.; Brown, M.; Clark, C.; Frangou, S.; White, T.; Micali, N. White matter alterations in anorexia nervosa: Evidence from a voxel-based meta-analysis. *Neurosc. Biobehav. Rev.* **2019**, *100*, 285–295. [CrossRef]
118. Connan, F.; Murphy, F.; Connor, S.E.; Rich, P.; Murphy, T.; Bara-Carill, N.; Morris, R.G. Hippocampal volume and cognitive function in anorexia nervosa. *Psychiatry Res. Neuroimaging* **2006**, *146*, 117–125. [CrossRef]
119. Cathomas, F.; Murrough, J.W.; Nestler, E.J.; Han, M.H.; Russo, S.J. Neurobiology of resilience: Interface between mind and body. *Biol. Psychiatry* **2019**, *86*, 410–420. [CrossRef]
120. Collo, G.; Pich, E.M. A human translational model based on neuroplasticity for pharmacological agents potentially effective in Treatment-Resistant Depression: Focus on dopaminergic system. *Neural Regen. Res.* **2020**, *15*, 1027. [CrossRef]
121. Schmidt, U.; Oldershaw, A.; Jichi, F.; Sternheim, L.; Startup, H.; McIntosh, V.; Landau, S. Out-patient psychological therapies for adults with anorexia nervosa: Randomised controlled trial. *Br. J. Psychiatry* **2012**, *201*, 392–399. [CrossRef]
122. Albano, G.; Hodsoll, J.; Kan, C.; Lo Coco, G.; Cardi, V. Task-sharing interventions for patients with anorexia nervosa or their carers: A systematic evaluation of the literature and meta-analysis of outcomes. *Int. Rev. Psychiatry* **2019**, *31*, 367–381. [CrossRef] [PubMed]

123. Schmidt, U.; Magill, N.; Renwick, B.; Keyes, A.; Kenyon, M.; Dejong, H.; Watson, C. The Maudsley Outpatient Study of Treatments for Anorexia Nervosa and Related Conditions (MOSAIC): Comparison of the Maudsley Model of Anorexia Nervosa Treatment for Adults (MANTRA) with specialist supportive clinical management (SSCM) in outpatients with broadly defined anorexia nervosa: A randomized controlled trial. *J. Consult. Clin. Psychol.* **2015**, *83*, 796. [PubMed]

124. Lipsman, N.; Woodside, D.B.; Giacobbe, P.; Hamani, C.; Carter, J.C.; Norwood, S.J.; Smith, G.S. Subcallosal cingulate deep brain stimulation for treatment-refractory anorexia nervosa: A phase 1 pilot trial. *Lancet* **2013**, *381*, 1361–1370. [CrossRef]

125. McClelland, J.; Kekic, M.; Bozhilova, N.; Nestler, S.; Dew, T.; Van den Eynde, F.; Schmidt, U. A randomised controlled trial of neuronavigated repetitive transcranial magnetic stimulation (rTMS) in anorexia nervosa. *PLoS ONE* **2016**, *11*, e0148606. [CrossRef]

126. Dalton, B.; Bartholdy, S.; McClelland, J.; Kekic, M.; Rennalls, S.J.; Werthmann, J.; Glennon, D. Randomised controlled feasibility trial of real versus sham repetitive transcranial magnetic stimulation treatment in adults with severe and enduring anorexia nervosa: The TIARA study. *BMJ Open* **2018**, *8*, e021531. [CrossRef]

127. Knyahnytska, Y.O.; Blumberger, D.M.; Daskalakis, Z.J.; Zomorrodi, R.; Kaplan, A.S. Insula H-coil deep transcranial magnetic stimulation in severe and enduring anorexia nervosa (SE-AN): A pilot study. *Neuropsychiatr. Dis. Treat.* **2019**, *15*, 2247. [CrossRef]

128. Lipsman, N.; Lam, E.; Volpini, M.; Sutandar, K.; Twose, R.; Giacobbe, P.; Lozano, A.M. Deep brain stimulation of the subcallosal cingulate for treatment-refractory anorexia nervosa: 1 year follow-up of an open-label trial. *Lancet Psychiatry* **2017**, *4*, 285–294. [CrossRef]

129. Himmerich, H.; Treasure, J. Psychopharmacological advances in eating disorders. *Expert Rev. Clin. Pharmacol.* **2018**, *11*, 95–108. [CrossRef]

130. Dold, M.; Aigner, M.; Klabunde, M.; Treasure, J.; Kasper, S. Second-generation antipsychotic drugs in anorexia nervosa: A meta-analysis of randomized controlled trials. *Psychother. Psychosom.* **2015**, *84*, 110–116. [CrossRef]

131. Attia, E.; Steinglass, J.E.; Walsh, B.T.; Wang, Y.; Wu, P.; Schreyer, C.; Marcus, M.D. Olanzapine versus placebo in adult outpatients with anorexia nervosa: A randomized clinical trial. *Am. J. Psychiatry* **2019**, *176*, 449–456. [CrossRef] [PubMed]

132. Hirschtritt, M.E.; Bloch, M.H.; Mathews, C.A. Obsessive-compulsive disorder: Advances in diagnosis and treatment. *JAMA* **2017**, *317*, 1358–1367. [CrossRef] [PubMed]

133. Fontenelle, L.F.; Yücel, M. A Clinical Staging Model for Obsessive–Compulsive Disorder: Is It Ready for Prime Time? *EClinicalMedicine* **2019**, *7*, 65–72. [CrossRef] [PubMed]

134. Rucker, J.J.; Iliff, J.; Nutt, D.J. Psychiatry & the psychedelic drugs. Past, present & future. *Neuropharmacology* **2018**, *142*, 200–218. [PubMed]

135. Mills, I.H.; Park, G.R.; Manara, A.R.; Merriman, R.J. Treatment of compulsive behaviour in eating disorders with intermittent ketamine infusions. *QJM Mon. J. Assoc. Physicians* **1998**, *91*, 493–503. [CrossRef]

136. Cardi, V.; Albano, G.; Ambwani, S.; Cao, L.; Crosby, R.D.; Macdonald, P.; Treasure, J. A randomised clinical trial to evaluate the acceptability and efficacy of an early phase, online, guided augmentation of outpatient care for adults with anorexia nervosa. *Psychol. Med.* **2019**, *16*, 1–12. [CrossRef]

137. Cardi, V.; Ambwani, S.; Robinson, E.; Albano, G.; MacDonald, P.; Aya, V.; Arcelus, J. Transition care in anorexia nervosa through guidance online from peer and carer expertise (TRIANGLE): Study protocol for a randomised controlled trial. *Eur. Eat. Disord. Rev.* **2017**, *25*, 512–523. [CrossRef]

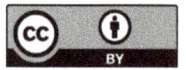

© 2020 by the authors. Licensee MDPI, Basel, Switzerland. This article is an open access article distributed under the terms and conditions of the Creative Commons Attribution (CC BY) license (http://creativecommons.org/licenses/by/4.0/).

MDPI
St. Alban-Anlage 66
4052 Basel
Switzerland
Tel. +41 61 683 77 34
Fax +41 61 302 89 18
www.mdpi.com

Journal of Clinical Medicine Editorial Office
E-mail: jcm@mdpi.com
www.mdpi.com/journal/jcm

www.ingramcontent.com/pod-product-compliance
Lightning Source LLC
LaVergne TN
LVHW070225100526
838202LV00015B/2090